HEMODYNAMICS AND CARDIOLOGY
Neonatology Questions and Controversies

HEMODYNAMICS AND CARDIOLOGY
Neonatology Questions and Controversies

Series Editor

Richard A. Polin, MD
Professor of Pediatrics
College of Physicians and Surgeons
Columbia University
Vice Chairman for Clinical and Academic Affairs
Department of Pediatrics
Director, Division of Neonatology
Morgan Stanley Children's Hospital of NewYork-Presbyterian
Columbia University Medical Center
New York, New York

Other Volumes in the Neonatology Questions and Controversies Series

GASTROENTEROLOGY AND NUTRITION

HEMATOLOGY, IMMUNOLOGY AND INFECTIOUS DISEASE

NEPHROLOGY AND FLUID/ELECTROLYTE PHYSIOLOGY

NEUROLOGY

THE NEWBORN LUNG

HEMODYNAMICS AND CARDIOLOGY

Neonatology Questions and Controversies

Charles S. Kleinman, MD
Formerly Professor of Clinical Pediatrics in Obstetrics and Gynecology
Columbia University College of Physicians and Surgeons
Weill Cornell Medical College of Cornell University
Director, Fetal Cardiology
Morgan Stanley Children's Hospital of NewYork-Presbyterian
New York, New York

Istvan Seri, MD, PhD, HonD
Professor of Pediatrics
Keck School of Medicine of the University of Southern California
Director, Center for Fetal and Neonatal Medicine
Head, USC Division of Neonatal Medicine
Children's Hospital Los Angeles
Los Angeles County and University of Southern California Medical Center
Los Angeles, California

Consulting Editor
Richard A. Polin, MD
Professor of Pediatrics
College of Physicians and Surgeons
Columbia University
Vice Chairman for Clinical and Academic Affairs
Department of Pediatrics
Director, Division of Neonatology
Morgan Stanley Children's Hospital of NewYork-Presbyterian
Columbia University Medical Center
New York, New York

SECOND EDITION

1600 John F. Kennedy Blvd.
Ste 1800
Philadelphia, PA 19103-2899

Notices

Knowledge and best practice in this field are constantly changing. As new research and experience
broaden our understanding, changes in research methods, professional practices, or medical treatment
may become necessary.

Practitioners and researchers must always rely on their own experience and knowledge in
evaluating and using any information, methods, compounds, or experiments described herein. In
using such information or methods they should be mindful of their own safety and the safety of
others, including parties for whom they have a professional responsibility.

With respect to any drug or pharmaceutical products identified, readers are advised to check the
most current information provided (i) on procedures featured or (ii) by the manufacturer of each
product to be administered to verify the recommended dose or formula, the method and duration
of administration, and contraindications. It is the responsibility of practitioners, relying on their own
experience and knowledge of their patients, to make diagnoses, to determine dosages and the best
treatment for each individual patient, and to take all appropriate safety precautions.

To the fullest extent of the law, neither the Publisher nor the authors, contributors, or editors
assume any liability for any injury and/or damage to persons or property as a matter of products
liability, negligence, or otherwise, or from any use or operation of any methods, products, instructions,
or ideas contained in the material herein.

Library of Congress Cataloging-in-Publication Data

Hemodynamics and cardiology : neonatology questions and controversies / [edited by] Charles S.
Kleinman, Istvan Seri.—2nd ed.
      p. ; cm.—(Neonatology questions and controversies)
   Includes bibliographical references and index.
   ISBN 978-1-4377-2763-0 (hardback)
   I. Kleinman, Charles S.   II. Seri, Istvan, MD.   III. Series: Neonatology questions and
controversies.
      [DNLM: 1. Cardiovascular Diseases.   2. Infant, Newborn, Diseases.   3. Infant, Newborn.
4. Neonatology—methods.   WS 290]
      618.92'12—dc23

                                                                      2012005557

Senior Content Strategist: Stefanie Jewell-Thomas
Content Development Specialist: Lisa Barnes
Publishing Services Manager: Anne Altepeter
Team Manager: Hemamalini Rajendrababu
Project Manager: Siva Raman Krishnamoorthy
Designer: Ellen Zanolle

Printed in the United States of America

Last digit is the print number: 9   8   7   6   5   4   3   2   1

This book is dedicated to my co-editor and respected colleague, Dr. Charles S. Kleinman, who passed away just before completing the final revision of the second part of this book, "Fetal and Neonatal Cardiology." During the completion of the second edition of this book, I wondered how Dr. Kleinman kept his focus, drive, and energy to continue working on this edition despite his battle with cancer. My admiration, utmost respect, and heart go out to Dr. Kleinman, who in my opinion is the true example of the inspiring clinician-scientist, colleague, mentor, and person many of us only dream about becoming.

Istvan Seri, MD, PhD, HonD

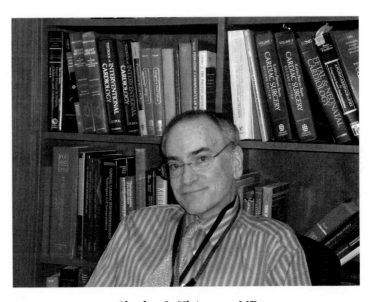

Charles S. Kleinman, MD

Contributors

Robert H. Anderson, MD, FRCPath
Institute of Medical Genetics
Newcastle University
Newcastle upon Tyne, United Kingdom
  *The Reappraisal of Normal and
  Abnormal Cardiac Development*

Kwame Anyane-Yeboa, MD
Professor of Clinical Pediatrics
Department of Pediatrics
Division of Clinical Genetics
Columbia University
Attending Pediatrician
Department of Pediatrics
Division of Clinical Genetics
Columbia University Medical Center
New York, New York
  *The Genetics of Fetal and Neonatal
  Cardiovascular Disease*

Emile Bacha, MD, FACS
Calvin F. Barber Professor and Chief
Division of Cardiothoracic Surgery
NewYork-Presbyterian
Columbia University Medical Center
Director, Pediatric Cardiac Surgery
Morgan Stanley Children's Hospital of
  NewYork-Presbyterian
New York, New York
  *Cardiac Surgery in the Neonate with
  Congenital Heart Disease*

Simon D. Bamforth, PhD
Institute of Human Genetics
Newcastle University
Newcastle upon Tyne, United Kingdom
  *The Reappraisal of Normal and
  Abnormal Cardiac Development*

Stefan Blüml, PhD
Department of Bioengineering
Viterbi School of Engineering
University of Southern California
Los Angeles, California;
Rudi Schulte Research Institute
Santa Barbara, California
  *Advanced Magnetic Resonance
  Neuroimaging Techniques in the
  Neonate with a Focus on Hemodynamic-
  Related Brain Injury*

Matthew Borzage, MS
Doctoral Student
Biomedical Engineering
University of Southern California
Doctoral Student Researcher
Center for Fetal and Neonatal Medicine
Children's Hospital Los Angeles
Los Angeles, California
  *Advanced Magnetic Resonance
  Neuroimaging Techniques in the
  Neonate with a Focus on Hemodynamic-
  Related Brain Injury*

Marko T. Boskovski, MD
Department of Pediatrics and Genetics
Yale University
New Haven, Connecticut
  *The Genetics of Fetal and Neonatal
  Cardiovascular Disease*

Martina Brueckner, MD
Associate Professor
Department of Pediatrics and Genetics
Yale University School of Medicine
New Haven, Connecticut
  *The Genetics of Fetal and Neonatal
  Cardiovascular Disease*

Nigel A. Brown, PhD
Head, Division of Biomedical Sciences
St. George's Hospital Medical School
University of London
London, United Kingdom
  *The Reappraisal of Normal and
  Abnormal Cardiac Development*

Bill Chaudhry, MB, PhD, ChB
Institute of Human Genetics
Newcastle University
Newcastle upon Tyne, United Kingdom
*The Reappraisal of Normal and
Abnormal Cardiac Development*

**John P. Cheatham, MD, FAAP,
FACC, FSCAI**
Professor, Pediatrics and Internal
  Medicine
Cardiology Division
The Ohio State University Medical
  Center;
Director, Cardiac Catheterization and
  Interventional Therapy
Co-Director, The Heart Center
Nationwide Children's Hospital
Columbus, Ohio
*Hybrid Management Techniques in the
Treatment of the Neonate with
Congenital Heart Disease*

Jonathan M. Chen, MD
David Wallace-Starr Foundation
  Professor
Cardiothoracic Surgery and Pediatrics
  Director
Pediatric Cardiovascular Services Chief
Pediatric Cardiac Surgery
NewYork-Presbyterian Hospital
New York, New York
*Cardiac Surgery in the Neonate with
Congenital Heart Disease*

Wendy Chung, MD, PhD
Herbert Irving Assistant Professor of
  Pediatrics and Medicine
Director of Clinical Genetics
Columbia University
New York, New York
*The Genetics of Fetal and Neonatal
Cardiovascular Disease*

Vicki L. Clifton, PhD
Associate Professor
Senior Research Fellow
Department of Pediatrics and
  Reproductive Health
University of Adelaide
Director of Clinical Research
  Development
Lyell McEwin Hospital
Adelaide, Australia
*Assessment of the Microcirculation in the
Neonate*

Ronald Clyman, MD
Professor of Pediatrics and Senior Staff
Cardiovascular Research Institute
University of California, San Francisco
San Francisco, California
*The Very Low Birth Weight Neonate
with Hemodynamically Significant
Ductus Arteriosus During the First
Postnatal Week*

Cynthia H. Cole, MD, MHP
Associate Professor of Pediatrics
Department of Pediatrics
Boston University
Boston Medical Center
Boston, Massachusetts
*The Preterm Neonate with
Cardiovascular and Adrenal
Insufficiency*

Preeta Dhanantwari, MD
Pediatric and Fetal Cardiologist
Department of Pediatric Cardiology
Children's Heart Center
Steven and Alexandra Cohen Children's
  Medical Center of New York
New Hyde Park, New York
*Human Cardiac Development in the
First Trimester*

**Mary T. Donofrio, MD, FAAP,
FACC, FASE**
Associate Professor
Pediatric Cardiology
George Washington University
Washington, District of Columbia
Director of the Fetal Heart Program
Pediatric Cardiology
Children's National Medical Center
Washington, District of Columbia
*Human Cardiac Development in the
First Trimester*

Adré J. du Plessis, MBChB, MPH
Chief
Division of Fetal and Transitional
  Medicine
Children's National Medical Center
Washington, District of Columbia
*Hemodynamics and Brain Injury in the
Preterm Neonate*

William D. Engle, MD
Professor of Pediatrics
The University of Texas Southwestern
  Medical Center at Dallas;
Attending Neonatologist
Department of Pediatrics
Parkland Health and Hospital System;
Attending Neonatologist
Department of Pediatrics
Children's Medical Center Dallas
Dallas, Texas
  *Definition of Normal Blood Pressure
  Range: The Elusive Target*

Nicholas J. Evans, DM, MRCPCH
Clinical Associate Professor
Department of Obstetrics, Gynecology
  and Neonatology
Sydney University;
Senior Staff Specialist and Head of
  Department
Newborn Care
Royal Prince Alfred Hospital
Sydney, Australia
  *Functional Echocardiography in the
  Neonatal Intensive Care Unit*

Erika F. Fernandez, MD
Assistant Professor
Department of Pediatrics
Division of Neonatology
University of New Mexico Health and
  Sciences Center;
Assistant Professor
Department of Pediatrics
Division of Neonatology
University of New Mexico Hospital
Albuquerque, New Mexico
  *The Preterm Neonate with
  Cardiovascular and Adrenal
  Insufficiency*

**Philippe S. Friedlich, MD, MS Epi,
MBA**
Associate Director
Center for Fetal and Neonatal Medicine
Children's Hospital Los Angeles;
Associate Professor of Pediatrics and
  Surgery
Division of Neonatal Medicine
Keck School of Medicine of the
  University of Southern California
Los Angeles, California
  Shock in the Surgical Neonate

Mark Galantowicz, MD
Murray D. Lincoln Endowed Chair in
  Cardiothoracic Surgery
Chief of Cardiothoracic Surgery
Co-Director
The Heart Center at Nationwide
  Children's Hospital
Associate Professor of Surgery
The Ohio State University College of
  Medicine
Columbus, Ohio
  *Hybrid Management Techniques in
  the Treatment of the Neonate with
  Congenital Heart Disease*

Arthur Garson, Jr., MD, MPH
Director, Center for Health Policy
Professor of Public Health Sciences
University of Virginia
Charlottesville, Virginia
  *New Concepts for Training the Pediatric
  Cardiology Workforce of the Future*

Julie S. Glickstein, MD
Associate Professor of Clinical
  Pediatrics
Department of Pediatrics
Columbia University Medical Center
Children's Hospital of
  NewYork-Presbyterian
New York, New York
  *The Current Role of Fetal
  Echocardiography*

Gorm Greisen, MD, PhD
Professor
Institute of Obstetrics, Gynecology and
  Pediatrics
University of Copenhagen;
Head
Department of Neonatology
Rigshospitalet
Copenhagen, Denmark
  *Autoregulation of Vital and Nonvital
  Organ Blood Flow in the Preterm and
  Term Neonate*
  *Methods to Assess Systemic and Organ
  Blood Flow in the Neonate*

Alan M. Groves, MD, FRCPCH
Clinical Senior Lecturer in Neonatal
  Medicine
Department of Pediatrics
Imperial College London
London, United Kingdom
  *Cardiovascular Magnetic Resonance in
  the Study of Neonatal Hemodynamics*

Punita Gupta, MD
Clinical Genetics
Columbia University Medical Center
Clinical Genetics Fellow
Department of Clinical Genetics
Children's Hospital of New York
New York, New York
*The Genetics of Fetal and Neonatal
Cardiovascular Disease*

William E. Hellenbrand, MD
Professor of Pediatrics and Cardiology
Section Chief
Yale University School of Medicine
New Haven, Connecticut
*Catheter-Based Therapy in the Neonate
with Congenital Heart Disease*

Deborah J. Henderson, PhD
Institute of Human Genetics
Newcastle University
Newcastle upon Tyne, United Kingdom
*The Reappraisal of Normal and
Abnormal Cardiac Development*

Ziyad M. Hijazi, MD, MPH
James A. Hunter, MD, University Chair
Professor of Pediatrics and Internal
   Medicine
Director, Rush Center for Congenital
   and Structural Heart Disease
Rush University Medical Center
Chicago, Illinois
*Catheter-Based Therapy in the Neonate
with Congenital Heart Disease
Hybrid Management Techniques in
the Treatment of the Neonate with
Congenital Heart Disease*

George M. Hoffman, MD
Professor
Departments of Anesthesiology and
   Pediatrics
Medical College of Wisconsin;
Director and Chief, Pediatric
   Anesthesiology
Associate Director, Pediatric Intensive
   Care
Children's Hospital of Wisconsin
Milwaukee, Wisconsin
*Regional Blood Flow Monitoring in the
Perioperative Period*

James Huhta, MD
Professor
Women's Health and Perinatology
   Research Group
Institute of Clinical Medicine
University of Tromso
Tromso, Norway;
Professor of Pediatrics
University of Florida
Gainesville, Florida;
Medical Director, Perinatal Cardiology
All Children's Hospital
St. Petersburg, Florida;
Lead Physician
Fetal Cardiology Working Group
Pediatrix Medical Group
Sunrise, Florida
*Clinical Evaluation of Cardiovascular
Function in the Human Fetus*

Damien Kenny, MD
Department of Congenital and
   Structural Heart Disease
Rush University Medical Center
Chicago, Illinois
*Hybrid Management Techniques in
the Treatment of the Neonate with
Congenital Heart Disease*

[†]Charles S. Kleinman, MD
Professor of Clinical Pediatrics in
   Obstetrics and Gynecology
Columbia University College of
   Physicians and Surgeons
Weill Cornell Medical College of
   Cornell University;
Director, Fetal Cardiology
Morgan Stanley Children's Hospital of
   NewYork-Presbyterian
New York, New York
*The Current Role of Fetal
Echocardiography*

**Martin Kluckow, PhD, MBBS,
FRACP**
Associate Professor
Department of Neonatology
University of Sydney;
Associate Professor and Senior Staff
   Specialist
Department of Neonatology
Royal North Shore Hospital
Sydney, Australia
*Clinical Presentations of Neonatal
Shock: The Very Low Birth Weight
Infant During the First Postnatal Day*

Ganga Krishnamurthy, MD
Assistant Professor of Pediatrics
Columbia University
Director of Neonatal Cardiac Care
Morgan Stanley Children's Hospital
  NewYork-Presbyterian
New York, New York
  *The Current Role of Fetal
  Echocardiography*

Linda Leatherbury, MD
Professor of Pediatrics
George Washington University School
  of Medicine and Health Sciences
Children's National Medical Center
Cardiology Principal Investigator
Children's Research Institute Center for
  Genetic Medicine Research
Washington, District of Columbia
  *Human Cardiac Development in the
  First Trimester*

Petra Lemmers, MD, PhD
Department of Neonatology
University Medical Center Utrecht/
  Wilhelmina Children's Hospital
Utrecht, The Netherlands
  *Clinical Applications of Near-Infrared
  Spectroscopy in Neonates*

Cecilia W. Lo, PhD
Department of Oncology
National Taiwan University Hospital
Institute of Toxicology
National Taiwan University College of
  Medicine
Nankang, Taiwan
  *Human Cardiac Development in the
  First Trimester*

Timothy J. Mohun, PhD
Division of Developmental Biology
MRC National Institute for Medical
  Research
London, United Kingdom
  *The Reappraisal of Normal and
  Abnormal Cardiac Development*

Antoon F. M. Moorman, PhD
Professor of Embryology and Molecular
  Biology of Cardiovascular Diseases
Department of Anatomy, Embryology,
  and Physiology
Academic Medical Center
University of Amsterdam
Director of the Netherlands Heart
  Foundation Molecular Cardiology
  Program of Heart Failure
Amsterdam, the Netherlands
  *The Reappraisal of Normal and
  Abnormal Cardiac Development*

Gunnar Naulaers, MD, PhD
Professor of Neonatology
Department of Pediatrics
University Hospital Leuven
Leuven, Belgium
  *Clinical Applications of Near-Infrared
  Spectroscopy in Neonates*

Shahab Noori, MD, RDCS
Associate Professor of Pediatrics
Department of Pediatrics
Keck School of Medicine of the
  University of Southern California
Attending Neonatologist
Division of Neonatology and the Center
  for Fetal and Neonatal Medicine
Department of Pediatrics
Children's Hospital Los Angeles
Los Angeles California and University
  of Southern California Medical
  Center
Los Angeles, California
  *Principles of Developmental
  Cardiovascular Physiology and
  Pathophysiology
  Assessment of Cardiac Output in
  Neonates: Techniques Using the Fick
  Principle, Pulse Wave Form Analysis,
  and Electrical Impedance
  The Very Low Birth Weight Neonate
  with Hemodynamically Significant
  Ductus Arteriosus During the First
  Postnatal Week*

Markus Osypka, PhD
President and CEO
Cardiotronic/Osypka Medical, Inc.
La Jolla, California
  *Assessment of Cardiac Output in
  Neonates: Techniques Using the Fick
  Principle, Pulse Wave Form Analysis,
  and Electrical Impedance*

Ashok Panigrahy, MD
Associate Professor of Radiology
University of Pittsburgh;
Radiologist-In-Chief
Associate Professor of Radiology
Department of Radiology
Children's Hospital of Pittsburgh
University of Pittsburgh Medical Center
Pittsburg, Pennsylvania;
Associate Professor of Radiology
Department of Radiology
Children's Hospital of Los Angeles
Los Angeles, California
  *Advanced Magnetic Resonance
  Neuroimaging Techniques in the
  Neonate with a Focus on Hemodynamic-
  Related Brain Injury*

Anthony N. Price, PhD
University College of London Centre
  for Advanced Biomedical Imaging
Department of Medicine and UCL
  Institute of Child Health
University College London, Medical
  School
The Hatter Cardiovascular Institute
University College London Hospital
London, United Kingdom
  *Cardiovascular Magnetic Resonance in
  the Study of Neonatal Hemodynamics*

Jan M. Quaegebeur, MD, PhD
Morris & Rose Milstein Professor of
  Surgery
Columbia University College of
  Physicians and Surgeons
Morgan Stanley Children's Hospital of
  NewYork-Presbyterian
New York, New York
  *Cardiac Surgery in the Neonate with
  Congenital Heart Disease*

Marc E. Richmond, MD
Assistant Professor of Clinical Pediatrics
Department of Pediatrics
Division of Pediatric Cardiology
Columbia University College of
  Physicians and Surgeons;
Assistant Attending
Pediatric Cardiology, Program for
  Pediatric Cardiomyopathy, Heart
  Failure, and Transplantation
Morgan Stanley Children's Hospital of
  NewYork-Presbyterian
New York, New York
  *Mechanical Pump Support and Cardiac
  Transplant in the Neonate*

Istvan Seri, MD, PhD, HonD
Professor of Pediatrics
Keck School of Medicine of the
  University of Southern California
Director, Center for Fetal and Neonatal
  Medicine;
Head, USC Division of Neonatal
  Medicine
Children's Hospital Los Angeles
Los Angeles County and University of
  Southern California Medical Center
Los Angeles, California
  *Principles of Developmental
  Cardiovascular Physiology and
  Pathophysiology
  Assessment of Cardiac Output in
  Neonates: Techniques Using the Fick
  Principle, Pulse Wave Form Analysis,
  and Electrical Impedance
  Clinical Presentations of Neonatal
  Shock: The Very Low Birth Weight
  Infant During the First Postnatal Day
  Shock in the Surgical Neonate*

Shabana Shahanavaz, MD
Pediatric Cardiologist
Division of Cardiology
St. Louis Children's Hospital
Saint Louis, Missouri
  *Catheter-Based Therapy in the Neonate
  with Congenital Heart Disease*

Cathy Shin, MD, FACS, FAAP
Assistant Professor of Surgery
University of Southern California
Attending Surgeon
Children's Hospital Los Angeles
Los Angeles, California
  Shock in the Surgical Neonate

Sadaf Soleymani, MS
Doctoral Student
Biomedical Engineering
University of Southern California
Doctoral Student Researcher
Center for Fetal and Neonatal Medicine
Children's Hospital Los Angeles
Los Angeles, California
  *Assessment of Cardiac Output in
  Neonates: Techniques Using the Fick
  Principle, Pulse Wave Form Analysis,
  and Electrical Impedance*

Michael J. Stark, PhD, MRCP
School of Pediatrics and Reproductive
  Health
The Robinson Institute
University of Adelaide
Adelaide, Australia
  *Assessment of the Microcirculation in the
  Neonate*

Theodora A. Stavroudis, MD
Assistant Professor of Pediatrics
Keck School of Medicine of the
  University of Southern California
Children's Hospital Los Angeles
Los Angeles, California
  *Principles of Developmental
  Cardiovascular Physiology and
  Pathophysiology*

James Stein, MD, FACS, FAAP
Associate Chief of Surgery
Chief Quality Officer
Children's Hospital Los Angeles
Assistant Professor of Surgery
Keck School of Medicine of the
  University of Southern California
Los Angeles, California
  Shock in the Surgical Neonate

James S. Tweddell, MD
Medical Director
Cardiothoracic Surgery
Children's Hospital of Wisconsin
Professor
Medical College of Wisconsin
Milwaukee, Wisconsin
  *Regional Blood Flow Monitoring in the
  Perioperative Period*

Frank van Bell, MD, PhD
Professor
Director, Department of Neonatology
University Medical Center Utrecht/
  Wilhelmina Children's Hospital
Utrecht, The Netherlands
  *Clinical Applications of Near-Infrared
  Spectroscopy in Neonates*

Suresh Victor, PhD, MRCPCH
Clinical Lecturer
School of Biomedicine
University of Manchester;
Honorary Consultant Neonatologist
Newborn Intensive Care Unit
Central Manchester University Hospital
  NHS Foundation Trust
Manchester, United Kingdom
  *Near-Infrared Spectroscopy and Its Use
  for the Assessment of Tissue Perfusion in
  the Neonate*

**Julie Anne Vincent, MD, FACC,
FAAP**
Associate Clinical Professor of Pediatrics
Department of Pediatrics
Columbia University, College of
  Physicians and Surgeons
Adjunct Assistant Professor of
  Pediatrics
Department of Pediatrics
Weill Cornell Medical College
Director, Pediatric Cardiac
  Catheterization Laboratories
Director, Pediatric Cardiology
  Fellowship Program
Department of Pediatrics
Morgan Stanley Children's Hospital of
  NewYork-Presbyterian
University Medical Center
Director, Pediatric Cardiac
  Catheterization Laboratories
Director, Pediatric Cardiology
  Fellowship Program
Department of Pediatrics
NewYork-Presbyterian Hospital/Weill
  Cornell Medical Center
New York, New York
  *Catheter-Based Therapy in the Neonate
  with Congenital Heart Disease*

Jodie K. Votava-Smith, MD
Advanced Fellow in Fetal Cardiology
Cincinnati Children's Hospital Medical
  Center
Cincinnati Ohio
  *The Current Role of Fetal
  Echocardiography*

Michael Weindling, MD, FRCP, FRCPCH, Hon FRCA
Professor of Perinatal Medicine
Department of Women's and Children's Health
University of Liverpool
Consultant Neonatologist
Neonatol Unit
Liverpool Women's Hospital
Liverpool, United Kingdom
Near-Infrared Spectroscopy and Its Use for the Assessment of Tissue Perfusion in the Neonate

Ian M. R. Wright, MBBS, DCH, MRCP(Paeds)UK, FRACP
Senior Staff Specialist in Neonatal Medicine
Kaleidoscope Neonatal Intensive Care Unit
John Hunter Children's Hospital
Associate Professor in Paediatrics and Child Health
University of Newcastle
Convenor of ABC Children's Research Network
Hunter Medical Research Centre
Newcastle, Australia
Assessment of the Microcirculation in the Neonate

Series Foreword

Richard A. Polin, MD

Medicine is a science of uncertainty and an art of probability.

—William Osler

Controversy is part of everyday practice in the NICU. Good practitioners strive to incorporate the best evidence into clinical care. However, for much of what we do, the evidence is either inconclusive or does not exist. In those circumstances, we have come to rely on the teachings of experienced practitioners who have taught us the importance of clinical expertise. This series, "Neonatology Questions and Controversies," provides clinical guidance by summarizing the best evidence and tempering those recommendations with the art of experience. To quote David Sackett, one of the founders of evidence-based medicine:

> Good doctors use both individual clinical expertise and the best available external evidence and neither alone is enough. Without clinical expertise, practice risks become tyrannized by evidence, for even excellent external evidence may be inapplicable to or inappropriate for an individual patient. Without current best evidence, practice risks become rapidly out of date to the detriment of patients.

This series focuses on the challenges faced by care providers who work in the NICU. When should we incorporate a new technology or therapy into everyday practice, and will it have positive impact on morbidity or mortality? For example, is the new generation of ventilators better than older technologies such as CPAP, or do they merely offer more choices with uncertain value? Similarly, the use of probiotics to prevent necrotizing enterocolitis is supported by sound scientific principles (and some clinical studies). However, at what point should we incorporate them into everyday practice given that the available preparations are not well characterized or proven safe? A more difficult and common question is when to use a new technology with uncertain value in a critically ill infant. As many clinicians have suggested, sometimes the best approach is to do nothing and "stand there."

The "Neonatology Questions and Controversies" series was developed to highlight the clinical problems of most concern to practitioners. The editors of each volume (Drs. Bancalari, Oh, Guignard, Baumgart, Kleinman, Seri, Ohls, Maheshwari, Neu, and Perlman) have done an extraordinary job selecting topics of clinical importance to everyday practice. When appropriate, less controversial topics have been eliminated and replaced by others thought to be of greater clinical importance. In total, there are 56 new chapters in the series. During the preparation of the *Hemodynamics and Cardiology* volume, Dr. Charles Kleinman died. Despite an illness that would have caused many to retire, Charlie worked until near the time of his death. He came to work each day, teaching students and young practitioners and offering his wisdom and expertise to families of infants with congenital heart disease. We dedicate the second edition of the series to his memory. As with the first edition, I am indebted to the exceptional group of editors who chose the content and edited each of the volumes. I also wish to thank Lisa Barnes (content development specialist at Elsevier) and Judy Fletcher (global content development director at Elsevier), who provided incredible assistance in bringing this project to fruition.

Preface

Cardiovascular compromise with or without congenital heart disease is a common finding in a large number of critically ill preterm and term neonates and is associated with a high incidence of mortality and significant short- and long-term morbidities. Therefore timely recognition and treatment of shock is of utmost importance. The diagnosis of shock is hampered by our inability to continuously assess systemic and organ blood flow in absolute numbers. As a result, treatment of cardiovascular compromise in neonates has rarely been based on a thorough understanding of the underlying cardiovascular pathophysiology. Instead, many of these neonates are routinely treated with volume boluses followed by the administration of vasopressors and/or inotropes with little regard to the etiology, phase, or pathophysiology of neonatal shock. It is not surprising therefore that there is very little evidence demonstrating that treatment of shock in neonates, especially without congenital heart disease, improves mortality or clinically meaningful short- and long-term outcomes.

However, since the publication of the first edition of *Hemodynamics and Cardiology* in the "Neonatology Questions and Controversies" series, some promising advances have been made in the ability to monitor neonatal hemodynamic parameters. In addition, recent studies have started to unravel some of the mysteries of the physiology and pathophysiology of cardiovascular transition to extrauterine life. The second edition of this series addresses these novel approaches and findings, making it both up-to-date and useful for the clinician and investigator who face uncertainty in clinical practice and study design and conduction.

The second edition has kept the major structure of the first edition and, accordingly, is divided into two parts.

The first part of this book, "Neonatal Hemodynamics," addresses the principles of developmental physiology and the pathophysiology of neonatal shock, the autoregulation of vital and nonvital organ blood flow, and the controversies surrounding the definition of normal blood pressure in the neonatal patient population. In addition to discussions on the use of functional echocardiography, near-infrared spectroscopy, and advanced magnetic resonance imaging, there are new chapters on available methods to assess cardiac output and microcirculation and the application of these technologies to preterm and term neonates. The ensuing section includes chapters that describe the different clinical presentations of neonatal shock with a focus on characteristic clinical features and pathophysiology. Reasonable approaches to treatment are also reviewed, with an emphasis on evidence-based approaches whenever evidence is available. The final chapter in this part of the book addresses the role of hemodynamics in brain injury, focusing on the preterm neonate during the transitional period.

The second part, "Fetal and Neonatal Cardiology," begins with a discussion of embryonic and fetal heart development. As the focus of pediatric cardiologists involved in the care of neonates with critical hemodynamic compromise has become more proactive, fetal diagnosis and management is becoming increasingly important, as has the role of fetal cardiology in the prenatal and postnatal management of neonates with congenital heart disease. Finally, the most recent therapeutic and imaging advances in the management of neonates with congenital heart disease are discussed in detail, providing novel information and conceptual framework for the clinician and researcher involved in the management and study of neonates with congenital heart disease.

Istvan Seri, MD, PhD, HonD

Contents

SECTION C

Clinical Presentations and Relevance of Neonatal Shock

PART II • FETAL AND NEONATAL CARDIOLOGY

SECTION D

Embryonic and Fetal Development

SECTION E

Fetal and Neonatal Cardiology

†Deceased.

SECTION A

Principles of Developmental Cardiovascular Physiology and Pathophysiology

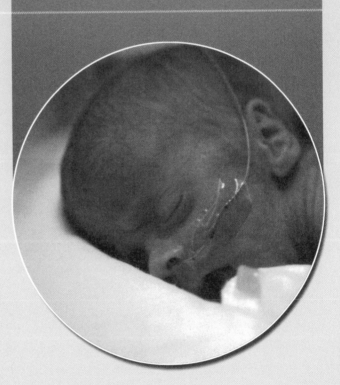

CHAPTER 1

Principles of Developmental Cardiovascular Physiology and Pathophysiology

Shahab Noori, MD, RDCS, Theodora A. Stavroudis, MD, Istvan Seri, MD, PhD, HonD

- **Principles of Developmental Physiology**
- **Developmental Cardiovascular Pathophysiology: Etiology and Pathophysiology of Neonatal Shock**
- **Case Study**
- **References**

This chapter first reviews fetal, transitional, and posttransitional hemodynamics with an emphasis on the principles of developmental cardiovascular physiology. Building on the physiologic principles reviewed, the second part of the chapter then discusses the etiology and pathophysiology of neonatal cardiovascular compromise. The major goals of this chapter are to help the reader appreciate the impact of immaturity and/or pathologic events on the physiology of neonatal cardiovascular transition and understand the primary factors leading to cardiovascular compromise in the preterm and term neonate. Only with this knowledge can one appropriately assess and manage hemodynamic disturbance in the immediate transitional period and beyond and potentially reduce the end-organ damage caused by the decrease in oxygen delivery to the organs, especially the immature brain of the affected neonate.

Principles of Developmental Physiology

Fetal Circulation

Fetal circulation is characterized by low systemic vascular resistance (SVR) with high systemic blood flow and high pulmonary vascular resistance with low pulmonary blood flow. Given the low oxygen tension in the fetus, fetal circulation allows for preferential flow of the most oxygenated blood to the heart and brain, two of the three "vital organs."[1] With the placenta rather than the lungs being the organ of gas exchange, most of the right ventricular output is diverted through the patent ductus arteriosus (PDA) to the systemic circulation. In fact, the pulmonary blood flow only constitutes about 7-8% of the combined cardiac output in fetal lambs.[2] However, the proportion of combined cardiac output that supplies the lungs is significantly higher in human fetus (11-25%), with some studies showing an increase in this proportion with advancing gestational age with the peak around 30 weeks.[3-5] During fetal life both ventricles contribute to the systemic blood flow and the circulation depends on the persistence of connections via the foramen ovale and PDA between the systemic and pulmonary circuits. Thus the two circulations function in "parallel" in the fetus. The right ventricle is the dominant pumping chamber and its contribution to the combined cardiac output is about 60%. The combined cardiac output is in the range of 400-450 mL/kg/min in the fetus and it is much higher than the systemic flow (about 200 mL/kg/min) after birth. Approximately one third of the combined cardiac output (150 mL/kg/min) perfuses the placenta via the umbilical vessels. However, placental blood flow decreases to 21% of the combined cardiac output near term.[6] The umbilical vein carries the oxygenated blood from the placenta though the portal veins and the ductus venosus to the inferior vena cava (IVC) and eventually to the heart. About 50% of oxygenated blood in the umbilical vein is shunted through ductus venosus and IVC to the right atrium where the oxygenated blood is preferentially directed to left atrium through the patent foramen ovale. This percentage decreases as gestation advances. One of the unique characteristics of the fetal circulation is that arterial oxygen saturation (SaO$_2$) is different between the upper and lower body. Having the most oxygenated blood in the left atrium ensures supply of adequate oxygen to the heart and brain. Furthermore, in response to hypoxemia, most of the blood flow in umbilical vein bypasses the portal circulation via ductus venosus and delivers the most oxygenated blood to the heart and brain.

Transitional Physiology

After birth, the circulation changes from parallel to series and thus the left and right ventricular outputs must become equal. However, this process, especially in very preterm infants, is not complete for days or even weeks after birth due to the inability of the fetal channels to close in a timely manner. The persistence of the PDA signifi-cantly alters the hemodynamics during transition and beyond. The impact of the PDA on pulmonary and systemic blood flow in the preterm infant is discussed in Chapter 13. At birth, the removal of low resistance placental circulation and the surge in catecholamines and other hormones increases the SVR. On the other hand, the pulmonary vascular resistance drops precipitously due to the act of breathing air and exposure of the pulmonary arteries to higher partial pressure of oxygen as compared to very low level in utero. Organ blood flow also changes significantly. In the newborn lamb, cerebral blood flow (CBF) drops in response to oxygen expo-sure.[7] Recently, a drop in CBF in the first few minutes after birth in normal term neonates was also reported.[8] This drop in CBF appears to be related, at least in part, to cerebral vasoconstriction in response to the increase in arterial blood oxygen content immediately after birth. In addition, the correlation between left-to-right PDA shunting and middle cerebral artery flow velocity (a surrogate for CBF) suggests a possible role of PDA in the observed reduction in CBF.[8] Finally, especially in some very preterm neonates, the inability of the immature myocardium to pump against the suddenly increased SVR might lead to a transient decrease in systemic blood flow, which in turn could also contribute to the decrease in CBF (Chapter 12).

Postnatal Circulation

Pressure, Flow, and Resistance

Poiseuille's equation ($Q = (\Delta P \times \pi r^4) / 8 \, \mu l$) describes the factors that determine the movement of fluid through a tube. This equation helps us understand how changes in cardiovascular parameters affect blood flow. Basically, flow (Q) is directly related to the pressure difference (ΔP) across the vessel and the fourth power of the radius (r) and inversely related to the length (l) of the vessel and the viscosity of the fluid (μ). Therefore blood pressure (BP) is the driving force behind moving blood through the vasculature. Because there are several differences between laminar flow of water through a tube and blood flow through the body, the relationship between the above factors in the body does not exactly follow the equation. In addition, because we do not measure all components of this equation, in clinical practice the interaction among BP, flow, and SVR is described by using an analogy of Ohm's law (cardiac output = pressure gradient/SVR). Therefore blood flow is directly related to BP and inversely related to SVR. Regulation of and changes in cardiac output and SVR determine the BP. In other words, systemic BP is the dependent variable of the interaction between the two independent variables: cardiac output (flow) and SVR. Because cardiac output is somewhat also affected by SVR, in theory, cardiac output cannot be considered as a completely independent variable.

    Cardiac output is determined by heart rate, preload, myocardial contractility, and afterload. Preload can be described in terms of pressure or volume, that is, central venous pressure or end-diastolic ventricular volume. Therefore preload is affected not only by the effective circulating blood volume but also by many other factors such as myocardial relaxation and compliance, contractility, and afterload. The limited data available on diastolic function in the newborn in general and in preterm infants in particular suggest lower myocardial compliance and relaxation function. On the other hand, baseline myocardial contractility is high or comparable to that in older children while the myocardial capacity to maintain contractility in the face of an increase in the afterload might be limited (see later). Afterload and SVR are related and usually change in the same direction. Yet, these two parameters are different and should not be used interchangeably. SVR is determined by the resistance of vascular system and regulated by changes in the diameter of the small resistance vessels, primarily the arterioles. In contrast, afterload is the force that myocardium has to overcome to pump blood out of the ventricles during the ejection period. Wall tension can be used as a measure of afterload. Therefore, based on La Place's law, left ventricular afterload is directly related to the intraventricular pressure and the left ventricular diameter at the end of systole and indirectly related to the myocardial wall thickness. Indeed, changes in SVR exert their effect on afterload indirectly by affecting BP.

Organ Blood Flow Distribution

Under resting physiologic conditions, blood flow to each organ is regulated by a baseline vascular tone under the influence of the autonomic nervous system. Changes in the baseline vascular tone regulate organ blood flow. Vascular tone is regulated by local tissue (e.g., H^+, CO_2, and O_2), paracrine (e.g., nitric oxide, prostacyclin, and endothelin-1), and neurohormonal factors as well as by the myogenic properties of the blood vessel. Under pathologic conditions such as hypoxia-ischemia, the relative organ distribution of cardiac output favors the "vital" organs (the brain, heart, and adrenal glands). In principle, vital organ designation is operational even in fetal life. However, the vascular bed of the forebrain (cortex) might only achieve the characteristic "vital organ" vasodilatory response to a decrease in perfusion pressure during late in the second trimester (see further discussion).

Microcirculatory Physiology

Other than being the site of exchange of oxygen and nutrients and the site of removal of metabolic by-products, microcirculation plays a significant role in regulating systemic and local hemodynamics. The small arteries and arterioles are the main regulators of peripheral vascular resistance, and the venules and small veins play an important role as capacitance vessels. Coupling of oxygen supply and demand is one of the primary functions of the microcirculation. Oxygen delivery (DO_2) depends on blood flow and oxygen content. The total oxygen content of the blood (hemoglobin-bound and dissolved) can be calculated based on the hemoglobin concentration (Hb; g/dL), SaO_2, and partial pressure of oxygen (PaO_2; mm Hg) in the arterial blood ([1.36 × Hb × SaO_2] + [0.003 × PaO_2]). Tissue blood flow is adjusted based on the oxygen consumption (VO_2) determined by the metabolic requirements. When the blood flow cannot be increased beyond a certain point, oxygen extraction is increased to meet the demand for VO_2. Therefore VO_2 is not affected by the decrease in blood flow until the tissue's capacity to extract more oxygen is exhausted. At this point, VO_2 becomes directly flow dependent.[9]

In healthy term infants, localized peripheral (buccal) perfusion assessed by capillary-weighted saturation using visible light spectroscopy has only a weak correlation with cardiac output during the transitional period.[10] Therefore it is possible that under physiologic conditions, peripheral blood flow is not affected by the variability in the systemic blood flow. In other words, blood flow (cardiac output) is regulated to meet VO_2. In ventilated preterm infants, limb blood flow assessed by near-infrared spectroscopy (NIRS) showed no correlation with BP.[11] Along with the poor correlation of buccal oxygen saturation with cardiac output in healthy term neonates, these findings suggest that regulation of the microcirculation and peripheral blood flow in hemodynamically relatively stable preterm and term neonates might be, at least to a certain point, independent of systemic blood flow.

Skin microcirculation has been more extensively studied in neonates. Orthogonal polarization spectral imaging studies of skin demonstrated that functional small vessel density, a measure of tissue perfusion and microcirculation, changes over the first postnatal month and directly correlates with hemoglobin concentration and environmental temperature in preterm infants.[12] In this study, functional small vessel density was also inversely related to BP. This finding indicates that evaluation of skin microcirculation may be useful in the indirect assessment of SVR. Findings of laser Doppler flowmetry studies of the skin indicate that the relationship between peripheral microvascular blood flow and cardiovascular function evolves during the first few days in preterm infants.[13] The inverse relationship between microvascular blood flow and calculated SVR and mean BP immediately after delivery was no longer present by the fifth day of postnatal life. In addition, preterm infants who died during the transitional period had higher baseline microvascular blood flow, that is, lower peripheral vascular resistance. These findings suggest that developmental changes in microcirculation also play a significant role in the regulation of transitional hemodynamics and that microcirculatory maladaptation is associated with and/or may increase the risk of mortality.

Given the limited data available and inconsistency of the findings, further studies of the regulation of microcirculation are needed to improve our understanding of the physiology and pathophysiology of the microcirculation during development and postnatal transition and characterizing its role in the regulation of systemic hemodynamics in the preterm and term neonate.

Myocardial Function—Developmental Aspects

There are significant differences in myocardial structure and function between the immature myocardium of the neonate and that of the older child and adult.[14,15] The immature myocardium of the preterm and term neonate has fewer contractile elements, higher water content, greater surface-to-volume ratio, and an underdeveloped sarcoplasmic reticulum. The immature myocardium primarily relies on the function of L-type calcium channels and thus on extracellular calcium concentration for calcium supply necessary for muscle contraction. In children and adults these channels only serve to trigger the release of calcium from its abundant intracellular sources in the sarcoplasmic reticulum. These characteristics of the immature myocardium explain the observed differences in myocardial compliance and contractility between preterm and term neonates and children and adults.

Echocardiographic studies have shown that the immature myocardium has a higher baseline contractile state and that contractility rapidly decreases in face of an increase in afterload.[16] The sensitivity of the immature myocardium to afterload means that for the same degree of rise in the afterload, the myocardium of the neonate has a more significant reduction in contractility compared to children or adults. With the rise in SVR after birth, left ventricular afterload increases. This, in turn, may lead to a significant decrease in myocardial contractility with possible clinical implications (see discussion under Myocardial Dysfunction).

Impact of the Immature Autonomic Nervous System on Regulating Cardiac Function and Vascular Tone

Circulatory function is mediated at the central and local levels through neural, hormonal, and metabolic mechanisms and reflex pathways (Fig. 1-1). Integral to the regulation of cardiac function and vascular tone is the central nervous system. The medulla generates complex patterns of sympathetic, parasympathetic, and cardiovascular responses that are essential for homeostasis as well as behavioral patterning of autonomic activity.[17,18] The balance between sympathetic and parasympathetic outflow to the heart and blood vessels is regulated by peripheral baroreceptors and chemoreceptors in the aortic arch and carotid sinus as well as by the mechanoreceptors in the heart and lungs.[19] Even though many of these pathways have been identified, much work remains to delineate the adaptation of cardiovascular control in the

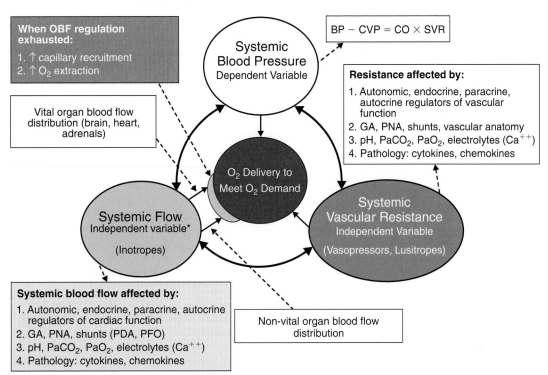

When OBF regulation exhausted:

1. ↑ capillary recruitment
2. ↑ O_2 extraction

Vital organ blood flow distribution (brain, heart, adrenals)

$$BP - CVP = CO \times SVR$$

Systemic Blood Pressure
Dependent Variable

Resistance affected by:

1. Autonomic, endocrine, paracrine, autocrine regulators of vascular function
2. GA, PNA, shunts, vascular anatomy
3. pH, $PaCO_2$, PaO_2, electrolytes (Ca^{++})
4. Pathology: cytokines, chemokines

O_2 Delivery to Meet O_2 Demand

Systemic Flow
Independent variable*

(Inotropes)

Systemic Vascular Resistance
Independent Variable

(Vasopressors, Lusitropes)

Systemic blood flow affected by:

1. Autonomic, endocrine, paracrine, autocrine regulators of cardiac function
2. GA, PNA, shunts (PDA, PFO)
3. pH, $PaCO_2$, PaO_2, electrolytes (Ca^{++})
4. Pathology: cytokines, chemokines

Non-vital organ blood flow distribution

Figure 1-1 To meet cellular metabolic demand, a complex interaction among blood flow, vascular resistance, and blood pressure takes place. Vascular resistance and blood flow are the independent variables and blood pressure is the dependent variable in this interaction characterized by the simplified equation using an analogy of Ohm's law: $BP - CVP = CO \times SVR$. However, as cardiac output is also affected by SVR, it cannot be considered a completely independent variable. In addition to the interaction among the major determinants of cardiovascular function, complex regulation of blood flow distribution to vital and nonvital organs, recruitment of capillaries and extraction of oxygen plays a fundamental role in the maintenance of hemodynamic homeostasis. BP, blood pressure; CO, cardiac output; CVP, central venous pressure; GA, gestational age; OBF, organ blood flow; $PaCO_2$, partial pressure of carbon dioxide in the arteries; PaO_2, partial pressure of oxygen in the arteries; PDA, patent ductus arteriosus; PFO, patent foramen ovale; PNA, postnatal age; SVR, systemic vascular resistance. (Modified with permission from Soleymani S, Borzage M, Seri I. Hemodynamic monitoring in neonates: advances and challenges. J Perinatol. 2010;30:S38-S45.)

immature infant where the maturation of the many components of this complex system is at varying pace and has been shown to lead to instability in autonomic function and maintenance of adequate organ blood flow and BP. The effect of the dynamic nature of the developing system on cardiovascular function is unclear but it may have short- and long-term implications for neonates born prematurely or with growth restriction.[20,21]

Heart rate variability analysis is a noninvasive tool employed to assess the sympathetic and parasympathetic modulation of the cardiovascular system over a relatively short period of time.[22-24] This method has been found useful in conditions where cardiac output has been impacted such as in patients with sepsis.[25,26] Heart rate variability analysis holds promise to further characterize the autonomic control of cardiovascular function in that the relationship among heart rate variability, sympathovagal balance, and the modulation of the renin-angiotensin-aldosterone system in various pathophysiologic states can be explored.

Developmental Cardiovascular Pathophysiology: Etiology and Pathophysiology of Neonatal Shock

To ensure normal cellular function and maintenance of structural integrity, delivery of oxygen must meet cellular oxygen demand. Oxygen delivery is determined by the oxygen content of the blood and cardiac output (see earlier). However, cardiac output can only deliver oxygen effectively to the organs if perfusion pressure (BP) is maintained in a range appropriate under the given condition of the cardiovascular system. Because BP is determined by the interaction between SVR and cardiac output (BP $\propto$ SVR $\times$ systemic blood flow; see Fig. 1-1), the complex interdependence between perfusion pressure and systemic blood flow mandates that, if possible, both be monitored in critically ill neonates.

Indeed, if SVR is too low, BP (perfusion pressure) may drop below a critical level where cellular oxygen delivery becomes compromised despite normal or even high cardiac output. However, if SVR is too high, cardiac output and thus organ perfusion may decrease to a critical level so that cellular oxygen delivery becomes compromised despite maintenance of BP in the perceived normal range. Therefore the use of BP or cardiac output alone for the assessment of the cardiovascular status is misleading, especially under certain critical circumstances in preterm and term neonates. Unfortunately, while BP can be continuously monitored, there are only few, recently developed and not yet fully validated invasive and noninvasive bedside techniques to use to continuously monitor systemic perfusion in absolute numbers in the critically ill neonate (see Chapter 6). Therefore, in most intensive care units, the clinician has been left with monitoring the indirect and rather insensitive and nonspecific measures of organ perfusion such as urine output, capillary refill time (CRT), and lactic acidosis. Among these measures, lactic acidosis is the most specific indirect measure of tissue hypoperfusion, and it has become available from small blood samples along with routine blood-gas analysis. However, this measure has its limitations as well, in that elevated serum lactic acid levels may represent an ongoing impairment in tissue oxygenation or a previous event with improvement in tissue perfusion (washout phenomenon). Thus serum lactic acid concentration needs to be sequentially monitored and a single value may not provide appropriate information on tissue perfusion. Furthermore, when epinephrine is being administered, epinephrine-induced specific increases in lactic acid levels occur independent of the state of tissue perfusion.[27]

Because it is a common practice to routinely measure BP in neonates, population-based normative data are available for the statistically defined normal ranges of BP in preterm and term neonates.[28-30] It is likely that the 5th or the 10th percentiles of these gestational- and postnatal-age-dependent normative data used to define hypotension do not represent BP values in every patient in whom autoregulation of organ blood flow or organ blood flow itself is necessarily compromised. Although recent findings have described the possible lower limits of BP below which autoregulation of CBF, cerebral function, and finally cerebral perfusion are impaired in very low birth weight (VLBW) preterm infants (Fig. 1-2), the true impact of gestational and postnatal age, the individual patient's ability to compensate with increased cardiac output and appropriate regulation of organ blood flow, and the underlying pathophysiology on the dependency of CBF on BP in this population remains to be determined.[31-36] Several epidemiologic studies have demonstrated that hypotension and/or low systemic perfusion are associated with increased mortality and morbidity in the neonatal patient population. Other studies found an increase in mortality and morbidity in preterm infants who received treatment for hypotension. Due to the retrospective and uncontrolled nature of these studies, it is hard to tease out the cause of adverse outcome associated with hypotension. It is possible that the poor outcome associated with hypotension is multifactorial and it may be due to the direct effect of hypotension on organ perfusion, the inappropriate use and titration of vasopressors/inotropes, coexistence of other pathologies with hypotension as a marker of disease severity, or a combination of all of these factors.[37]

Definition and Phases of Shock

Shock is defined as a condition in which supply of oxygen to the tissues does not meet oxygen demand. In the initial *compensated phase* of shock, neuroendocrine compensatory mechanisms and increased tissue oxygen extraction maintain perfusion pressure, blood flow, and oxygen supply to the vital organs (heart, brain, and adrenal glands) at the expense of blood flow to the rest of the body. This is achieved

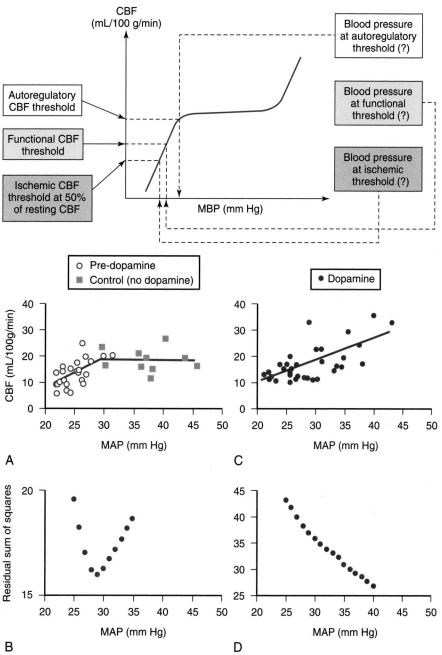

Figure 1-2 A, Definition of hypotension by three pathophysiologic phenomena of increasing severity: the "autoregulatory, functional and ischemic thresholds" of hypotension. Cerebral blood flow (CBF) is compromised when blood pressure decreases to below autoregulatory threshold. With further decrease in blood pressure, first brain function is impaired followed by tissue injury as ischemic threshold is crossed. **B,** Panel A and C. Serial measurements of CBF and mean arterial pressure (MAP) in a normotensive and untreated hypotensive extremely low birth weight (ELBW) neonates at 13 to 40 hours after birth. Note that there appears to be a breakpoint at 30 mm Hg in the CBF-MAP autoregulation curve. Panel B and D. Note the close relationship between CBF with MAP after the initiation of dopamine infusion (10 μg • kg−1 per min) in hypotensive ELBW neonates. Thus dopamine normalizes MAP and CBF but does not immediately restore CBF autoregulation. Plot of CBF versus MAP (Panel D) using the data of Panel B reveals a positive linear correlation (R = .88; P < .001).

Continued

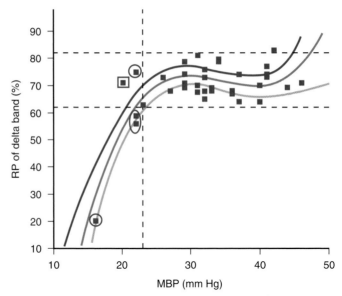

Figure 1-2, cont'd   C, Relationship between mean blood pressure (MBP) and the relative power (RP) of the delta band of the amplitude-integrated EEG, showing line of best fit with 95% confidence interval in VLBW neonates. Horizontal dotted lines represent the normal range of the relative power of the delta band (10th-90th percentile). Vertical dotted line represents the point of intercept. Circled squares indicate infants with abnormal cerebral fractional oxygen extraction (CFOE). (**A,** From McLean CW, Cayabyab RG, Noori S, et al. Cerebral circulation and hypotension in the premature infant—diagnosis and treatment. In: Perlman JM, ed. Neonatology questions and controversies: neurology. Philadelphia: Saunders/Elsevier; 2008:3-26. **B,** Adapted with permission from Munro MJ, Walker AM, Barfield CP. Hypotensive extremely low birth weight infants have reduced cerebral blood flow. Pediatrics 2004;114:1591-1596. **C,** Adapted with permission from Victor S, Marson AG, Appleton RE, et al. Relationship between blood pressure, cerebral electrical activity, cerebral fractional oxygen extraction, and peripheral blood flow in very low birth weight newborn infants. Pediatr Res. 2006;59:314-319.)

by selective vasoconstriction of the resistance vessels in the nonvital organs leading to maintenance of BP in the normal range and redistribution of blood flow to the vital organs. Low-normal to normal BP, increased heart rate, cold extremities, delayed CRT, and oliguria are the hallmarks of this phase. However, whereas these clinical signs are useful in detecting early shock in pediatric and adult patients, they are of limited value in neonates, especially in preterm infants in the immediate postnatal period. Indeed, in preterm infants immediately after birth, shock is rarely diagnosed in this phase and it is usually only recognized in the second uncompensated phase. In the *uncompensated phase* of shock, the neuroendocrine compensatory mechanisms fail and hypotension and decreased vital and nonvital organ perfusion and oxygen delivery develop. These events first result in the loss of vital organ blood flow auto-regulation and the development of lactic acidosis; if the process progresses, cellular function and then structural integrity become compromised. Even in the compensated phase, however, recognition of shock may be delayed because of the uncertainty about the definition of hypotension in preterm infants.[38,39] Finally, if treatment is delayed or ineffective, shock progresses to its final *irreversible phase*. In this phase, irreparable cellular damage occurs in all organs and therapeutic interventions will fail to sustain life.

Etiology of Neonatal Shock

Neonatal shock may develop because of volume loss (absolute hypovolemia), myocardial dysfunction, abnormal peripheral vasoregulation, or a combination of two or all of these factors.

Hypovolemia

Adequate preload is essential for maintaining normal cardiac output and organ blood flow. Therefore pathologic conditions associated with absolute or relative hypovolemia can lead to a decrease in cardiac output, poor tissue perfusion, and shock. Although absolute hypovolemia is a common cause of shock in the pediatric population, in neonates in the immediate postnatal period it is rarely the primary cause. Neonates are born with approximately 80-100 mL/kg of blood volume and only a significant drop in blood volume leads to hypotension. Perinatal events that can cause hypovolemia include a tight nuchal cord, cord avulsion, cord prolapse, placental abruption, fetomaternal transfusion, and birth trauma such as subgaleal hemorrhage. Fortunately, these perinatal events either do not result in significant hypovolemia and shock in most instances (e.g., placental abruption) or their occurrence is very rare (e.g., cord avulsion). Another cause of absolute hypovolemia is transepidermal water loss in extremely low birth weight (ELBW) infants in the immediate postnatal period.

To explore the role of intravascular volume status in the occurrence of hypotension, several investigators have evaluated the relationship between blood volume and systemic arterial BP in normotensive and hypotensive preterm infants. Bauer and colleagues measured blood volume in 43 preterm neonates during the first 2 postnatal days and found a weak but statistically significant positive correlation between BP and blood volume (Fig. 1-3A).[40] However, there was no correlation between blood volume and BP until blood volume exceeded 100 mL/kg.[40] Barr and colleagues found no relationship between arterial mean BP and blood volume in preterm infants (see Fig. 1-3B) and no difference in blood volume between hypotensive and normotensive infants.[41] Similarly, Wright and Goodall reported no relationship between blood volume and BP in preterm neonates in the immediate postnatal period (see Fig. 1-3C).[42] Therefore absolute hypovolemia is thought to be an unlikely primary cause of hypotension in preterm infants in the immediate postnatal period. This notion is further supported by the fact that dopamine is more effective than volume administration in improving BP in preterm infants during the first days after delivery.[43,44] On the other hand, increase in blood volume as a result of delayed cord clamping has been shown to confer some short-term hemodynamic benefits.[45-48]

Myocardial Dysfunction

As discussed earlier, there are considerable differences in the structure and function of the myocardium among preterm and term infants and children. The significant immaturity of the myocardium of the preterm infant, at least in part, accounts for why these patients are susceptible to development of myocardial failure following delivery.[14,15]

The limited capacity to increase contractility above the baseline makes the immature myocardium susceptible to fail when SVR abruptly increases. This disadvantage associated with myocardial immaturity is especially important during the initial transitional period. As the low resistance placental circulation is removed, SVR suddenly increases. This acute rise in the SVR and afterload may compromise left cardiac output and systemic blood flow. Indeed, superior vena cava (SVC) flow, used as a surrogate for systemic blood flow (left cardiac output), is low in a large proportion of VLBW infants during the first 6-12 postnatal hours.[49] The exaggerated decrease in myocardial contractility in response to increase in left ventricular afterload may play a role in development of low SVC flow.[50] However, this low flow state appears to be transient as the majority of the patients recover by 24-36 hours after delivery. Similarly, findings of Doppler studies of CBF suggest an increase in CBF shortly after delivery.[51] Therefore, although the myocardium of the preterm neonate undergoes structural and functional maturation over many months, it appears that, after a transient dysfunction of varying severity immediately after delivery, it can relatively rapidly adapt to the postnatal changes in systemic hemodynamics.

In addition to the developmentally regulated susceptibility to dysfunction, a decrease in the oxygen supply associated with perinatal depression is a major cause of poor myocardial function and low cardiac output in preterm and term neonates immediately following delivery. During fetal life, despite being in a "hypoxic" environment by postnatal norms, neuroendocrine and other compensatory mechanisms

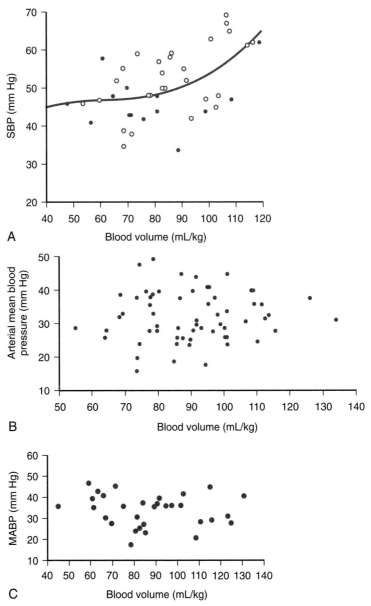

Figure 1-3   **A,** Relationship between blood volume and systemic blood pressure. Open and closed circles represent systolic blood pressure (SBP) measured by oscillometry or an umbilical artery catheter, respectively (see text for details). **B and C,** Relationship between blood volume and mean arterial blood pressure (MABP). There is no significant association (see text for details). (**A,** Adapted with permission from Bauer K, Linderkamp O, Versmold HT. Systolic blood pressure and blood volume in preterm infants. Arch Dis Child Fetal Neonatal Ed. 1994;69:521-522. **B,** Adapted with permission from Barr PA, Bailey PE, Sumners J. Relation between arterial blood pressure and blood volume and effect of infused albumin in sick preterm infants. Pediatrics. 1977;60:282-289. **C,** Adapted with permission from and Wright IM, Goodall SR. Blood pressure and blood volume in preterm infants. Arch Dis Child Fetal Neonatal Ed. 1994;70: F230-F231.)

and the unique fetal circulation enable the fetus to tolerate the "relative" hypoxemia and even brief episodes of true fetal hypoxemia. As mentioned earlier, during fetal hypoxemia the distribution of blood flow is altered to maintain perfusion and oxygen supply to the vital organs including the heart.[52-54] However, a significant degree of hypoxemia, especially when associated with metabolic acidosis, can rapidly exhaust the compensatory mechanisms and result in myocardial dysfunction. The critical threshold of fetal arterial oxygen saturation below which metabolic acidosis develops varies depending on the cause of fetal hypoxia. In the animal model of maternal hypoxia-induced fetal hypoxia, fetal arterial oxygen saturations below 30% are associated with metabolic acidosis. In addition, it appears that the fetus is more or less susceptible to hypoxia if the cause of hypoxia is umbilical cord occlusion or decreased uterine blood flow, respectively. Human data obtained by fetal pulse oximetry are consistent with the results of animal studies and indicate that the oxygen saturation of 30% is indeed the threshold for the development of fetal metabolic acidosis.[55]

An increase in cardiac enzymes and cardiac troponin T and I are useful in the assessment of the degree of myocardial injury associated with perinatal asphyxia.[56-59] In addition, increases in cardiac troponin T and I have been shown to be helpful in diagnosing myocardial injury even in the mildly depressed neonate. Whereas cardiac troponin T and I may be more sensitive than echocardiographic findings in detecting myocardial injury, the cardiovascular significance of the elevation of troponins in the absence of myocardial dysfunction remains unclear.[60]

Modifications of the cardiac contractile protein, myosin regulatory light chain 2 (MLC2) have also been implicated in the development of cardiac systolic dysfunction following newborn asphyxia. In a piglet model of perinatal asphyxia, a decrease in MLC2 phosphorylation and an increase in MLC2 degradation via nitration were observed suggesting that these are potential targets for therapeutic interventions to reduce myocardial damage in perinatal depression.[61] Nevertheless, documentation of clinical relevance of these findings is necessary to determine the future utility of such therapies.

Tricuspid regurgitation is the most common echocardiographic finding in neonates with perinatal depression and myocardial dysfunction. In cases with severe perinatal depression and myocardial injury, myocardial dysfunction frequently leads to decreases in cardiac output and the development of full-blown cardiogenic shock.[62,63] Finally, if the myocardium is not appropriately supported by inotropes, the ensuing low cardiac output will exacerbate the existing metabolic acidosis.[64]

Cardiogenic shock due to congenital heart defect, arrhythmia, cardiomyopathy, and PDA is discussed in other chapters in this book.

Vasodilation

The regulation of vascular smooth muscle tone is complex and involves neuronal, endocrine, paracrine, and autocrine factors (Fig. 1-4). Regardless of the regulatory stimuli, intracellular calcium availability plays the central role in regulating vascular smooth muscle tone. In the process of smooth muscle cell contraction, the regulatory protein calmodulin combines with calcium to activate myosin kinase. This enzyme phosphorylates the myosin light chain, facilitating its binding with actin and thus resulting in contraction. As for vasodilation, in addition to the reduction in intracellular calcium availability, myosin phosphatase generates muscle relaxation by dephosphorylation of the myosin light chain.

Maintenance of the vascular tone depends on the balance between the opposing forces of vasodilation and vasoconstriction. The vasodilatory and vasoconstricting mediators exert their effects by inducing alteration in cytosolic calcium concentration and/or by direct activation of the enzymes involved in the process. Influx of calcium through cell membrane voltage-gated calcium channels and release of calcium from sarcoplasmic reticulum are the two sources responsible for the rise in cytosolic calcium required for muscle contraction.

Recently, the role of various potassium channels has been identified in the regulation of vascular tone. Among these, the adenosine triphosphate (ATP)-dependent potassium channel (K_{ATP}) emerged as the key channel through which many modulators exert their action on vascular smooth muscle tone. In addition, the K_{ATP} channel has been implicated in pathogenesis of vasodilatory shock.[65] K_{ATP} channels are located on the smooth muscle cell membrane and opening of these channels leads to K^+ efflux with resultant hyperpolarization of the cell membrane. Cell membrane hyperpolarization in turn causes the closure of the voltage-gated calcium channels in the cell membrane and thus a reduction in cytosolic calcium and a decreased vascular tone.

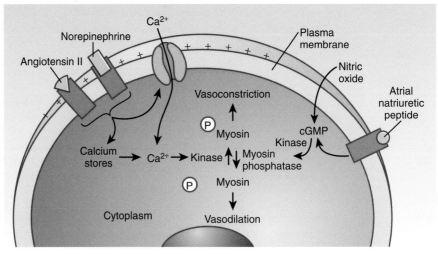

Figure 1-4 Regulation of vascular smooth muscle tone. The steps involved in vasoconstriction and vasodilation are shown in blue and red, respectively. Phosphorylation (P) of myosin is the critical step in the contraction of vascular smooth muscle. The action of vasoconstrictors such as angiotensin II and norepinephrine result in an increase in cytosolic calcium concentration, which activates myosin kinase. Vasodilators such as atrial natriuretic peptide and nitric oxide activate myosin phosphatase and, by dephosphorylating myosin, cause vasorelaxation. The plasma membrane is shown at resting potential (plus signs). cGMP, denotes cyclic guanosine monophosphate. (Adapted with permission from Landry DW, Oliver JA. The pathogenesis of vasodilatory shock. N Engl J Med. 2001;345:588-595.)

Under normal conditions, the K_{ATP} channels are closed for the most part. However, under pathologic conditions a number of stimuli may activate these channels and thus affect tissue perfusion. For instance, via the associated reduction in ATP and the increase in H^+ concentration and lactate levels, tissue hypoxia activates K_{ATP} channels, resulting in vasodilation and a compensatory increase in tissue perfusion.[66]

As mentioned earlier, a number of vasodilators and vasoconstrictors exert their effects through the K_{ATP} channels. For example, in septic shock, several endocrine and paracrine factors such as atrial natriuretic peptide, adenosine, and nitric oxide are released, resulting in activation of K_{ATP} channels.[66,67] Thus K_{ATP} channels are thought to play an important role in pathogenesis of vasodilatory shock. Indeed, animal studies have shown an improvement in BP following administration of K_{ATP} channel blockers.[68,69] However, a small human trial failed to show any benefit of the administration of the K_{ATP} channel inhibitor glibenclamide in adults with septic shock.[70] Although the sample size was small and several problems have been identified with the methodology, the findings of this study suggest that the mechanism of vasodilation in septic shock is more complex than initially believed.[71]

Eicosanoids are derived from cell membrane phospholipids through metabolism of arachidonic acid by the cyclooxygenase or lipoxygenase enzymes and have a wide range of effects on vascular tone. For example, prostacyclin and prostaglandin (PG)E_2 are vasodilators while thromboxane A_2 is a vasoconstrictor. Apart from their involvement in the physiologic regulation of vascular tone, these eicosanoids also play a role in pathogenesis of shock. Both human and animal studies have shown a beneficial effect of cyclooxygenase inhibition in septic shock.[72,73] In addition, rats deficient in essential fatty acid and thus unable to produce significant amounts of eicosanoids are less susceptible to endotoxic shock than their wild-type counterparts. However, the role of eicosanoids in the pathogenesis of shock is also more complex and some studies suggest that, under different conditions, they may actually have a beneficial role. For example, administration of PGI_2, PGE_1, and PGE_2 improves the cardiovascular status in animals with hypovolemic shock.[74,75] Another layer of complexity is revealed by the observation that production of both the vasodilator and vasoconstrictor prostanoids is increased in shock.[76,77]

Nitric oxide (NO) is another paracrine substance, which plays an important role in the regulation of vascular tone. Normally, NO is produced in vascular endothelial cells by the constitutive enzyme endothelial NO synthase (eNOS). NO then diffuses to the adjacent smooth muscle cells where it activates guanylyl cyclase, resulting in increased cyclic guanosine monophosphate (cGMP) formation. Cyclic GMP then induces vasodilation by the activation of cGMP-dependent protein kinase and the different K^+ channels as well as by the inhibition of inositol triphosphate formation and calcium entry into the vascular smooth muscle cells.

In septic shock, endotoxin, and cytokines such as tumor necrosis factor alpha, result in increased expression of inducible NO synthase (iNOS).[78-81] Studies in animals and humans have shown that NO level significantly increases in various forms of shock especially in septic shock.[82,83] This excessive and dysregulated production of NO then leads to severe vasodilation, hypotension, and vasopressor resistance (see later and Chapters 12 and 14). Because of the role of NO in the pathogenesis of vasodilatory shock, a number of studies have looked at the NO production pathway as a potential target of therapeutic interventions. However, studies using a nonselective NOS inhibitor in patients with septic shock have found significant side effects and increased mortality associated with this treatment modality.[84-86] The deleterious effects were likely due to inhibition of eNOS, the constitutive NOS that plays an important role in the physiologic regulation of vascular tone. Indeed, subsequent studies using a selective iNOS inhibitor found an improvement of BP and a reduction in lactic acidosis.[87] Whether the use of selective iNOS inhibitors is beneficial in neonatal vasodilatory shock remains unknown.

Recently there has been a renewed interest in the cardiovascular effects of vasopressin.[88,89] Although in postnatal life and under physiologic conditions, this hormone is primarily involved in the regulation of osmolality, there is accumulating evidence suggesting a role of vasopressin in the pathogenesis of vasodilatory shock. Vasopressin exerts its vascular effects through the two isoforms of V_1 receptors. V_{1a} receptor is expressed in all vessels while V_{1b} is only present in pituitary gland. The renal epithelial effects of vasopressin are mediated through V_2 receptors.

Postnatally and under physiologic conditions, vasopressin contributes little if any to the maintenance of vascular smooth muscle tone. However, under pathologic conditions such as in shock, with the decrease in BP vasopressin production increases attenuating the further decline in BP. With progression of the circulatory compromise, however, vasopressin levels decline as pituitary vasopressin stores become depleted. The decline in vasopressin production leads to further losses of vascular tone and contributes to the development of refractory hypotension.[90] Findings on the effectiveness of vasopressin replacement therapy in reversing refractory hypotension further support the role of vasopressin in the pathogenesis of vasodilatory shock.[91,92] The vasoconstrictor effects of vasopressin appear to be dose-dependent.[93] As mentioned earlier, excessive production of NO and activation of K_{ATP} channels are some of the major mechanisms involved in the pathogenesis of vasodilatory shock. Under these circumstances, vasopressin inhibits NO-induced cGMP production and inactivates the K_{ATP} channels resulting in improvement in vascular tone. In addition, vasopressin releases calcium from sarcoplasmic reticulum and augments the vasoconstrictive effects of norepinephrine. As for its clinical use, vasopressin has been shown to improve cardiovascular function in neonates and children presenting with vasopressor-resistant vasodilatory shock after cardiac surgery.[94] However, the few published case series on preterm infants with refractory hypotension show variable effects of vasopressin treatment with improvement in BP and urine output only in some patients.[95,96]

In general, vasodilation with or without decreased myocardial contractility is the dominant underlying cause of hemodynamic disturbances in septic shock. However, there are very limited data on changes in cardiovascular function in neonates with septic shock. A recent study in preterm infants with late-onset sepsis found that the high cardiac output characteristic for the earlier stages of septic shock diminished and SVR sharply increased before death in nonsurviving patients while there was only a mild increase in the SVR during the course of the cardiovascular disturbance in patients who survived. The authors also described a significant variability in hemodynamic response among the survivors.[97] Another study in children with fluid resistant shock found different patterns of hemodynamic derangement in central venous catheter-related (CVCR) versus community acquired (CA) infections. Low SVR and low cardiac output were the dominant pathophysiologic findings in patients with CVCR and CA septic shock, respectively. These findings suggest that the hemodynamic response may be different depending on the type of bacterial pathogen and/or represent the fact that patients with CA septic shock are usually diagnosed at a later stage and thus myocardial dysfunction might have already set in at the time of the diagnosis.[98] The results of the above studies underscore the importance of direct assessment of cardiac function by echocardiography and tailoring the treatment strategy according to the hemodynamic finding in each individual patient.

The case study presented here underscores this point and illustrates that the population-based BP values defining hypotension must be viewed as guidelines only that do not necessarily apply to the given patient. This is explained by the fact that a number of factors including gestational and postnatal age, preexisting insults, $PaCO_2$ and PaO_2 levels, acidosis, and the underlying pathophysiology all impact the critical BP value in the given patient at which perfusion pressure becomes progressively inadequate to first sustain vital organ (brain, heart, adrenal glands) perfusion and blood flow autoregulation, then brain function and, finally structural integrity of the organs.

Case Study

A preterm infant (twin A) was born at $31\frac{1}{7}$ weeks' gestation (BW 1180 g, 8th percentile) via cesarean section due to abnormal umbilical cord Doppler findings. There was no evidence of chorioamnionitis, and Apgar scores were 4 and 7 at 1 and 5 minutes, respectively. The patient was in room air without any respiratory support and blood gases and CRT had been normal during the first 3 postnatal hours in the neonatal intensive care unit. However, the neonate's mean arterial BP had been low and at 3 hours of age was 21 mm Hg with systolic and diastolic BPs at 34 and 14 mm Hg, respectively.

What would be the best course of action? Should one increase BP by increasing SVR and cardiac output using a vasopressor with inotropic property such as dopamine or epinephrine? Or, is increasing cardiac output using a primarily inotropic agent such as dobutamine more appropriate in hypotensive preterm neonates during the early postnatal transitional period? Or, should one attempt to further increase preload by giving additional boluses of physiologic saline? Or, should we ignore the mean arterial BP value as the clinical exam and laboratory findings were not suggestive of poor perfusion and there was no metabolic acidosis? Most neonatologists would choose one of the above listed options and, in the absence of additional information on the hemodynamic status, it is indeed impossible to know what to do and whether the treatment choice chosen was the right one.

Therefore, before choosing a treatment option, we had obtained additional information on the cardiovascular status by assessing cardiac function, systemic perfusion, and CBF using targeted neonatal echocardiography (Fig. 1-5). Myocardial contractility, assessed by the shortening fraction, was 35% (normal 28-42%) and left ventricular output was 377 mL/kg/min (normal 150-300 mL/kg/min) in the presence of an equally bidirectional PDA flow. Middle cerebral artery (MCA) blood flow, assessed by MCA mean velocity and flow pattern, was normal. Using the additional hemodynamic information obtained by echocardiography and ultrasonography, it was clear that the cause of the low BP was the low SVR with a compensatory increase in the cardiac output (BP ∝ Cardiac output × SVR). Given the normal myocardial contractility, the high cardiac output and the normal CBF along with the lack of clinical or laboratory signs of systemic hypoperfusion, we opted to closely monitor the patient without any intervention to attempt to increase the BP. By 9 hours of age, mean BP spontaneously increased to 29 mm Hg and the repeat echocardiogram

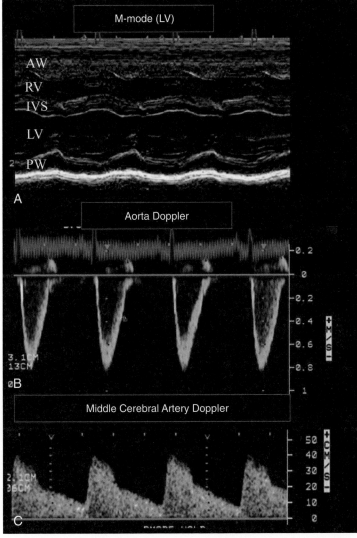

Figure 1-5   Direct assessment of hemodynamic by echocardiography and Doppler. **A,** The changes in cardiac wall motions are shown in this M-mode image; note the normal motion of the IVS and PW resulting in normal shortening fraction. **B,** The spectral Doppler at the aortic valve is shown here, which along with the diameter of aorta is used to estimate the left ventricular output. **C,** The middle cerebral artery flow Doppler depicts a normal pattern. AW, anterior wall; IVS, intraventricular septum; LV, left ventricle; PW, posterior Wall; RV, right ventricle.

revealed a mild decrease in left ventricular output. Accordingly, a significant increase in the calculated SVR had occurred (Fig. 1-6). After another 24 hours had passed, mean BP increased to 31 mm Hg and, because cardiac output did not change, calculated SVR continued to rise. The patient remained clinically stable during the entire hospital course and was discharged home without evidence of early brain morbidity.

This case study illustrates several important points. First, without appropriate assessment of systemic and organ blood flow while relying on BP and the indirect clinical and laboratory signs of tissue perfusion, it would have been impossible to ascertain the adequacy of systemic and brain perfusion *at the time of presentation*. Secondly, assessment of cardiac output and the calculation of the SVR did aid in choosing the most appropriate course of action. Thirdly, in addition to the evaluation of cardiac output and calculation of SVR, information on systemic blood flow distribution to the organs, especially the brain, may help in formulating a

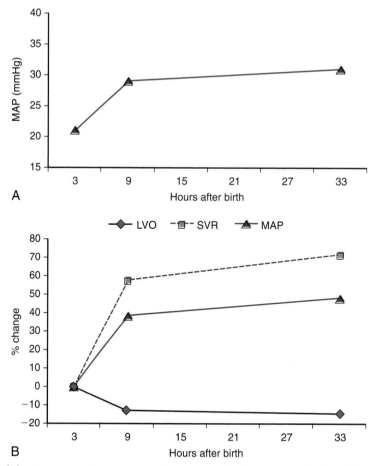

Figure 1-6 The changes in hemodynamics are shown in these graphs. **A,** Mean BP gradually increased from 21 mm Hg to 31 mm Hg over 30 hours. **B,** The 38% increase in mean BP at 9 hours after birth was the result of an increase in SVR (57%) and a mild decrease in left ventricular output (LVO) (13%). SVR continued to rise without a significant change in LVO at 33 hours.

pathophysiology-based treatment strategy in neonates with suspected hemodynamic derangement.

In this case, we chose to closely monitor the infants rather than to treat the hypotension as we documented a compensatory increase in cardiac output and one of the surrogate measures of CBF (MCA Doppler and flow pattern) was normal. In this case, it took 6 hours for the vascular tone to spontaneously improve to the degree where mean BP reached the lower limit of the population-based normal value. One may argue for the careful titration of low-dose vasopressor support even in this situation so that normalization of SVR can be facilitated and hence mean BP would have "normalized" faster. However, in a patient with evidence of adequate systemic and cerebral blood flow, the potential side effects of vasopressor use likely outweigh its benefits. This is especially true if vasopressors, when used, are not carefully titrated to achieve an appropriate hemodynamic target beyond the "normalization" of the BP. Because CBF autoregulation is impaired during hypotension, a significant and rapid rise in BP results in an abrupt increase in CBF with a potential for cerebral injury, possibly a hemorrhage.[34] However, in patients in whom cardiac output does not compensate for the decreased SVR, hypotension will lead to decreased CBF with a potential for cerebral injury, possibly ischemic lesions especially in the white matter with or without a secondary hemorrhage.[34] In addition and as discussed earlier, because our ability to clinically assess the adequacy of circulation is inaccurate, it is very important that low BP values are not disregarded without additional direct assessment of systemic hemodynamics and CBF and close and careful monitoring of the patient.[99]

Adrenal Insufficiency (See Chapters 12 and 14)

The adrenal glands play a crucial role in cardiovascular homeostasis. *Mineralocorticoids* regulate intravascular volume through their effects on maintaining adequate extracellular sodium concentration. In cases of mineralocorticoid deficiency such as the salt-wasting type of congenital adrenal hyperplasia, the renal loss of sodium is associated with volume depletion and leads to a decrease in circulating blood volume resulting in low cardiac output and shock. In addition to their role in the maintenance of circulating blood volume, physiologic levels of mineralocorticoids play an important role in the regulation of cytosolic calcium availability in the myocardium and vascular smooth muscle cells.[100] *Glucocorticoids* exert their cardiovascular effects mainly by enhancing the sensitivity of the cardiovascular system to catecholamines. The rapid rise of BP in the early postnatal period has been attributed to maturation of glucocorticoid-regulated vascular smooth muscle cell response to central and local stimulatory mechanisms, changes in the expression of the vascular angiotensin II receptor subtypes, and accumulation of elastin and collagen in large arteries.[101-103] Glucocorticoids play a role in the latter mechanism via their stimulatory effect on collagen synthesis in the vascular wall.[104] Given the importance of corticosteroids in cardiovascular stability, it is not surprising that deficiency of these hormones plays a role in the pathogenesis of certain forms of neonatal shock.

Preterm infants are born with an immature hypothalamic-pituitary-adrenal axis. Several indirect pieces of evidence suggest that immature preterm infants are only capable of producing enough corticosteroids to meet their metabolic demand and support their growth during well state (Chapter 14). When critically ill, a number of these patients cannot mount an adequate stress response. This condition has been referred to as relative adrenal insufficiency. However, the cause of this condition remains unclear. Hanna et al reported normal adrenal response to both corticotropin-releasing hormone (CRH) and adrenocorticotropic hormone (ACTH) stimulation tests in ELBW infants, and these authors concluded that failure of mounting an adequate stress response in sick preterm neonates may be related to the inability if the immature hypothalamus to recognize stress and/or because of inadequate hypothalamic secretion of CRH in response to stress.[105] In contrast, Ng and colleagues reported a severely reduced cortisol (adrenal) response to human CRH in premature infants with vasopressor-resistant hypotension during the first postnatal week.[106] The same group of investigators using CRH stimulation test also studied the characteristics of pituitary-adrenal response in a large group of VLBW infants.[107] Compared with normotensive infants, hypotensive patients receiving vasopressors/inotropes had higher ACTH but lower cortisol responses. Similarly, Masumoto and colleagues found that while cortisol precursors were elevated in preterm infants with late onset circulatory collapse, their serum cortisol concentrations were similar to those of the control group suggesting immaturity of the adrenal gland.[108] In contrast to the findings of Hanna and colleagues, the more recent data suggest that the pituitary gland of the VLBW infant is mature enough to mount adequate ACTH response and that the primary problem of relative adrenal insufficiency is the immaturity of the adrenal glands.[105,107,108]

Even though absolute adrenal insufficiency is a rare diagnosis in neonatal period, as mentioned earlier, there is accumulating evidence that relative adrenal insufficiency is a rather common entity in preterm infants (Chapter 14). Relative adrenal insufficiency is defined as a low baseline total serum cortisol level considered inappropriate for the degree of severity of the patient's illness. However, there is no agreement on what this level might be. For the purpose of replacement therapy in adults, a cortisol level below 15 mcg/dL is usually considered diagnostic for relative adrenal insufficiency.[109] To establish the presumptive diagnosis of relative adrenal insufficiency for the neonatal patient population, some authors have suggested the use of a total serum cortisol cutoff value of 5 mcg/dL while others have used the cutoff value established for adults (15 mcg/dL).[110,111] However, use of an arbitrary

A

single serum cortisol level to define relative adrenal insufficiency may not be appropriate especially in the neonatal period primarily because there is a large variation in total serum cortisol levels in neonates.[105,107,112-118] In addition, during the first 3 months of postnatal life, total serum cortisol levels progressively decrease with advancing postnatal age.[119,120] Furthermore, most studies have shown an inverse relationship between total serum cortisol levels and gestational age.[119-122] The study by Ng and colleagues discussed earlier has also demonstrated a gestational age-independent correlation between serum cortisol level and the lowest BP registered in the immediate postnatal period in VLBW infants.[107] These authors also found that serum cortisol levels inversely correlate with the maximum and cumulative dose of vasopressor/inotropes. However, despite these correlations, they found an overlap of serum cortisol levels between normotensive and hypotensive VLBW infants thus making it difficult to define a single serum cortisol level below which adrenal insufficiency can be diagnosed with certainty. A large prospective study of low-dose hydrocortisone therapy for prophylaxis of early adrenal insufficiency showed that low cortisol values at 12-48 hours or postnatal days 5-7 were not predictive of increased rates of morbidity or mortality.[123] This casts further doubt on the utility of low cortisol level on a single random blood draw for the diagnosis of relative adrenal insufficiency.

Another important factor to consider is that free rather than bound cortisol is the active form of the hormone. Most of the circulating cortisol is bound to corticosteroid binding globulin and albumin. Therefore, with changes in the concentrations of these binding proteins, total serum cortisol level may change without a significant change in the availability of the biologically active form (i.e., free cortisol).[124] In addition, the fraction of free cortisol is different in neonates from that in adults. In adults, free cortisol constitutes about 10% of total serum cortisol but in neonates free cortisol is 20 to 30% of their total serum cortisol.[119] Finally, disease severity also appears to influence the ratio of free-to-total serum cortisol concentration as in critically ill adults, the percentage of free cortisol can be almost three times as high as in healthy subjects.[124] There is no information on the potential impact of critical condition on the ratio of free-to-total serum cortisol concentration in neonates.

Regardless of the pathogenesis of relative adrenal insufficiency, immaturity of the hypothalamus-pituitary-adrenal axis in general has been linked to susceptibility to common complication of prematurity such as PDA and bronchopulmonary dysplasia.[113,125,126] In addition, due to the role of corticosteroids in the regulation of BP and cardiovascular homeostasis, it is not surprising that adrenal insufficiency is commonly identified as a cause of hypotension especially when hypotension is resistant to vasopressor/inotropes (Chapter 14). Indeed, it has been demonstrated that more than half of the mechanically ventilated near term and term infants receiving vasopressor/inotropes have total serum cortisol levels below 15 mcg/dL.[73] In more immature preterm infants, even a larger proportion of the patients has low serum cortisol levels. Korte and colleagues have found that 76% of sick VLBW infants have serum cortisol levels less than 15 mcg/dL.[110] Finally, recent studies demonstrating an improvement in the cardiovascular status in response to low dose steroid administration to preterm and term neonates indirectly support the role of relative adrenal insufficiency in the pathogenesis of hypotension (Chapter 14).[106,127-135]

Downregulation of Adrenergic Receptors

With exposure to agonists, stimulation of receptors generally results in desensitization, sequestration, and, finally, downregulation of the receptor. This process has been extensively studied in beta- and alpha-adrenergic receptors. For beta-adrenergic receptors, desensitization of receptor signaling occurs within seconds to minutes of the ligand-induced activation of the receptor. Desensitization involves uncoupling of the receptor-G-protein compound caused by a conformational change of the receptor following phosphorylation of its cytoplasmic loops. If stimulation of the beta-adrenergic receptor is sustained, the process leads to endocytosis of the intact phosphorylated receptor (sequestration). Both receptor desensitization and

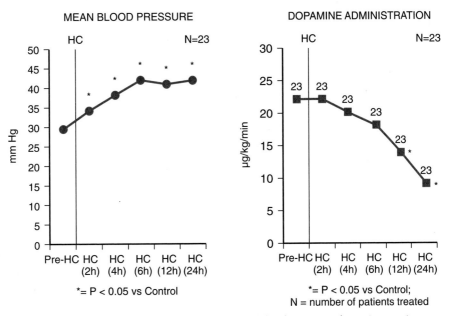

Figure 1-7 The increase in mean blood pressure and the decrease in dopamine requirement in response to low-dose hydrocortisone (HC) treatment in preterm infants with vasopressor-resistant hypotension. (Adapted with permission from Seri I, Tan R, Evans J. Cardiovascular effects of hydrocortisone in preterm infants with pressor-resistant hypotension. Pediatrics. 2001;107:1070-1074.)

sequestration are rapidly reversible. However, with continued prolonged exposure to its ligand, downregulation of the adrenergic receptor occurs. This process involves lysosomal degradation of the receptor protein. Recovery from down-regulation requires biosynthesis of new receptor protein, which takes several hours and is enhanced in the presence of corticosteroids.[130,136]

Recently, downregulation of adrenergic receptors has been implicated in the pathogenesis of vasopressor-resistant hypotension. Improvement in the cardiovascular status in patients with refractory hypotension following administration of corticosteroids supports this notion as glucocorticoids upregulate adrenergic receptor gene function and result in enhanced expression of adrenergic receptors.[137,138] These "genomic" effects of corticosteroids may explain why vasopressor requirement decreases within 6 to 12 hours following corticosteroid administration (Fig. 1-7).[130,131] However, it is important to point out that the beneficial steroidal effects on the cardiovascular system are not limited to adrenergic receptor upregulation. Other genomic mechanisms include inhibition of inducible nitric oxide synthase, and upregulation of myocardial angiotensin II receptors.[130,139-141] Nongenomic steroidal actions include the immediate increase in cytosolic calcium availability in vascular smooth muscle and myocardial cells, inhibition of degradation and reuptake of catecholamines, and inhibition of prostacyclin production.[130,140] The wide range of genomic and nongenomic effects of steroids explains the rapid and often sustained improvement in all components of the cardiovascular status (Fig. 1-8) of the critically ill neonate treated with low-dose hydrocortisone.[130,132]

While downregulation of the cardiovascular adrenergic receptors is well described in critically ill adults and many clinical observations support its occurrence in neonates, findings of one study in the newborn rat question the importance of this phenomenon during the early neonatal period.[142] By studying the effects of acute and chronic stimulation of beta-adrenergic receptors in newborn rats, the authors found that neonatal beta-adrenergic receptors are inherently capable of desensitization in some, but not all, tissues. For example, while beta-adrenergic receptors in the liver became desensitized, beta-agonists did not seem to elicit

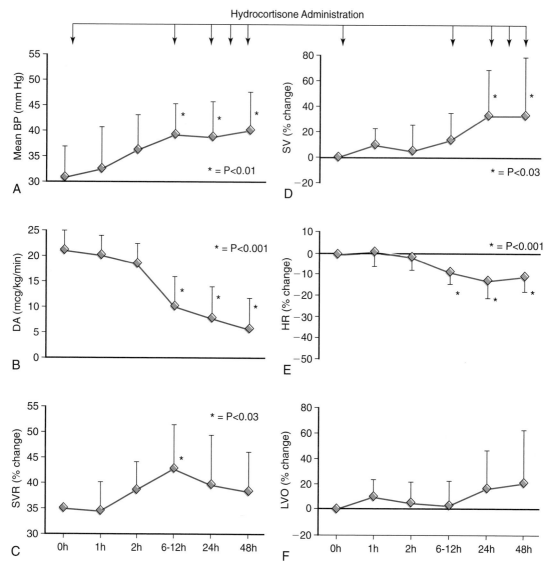

Figure 1-8 Changes in cardiovascular function in response to hydrocortisone (HC) in vasopressor-treated preterm neonates. **A** and **B** depict changes in mean BP and dopamine dosage (DA), respectively. The percentage changes relative to baseline (0 hour) in systemic vascular resistance (SVR) **(C)**, stroke volume (SV) **(D)**, heart rate (HR) **(E)**, and left ventricular output (LVO) **(F)**. (Adapted with permission from Noori S, Friedlich P, Wong P, et al. Hemodynamic changes after low-dosage hydrocortisone administration in vasopressor-treated preterm and term neonates. Pediatrics. 2006;118:1456-1466.)

desensitization of the beta-adrenergic receptor and adenylyl cyclase signaling in the myocardium of the newborn rat. Obviously, further studies are needed to gain a better understanding of the potential developmentally regulated differences in the response of the cardiovascular adrenergic receptors to prolonged agonist exposure. Chapter 14 also addresses these questions in the context of relative adrenal insufficiency of the preterm and term neonate.

In summary, this chapter reviews the principles of developmental hemodynamics during fetal life, postnatal transition, and the neonatal period as well as the etiology and pathophysiology of neonatal cardiovascular compromise. Although significant advances have recently been made in these areas, much more needs to be understood before we can accurately diagnose and appropriately treat preterm and term neonates with cardiovascular compromise during transition and beyond (see also Chapters 12, 15, and 16).

References

1. Kiserud T. Physiology of the fetal circulation. Semin Fetal Neonatal Med. 2005;10:493-503.
2. Rudolph AM. Distribution and regulation of blood flow in the fetal and neonatal lamb. Circ Res. 1985;57:811-821.
3. Sutton MS, Groves A, MacNeill A, et al. Assessment of changes in blood flow through the lungs and foramen ovale in the normal human fetus with gestational age: a prospective Doppler echocardiographic study. Br Heart J. 1994;71:232-237.
4. Rasanen J, Wood DC, Weiner S, et al. Role of the pulmonary circulation in the distribution of human fetal cardiac output during the second half of pregnancy. Circulation. 1996;94:1068-1073.
5. Mielke G, Benda N. Cardiac output and central distribution of blood flow in the human fetus. Circulation. 2001;103:1662-1668.
6. Kiserud T, Ebbing C, Kessler J, et al. Fetal cardiac output, distribution to the placenta and impact of placental compromise. Ultrasound Obstet Gynecol. 2006;28:126-136.
7. Iwamoto HS, Teitel D, Rudolph AM. Effects of birth-related events on blood flow distribution. Pediatr Res. 1987;22:634-640.
8. Noori S, Wlodaver A, Gottipati V, et al. Transitional changes in cardiac and cerebral hemodynamics in term neonates at birth. J Pediatr. 2012 (in press).
9. Weindling AM. Peripheral oxygenation and management in the perinatal period. Semin Fetal Neonatal Med. 2010;15:208-215.
10. Noori S, Drabu B, McCoy M, et al. Non-invasive measurement of local tissue perfusion and its correlation with hemodynamic indices during the early postnatal period in term neonates. J Perinatol. 2011 Apr 28. [Epub ahead of print]
11. Kissack CM, Weindling AM. Peripheral blood flow and oxygen extraction in the sick, newborn very low birth weight infant shortly after birth. Pediatr Res. 2009;65:462-467.
12. Kroth J, Weidlich K, Hiedl S, et al. Functional vessel density in the first month of life in preterm neonates. Pediatr Res. 2008;64:567-571.
13. Stark MJ, Clifton VL, Wright IM. Microvascular flow, clinical illness severity and cardiovascular function in the preterm infant. Arch Dis Child Fetal Neonatal Ed. 2008;93:F271-F274.
14. Anderson PA. The heart and development. Semin Perinatol. 1996;20:482-509.
15. Noori S, Seri I. Pathophysiology of newborn hypotension outside the transitional period. Early Hum Dev. 2005;81:399-404.
16. Rowland DG, Gutgesell HP. Noninvasive assessment of myocardial contractility, preload, and afterload in healthy newborn infants. Am J Cardiol. 1995;75:818-821.
17. Gilbey MP, Spyer KM. Physiological aspects of autonomic nervous system function. Curr Opin Neurol Neurosurg. 1993;6:518-523.
18. Spyer KM. Annual review prize lecture. Central nervous mechanisms contributing to cardiovascular control. J Physiol. 1994;474:1-19.
19. Segar JL. Neural regulation of blood pressure during fetal and newborn life. In: Polin RA, Fox WW, Abman SH, eds. Fetal and neonatal physiology, 3rd ed. Philadelphia: Pennsylvania; 2004, Saunders.
20. Galland BC, Taylor BJ, Bolton DP, et al. Heart rate variability and cardiac reflexes in small for gestational age infants. J Appl Physiol. 2006;100:933-939.
21. Patural H, Pichot V, Jaziri F, et al. Autonomic cardiac control of very preterm newborns: a prolonged dysfunction. Early Hum Dev. 2008;84:681-687.
22. Pomeranz B, Macaulay RJ, Caudill MA, et al. Assessment of autonomic function in humans by heart rate spectral analysis, Am J Physiol. 1985;248:H151-H153.
23. Heart rate variability: Standards of measurement, physiological interpretation, and clinical use. Task Force of the European Society of Cardiology and the North American Society of Pacing and Electrophysiology. Circulation. 1996;93:1043-1065.
24. Kleiger RE, Stein PK, Bigger JT Jr. Heart rate variability: measurement and clinical utility. Ann Noninvasive Electrocardiol. 2005;10:88-101.
25. Griffin MP, Lake DE, Bissonette EA, et al. Heart rate characteristics: novel physiomarkers to predict neonatal infection and death. Pediatrics. 2005;116:1070-1074.
26. Fairchild KD, O'Shea TM. Heart rate characteristics: physiomarkers for detection of late-onset neonatal sepsis. Clin Perinatol. 2010;37:581-598.
27. Valverde E, Pellicer A, Madero R, et al. Dopamine versus epinephrine for cardiovascular support in low birth weight infants: analysis of systemic effects and neonatal clinical outcomes. Pediatrics. 2006;117:e1213-e1222.
28. Seri I. Circulatory support of the sick newborn infant. In: Levene MI, Evans N, Archer N, eds. Seminars in neonatology: perinatal cardiology. London: WB Saunders; 2001:85-95.
29. Nuntnarumit P, Yang W, Bada-Ellzey HS. Blood pressure measurements in the newborn. Clin Perinatol. 1999;26:981-996.
30. Zubrow AB, Hulman S, Kushner H, et al. Determinants of blood pressure in infants admitted to neonatal intensive care units: a prospective multicenter study. J Perinatol. 1995;15:470-479.
31. Munro MJ, Walker AM, Barfield CP. Hypotensive extremely low birth weight infants have reduced cerebral blood flow. Pediatrics. 2004;114:1591-1596.
32. Victor S, Marson AG, Appleton RE, et al. Relationship between blood pressure, cerebral electrical activity, cerebral fractional oxygen extraction, and peripheral blood flow in very low birth weight newborn infants. Pediatr Res. 2006:314-319.

33. Børch K, Lou HC, Greisen G. Cerebral white matter blood flow and arterial blood pressure in preterm infants. Acta Pædiatrica. 2010;99:1489-1492.
34. Tsuji M, Saul JP, du Plessis A, et al. Cerebral intravascular oxygenation correlates with mean arterial pressure in critically ill premature infants. Pediatrics. 2000;106:625-632.
35. Tyszczuk L, Meek J, Elwell C, et al. Cerebral blood flow is independent of mean arterial blood pressure in preterm infants undergoing intensive care. Pediatrics. 1998;102:337-341.
36. Kissack CM, Garr R, Wardle SP, et al. Cerebral fractional oxygen extraction in very low birth weight infants is high when there is low left ventricular output and hypocarbia but is unaffected by hypotension. Pediatr Res. 2004;55:400-405.
37. Noori S, Stavroudis TA, Seri I. Systemic and cerebral hemodynamics during the transitional period after premature birth. Clin Perinatol. 2009;36:723-736.
38. Seri I, Evans J. Controversies in the diagnosis and management of hypotension in the newborn infant. Curr Opin Pediatr. 2001;13:116-123.
39. Al-Aweel I, Pursley DM, Rubin LP, et al. Variations in prevalence of hypotension, hypertension, and vasopressor use in NICUs. J Perinatol. 2001;21:272-278.
40. Bauer K, Linderkamp O, Versmold HT. Systolic blood pressure and blood volume in preterm infants. Arch Dis Child Fetal Neonatal Ed. 1994;70:F230-F231.
41. Barr PA, Bailey PE, Sumners J, et al. Relation between arterial blood pressure and blood volume and effect of infused albumin in sick preterm infants. Pediatrics. 1977;60: 282-289.
42. Wright IM, Goodall SR. Blood pressure and blood volume in preterm infants. Arch Dis Child Fetal Neonatal Ed. 1994;70:F230-F231.
43. Gill AB, Weindling AM. Randomised controlled trial of plasma protein fraction versus dopamine in hypotensive very low birthweight infants. Arch Dis Child. 1993;69:284-287.
44. Lundstrom K, Pryds O, Greisen G. The haemodynamic effects of dopamine and volume expansion in sick preterm infants. Early Hum Dev. 2000;57:157-163.
45. Zaramella P, Freato F, Quaresima V, et al. Early versus late cord clamping: Effects on peripheral blood flow and cardiac function in term infants. Earl Hum Develop. 2008;84:195-200.
46. Baenziger O, Stolkin F, Keel M, et al. The influence of the timing of cord clamping on postnatal cerebral oxygenation in preterm neonates: a randomized, controlled trial. Pediatrics. 2007;119: 445-449.
47. Nelle M, Fisher S, Conze S, et al. Effects of late cord clamping on circulation in prematures (VLBWI). Pediatr Res. 1998;44:454 [abstract].
48. Rabe H, Reynolds G, Diaz-Rossello J. A systematic review and meta-analysis of a brief delay in clamping the umbilical cord of preterm infants. Neonatology. 2008;93:138-144.
49. Kluckow M, Evans N. Low superior vena cava flow and intraventricular haemorrhage in preterm infants. Arch Dis Child Fetal Neonatal Ed. 2000;82:F188-F194.
50. Osborn DA, Evans N, Kluckow M. Left ventricular contractility in extremely premature infants in the first day and response to inotropes. Pediatr Res. 2007;61:335-340.
51. Kehrer M, Blumenstock G, Ehehalt S, et al. Development of cerebral blood flow volume in preterm neonates during the first two weeks of life. Pediatr Res. 2005;58:927-930.
52. Noori S, Friedlich P, Seri I. Pathophysiology of neonatal shock. In: Polin RA, Fox WW, Abman S, eds. Fetal and neonatal physiology, 3rd ed. Philadelphia: WB Saunders; 2003:772-782.
53. Reuss ML, Rudolph AM. Distribution and recirculation of umbilical and systemic venous blood flow in fetal lambs during hypoxia. J Dev Physiol. 1980;2:71-84.
54. Davies JM, Tweed WA. The regional distribution and determinants of myocardial blood flow during asphyxia in the fetal lamb. Pediatr Res. 1984;18:764-767.
55. Kuhnert M, Seelbach-Goebel B, Butterwegge M. Predictive agreement between the fetal arterial oxygen saturation and scalp pH: results of the German multicenter study. Am J Obstet Gynecol. 1998;178:330-335.
56. Gunes T, Ozturk MA, Koklu SM, et al. Troponin-T levels in perinatally asphyxiated infants during the first 15 days of life. Acta Paediatr. 2005;94:1638-1643.
57. Trevisanuto D, Picco G, Golin R, et al. Cardiac troponin I in asphyxiated neonates. Biol Neonate. 2006;89:190-193.
58. Gaze DC, Collinson PO. Interpretation of cardiac troponin measurements in neonates—the devil is in the details. Biol Neonate. 2006;89:194-196.
59. El-Khuffash A, Davis PG, Walsh K, et al. Cardiac troponin T and N-terminal-pro-B type natriuretic peptide reflect myocardial function in preterm infants. J Perinatol. 2008;28:82-86.
60. Szymankiewicz M, Matuszczak-Wleklak M, Hodgman JE, et al. Usefulness of cardiac troponin T and echocardiography in the diagnosis of hypoxic myocardial injury of full-term neonates. Biol Neonate. 2005;88:19-23.
61. Doroszko A, Polewicz D, Cadete VJ, et al. Neonatal asphyxia induces the nitration of cardiac myosin light chain 2 that is associated with cardiac systolic dysfunction. Shock. 2010;34:592-600.
62. Walther FJ, Siassi B, Ramadan NA, et al. Cardiac output in newborn infants with transient myocardial dysfunction. J Pediatr. 1985;107:781-785.
63. Barberi I, Calabro MP, Cordaro S, et al. Myocardial ischaemia in neonates with perinatal asphyxia. Electrocardiographic, echocardiographic and enzymatic correlations. Eur J Pediatr. 1999;158: 742-747.
64. Seri I, Noori S. Diagnosis and treatment of neonatal hypotension outside the transitional period. Early Hum Dev. 2005;81:405-411.

65. Landry DW, Oliver JA. The pathogenesis of vasodilatory shock. N Engl J Med. 2001;345:588-595.
66. Quayle JM, Nelson MT, Standen NB. ATP-sensitive and inwardly rectifying potassium channels in smooth muscle. Physiol Rev. 1997;77:1165-1232.
67. Murphy ME, Brayden JE. Nitric oxide hyperpolarizes rabbit mesenteric arteries via ATP-sensitive potassium channels. J Physio. 1995;486:47-58.
68. Vanelli G, Hussain SN, Dimori M, et al. Cardiovascular responses to glibenclamide during endotoxaemia in the pig. Vet Res Commun. 1997;21:187-200.
69. Gardiner SM, Kemp PA, March JE, et al. Regional haemodynamic responses to infusion of lipopolysaccharide in conscious rats: effects of pre- or post-treatment with glibenclamide. Br J Pharmacol. 1999;128:1772-1778.
70. Warrillow S, Egi M, Bellomo R. Randomized, double-blind, placebo-controlled crossover pilot study of a potassium channel blocker in patients with septic shock. Crit Care Med. 2006;34:980-985.
71. Oliver JA, Landry DW. Potassium channels and septic shock. Crit Care Med. 2006;34:1255-1257.
72. Fink MP. Therapeutic options directed against platelet activating factor, eicosanoids and bradykinin in sepsis. J Antimicrob Chemother. 1998;41:81-94.
73. Arons MM, Wheeler AP, Bernard GR, et al. Effects of ibuprofen on the physiology and survival of hypothermic sepsis. Ibuprofen in Sepsis Study Group. Crit Care Med. 1999;27:699-707.
74. Feuerstein G, Zerbe RL, Meyer DK, et al. Alteration of cardiovascular, neurogenic, and humoral responses to acute hypovolemic hypotension by administered prostacyclin. J Cardiovasc Pharmacol. 1982;4:246-253.
75. Machiedo GW, Warden MJ, LoVerme PJ, et al. Hemodynamic effects of prolonged infusion of prostaglandin E1 (PGE1) after hemorrhagic shock. Adv Shock Res. 1982;8:171-176.
76. Reines HD, Halushka PV, Cook JA, et al. Plasma thromboxane concentrations are raised in patients dying with septic shock. Lancet. 1982;2:174-175.
77. Ball HA, Cook JA, Wise WC, et al. Role of thromboxane, prostaglandins and leukotrienes in endotoxic and septic shock. Intensive Care Med. 1986;12:116-1126.
78. Rubanyi GM. Nitric oxide and circulatory shock. Adv Exp Med Biol. 1998;454:165-172.
79. Liu S, Adcock IM, Old RW, et al. Lipopolysaccharide treatment in vivo induces widespread tissue expression of inducible nitric oxide synthase mRNA. Biochem Biophys Res Commun. 1993;196:1208-1213.
80. Taylor BS, Geller DA. Molecular regulation of the human inducible nitric oxide synthase (iNOS) gene. Shock. 2000;13:413-424.
81. Titheradge MA. Nitric oxide in septic shock. Biochim Biophys Acta. 1999;1411:437-455.
82. Doughty L, Carcillo JA, Kaplan S, et al. Plasma nitrite and nitrate concentrations and multiple organ failure in pediatric sepsis. Crit Care Med. 1998;26:157-162.
83. Carcillo JA. Nitric oxide production in neonatal and pediatric sepsis. Crit Care Med. 1999;27:1063-1065.
84. Barrington KJ, Etches PC, Schulz R, et al. The hemodynamic effects of inhaled nitric oxide and endogenous nitric oxide synthesis blockade in newborn piglets during infusion of heat-killed group B streptococci. Crit Care Med. 2000;28:800-808.
85. Mitaka C, Hirata Y, Ichikawa K, et al. Effects of nitric oxide synthase inhibitor on hemodynamic change and O2 delivery in septic dogs. Am J Physiol. 1995;268:H2017H201-H2017H223.
86. Grover R, Zaccardelli D, Colice G, et al. An open-label dose escalation study of the nitric oxide synthase inhibitor, N(G)-methyl-L-arginine hydrochloride (546C88), in patients with septic shock. Glaxo Wellcome International Septic Shock Study Group. Crit Care Med. 1999;27:913-922.
87. Mitaka C, Hirata Y, Yokoyama K, et al. A selective inhibitor for inducible nitric oxide synthase improves hypotension and lactic acidosis in canine endotoxic shock. Crit Care Med. 2001;29:2156-2161.
88. Rozenfeld V, Cheng JW. The role of vasopressin in the treatment of vasodilation in shock states. Ann Pharmacother. 2000;34:250-254.
89. Robin JK, Oliver JA, Landry DW. Vasopressin deficiency in the syndrome of irreversible shock. J Trauma. 2003;54:S149-S154.
90. Landry DW, Oliver JA. The pathogenesis of vasodilatory shock. N Engl J Med. 2001;345:588-595.
91. Landry DW, Levin HR, Gallant EM, et al. Vasopressin deficiency contributes to the vasodilation of septic shock. Circulation. 1997;95:1122-1125.
92. Liedel JL, Meadow W, Nachman J, et al. Use of vasopressin in refractory hypotension in children with vasodilatory shock: five cases and a review of the literature. Pediatr Crit Care Med. 2002;3:15-18.
93. Malay MB, Ashton JL, Dahl K, et al. Heterogeneity of the vasoconstrictor effect of vasopressin in septic shock. Crit Care Med. 2004;32:1327-1331.
94. Rosenzweig EB, Starc TJ, Chen JM, et al. Intravenous arginine-vasopressin in children with vasodilatory shock after cardiac surgery. Circulation. 1999;100:II182-II186.
95. Meyer S, Gottschling S, Baghai A, et al. Arginine-vasopressin in catecholamine-refractory septic versus non-septic shock in extremely low birth weight infants with acute renal injury. Crit Care. 2006;10:R71.
96. Bidegain M, Greenberg R, Simmons C, et al. Vasopressin for refractory hypotension in extremely low birth weight infants. J Pediatr. 2010;157:502-504.

97. de Waal K, Evans N. Hemodynamics in preterm infants with late-onset sepsis. J Pediatr. 2010;156:918-922.

98. Brierley J, Peters MJ. Distinct hemodynamic patterns of septic shock at presentation to pediatric intensive care. Pediatrics. 2008;122:752-759.

99. de Boode WP. Clinical monitoring of systemic hemodynamics in critically ill newborns. Early Hum Dev. 2010;86:137-141.

100. Wehling M. Looking beyond the dogma of genomic steroid action: insights and facts of the 1990s. J Mol Med. 1995;73:439-447.

101. Cox BE, Rosenfeld CR. Ontogeny of vascular angiotensin II receptor subtype expression in ovine development. Pediatr Res. 1999;45:414-424.

102. Kaiser JR, Cox BE, Roy TA, et al. Differential development of umbilical and systemic arteries. I. ANG II receptor subtype expression. Am J Physiol. 1998;274:R797-807.

103. Bendeck MP, Langille BL. Rapid accumulation of elastin and collagen in the aortas of sheep in the immediate perinatal period. Circ Res. 1991;69:1165-1169.

104. Leitman DC, Benson SC, Johnson LK. Glucocorticoids stimulate collagen and noncollagen protein synthesis in cultured vascular smooth muscle cells. J Cell Biol. 1984;98:541-549.

105. Hanna CE, Keith LD, Colasurdo MA, et al. Hypothalamic pituitary adrenal function in the extremely low birth weight infant. J Clin Endocrinol Metab. 1993;76:384-387.

106. Ng PC, Lam CWK, Fok TF, et al. Refractory hypotension in preterm infants with adrenocortical insufficiency. Arch Dis Child Fetal Neonatal Ed. 2001;84:F122-F124.

107. Ng PC, Lee CH, Lam CWK, et al. Transient adrenocortical insufficiency of prematurity and systemic hypotension in very low birthweight infants. Arch Dis Child, Fetal Neonatal Ed. 2004;89:F119-F126.

108. Masumoto K, Kusuda S, Aoyagi H, et al. Comparison of serum cortisol concentrations in preterm infants with or without late-onset circulatory collapse due to adrenal insufficiency of prematurity. Pediatr Res. 2008;63:686-690.

109. Cooper MS, Stewart PM. Corticosteroid insufficiency in acutely ill patients. N Engl J Med. 2003;348:727-734.

110. Korte C, Styne D, Merritt TA, et al. Adrenocortical function in the very low birth weight infant: improved testing sensitivity and association with neonatal outcome. J Pediatr. 1996;128:257-263.

111. Fernandez E, Schrader R, Watterberg K. Prevalence of low cortisol value in term and nearterm infants with vasopressor-resistant hypotension. J Perinatol. 2005;25:114-118.

112. Hingre RV, Gross SJ, Hingre KS, et al. Adrenal steroidogenesis in very low birth weight preterm infants. J Clin Endocrinol Metab. 1994;78:266-270.

113. Watterberg KL, Scott SM. Evidence of early adrenal insufficiency in babies who develop bronchopulmonary dysplasia. Pediatrics. 1995;95:120-125.

114. Jett PL, Samuels MH, McDaniel PA, et al. Variability of plasma cortisol levels in extremely low birth weight infants. J Clin Endocrinol Metab. 1997;82:2921-2925.

115. Hanna CE, Jett PL, Laird MR, et al. Corticosteroid binding globulin, total serum cortisol, and stress in extremely low-birth-weight infants. A J Perinatol. 1997;14:201-204.

116. Ng PC, Wong GWK, Lam CWK, et al. The pituitary-adrenal responses to exogenous human corticotropin-releasing hormone in preterm, very low birth weight infants. J Clin Endocrinol Metab. 1997;82:797-799.

117. Procianoy RS, Cecin SKG, Pinheiro CEA. Umbilical cord cortisol and prolactin levels in preterm infants; relation to labor and delivery. Acta Paediatr Scand. 1983;72:713-716.

118. Terrone DA, Smith LG, Wolf EJ, et al. Neonatal effects and serum cortisol levels after multiple courses of maternal corticosteroids. Obstet Gynecol. 1997;90:819-823.

119. Rokicki W, Forest MG, Loras B, et al. Free cortisol of human plasma in the first three months of life. Biol Neonate. 1990;57:21-29.

120. Wittekind CA, Arnold JD, Leslie GI, et al. Longitudinal study of plasma ACTH and cortisol in very low birth weight infants in the first 8 weeks of life. Early Hum Dev. 1993;33:191-200.

121. Goldkrand JW, Schulte RL, Messer RH. Maternal and fetal plasma cortisol levels at parturition. Obstet Gynecol. 1976;47:41-45.

122. Scott SM, Watterberg KL. Effect of gestational age, postnatal age, and illness on plasma cortisol concentrations in premature infants. Pediatr Res. 1995;37:112-116.

123. Aucott SW, Watterberg KL, Shaffer ML, et al; PROPHET Study Group. Do cortisol concentrations predict short-term outcomes in extremely low birth weight infants? Pediatrics. 2008;122:775-781.

124. Hamrahian AH, Oseni TS, Arafah BM. Measurements of serum free cortisol in critically ill patients. N Engl J Med. 2004;350:1629-1638.

125. Watterberg KL, Scott SM, Backstrom C, et al. Links between early adrenal function and respiratory outcome in preterm infants: airway inflammation and patent ductus arteriosus. Pediatrics. 2000;105:320-324.

126. Watterberg KL, Gerdes JS, Cole CH, et al. Prophylaxis of early adrenal insufficiency to prevent bronchopulmonary dysplasia: a multicenter trial. Pediatrics. 2004;114:1649-1657.

127. Helbock HJ, Insoft RM, Conte FA. Glucocorticoid-responsive hypotension in extremely low birth weight newborns. Pediatrics. 1993;92:715-717.

128. Fauser A, Pohlandt F, Bartmann P, et al. Rapid increase of blood pressure in extremely low birth weight infants after a single dose of dexamethasone. Eur J Pediatr. 1993;152:354-356.

129. Gaissmaier RE, Pohlandt F. Single dose dexamethasone treatment of hypotension in preterm infants. J Pediatr. 1999;134:701-705.
130. Seri I, Tan R, Evans J. Cardiovascular effects of hydrocortisone in preterm infants with pressor-resistant hypotension. Pediatrics. 2001;107:1070-1074.
131. Noori S, Siassi B, Durand M, et al. Cardiovascular effects of low-dose dexamethasone in very low birth weight neonates with refractory hypotension. Biol Neonate. 2006;89:82-87.
132. Noori S, Friedlich P, Wong P, et al. Hemodynamic changes following low-dose hydrocortisone administration in vasopressor-treated neonates. Pediatrics. 2006;118:1456-1466.
133. Ng PC, Lee CH, Bnur FL, et al. A double-blind, randomized, controlled study of a "stress dose" of hydrocortisone for rescue treatment of refractory hypotension in preterm infants. Pediatrics. 2006;117:367-375.
134. Baker CF, Barks JD, Engmann C, et al. Hydrocortisone administration for the treatment of refractory hypotension in critically ill newborns. J Perinatol. 2008;28:412-419.
135. Higgins S, Friedlich P, Seri I. Hydrocortisone for hypotension and vasopressor dependence in preterm neonates: a meta-analysis. J Perinatol. 2010;30:373-378.
136. Tsao P, von Zastrow M. Downregulation of G protein-coupled receptors. Curr Opin Neurobiol. 2000;10:365-369.
137. Davies AO, Lefkowitz RJ. Regulation of beta adrenergic receptors by steroid hormones. Annu Rev Physiol. 1984;46:119-130.
138. Hadcock JR, Malbon CC. Regulation of beta adrenergic receptor by permissive hormones: gluco-corticoids increase steady-state levels of receptor mRNA. Proc Natl Acad Sci U S A. 1988;85:8415-8419.
139. Radomski MW, Palmer RMJ, Moncada S. Glucocorticoids inhibit the expression of an inducible, but not the constitutive, nitric oxide synthase in vascular endothelial cells. Proc Natl Acad Sci U S A. 1990;87:10043-10047.
140. Wehling M. Specific, nongenomic actions of steroid hormones. Annu Rev Physiol. 1997;59:365-393.
141. Segar JL, Bedell K, Page WV, et al. Effect of cortisol on gene expression of the renin-angiotensin system in fetal sheep. Pediatr Res. 1995;37:741-746.
142. Auman JT, Seidler FJ, Tate CA, et al. Are developing beta-adrenoceptors able to desensitize? Acute and chronic effects of beta-agonists in neonatal heart and liver. Am J Physiol Regul Integr Comp Physiol. 2002;283:R205-R217.

CHAPTER 2

Autoregulation of Vital and Nonvital Organ Blood Flow in the Preterm and Term Neonate

Gorm Greisen, MD, PhD

- Regulation of Arterial Tone
- Blood Flow to the Brain
- Blood Flow to Other Organs
- Distribution of Cardiac Output in the Healthy Human Neonate
- Mechanisms Governing the Redistribution of Cardiac Output in the Fetal "Dive" Reflex
- Distribution of Cardiac Output in the Shocked Newborn
- Conclusion
- References

In most organs the principal role of perfusion is to provide substrates for cellular energy metabolism, with the final purpose of maintaining normal intracellular concentrations of the high-energy phosphate metabolites adenosine triphosphate (ATP) and phosphocreatine (PCr). The critical substrate is usually oxygen. Accordingly, organ blood flow is regulated by the energy demand of the given tissue. For instance in the brain, during maximal activation by seizures, cerebral blood flow increases 3-fold while in the muscle during maximal exercise, blood flow increases up to 8-fold. In addition, some organs such as the brain, heart, and liver have higher baseline oxygen and thus higher blood flow demand than others. Finally, in the skin, perfusion may be considerably above the metabolic needs as the increase in skin blood flow plays an important role in thermoregulation. Indeed, during heating, skin blood flow may increase by as much as 4-fold without any increase in energy demand.

In the developing organism metabolic requirements are increased by as much as 40% due to the expenditures of growth. Since growth involves deposition of protein and fat, energy metabolism and, in particular, tissue oxygen requirement are not increased as much as the requirements of protein and energy.

When blood flow is failing there are several lines of defense mechanisms before the tissue is damaged. First, more oxygen is extracted from the blood. Normal oxygen extraction is about 30%, resulting in a venous oxygen saturation of 65-70%. Oxygen extraction can increase up to 50-60%, resulting in a venous oxygen saturation of 40-50%, which corresponds to a venous, that is, end-capillary, oxygen tension of 3-4 kPa. This is the critical value for oxygen tension for driving the diffusion of molecular oxygen from the capillary into the cell and to the mitochondrion (Fig. 2-1). Second, microvascular anatomy and the pathophysiology of the underlying disease process are both important for the final steps of oxygen delivery to tissue. When the cell senses oxygen insufficiency, its function is affected as growth stops, organ function fails, and finally cellular and thus organ survival are threatened (Fig. 2-2). *Ischemia* is the term used for inadequate blood flow to maintain appropriate cellular function and integrity. Since there are several steps in the cellular reaction to oxygen insufficiency, more than one ischemic threshold may be defined. It is

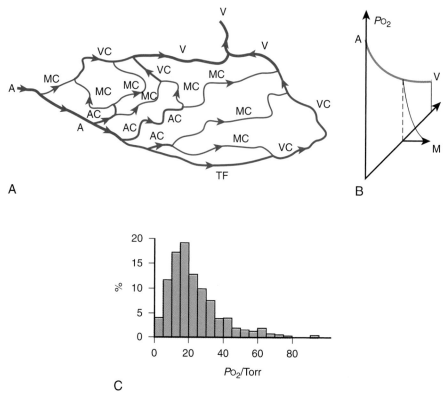

Figure 2-1   A, Draft of a capillary network. **B,** A three-dimensional graph illustrating the Po_2 gradients from the arterial (A) to the venous (V) end of the capillaries and the radial gradient of Po_2 in surrounding tissue to the mitochondrion (M). Y-axis: Po_2; X-axis: distance along the capillary (typically 1000 μm); Z-axis: distance into tissue (typically 50 μm). **C,** The wide distribution of tissue Po_2 as recorded by microelectrode. Y-axis: frequency of measurements; X-axis: Po_2. Po_2 values in tissue are typically 10-30 Torr (1.5-4.5 kPa), but range from near-arterial levels to near zero. The cells with the lowest Po_2 determine the ischemic threshold, that is, the most remote cells at the venous end of capillaries. Microvascular factors, such as capillary density, and distribution of blood flow among capillaries are very important for oxygen transport to tissue.

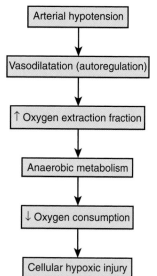

Figure 2-2   The lines of defense against oxygen insufficiency. First, when blood pressure falls, autoregulation of organ blood flow will reduce vascular resistance and keep blood flow nearly unaffected. If the blood pressure falls below the lower limit of the autoregulation, or if autoregulation is impaired by vascular pathology or immaturity, blood flow to the tissue falls. At this point, oxygen extraction increases from each milliliter of blood. The limit of this compensation is when the minimal venous oxygen saturation, or rather the minimal end-capillary oxygen tension, has been reached. This process is determined by microvascular factors as illustrated in Figure 2-1. When the limits of oxygen extraction have been reached, the marginal cells resort to anaerobic metabolism (increase glucose consumption to produce lactate) to meet their metabolic needs. If this is insufficient, oxygen consumption decreases as metabolic functions related to growth and to organ function are shut down. However, in vital organs, such as the brain, heart, and adrenal glands, loss of function is life threatening. In nonvital organs, development may be affected if this critical state is long lasting. Acute cellular death by necrosis occurs only when vital cellular functions break down and membrane potentials and integrity cannot be maintained. In newborn mammals, "hypoxic hypometabolism" is a mechanism that reduces the sensitivity to hypoxic-ischemic injury

possible that newborn infants can be partly protected against hypoxic-ischemic injury by mechanisms akin to hibernation by "hypoxic hypometabolism."[1]

The immature mammal is able to "centralize" blood flow during periods of stress. This pattern of flow distribution is often called the "dive reflex," since it is qualitatively similar to the adaptation of circulation in seals during diving, a process that allows sea mammals to stay under water for 20 min or more. Blood flow to the skin, muscle, kidneys, liver, and other nonvital organs is reduced to spare the oxygen reserve for the vital organs. The brain, heart, and adrenals. This reaction is relevant during birth with the limitations on placental oxygen transport imposed by uterine contractions and has been studied intensively in the fetal lamb. It has the potential of prolonging passive survival at a critical moment in the individual's life. For comparison, the "fight-or-flight" response of the mature terrestrial mammal supports sustained maximal muscle work.

Blood flows toward the point of lowest resistance. While flow velocities in the heart are high enough to allow kinetic energy of the blood to play an additional role, this role is minimal in the peripheral circulation. Organs and tissues are perfused in parallel and the blood flow through the tissue is the result of the pressure gradient from artery to vein, the so-called perfusion pressure. Vascular resistance is due to the limited diameter of blood vessels, particularly the smaller arteries and arterioles, and blood viscosity. Regulation of organ blood flow takes place by modifying arterial diameter, that is by varying the tone of the smooth muscle cells of the arterial wall. Factors that influence vascular resistance are usually divided into four categories: blood pressure, chemical (PCO_2 and PO_2), metabolic (functional activation), and neurogenic. Most studies have been done on cerebral vessels. The following account therefore refers to cerebral vessels from mature animals, unless stated otherwise.

Regulation of Arterial Tone

The Role of Conduit Arteries in Regulating Vascular Resistance

It is usually assumed that the arteriole—the precapillary muscular vessel with a diameter of 20-50 μm—is the primary determinant of vascular resistance and the larger arteries are more or less considered as passive conduits. However, this is not the case. For instance, in the adult cat the pressure in the small cerebral arteries (150-200 μm) is only 50-60% of the aortic pressure.[2] Thus the reactivity of the entire muscular arterial tree is of relevance in regulating organ blood flow. The role of the pre-arteriolar vessels is likely more important in the newborn than in the adult. First, the smaller body size translates to smaller conduit arteries. The resistance is proportional to length but inversely proportional to the diameter to the power of four. Therefore the conduit arteries of the newborn will make an even more important contribution to the vascular resistance. Second, conduit arteries in the newborn are very reactive. The diameter of the carotid artery increases by 75% during acute asphyxia in term lambs, whereas the diameter of the descending aorta decreases by 15%.[3] The latter change may just reflect a passive elastic reaction to the decreased blood pressure, whereas the former indicates active vasodilation translating into reduced vascular tone. For comparison, flow-induced vasodilatation in the forearm in adults is in the order of 5% or so. As resistance is proportional to the diameter to the power of four, the findings in asphyxiated lambs indicate a roughly 90% reduction of the arterial component of the cerebrovascular resistance with a near doubling of the arterial component of vascular resistance in the lower body. Incidentally, these observations also suggest that blood flow velocity as recorded from conduit arteries by Doppler ultrasound may be potentially misleading in the neonatal patient population.

Arterial Reaction to Pressure (Autoregulation)

Smooth muscle cells of the arterial wall contract in response to increased intravascular pressure in the local arterial segment to a degree that more than compensates for the passive stretching of the vessel wall by the increased pressure. The net result is that arteries constrict when pressure increases and dilate when pressure drops.

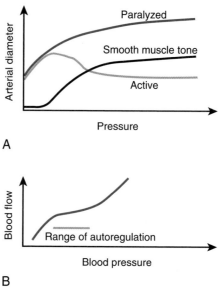

Figure 2-3 Increasing pressure leads to progressive dilatation of a paralyzed artery. As pressure increases more, the elastic capacity is exhausted and vasodilation decreases as collagen restricts further dilation limiting risk of rupture **(A)**. A certain range of pressures is associated with a proportional variation in smooth muscle tone. The precise mechanism of this mechanochemical coupling is not known but it is endogenous to all vascular smooth muscle cells. As a result, in an active artery, the diameter varies inversely with pressure over a certain range. This phenomenon constitutes the basis of arterial "autoregulation" **(B)**.

This phenomenon is called the autoregulation of blood flow (Fig. 2-3). The response time in isolated, cannulated arterial segments is in the order of 10 seconds.[4] The cellular mechanisms of this process are now better understood. Vessel wall constriction constitutes an intrinsic myogenic reflex and is independent of endothelial function. Rather, pressure induces an increase in the smooth muscle cell membrane potential, which regulates vascular smooth muscle cell activity through the action of voltage-gated calcium channels. Although the precise mechanism of the mechanochemical coupling is unknown, the calcium signal is modulated in many ways.[5] It is beyond the scope of this chapter to discuss the modulation of the calcium signal in detail. Suffice it to mention that phospholipases and activation of protein kinase C are involved, and, at least in the rat middle cerebral artery, the arachidonic acid metabolite 20-HETE has also been implicated.[6] Furthermore, a different modulation of intracellular calcium concentration by alternative sources such as the calcium-dependent K^+ channels also exists. The role of the different K^+ channels in modifying smooth cell membrane potential may, at least in part, explain the various arterial responses to pressure in different vascular beds. These vascular bed–specific responses result in the unique blood flow distribution between vital and nonvital organs.[7]

Interaction of Autoregulation and Hypoxic Vasodilatation

As described earlier, arterial smooth muscle tone is affected by a number of factors, all contributing to determine the incident level of vascular resistance. Among the vasodilators, hypoxia is one of the more potent and physiologically relevant factors. Vascular reactivity to O_2 depends, in part, on intact endothelial function ensuring appropriate local nitric oxide (NO) production. Hypoxia also induces tissue lactic acidosis. The decreased pH constitutes a point of interaction between the O_2 reactivity and the CO_2 reactivity (see later). In addition, hypoxia decreases smooth muscle membrane potential by the direct and selective opening of both the calcium-activated and ATP-sensitive K^+ channels in the cell membrane.[8] In the immature brain, adenosine is also an important regulator of the vascular response to hypoxia.[9] The

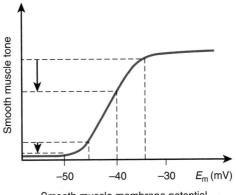

Smooth muscle membrane potential

Figure 2-4 The relationship between smooth muscle cell membrane potential (E_m) and tone. Pressure affects smooth muscle tone through membrane potential. Increased pressure increases membrane potential (i.e., makes it less negative), whereas decreased pressure induces hyperpolarization (membrane potential more negative). Hyperpolarization induces relaxation and hence vasodilatation. The modifying effect of hypoxia is illustrated by the dashed lines and arrows. At high membrane potential (–35 mV), a decrease in membrane potential by 5 mV induces a marked reduction in muscular tone. Thus at high pressures hypoxemia can be compensated by vasodilatation. However, at low membrane potential (hyperpolarization) a similar hypoxia-induced decrease in membrane potential has much less effect on muscular tone. This predicts that at low blood pressure, hypoxemia cannot be well compensated by increased blood flow. Many other factors may influence muscle tone by modifying membrane potential, and the magnitude of effects can be predicted to be interdependent.

membrane potential response to hypoxia is independent of the existing intravascular pressure.[10] However, at lower pressures, the decrease in membrane potential only leads to minimal further arterial dilation because, at low vascular tone, the membrane potential/muscular tone relationship is outside the steep part of the slope (Fig. 2-4). In other words, at low perfusion pressures the dilator pathway has already been near maximally activated. Therefore in a hypotensive neonate, a superimposed hypoxic event cannot be appropriately compensated due to the low perfusion pressure. The end-result is tissue hypoxia-ischemia with the potential of causing irreversible damage to organs especially to the brain.

Interaction of Autoregulation and PCO$_2$

Arteries and arterioles constrict with hypocapnia and dilate with hypercapnia. The principal part of this reaction is mediated through changes in pH, that is, H^+ concentration. Perivascular pH has a direct effect on the membrane potential of arterial smooth muscle cells since the extracellular H^+ concentration is one of the main determinants of the potassium conductance of the plasma membrane in arterial smooth muscle cells regulating the outward K^+ current.[8] Therefore when the pH decreases, the K^+ outflow from the vascular smooth muscle cell increases, resulting in hyperpolarization of the cell membrane and thus vasodilatation. Furthermore, increased extracellular and, to a lesser degree, intracellular H^+ concentrations reduce the conductance of the voltage-dependent calcium channels further enhancing vasorelaxation.[11]

Hypercapnic vasodilatation is reduced by up to 50% when NO synthase (NOS) activity is blocked in the brain of the adult rat.[12] The hypercapnic response is restituted by the addition of an NO donor.[13] This finding suggests that unhindered local NO production is necessary for the pH to exert its vasoregulatory effects. It has recently been suggested that, although the calcium-activated and ATP-sensitive K^+ channels play the primary role in the vascular response to changes in PCO$_2$, the function of these channels is regulated by local NO production.[14]

The role of prostanoids in mediating the vascular response to PCO$_2$ is less clear.[15,16] The fact that indomethacin abolishes the normal cerebral (or other organ) blood flow–CO_2 response in preterm infants is likely a direct effect of the drug independent of its inhibitory action on prostanoid synthesis.[17] This notion is supported by the finding that ibuprofen is devoid of such effects on the organ blood flow–CO_2 response.[18]

Interaction of Autoregulation and Functional Activation (Metabolic Blood Flow Control)

Several mechanisms operate to match local blood flow to metabolic requirements, including changes in pH, local production of adenosine, ATP and NO, and local neural mechanisms. In muscle it appears that there is not a single factor dominating, since the robust and very fast coupling of activity and blood flow is almost unaffected by blocking any of these mechanisms one by one.[19] In brain, astrocytes may be the central sites of regulation of this response in the neurovascular unit via their perivascular end-feet and by utilizing many of the aforementioned cellular mechanisms such as changes in K^+ ion flux and local production of prostanoids, ATP, and adenosine.[20] Among these cellular regulators, adenosine has been proposed to play a principal role.[21] Adenosine works by regulating the activity of the calcium-activated and ATP-sensitive K^+ channels.

Flow-mediated Vasodilatation

Endothelial cells sense flow by shear stress, and produce NO in reaction to high shear stress at high flow velocities. NO diffuses freely, and reaches the smooth muscle cell underneath the endothelium. NO acts on smooth muscle K^+ channels using cyclic guanosine monophosphate (GMP) as the secondary messenger and then a series of intermediate steps. Since NO is a vasodilator, the basic arterial reflex to high flow is vasodilation. Thus when a tissue is activated (e.g., a muscle contracts), the local vessels first dilate, as directed by the mechanisms of the metabolic flow control described earlier, and blood flow increases. This initial increase in blood flow is then sensed in the conduit arteries through the shear stress–induced increase in local NO production and vascular resistance is further reduced allowing flow to increase yet again. The action remains local as the generated NO diffusing into the bloodstream is largely inactivated by hemoglobin.

Sympathetic Nervous System

Epinephrine in the blood originates from the adrenal glands, whereas norepinephrine is produced by the sympathetic nerve endings and the extraadrenal chromaffin tissue. Sympathetic nerves are present in nearly all vessels located in the adventitia and on the smooth muscle cells. Adrenoreceptors are widely distributed in the cardiovascular system, located on smooth muscle and endothelial cells. Several different adrenoreceptors exist; alpha-1 receptors with at least three subtypes are present primarily in the arteries and the myocardium, while alpha-2, beta-1, and beta-2 receptors are expressed in all types of vessels and the myocardium. In the arteries and veins alpha-receptor stimulation causes vasoconstriction, and beta-receptor stimulation results in vasodilatation. Both alpha- and beta-adrenoreceptors are frequently expressed in the membrane of the same cell. Therefore the response of the given cell to epinephrine or norepinephrine depends on the relative abundance of the receptor types expressed.[22] Of clinical importance is the regulation of the expression of the cardiovascular adrenergic receptors by corticosteroids, the high incidence of relative adrenal insufficiency in preterm neonates and critically ill term infants, the role of glucocorticoids and mineralocorticoids in maintaining the sensitivity of the cardiovascular system to endogenous and exogenous catecholamines and the down-regulation of the cardiovascular adrenergic receptors in response to increased release of endogenous catecholamines or administration of exogenous catecholamines in critical illness.[23-25] Typically, arteries and arterioles of the skin, gut, and muscle constrict in response to increases in endogenous catecholamine production, whereas those of the heart and brain either do not constrict or dilate (see later). The response also depends on the resting tone of the given vessel. Furthermore, the sensitivity of a vessel to circulating norepinephrine may be less than the sensitivity to norepinephrine produced by increased sympathetic nerve activity, since alpha-1 receptors may be particularly abundant in the membrane regions close to the nerve terminals. The signaling pathways of the adrenoreceptors are complex and dependent on the receptor subtype. Activation of alpha-adrenoreceptors generally results in vasoconstriction mediated by increased release of calcium from intracellular stores as a first step, while beta-receptor–induced vasodilation is mediated by increased cyclic adenosine monophosphate (AMP) generation. However, the system is far more complex and, among other mechanisms, receptor activation-associated changes in K^+ conductance and local NO synthesis are also involved. Finally, the sympathetic nervous system is activated during hypoxia, hypotension, or hypovolemia via stimulation of different chemoreceptors and baroreceptors in vessel walls and the vasomotor centers in the medulla. Activation of the sympathetic nervous system plays a central role in the cardiovascular response to stress and it is the mainstay of the dive reflex response during hypoxia-ischemia.

Humoral Factors in General Circulation

A large number of endogenous vasoactive factors other than those mentioned earlier also play a role in the extremely complex process of organ blood flow regulation such as angiotensin II, arginine-vasopressin, vasointestinal peptide, neuropeptide gamma, and endothelin-1. However, none of these vasoactive factors has been shown to have a significant importance in isolation under normal conditions except for the role of angiotensin II in regulating renal microhemodynamics.

Summary

In summary, a great many factors have an input and interact to define the degree of contraction of the vascular smooth muscle cells and hence regulate arterial and arteriolar tone (see Fig. 2-4). Although many details are unknown, especially in the developing immature animal or human, the final common pathway appears to involve the smooth-cell membrane potential, cytoplasmic calcium concentration, and the calcium/calmodulin myosin light chain kinase-mediated phosphorylation of the regulatory light chains of myosin resulting in the interaction of actin and myosin (Fig. 2-5). However, the complexity of the known factors and their interplay as well as the differences in the response among the different organs are overwhelming and no simple or unifying principle of vascular tone regulation has gained a foothold. Indeed, the complexity predicts that vascular tone and reactivity in a particular arterial segment in a particular tissue may differ markedly from that in other segments or other tissues. Unfortunately, the insights are as yet insufficient to allow any quantitative predictions for different organs or vascular tree segments.

Blood Flow to the Brain

Brain injury is common in newborn infants. It can occur rapidly, is frequently irreversible, and rarely, in itself, prevents survival. Injury to no other organs in the neonatal period has the same clinical importance as the other organs have a better capacity to recover even from severe hypoxic-ischemic damage. Disturbances in blood flow and inflammation have been proposed as the major factors in the development of neonatal brain injury.

Autoregulation of Cerebral Blood Flow in the Immature Brain

Pressure-flow autoregulation has been widely investigated in the immature cerebral vasculature since the original observation of direct proportionality of cerebral blood flow (CBF) to systolic blood pressure in a group of neonates during stabilization after birth.[26]

An adequate autoregulatory plateau, shifted to the left to match the lower perinatal blood pressure, has been demonstrated in several animal species shortly after birth, including dogs, lambs, and rats.[27-31] In fetal lambs, autoregulation is not present at 0.6 gestation but is functional at 0.9 gestation.[32] The lower threshold of

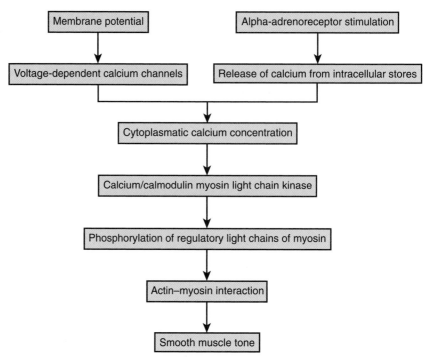

Figure 2-5 A scheme of the pathway from smooth muscle cell membrane potential and alpha-adrenoreceptor stimulation to changes in muscle tone.

the autoregulation is developmentally regulated and it is closer to the normal resting systemic blood pressure at 0.75 gestation compared with 0.9 gestation.[33] Thus in the more immature subject there is less vasodilator reserve, which limits the effectiveness of CBF autoregulation at earlier stages of development. In newborn lambs, autoregulation could be completely abolished for 4 to 7 hours by 20 minutes of hypoxemia with arterial oxygen saturations about 50%.[34]

Unfortunately, the response of CBF autoregulation to pathologic conditions and the impact of immaturity on the process are much less well investigated in the human neonate. However, observational studies of global CBF in stable neonates without evidence of major brain injury suggest that autoregulation is intact.[35-40] More recently, in a group of premature neonates of 24 to 34 weeks' gestation (median gestational age, 27.5 weeks) absolute cerebral blood flow was measured by near-infrared spectroscopy (NIRS) using the oxygen transient method and the findings in 14 hypotensive subjects (mean blood pressure <30 mm Hg) were compared with those in 16 patients with mean blood pressures of 30 mm Hg or more. CBF was 13.9 vs. 12.3 mL/100 g/min, suggesting that the lower pressure threshold of autoregulation in these babies was less than 30 mm Hg.[41] In a group of 13 extremely preterm babies with a median gestational age of 24 weeks (60% of gestation) CBF measured by NIRS was found to be very low at 6.7 mL/100 g/min (range, 4.4 to 11 mL/100 g/min). However, there was no association between CBF and mean blood pressure in these patients suggesting that autoregulation in the human may develop earlier than in the lamb.[42] These latter findings were supported by another study using NIRS to estimate fractional oxygen extraction by the jugular venous occlusion method in very preterm babies as fractional oxygen extraction in 14 babies of 27 weeks' gestation and with a mean arterial blood pressure of 25 mm Hg did not differ from that in the controls.[43] In contrast to these findings, evidence of absent autoregulation has been found under pathologic conditions such as following severe birth asphyxia in term infants, and in preterm infants in association with brain injury or death.[38,40,44-47]

Based on imaging of flow using single photon emission computed tomography (SPECT) during arterial hypotension in 24 preterm infants with persistently normal brain ultrasound it has been suggested that CBF to the periventricular white matter may be selectively reduced at blood pressures less than 30 mm Hg.[48] Although these data support the notion that the periventricular white matter represents a "watershed area," the statistical relation in this study was based on differences among different infants and thus there may be alternative explanations for the findings. However, in support of the findings of this study, a recent study using NIRS to assess absolute CBF in very preterm neonates during the first postnatal day found some evidence for the lower threshold of the autoregulatory curve being around 29 mm Hg.[49]

In conclusion, the lower threshold for CBF autoregulation may be around 30 mm Hg or somewhat below and autoregulation can be assumed to operate in most newborn infants, even the most immature. When blood pressure falls below the threshold, CBF will fall more than proportionally due to the elastic reduction in vascular diameter. However, significant blood flow is believed to be present until the blood pressure is less than 20 mm Hg.

Effect of Carbon Dioxide on Cerebral Blood Flow

Changes in carbon dioxide tension (PCO_2) have more pronounced effects on CBF than on blood flow in other organs due to the presence of the blood-brain barrier. The blood-brain barrier is an endothelium with tight junctions, which does not allow HCO_3^- to pass through readily. The restricted diffusion of HCO_3^- means that hypercapnia decreases pH in the perivascular space in the brain more readily than elsewhere in blood where the buffering is more effective due to the presence of hemoglobin. This difference in response to a change in PCO_2 continues until HCO_3^- equilibrates over the course of hours.

In normocapnic adults small acute changes in arterial PCO_2 ($PaCO_2$) result in a change in CBF by 30% per kPa (4% per mm Hg $PaCO_2$). Similar reactivity has been demonstrated in the normal human neonate by venous occlusion plethysmography and in stable preterm ventilated infants without major germinal layer hemorrhage by using the ^{133}Xe clearance technique.[37,50,51] However, $PaCO_2$ reactivity is less than 30% per kPa during the first 24 hours.[38]

Contrary to the vasodilation induced by increases in the PCO_2, a hyperventilation-related decrease in $PaCO_2$ causes hypocapnic cerebral vasoconstriction and has been found to be associated with brain injury in preterm but not in term infants or adults.[37,52-54] It is an open question whether hypocapnia alone can cause ischemia, or if it works in combination with other factors, such as hypoxemia, hypoglycemia, the presence of high levels of cytokines, sympathetic activation, or seizures.

Metabolic Control of Blood Flow to the Brain

CBF in term infants, estimated by venous occlusion plethysmography, is greater during active sleep than during quiet sleep, and in preterm infants of 32 to 35 weeks' postmenstrual age, in the wake state compared with sleep.[55-58] Thus there is flow-metabolism coupling even before term gestation in the brain. This finding is further supported by the documented increase in CBF seen during seizure activity and by the strong relation between CBF and blood hemoglobin concentration.[35,39]

Recently, the cerebrovascular response to functional activation by visual stimulation has been studied by magnetic resonance imaging (MRI) and NIRS.[59-61] The findings suggest a non-existent or inconsistent response in infants before term or within the first weeks after birth. The authors explained their findings by the presence of underdeveloped visual cortical projections even at term. Recent studies on the cerebrovascular response to sensorimotor stimulation using functional MRI also found an inconsistent pattern of responses in former very preterm and preterm neonates at near-term postmenstrual age.[62,63] These findings can also be explained by the developmentally regulated delay in the maturation of the sensorimotor cortex. The field of functional activation using near-infrared spectroscopy in newborn infants is rapidly evolving and has recently been reviewed.[64]

Cerebrovenous oxygen saturation was entirely normal (64% ± 5%) as estimated by NIRS and jugular occlusion technique in 11 healthy, term infants 3 days after birth.[65] This indicates that there is a balance between blood flow and cerebral oxygen consumption at term. The average value of global CBF measured by ^{133}Xe clearance in 11 preterm, healthy infants during the first postnatal week was 20 mL/100 g/min.[36] However, the contrast between flow to gray and white matter is high compared with the findings in immature animals.[66]

Adrenergic Mechanisms Affecting Cerebral Blood Flow

Based on findings of animal studies, the sympathetic system appears to play a greater role affecting CBF and its autoregulation in the perinatal period than it does later in life.[67-71] This finding has been attributed to the relative immaturity of the nitric oxide–induced vasodilatory mechanisms during early development.[72] The adrenergic effect results, at least in part, to enhanced constriction of conduit arteries.

A rare study of human neonatal arteries in vitro (obtained postmortem from preterm neonates with gestational age of 23 to 34 weeks) showed basal tone and a pressure-diameter relation quite similar to those seen in adult pial arteries.[73] The neonatal arteries, however, were significantly more sensitive to exogenous norepinephrine and electrical field activation of adventitial sympathetic nerve fibers and had a much higher sympathetic nerve density compared with those in the adult pial arteries.[74,75]

Effect of Medications on Cerebral Blood Flow

Indomethacin reduces CBF in experimental animals, adults, and preterm neonates.[76] As mentioned earlier, a loss of the normal CBF-CO_2 reactivity has also been demonstrated in preterm infants.[17] The crucial question concerning the use of indomethacin in preterm neonates and its effect on CBF is whether indomethacin reduces CBF to ischemic levels resulting in brain injury. Interestingly, although indomethacin decreases the incidence of severe peri-intraventricular hemorrhage (PIVH), this early effect does not translate to better long-term neurodevelopmental outcomes.[77] This raises the possibility that the indomethacin-induced global decrease in CBF may represent a double-edged sword. Contrary to indomethacin, ibuprofen does not have significant cerebrovascular effects.[18,78] However, it is not known whether the use of ibuprofen rather than indomethacin for the treatment of patent ductus arteriosus (PDA) results in improved long-term neurodevelopmental outcome.

Among the methylxanthines, aminophylline reduces CBF and $PaCO_2$ in experimental animals, adults, and preterm infants but caffeine has less effect on CBF.[79,80] Methylxanthines are potent adenosine receptor antagonists. However, it is not entirely clear whether the reduction of CBF is the direct effect of methylxanthines, a result of the decrease in $PaCO_2$, or a combination of these two actions.

Dopamine increases blood pressure and thereby may affect CBF. However, it does not appear to have a selective (dilatory) effect on brain vessels.[81,82]

In babies with blood pressure over 30 mm Hg, dopamine infusion at 0.3 mg/kg/hr was effective in increasing arterial blood pressure and left ventricular output, and did not increase CBF.[83] In babies with hypotension, however, a positive pressure-flow relation was found at 1.9% per mm Hg (95% confidence interval [CI], 0.8 to 3.0) and 6% per mm Hg.[44,84] It is unclear whether the discrepancy between the findings of these two studies and those cited earlier can be explained by the presence or absence of hypotension, by the statistical uncertainty of small studies, or by differences in the methodology and the clinical status of the patients.[81,82]

Ischemic Thresholds in the Brain

In the newborn puppy, venous oxygen saturation (SvO_2) may decrease from 75% to 40% without provoking significant lactate production.[85] The exact minimum value of "normal" SvO_2 depends on, among other things, the oxygen dissociation curve. Therefore it may be affected by changes in pH and the proportion of fetal hemoglobin present in the blood.

In the cerebral cortex of the adult baboon and man, the threshold of blood flow sufficient to maintain tissue integrity depends on the duration of the low flow.

For instance, if the low flow lasts for a few hours, the limit of minimal CBF to maintain tissue integrity is around 10 mL/100 g/min.[86] In acute localized brain ischemia, blood flow may remain sufficient to maintain structural integrity but fail to sustain electrical activity, a phenomenon called "border zone" or "penumbra."[87] Indeed, in progressing ischemia electrical failure is a warning for the development of permanent tissue injury. In the adult human brain cortex, electrical function ceases at about 20 mL/100 g/min of blood flow, while in the subcortical gray matter and brainstem of the adult baboon the blood flow threshold is around 10 to 15 mL/100 g/min.[88]

The threshold values of CBF for neonates are not known. However, in view of the low resting levels of CBF and the comparatively longer survival in total ischemia or anoxia, neonatal CBF thresholds are likely to be considerably less than 10 mL/100 g/min. Indeed, in ventilated preterm infants visual evoked responses were unaffected at global CBF levels below 10 mL/100 g/min corresponding to a cerebral oxygen delivery of 50 μmol/100 g/min.[37,89]

However, low CBF and cerebral oxygen delivery estimated by ^{133}Xe clearance carry a risk of later death, cerebral atrophy, or neurodevelopmental deficit.[90-93] As mentioned earlier though, the lower limit of acceptable CBF is unknown in the neonate and it is also unclear whether treatment modalities aimed at increasing CBF can improve the outcome.

Periventricular white matter is believed to be particularly vulnerable to hypoxic-ischemic injury especially in preterm infants. However, the pathogenesis of white matter injury is likely to be more complex as interactions among decreased perfusion and increased cytokine production and oxidative damage have recently been postulated to be of importance. The only direct evidence indicating that periventricular leukomalacia (PVL) is primarily a hypoxic-ischemic lesion comes from the findings identifying hyperventilation with the associated cerebral vasoconstriction as a robust risk factor for PVL and cerebral palsy.

Blood Flow to Other Organs

Based on studies on the distribution of cardiac output in term fetal lambs and newborn piglets, the typical abdominal organ blood flow appears to be around 100 to 350 mL/100 g/min.[94-95] In the fetus, abdominal organ blood flow is higher than in the newborn with the exception of the intestine.

Kidney

The adult kidneys constitute 0.5% of body weight but represent 25% of resting cardiac output, making them the most richly perfused organ of the body. In the newborn, although the kidneys are relatively larger, they receive less blood flow probably due to the immature renal function. Renal arteries display appropriate autoregulation with a lower threshold adjusted to the prevailing lower blood pressure.[96] In addition to structural immaturity, high levels of circulating vasoactive mediators such as angiotensin II, vasopressin, and endogenous catecholamines explain the relatively low renal blood flow in the immediate postnatal period. Indeed, after alpha-adrenergic receptor blockade, renal nerve stimulation results in increased blood flow. To counterbalance the renal vasoconstriction and increased sodium reabsorption caused by the aforementioned hormones, the neonatal kidney is more dependent on the local production of vasodilatory prostaglandins compared to later in life. This explains why indomethacin, a cyclooxygenase (COX) inhibitor, readily reduces renal blood flow and urinary output in the neonate but not in the euvolemic child or adult. Interestingly, the renal side effects of another COX inhibitor, ibuprofen, are less pronounced in the neonate.[97] Finally, dopamine increases renal blood flow at a dose with minimal effect on blood pressure.[81]

Liver

The liver is a large organ that has a double blood supply with blood originating from the stomach and intestines through the portal system and also from the hepatic branch of the celiac artery through the hepatic artery. The proportion of blood flow from these sources in the normal adult is 3 : 1, respectively. Hepatic vessels are richly innervated with sympathetic and parasympathetic nerves. The hepatic artery constricts in response to sympathetic nerve stimulation and exogenous norepinephrine while the response of the portal vein is less well characterized. Angiotensin II is a potent vasoconstrictor of the hepatic vascular beds. During the first days after birth, a portion of the portal blood flow remains shunted past the liver through the ductus venosus until it closes. Portal liver blood flow in lambs is 100 to 150 mL/100 g/min during the first postnatal day and increases to over 200 mL/100 g/min by the end of the first week.[98]

Stomach and Intestines

The stomach and intestines are motile organs, and variation in intestinal wall tension influences vascular resistance.[99] For example, stimulation of sympathetic nerves results in constriction of the intestinal arteries and arterioles and in the relaxation of the intestinal wall. Thus the effects on vascular resistance and intestinal wall tension are opposite. Furthermore, a number of gastrointestinal hormones and paracrine substances such as gastrin, glucagon, and cholecystokinin dilate intestinal vessels likely contributing to the increase in intestinal blood flow during digestion. Local metabolic coupling also contributes to the digestion-associated increase in intestinal blood flow. Intestinal blood flow also shows well-developed autoregulation, and responses to sympathetic nerve stimulation, exogenous catecholamines, and angiotensin II similar to that of the other abdominal organs in the immature animal.

Distribution of Cardiac Output in the Healthy Human Neonate

If the heart fails to increase cardiac output to maintain systemic blood pressure, a selective and marked increase in the flow to one organ can in principle compromise blood flow to other organs ("steal" phenomenon). No single organ of critical importance is large in itself at birth (Table 2-1).

Blood Flow to the Upper Part of the Body

Blood flow to various organs differs considerably at the resting state. The data from recent Doppler flow volumetric studies allows some comparisons for the upper part of the body in healthy term infants. Blood flow to the brain, defined as the sum of

Table 2-1 ORGAN WEIGHTS IN TERM AND EXTREMELY LOW BIRTH WEIGHT NEONATES*

Organ or Tissue	Body Weight (g)	
	3500	1000
Brain	411 (12%)	143 (15%)
Heart	23 (1%)	8 (1%)
Liver	153 (4%)	47 (5%)
Kidney	28 (1%)	10 (1%)
Fat	23%**	<5%

Data from Charles AD, Smith NM. Perinatal postmortem. In: Rennie JM, ed. Roberton's textbook of neonatology. Beijing: Elsevier; 2005:1207-1215.
*Total body water is around 75% and 85-90% of body weight in term neonates and extremely low birth weight neonates, respectively.
**Data from Uthaya S, Bell J, Modi N. Adipose tissue magnetic resonance imaging in the newborn. Horm Res 2004;62(Suppl 3):1430-1438.

Table 2-2 VOLUMETRIC BLOOD FLOW BY DOPPLER ULTRASOUND MEASUREMENT FOR THE UPPER PART OF THE BODY IN HEALTHY TERM INFANTS

Vessel	n	Age	Flow (mL/kg/min)	Flow (mL/min)	Reference
Vertebral arteries	22	39-40 (weeks)	—	19*	Kehrer[111]
Internal carotid arteries	—		51*		
Right common carotid	21	Day 1-3	17.7	117**	Sinha[112]
Superior vena cava	14	Day 1	76	258	Kluckow[101]
Ascending aorta	147	500			

Newborn infants born at term were mixed with former preterm infants reaching 39-40 postmenstrual weeks.[111]
*Values for sum of right and left.
**Value multiplied by 2 for comparison.

the blood flowing through the two internal carotid and two vertebral arteries, corresponds to 18 mL/100 g/min using a mean brain weight of 385 g for the term infant. This blood flow is close to what is expected from the data on CBF in the literature assessed by NIRS and ^{133}Xe clearance (Table 2-2).

Blood Flow to the Lower Part of the Body

Lower body blood flows are less well studied in the human neonate. In a recent study in extremely low–birth weight infants with no ductal shunt and a cardiac output of 200 mL/kg/min, aortic blood flow was found to be 90 mL/kg/min at the level of the diaphragm.[100] Although this finding is in good agreement with the data by Kluckow and Evans showing that approximately 50% of left ventricular output returns through the superior vena cava (SVC) in preterm neonates, some caution is warranted because most preterm infants enrolled in the studies on SVC blood flow measurements had a PDA.[101]

The data on individual abdominal organ flows in neonates are less current but available with a renal blood flow (right + left) of 21 mL/kg/min, a superior mesenteric artery blood flow of 43 mL/kg/min, and a celiac artery blood flow of 70 mL/kg/min.[102-104] In the study by Agata and colleagues, the results were divided by two to account for the parabolic arterial flow profile.[104] However, since the sum of these abdominal organ blood flows exceeds the blood flow in the descending aorta and since blood flow from other organ systems in the lower body such as bones, muscle, and skin has not been taken into consideration, it is clear that blood flows to the abdominal organs have been overestimated in the neonate. The reasons for this discrepancy are unclear but they may, at least in part, be related to the use of less sophisticated color Doppler equipment using lower ultrasound frequencies in the studies performed in the early 1990s. In terms of perfusion rate, the renal blood flow of 21 mL/min/kg body weight transforms to 210 mL/min/100 g kidney weight. Again, this is higher than that expected from studies using hippuric acid clearance.[105] Taking all these findings into consideration, it is reasonable to conclude that normal organ flow in the human neonate is likely to be comparable to that in different animal species and is around 100 to 300 mL/100 g/min. For comparison, lower limb blood flow in the human infant has been estimated by NIRS and the venous occlusion technique to be around 3.5 mL/100 g/min.[106]

In summary, cardiac output is distributed approximately equally to the upper and lower body in the normal healthy newborn infant at gestational ages from 28 to 40 weeks. It may come as a surprise to many readers that only 25-30% of the blood flow to the upper part of the body goes to the brain, whereas the abdominal organs can be assumed to account for the largest part of the blood flow to the lower part of the body. Although good estimates of abdominal organ perfusion rates are not available, they appear to be higher than the perfusion rate of the brain. Therefore a relative hyperperfusion of the abdominal organs could result in a significant "steal" of cardiac output from the brain.

Mechanisms Governing the Redistribution of Cardiac Output in the Fetal '"Dive" Reflex

Aerobic Diving

The diving reflex of sea mammals occurs within the "aerobic diving limit," that is, without hypoxia severe enough to lead to the production of lactic acid. The key components are reflex bradycardia mediated through the carotid chemoreceptors and the vagal nerve, reflex vasoconstriction of the vascular beds of "nonvital" organs, and recruitment of blood from the spleen. All of this results in a reduced cardiac output, a dramatically increased circulation time, and hence a lag between tissue oxygen consumption and CO_2 production.[107]

Reactions to Hypoxia

Similarly, the immediate reaction to hypoxia in the perinatal mammal is bradycardia and peripheral vasoconstriction. Since the reaction to fetal distress is of great clinical interest, it has been extensively studied in the fetal lamb. The response to fetal distress is qualitatively similar but quantitatively different among the different modes of induction of fetal distress such as maternal hypoxemia, graded reduction of umbilical blood flow, repeated or graded reduction or complete arrest of uterine blood flow, and reduction of fetal blood volume.[108] Among the vital organs, adrenal blood flow increases in all situations and, whereas the typical response also includes an increase in the blood flow to the heart and the brain, this is not the case when fetal distress is caused by reduction of fetal blood volume (heart) or the arrest of uterine blood flow (brain). As for the nonvital organs, although the typical response is a reduction in blood flow to the gut, liver, kidneys, muscle, and skin, this is not the case when fetal distress is caused by the graded reduction of umbilical blood flow. The fetal circulation is unique and significantly different from the circulation following the transitional adaptation of the newborn and includes the presence of the umbilical vascular bed, the shunting of oxygenated umbilical venous blood past the liver through the ductus venosus, and streaming of this blood through the foramen ovale to the left side of the heart and upper part of the body. These peculiar features may explain some of the aforementioned differences between fetal and postnatal hemodynamic responses to stress.

Modifying Effects

Preterm lambs appear less able to produce a strong epinephrine and norepinephrine response to stress and the blood pressure rise is accordingly less than at term.[108] Since carotid sinus denervation does not abolish the redistribution of cardiac output, supplementary mechanisms must be operational in the fetus.[109] Indeed, at least in the later phase (after 15 min) of the hemodynamic response, the renin-angiotensin system seems to play an important role. Importantly, recent findings indicate that a systemic inflammatory response significantly interferes with the redistribution of cardiac output during arrest of uterine blood flow in the fetal sheep and compromises cardiac function and the chance of successful resuscitation.[110] This hemodynamic response to inflammation in the fetal sheep appears to be, at least in part, regulated by locally generated NO as it could be prevented by the administration of the non-selective NO synthase inhibitor, L-NAME.

Distribution of Cardiac Output in the Shocked Newborn

The Term Neonate with Low Cardiac Output

The pale gray, yet awake term baby with poor systemic perfusion due to congenital heart disease resulting in decreased cardiac output (systemic blood flow) may be the best example for the operation of efficient cardiovascular centralization mechanisms in the human newborn. This baby may have very low central venous oxygen saturation, but will still produce urine, have bowel motility, and, in the initial phase of the cardiovascular compromise, a normal blood lactate. There is little we may be able to do—short of the appropriate cardiac surgical procedure—to help this baby improve the distribution of the limited systemic blood flow. Attempts to increase blood pressure or, conversely, to reduce cardiac afterload may, in fact, interfere with the precarious blood flow distribution and lead to further decreases in blood flow to the organs despite "normal" blood pressure readings, or to a decrease in perfusion pressure resulting in further impairment in tissue perfusion, respectively. In this situation, treatment resulting in increased systemic blood flow without decreasing the perfusion pressure is the only appropriate approach.

The Very Preterm Neonate During Immediate Postnatal Adaptation

In the very preterm neonate with poor systemic perfusion during the period of immediate postnatal transition with the fetal channels still open, the situation is likely to be different. This baby may present with a better color and capillary refill suggesting appropriate peripheral perfusion. Yet, motor activity is likely to be reduced, urinary output low, and blood lactate slightly high. Based on the findings discussed earlier, this baby may have immature and insufficient adrenergic mechanisms to rely on for maintaining sufficient perfusion pressure to the vital organs. In addition, owing to the immaturity of the myocardium, this patient may initially be unable to adapt to the sudden increase in the systemic vascular resistance following separation from the placenta. Regulation of CBF and the sensitivity of the cerebral arteries and arterioles are likely also affected by the immaturity. This would result in the presence of a very narrow CBF autoregulatory plateau and, due to the enhanced expression of alpha-adrenergic receptors during early development, an increased vasoconstrictive response to the administration of exogenous sympathomimetic amines resulting in further decreases in CBF despite improvement in the blood pressure. Again, maintenance of both an appropriate systemic blood flow and perfusion pressure must be the goal of the intervention (see Chapters 1 and 12).

Other Scenarios

Other scenarios relevant to the neonatologist are shock due to low peripheral vascular resistance in sepsis and loss of blood volume. The inflammatory vascular pathology associated with infection cannot be directly treated, and the effectiveness of available supportive treatment modalities of the critically ill septic neonate has not been systematically studied. In addition, microvascular pathophysiology, oxygen radical damage, and disturbances in the oxidative metabolism may be as important as the issues of distribution of blood flow. Therefore this is a difficult-to-manage situation, as also suggested by the poor prognosis for intact survival.

In contrast, the management of acute loss of circulating volume by hemorrhage or rapid fluid loss is simple. Timely administration of adequate volumes of blood or saline may be as lifesaving as for any other patient. The refilling of the circulation should not be delayed by concerns over specific peculiarities of the newborn.

Conclusion

A significant body of knowledge of the physiology and pathophysiology of human neonatal organ blood flow has been accumulated in the literature over the last 40 years. The multiple mechanisms of regulation of blood flow to the organs also operate in the newborn. Accordingly, the distribution of cardiac output to specific organs is actively regulated. Unfortunately, the cerebral hemispheres are not always privileged, especially in the preterm neonate.

References

1. Mortola JP. Implications of hypoxic hypometabolism during mammalian ontogenesis. Respir Physiol Neurobiol. 2004:141;345-356.
2. Heistad DD. What is new in cerebral microcirculation. Landis award lecture. Microcirculation. 2001;8;365-375.

3. Malcus P, Kjellmer I, Lingman G, et al. Diameters of the common carotid artery and aorta change in different directions during acute asphyxia in the fetal lamb. J Perinat Med. 1991;19;259-267.

4. Lagaud G, Gaudreault N, Moore ED, et al. Pressure-dependent myogenic constriction of cerebral arteries occurs independently of voltage-dependent activation. Am J Physiol Heart Circ Physiol. 2002;283:H2187-H2195.

5. Hill MA, Zou H, Potocnik SJ, et al. Invited review. Arteriolar smooth muscle mechanotransduction. Ca2 signaling pathways underlying myogenic reactivity. J Appl Physiol. 2001;91:973-983.

6. Gebremedin A, Lange AR, Lowry TF, et al. Production of 20-HETE and its role in autoregulation of cerebral blood flow. Circ Res. 2000;87:60-65.

7. Dora KA. Does arterial myogenic tone determine blood distribution in vivo? Am J Physiol Heart Circ Physiol. 2005;289:1323-1325.

8. Pearce WJ, Harder DR. Cerebrovascular smooth muscle and endothelium. In: Mraovitch S, Sercombe R, eds. Neurophysiological basis of cerebral blood flow control. An introduction. London: John Libbey; 1996:153-158.

9. Pearce WJ. Hypoxic regulation of the fetal cerebral circulation. J Appl Physiol. 2006;100:731-738.

10. Liu Y, Harder DR, Lombard JH. Interaction of myogenic mechanisms and hypoxic dilation in rat middle cerebral arteries. Am J Physiol Heart Circ Physiol. 2002;283:H2276-H2281.

11. Aalkjær C, Poston L. Effects of pH on vascular tension. Which are the important mechanisms? J Vasc Res. 1996;33;347-359.

12. Wang Q, Pelligrino DA, Baughman VL, et al. The role of neuronal nitric oxide synthetase in regulation of cerebral blood flow in normocapnia and hypercapnia in rats. J Cereb Blood Flow Metab. 1995;15:774-778.

13. Iadecola C, Zhang F. Permissive and obligatory roles of NO in cerebrovascular responses to hypercapnia and acetylcholine. Am J Physiol. 1996;271:R990-R1001.

14. Lindauer U, Vogt J, Schuh-Hofer S, et al. Cerebrovascular vasodilation to extraluminal acidosis occurs via combined activation of ATP-sensitive and Ca2+-activated potassium channels. J Cereb Blood Flow Metab. 2003;23:1227-1238.

15. Wagerle LC, Mishra OP. Mechanism of CO2 response in cerebral arteries of the newborn pig: role of phospholipase, cyclooxygenase, and lipooxygenase pathways. Circ Res. 1988;62:1019-1026.

16. Rama GP, Parfenova H, Leffler CW. Protein kinase Cs and tyrosine kinases in permissive action of prostacyclin on cerebrovascular regulation in newborn pigs. Pediatr Res. 1996;41:83-89.

17. Edwards AD, Wyatt JS, Ricardsson C, et al. Effects of indomethacin on cerebral haemodynamics in very preterm infants. Lancet. 1992;i:1491-1495.

18. Patel J, Roberts I, Azzopardi D, et al. Randomized double-blind controlled trial comparing the effects of ibuprofen with indomethacin on cerebral hemodynamics in preterm infants with patent ductus arteriosus. Pediatr Res. 2000;47:36-42.

19. Clifford PS, Hellsten Y. Vasodilatory mechanisms in contracting skeletal muscle. J Appl Physiol. 2004;97:393-403.

20. Koehler RC, Gebremedhin D, Harder DR. Role of astrocytes in cerebrovascular regulation. J Appl Physiol. 2006;100:307-317.

21. Phillis JW. Adenosine and adenine nucleotides as regulators of cerebral blood flow: roles of acidosis, cell swelling, and KATP channels. Crit Rev Neurobiol. 2004;16:237-270.

22. Guimaraes S, Moura D. Vascular adrenoreceptors. an update. Pharm Rev. 2001;53:319-356.

23. Seri I, Tan R, Evans J. The effect of hydrocortisone on blood pressure in preterm neonates with vasopressor-resistant hypotension. Pediatrics. 2001;107:1070-1074.

24. Watterberg KL. Adrenal insufficiency and cardiac dysfunction in the preterm infant. Pediatr Res. 2002;51:422-424.

25. Noori S, Seri I. Pathophysiology of newborn hypotension outside the transitional period. Early Hum Dev. 2005;81:399-404.

26. Lou HC, Lassen NA, Friis-Hansen B. Low cerebral blood flow in hypotensive perinatal distress. Acta Neurol Scand. 1977;56:343-352.

27. Hernandez MJ, Brennan RW, Bowman GS. Autoregulation of cerebral blood flow in the newborn dog. Brain Res. 1980;184:199-201.

28. Pasternak JF, Groothuis DR. Autoregulation of cerebral blood flow in the newborn beagle puppy. Biol Neonate. 1985;48:100-109.

29. Tweed WA, Cote J, Pash M, et al. Arterial oxygenation determines autoregulation of cerebral blood flow in the fetal lamb. Pediatr Res. 1983;17:246-249.

30. Papile LA, Rudolph AM, Heyman MA. Autoregulation of cerebral blood flow in the preterm fetal lamb. Pediatr Res. 1985;19:59-161.

31. Pryds A, Pryds O, Greisen G. Cerebral pressure autoregulation and vasoreactivity in the newborn rat. Pediatr Res. 2005;57:294-298.

32. Helau S, Koehler RC, Gleason CA, et al. Cerebrovascular autoregulation during fetal development in sheep. Am J Physiol Heart Circ Physiol. 1994;266:H1069-H1074.

33. Müller T, Löhle M, Schubert H, et al. Developmental changes in cerebral autoregulatory capacity in the fetal sheep parietal cortex. J Physiol. 2002;539:957-967.

34. Tweed WA, Cote J, Lou H, et al. Impairment of cerebral blood flow autoregulation in the newborn lamb by hypoxia. Pediatr Res. 1986;20:516-519.

35. Younkin DP, Reivich M, Jaggi JL, et al. The effect of haematocrit and systolic blood pressure on cerebral blood flow in newborn infants. J Cereb Blood Flow Metab. 1987;7:295-299.

36. Greisen G. Cerebral blood flow in preterm infants during the first week of life. Acta Paediatr Scand. 1986;75:43-51.

37. Greisen G, Trojaborg W. Cerebral blood flow, PaCO2 changes, and visual evoked potentials in mechanically ventilated, preterm infants. Acta Paediatr Scand. 1987;76:394-400.
38. Pryds O, Greisen G, Lou H, et al. Heterogeneity of cerebral vasoreactivity in preterm infants supported by mechanical ventilation. J Pediatr. 1989;115:638-645.
39. Pryds O, Andersen GE, Friis-Hansen B. Cerebral blood flow reactivity in spontaneously breathing, preterm infants shortly after birth. Acta Paediatr Scand. 1990;79:391-396.
40. Pryds O, Greisen G, Lou H, et al. Vasoparalysis is associated with brain damage in asphyxiated term infants. J Pediatr. 1990;117:119-125.
41. Tyszczuk L, Meek J, Elwell C, et al. Cerebral blood flow is independent of mean arterial blood pressure in preterm infants undergoing intensive care. Pediatrics. 1998;102:337-341.
42. Noone MA, Sellwood M, Meek JH, et al. Postnatal adaptation of cerebral blood flow using near infrared spectroscopy in extremely preterm infants undergoing high-frequency oscillatory ventilation. Acta Paediatr. 2003;92:1079-1084.
43. Wardle SP, Yoxall CW, Weindling AM. Determinants of cerebral fractional oxygen extraction using near-infrared spectroscopy in preterm neonates. J Cereb Blood Flow Metab. 2000;20:272-279.
44. Milligan DWA. Failure of autoregulation and intraventricular haemorrhage in preterm infants. Lancet. 1980;i:896-899.
45. Tsuji M, Saul JP, du Plessis A, et al. Cerebral intravascular oxygenation correlates with mean arterial pressure in critically ill premature infants. Pediatrics. 2000;106;625-632.
46. Wong FY, Leung TS, Austin T, et al. Impaired autoregulation in preterm infants identified by using spatially resolved spectroscopy. Pediatrics. 2008;121:e604-e611.
47. O'Leary H, Gregas MC, Limperopoulos C, et al. Elevated cerebral pressure passivity is associated with prematurity-related intracranial hemorrhage. Pediatrics. 2009;124:302-309.
48. Børch K, Lou HC, Greisen G. Cerebral white matter flow and arterial blood pressure in preterm infants. Acta Paediatr. 2010;99:1489-1492.
49. Munro MJ, Walker AM, Barfield CP. Hypotensive extremely low birth weight infants have reduced cerebral blood flow. Pediatrics. 2004;114:1591-1596.
50. Leahy FAN, Cates D, MacCallum M, et al. Effect of CO2 and 100% O2 on cerebral blood flow in preterm infants. J Appl Physiol. 1980;48:468-472.
51. Rahilly PM. Effects of 2% carbon dioxide, 0.5% carbon dioxide, and 100% oxygen on cranial blood flow of the human neonate. Pediatrics. 1980;66:685-689.
52. Calvert SA, Hoskins EM, Fong KW, et al. Aetiological factors associated with the development of periventricular leucomalacia. Acta Paediatr Scand. 1987;76:254-259.
53. Graziani LJ, Spitzer AR, Mitchell DG, et al. Mechanical ventilation in preterm infants. Neurosonographic and developmental studies. Pediatrics. 1992;90:515-522.
54. Ferrara B, Johnson DE, Chang P-N, et al. Efficacy and neurologic outcome of profound hypocapneic alkalosis for the treatment of persistent pulmonary hypertension in infancy. J Pediatr. 1984;105:457-461.
55. Milligan DWA. Cerebral blood flow and sleep state in the normal newborn infant. Early Hum Develop. 1979;3:321-328.
56. Rahilly PM. Effects of sleep state and feeding on cranial blood flow of the human neonate. Arch Dis Child. 1980;55:265-270.
57. Mukhtar AI, Cowan FM, Stothers JK. Cranial blood flow and blood pressure changes during sleep in the human neonate. Early Hum Develop. 1982;6:59-64.
58. Greisen G, Hellstrom-Westas L, Lou H, et al. Sleep-waking shifts and cerebral blood flow in stable preterm infants. Pediatr Res. 1985;19:1156-1159.
59. Born P, Leth H, Miranda MJ, et al. Visual activation in infants and young children studied by functional magnetic resonance imaging. Pediatr Res. 1998;44:578-583.
60. Martin E, Joeri P, Loenneker T, et al. Visual processing in infants and children studied using functional MRI. Pediatr Res. 1999;46:135-140.
61. Meek JH, Firbank M, Elwell CE, et al. Regional hemodynamic responses to visual stimulation in awake infants. Pediatr Res. 1998;43:840-843.
62. Erberich GS, Friedlich P, Seri I, et al. Brain activation detected by functional MRI in preterm neonates using an integrated radiofrequency neonatal head coil and MR compatible incubator. Neuroimage. 2003;20:683-692.
63. Erberich SG, Panigrahy A, Friedlich P, et al. Somatosensory lateralization in the newborn brain. Neuroimage. 2006;29:155-161.
64. Wolf M, Greisen G. Advances in near-infrared spectroscopy to study the brain of the preterm and term neonate. Clin Perinatol. 2009;36;807-834.
65. Buchvald FF, Keshe K, Greisen G. Measurement of cerebral oxyhaemoglobin saturation and jugular blood flow in term healthy newborn infants by near-infrared spectroscopy and jugular venous occlusion. Biol Neonate. 1999;75:97-103.
66. Børch K, Greisen G. Blood flow distribution in the normal human preterm brain. Pediatr Res. 1998;43:28-33.
67. Hernandez MJ, Hawkins RA, Brennan RW. Sympathetic control of regional cerebral blood flow in the asphyxiated newborn dog. In: Heistad DD, Marcus ML, eds. Cerebral blood flow, effects of nerves and neurotransmitters. New York: Elsevier; 1982:359-366.
68. Hayashi S, Park MK, Kuelh TJ. Higher sensitivity of cerebral arteries isolated from premature and newborn baboons to adrenergic and cholinergic stimulation. Life Sciences. 1984;35:253-260.
69. Wagerle LC, Kumar SP, Delivoria-Papadopoulos M. Effect of sympathetic nerve stimulation on cerebral blood flow in newborn piglets. Pediatr Res. 1986;20:131-135.

70. Kurth CD, Wagerle LC, Delivoria-Papadopoulos M. Sympathetic regulation of cerebral blood flow during seizures in newborn lambs. Am J Physiol. 1988;255:H563-H568.
71. Goplerud JM, Wagerle LC, Delivoria-Papadopoulos M. Sympathetic nerve modulation of regional cerebral blood flow during asphyxia in newborn piglets. Am J Physiol. 1991;260:H1575-H1580.
72. Wagerle LC, Moliken W, Russo P. Nitric oxide and alpha-adrenergic mechanisms modify contractile responses to norepinephrine in ovine fetal and newborn cerebral arteries. Pediatr Res. 1995; 38:237-242.
73. Bevan RD, Vijayakumaran E, Gentry A, et al. Intrinsic tone of cerebral artery segments of human infants between 23 weeks of gestation and term. Pediatr Res. 1998;43:20-27.
74. Bevan R, Dodge J, Nichols P, et al. Responsiveness of human infant cerebral arteries to sympathetic nerve stimulation and vasoactive agents. Pediatr Res. 1998;44:730-739.
75. Bevan RD, Dodge J, Nichols P, et al. Weakness of sympathetic neural control of human pial compared with superficial temporal arteries reflects low innervation density and poor sympathetic responsiveness. Stroke. 1998;29:212-221.
76. Pryds O, Greisen G, Johansen K. Indomethacin and cerebral blood flow in preterm infants treated for patent ductus arteriosus. Eur J Pediatr. 1988;147:315-316.
77. Schmidt B, Davis P, Moddemann D, et al, and Trial of Indomethacin Prophylaxis in Preterms Investigators. Long-term effects of indomethacin prophylaxis in extremely-low-birth-weight infants. N Engl J Med. 2001;344:1966-1972.
78. Mosca F, Bray M, Lattanzio M, et al. Comparative evaluation of the effects of indomethacin and ibuprofen on cerebral perfusion and oxygenation in preterm infants with patent ductus arteriosus. J Pediatr. 1997;131:549-554.
79. Pryds O, Schneider S. Aminophylline induces cerebral vasoconstriction in stable, preterm infants without affecting the visual evoked potential. Eur J Pediatr. 1991;150:366-369.
80. Lundstrøm KE, Larsen PB, Brendstrup L, et al. Cerebral blood flow and left ventricular output in spontaneously breathing, newborn preterm infants treated with caffeine or aminophylline. Acta Paediatr. 1995;84:6-9.
81. Seri I, Abbasi S, Wood DC, et al. Regional hemodynamic effects of dopamine in the sick preterm neonate. J Pediatr. 1998;133:728-734.
82. Zhang J, Penny DJ, Kim NS, et al. Mechanisms of blood pressure increase induced by dopamine in hypotensive preterm neonates. Arch Dis Child. 1999;81:F99-F104.
83. Lundstrøm KE, Pryds O, Greisen G. The haemodynamic effect of dopamine and volume expansion in sick preterm infants. Early Hum Develop. 2000;57:157-163.
84. Jayasinghe D, Gill AB, Levene MI. CBF reactivity in hypotensive and normotensive preterm infants. Pediatr Res. 2003;54:848-853.
85. Reuter JH, Disney TA. Regional cerebral blood flow and cerebral metabolic rate of oxygen during hyperventilation in the newborn dog. Pediatr Res. 1986;20:1102-1106.
86. Jones TH, Morawetz RB, Crowell RM, et al. Thresholds of focal cerebral ischaemia in awake monkeys. J Neurosurg. 1981;54:773-782.
87. Astrup J. Energy-requiring cell functions in the ischaemic brain. J Neurosurg. 1982;56:482-497.
88. Branston NM, Ladds A, Symon L, et al. Comparison of the effects of ischaemia on early components of somatosensory evoked potentials in brainstem, thalamus, and cerebral cortex. J Cereb Blood Flow Metab. 1984;4:68-81.
89. Pryds O, Greisen G. Preservation of single flash visual evoked potentials at very low cerebral oxygen delivery in sick, newborn, preterm infants. Pediatr Neurol. 1990;6:151-158.
90. Lou HC, Skov H. Low cerebral blood flow: a risk factor in the neonate. J Pediatr. 1979;95: 606-609.
91. Ment RL, Scott DT, Lange RC, et al. Postpartum perfusion of the preterm brain; relationship to neurodevelopmental outcome Childs Brain. 1983;10:266-272.
92. Pryds O. Low neonatal cerebral oxygen delivery is associated with brain injury in preterm infants. Acta Paediatr. 1994;83:1233-1236.
93. Krageloh-Mann I, Toft P, Lunding J, et al. Brain lesions in preterms: origin, consequences and compensation. Acta Paediatrica. 1999;88:897-908.
94. Fujimori K, Honda S, Sanpei M, et al. Effects of exogenous big endothelin-1 on regional blood flow in fetal lambs. Obstet Gynecol. 2005;106:818-823.
95. Powell RW, Dyess DL, Collins JN, et al. Regional blood flow response to hypothermia in premature, newborn, and neonatal piglets. J Pediatr Surg. 1999;34:193-198.
96. Jose PA, Haramati A, Fildes RD. Postnatal maturation of renal blood flow. In: Polin RA, Fox WW, eds. Fetal and neonatal physiology. Philadelphia: WB Saunders; 1998:1573-1578.
97. Pezzati M, Vangi V, Biagiotti R, et al. Effects of indomethacin and ibuprofen on mesenteric and renal blood flow in preterm infants with patent ductus arteriosus. J Pediatr. 1999;135: 733-738.
98. Rudolph CD, Rudolph AM. Fetal and postnatal hepatic vasculature and blood flow. In: Polin RA, Fox WW, eds. Fetal and neonatal physiology. Philadelphia: WB Saunders; 1998:1442-1449.
99. Clark DA, Miller MJS. Development of the gastrointestinal circulation in the fetus and newborn. In: Polin RA, Fox WW, eds. Fetal and neonatal physiology. Philadelphia: WB Saunders; 1998:929-933.
100. Shimada S, Kasai T, Hoshi A, et al. Cardiocirculatory effects of patent ductus arteriosus in extremely low-birth-weight infants with respiratory distress syndrome. Pediatr Int. 2003;45:255-262.
101. Kluckow M, Evans N. Superior vena cava flow. A novel marker of systemic blood flow. Arch Dis Child. 2000;82:F182-F187.

102. Visser MO, Leighton JO, van de Bor M, et al. Renal blood flow in the neonate; quantitation with color and pulsed Doppler ultrasound. Radiology. 1992;183:441-444.
103. Van Bel F, van Zwieten PH, Guit GL, et al. Superior mesenteric artery blood flow velocity and estimated volume flow. duplex Doppler US study of preterm and term neonates. Radiology. 1990;174:165-169.
104. Agata Y, Hiraishi S, Misawa H, et al. Regional blood flow distribution and left ventricular output during early neonatal life: a quantitative ultrasonographic assessment. Pediatr Res. 1994;36: 805-810.
105. Yao LP, Jose PA. Developmental renal hemodynamics. Pediatr Nephrol. 1995;9:632-637.
106. Bay-Hansen R, Elfving B, Greisen G. Use of near infrared spectroscopy for estimation of peripheral venous saturation in newborns; comparison with co-oximetry of central venous blood. Biol Neonate. 2002;82:1-8.
107. Stephenson R. Physiological control of diving behaviour in the Weddell seal Leptonychotes weddelli; a model based on cardiorespiratory control theory. J Exp Biol. 2005;208:1971-1991.
108. Jensen A, Garnier Y, Berger R. Dynamics of fetal circulatory responses to hypoxia and asphyxia. Eur J Obstet Gynecol Reprod Biol. 1999;84:155-172.
109. Green LR, McGarrigle HHG, Bennet L, et al. Angiotensin II and cardiovascular chemoreflex responses to acute hypoxia in late gestation fetal sheep. J Physiol. 1998;507:857-867.
110. Coumans ABC, Garnier Y, Supcun S, et al. Nitric oxide and fetal organ blood flow during normoxia and hypoxemia in endotoxin-treated fetal sheep. Obstet Gynecol. 2005;105:145-155.
111. Kehrer M, Krägeloh-Mann L, Goelz R, et al. The development of cerebral perfusion in healthy preterm and term neonates. Neuropediatrics. 2003;34:281-286.
112. Sinha AK, Cane C, Kempley ST. Blood flow in the common carotid artery in term and preterm infants; reproducibility and relation to cardiac output. Arch Dis Child. 2006;91:31-35.

2

CHAPTER 3

Definition of Normal Blood Pressure Range: The Elusive Target

William D. Engle, MD

- ● **Case Study**
- ● **Measuring Blood Pressure**
- ● **Normative Data for Blood Pressure in Neonates**
- ● **Adjuncts to Blood Pressure Measurement in the Diagnosis of Compromised Circulatory Function**
- ● **Clinical Factors that may Affect Blood Pressure**
- ● **Conclusion**
- ● **References**

Few aspects of the management of high-risk neonates have generated as much controversy as the assessment of blood pressure, and this is particularly true of preterm neonates. The approach to this problem may differ greatly among various institutions and between clinicians within a given center. The variation may relate to training, but also it is a reflection of the need for further data that would provide the clinician with a better understanding of the relationship between blood pressure and meaningful clinical outcomes.

Case Study

An 820-g male infant was born at 27 weeks' gestation. The pregnancy was complicated by placenta previa, and delivery was by cesarean section (C/S) after preterm, premature rupture of membranes, and subsequent onset of labor. There was no significant vaginal bleeding. The infant was apneic initially but he responded well to positive-pressure ventilation. He developed retractions and grunting, and was intubated. Apgars were 5 and 8 and 1 and 5 minutes, respectively.

In the neonatal intensive care unit (NICU), the chest x-ray (CXR) was consistent with surfactant deficiency (respiratory distress syndrome, RDS), and he received surfactant replacement therapy. Subsequently, the FiO_2 requirement to maintain oxygen saturation in the 88-94% range decreased from 0.70 to 0.30, and ventilatory pressures were weaned appropriately. Attempts to place an umbilical artery catheter (UAC) were unsuccessful; an umbilical venous catheter (UVC) was placed. He was begun on a dextrose and amino acid solution at 60 mL/kg/day, and ampicillin and gentamicin were given. The hematocrit was 47% and serum glucose was 97 to 125 mg/dL.

Mean blood pressure on admission was 31 mm Hg (determined by oscillometry). At 2 hours of postnatal life, mean blood pressure had decreased to 25 mm Hg. Heart rate varied between 135 and 160 bpm. The infant was moving spontaneously, and capillary refill time was approximately 2 sec. He had not voided.

This case is similar to those seen frequently in any NICU: the very small neonate who seems to be doing fairly well from a cardiorespiratory standpoint, but whose

49

mean blood pressure engenders acute discomfort in the staff. Various issues involving whether or how to treat the blood pressure in the very low birth weight (VLBW) neonate during the immediate postnatal period are discussed in Chapter 12. Here we might ask:

1. Should a preterm neonate who requires mechanical ventilation, and in whom a UAC is unsuccessful, have a peripheral arterial line?
2. If so, should this be attempted immediately after the failed UAC attempt, or only after it appears that the blood pressure will be a problem?
3. What evidence is available to determine when a "problem" blood pressure exists?
4. What is the role of heart rate, capillary refill time, urine output, and other nonspecific indicators of the cardiovascular status in the decision-making process as one attempts to determine whether or not this is an adequate blood pressure?

To address these questions, this chapter reviews the methods of measurement of blood pressure, normative values for blood pressure in preterm and term neonates, clinical assessments used often in conjunction with blood pressure measurement, and clinical factors that can influence blood pressure (see also Chapters 1 and 12).[1-4]

Measuring Blood Pressure

It is appropriate to ask why there is so much attention paid to assessment of blood pressure. Clearly, the primary issue regarding possible hypotension in neonates is the concern that impaired central nervous system perfusion may lead to ischemic damage[1,2] (Chapter 16). Arterial pressure is determined by two factors: the propulsion of blood by the heart and the resistance to flow of this blood through the blood vessels.[3] Thus *flow = pressure/resistance* and, consequently, *pressure = flow × resistance*. In the case of the normal systemic circulation, the left ventricle serves as the pump, which generates sufficient pressure to overcome vascular resistance and create systemic arterial flow and maintain appropriate perfusion pressure in the organs. From a clinical standpoint, blood flow resulting in adequate tissue perfusion is the variable of critical interest, and disturbances of perfusion represent some position on the continuum of the complex disorder of shock.[3] However, since, despite recent advances (Chapter 6), it is not practical to measure flow routinely, and resistance can only be calculated but not measured, we rely greatly on blood pressure determinations to gauge the adequacy of cardiac output and systemic perfusion. It is obvious from the equations that significant changes in vascular resistance might result in changes in blood flow (and thus changes in tissue perfusion) without recognizable alterations in blood pressure. This suggests that blood pressure is not the only physiologic variable of primary interest. This issue becomes even more complicated in the transitional circulation of the VLBW neonate with shunting across the fetal channels, where neither mean blood pressure nor cardiac output alone is necessarily a good predictor of systemic blood flow.[4] The complex interaction among pressure, flow, and resistance along with possibilities for improved monitoring of circulatory status is shown in Figure 3-1.[5]

The "gold standard" for determination of blood pressure in the critically ill neonate is a direct continuous reading from an indwelling arterial line, and generally this method is used whenever arterial access is available. The ability to measure blood pressure noninvasively represents a major advance in neonatal care, although a major drawback associated with these methods is the inability to obtain continuous measurements.[6] Detailed recent reviews of blood pressure measurement and monitoring in the neonate are available.[7,8]

Direct Measurement of Blood Pressure

Using a catheter–transducer fluid-filled system, blood pressure is measured directly most frequently by utilizing a UAC with its tip in the thoracic or distal aorta or a catheter placed in a peripheral artery. The purpose of this section is to point out common issues related to direct measurement of blood pressure in neonates. For a

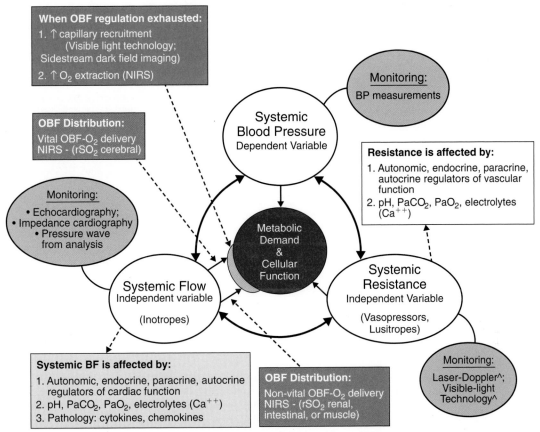

When OBF regulation exhausted:
1. ↑ capillary recruitment
   (Visible light technology;
Sidestream dark field imaging)
2. ↑ O_2 extraction (NIRS)

OBF Distribution:
Vital OBF-O_2 delivery
NIRS - (rSO_2 cerebral)

Monitoring:
BP measurements

Systemic Blood Pressure
Dependent Variable

Resistance is affected by:
1. Autonomic, endocrine, paracrine, autocrine regulators of vascular function
2. pH, $PaCO_2$, PaO_2, electrolytes (Ca^{++})

Monitoring:
• Echocardiography;
• Impedance cardiography
• Pressure wave from analysis

Metabolic Demand & Cellular Function

Systemic Flow
Independent variable
(Inotropes)

Systemic Resistance
Independent Variable
(Vasopressors, Lusitropes)

Systemic BF is affected by:
1. Autonomic, endocrine, paracrine, autocrine regulators of cardiac function
2. pH, $PaCO_2$, PaO_2, electrolytes (Ca^{++})
3. Pathology: cytokines, chemokines

OBF Distribution:
Non-vital OBF-O_2 delivery
NIRS - (rSO_2 renal, intestinal, or muscle)

Monitoring:
Laser-Doppler^;
Visible-light Technology^

Figure 3-1   Interaction among and monitoring of blood pressure (BP), blood flow, blood flow distribution, and vascular resistance. To satisfy cellular metabolic demand, an intricate interplay among blood flow, vascular resistance, and BP take place. Regulation of organ blood flow distribution, capillary recruitment, and oxygen extraction is also essential for the maintenance of hemodynamic homeostasis. Monitoring methods depicted have mostly been used for clinical research purposes at this time. It is unknown whether laser Doppler and/or visible light technologies can reliably monitor changes in systemic vascular resistance. NIRS, near-infrared spectroscopy; OBF, organ blood flow; rSO2, regional tissue oxygen saturation. (From Soleymani S, Borzage M, Seri I. Hemodynamic monitoring in neonates: advances and challenges. J Perinatol. 2010;30:S38-S45. Used with permission from Nature Publishing Group.)

more extensive review of direct measurement of blood pressure, the reader is referred to several excellent publications.[7-10]

The first direct measurement of blood pressure was made in the eighteenth century and is credited to Hales. He attached a long vertical tube to a cannula that was inserted into the crural artery of a horse, and demonstrated reduction in blood pressure following hemorrhage.

A wave can be defined as a traveling disturbance carrying energy, and it can be characterized by frequency, intensity or amplitude, direction, and velocity.[8,9] The pressure pulse is a complex waveform that is dependent on site of measurement (see later). It should be noted that the speed of the pressure pulse greatly exceeds that of the actual blood flow, and the fundamental frequencies of the pressure pulse bear little relationship to the repetition rate of the initiating event.[8,11] The pressure pulse should not be confused with the pulse pressure, which refers to the difference between systolic and diastolic blood pressure.

The system used for continuous, direct blood pressure monitoring in today's NICU generally is referred to as "under-damped and second order".[8] Instead of a column of mercury, modern systems for measuring blood pressure have several components, the most important of which is the transducer. The transducer converts mechanical energy (pressure) to electrical energy (current or voltage). Compared with older strain gauge pressure transducers, today's transducers have a silicon chip, and they are inexpensive, accurate, and disposable.[12] The transducer must be positioned at the level of the catheter opening, and correctly "zeroing" the system (stopcock connected to transducer open to atmospheric pressure) is a critical step in obtaining accurate blood pressure values. This process should be performed at least every 12 hours to ensure the accuracy of blood pressure measurements over time.

An ideal pressure-monitoring system should reflect the pressure pulse accurately so that the monitor waveform is similar to that at the site of measurement, and to do this it must have an appropriate frequency response.[8] A method for determining the resonant frequency and damping coefficient has been described by Gardner.[10] Systems in clinical use generally have a resonant frequency of 15 to 25 Hz and a coefficient of 0.1 to 0.4.[7]

Generally, direct readings of blood pressure in the neonate are considered to be accurate, although several problems may occur. A small-diameter catheter may cause the systolic reading to be low. Excessive damping secondary to the introduction of small air bubbles or clots into the system may result in decreased systolic but increased diastolic readings.[7,13] Since mean blood pressure, which is considered more reflective of perfusion pressure than systolic or diastolic pressure, has generally been considered to be unaffected by damping, this potential inaccuracy may not be a significant clinical problem. However, Cunningham and colleagues reported that damping (defined as a sudden reduction of pulse pressure by more than 8 mm Hg or complete loss of the systolic and diastolic differential) also might affect mean blood pressure.[14] In 24% of damping episodes studied, the difference was ≥4.1 mm Hg.[14]

Conversely, as the pressure pulse travels from aortic root to peripheral arteries, amplification of some components may occur, and somewhat counter-intuitively, measured systolic pressure may be higher in the dorsalis pedis or radial artery versus the aorta.[7,8] This is caused by a gradual increase in impedance as the pressure pulse travels distally through more narrow channels, and the observed waveform may appear narrower and taller than observed more proximally. Diastolic and mean blood pressures are less affected by this phenomenon, but mean blood pressure calculated using the formula "diastolic pressure plus one third of pulse pressure" would be falsely high.[7] Generally, the difference is not clinically significant, and a very strong correlation between blood pressures obtained via umbilical and peripheral artery catheters was reported by Butt and Whyte.[15]

Although direct measurement of blood pressure is considered the gold standard and generally is felt to be the most appropriate method for monitoring a critically ill neonate (see later), it is important to minimize distortions if one is to obtain accurate values. Use of tubing that is as short as possible, large-bore, stiff, and noncompliant as well as minimizing the number of stopcocks and manifolds will help in this regard.[16]

Noninvasive Measurement of Blood Pressure

Manufacturers of noninvasive blood pressure monitors must provide accuracy data to the Food and Drug Administration (FDA) before they may be marketed.[17] Guidelines followed in generating this data must conform to the requirements of the American National Standard for Manual, Electronic, or Automated Sphygmomanometers (ANSI/AAMI SP10). The mean difference of paired comparisons between direct and noninvasive methods must be within ±5 mm Hg with a standard deviation ≤ 8 mm Hg.[18] In considering studies that have examined agreement between invasive and noninvasive methods, it is important to consider the impact of more recent technological improvements. For example, Nelson and colleagues found that an improved algorithm for the DINAMAP MPS oscillometric device resulted in agreement that met the standards noted earlier.[19]

All noninvasive techniques for estimating blood pressure analyze changes in blood flow and, since direct methods measure pressure, one would not necessarily expect the results obtained with noninvasive and direct methods to be identical.[16]

Of the common noninvasive techniques (palpation, auscultation, Doppler, and oscillometry), oscillometry is used most often.[20] An additional method that utilizes a photoelectric principle and provides a continuous arterial waveform through a finger cuff also has been described. The Finapres (FINger Arterial PRESsure) method uses a photoplethysmographic system applied to the finger and provides a continuous beat-to-beat waveform. Because of the cuff size, previous investigators placed the finger cuff around the wrist of the baby. More recently, Andriessen and colleagues developed a miniature cuff, and in a small study of neonates, infants and young children, demonstrated good agreement between this technique and arterial blood pressure determined invasively.[21] Another method of determining blood pressure has been by measurement of pulse oximetry.[22] Measurements were made in 50 patients by gradually inflating an appropriately sized cuff until the plethysmographic waveform disappeared, then inflating the cuff another 20 mm Hg, then gradually deflating the cuff until the waveform reappeared. Systolic pressure was calculated as the average of the blood pressures at which the waveform disappeared and reappeared. Although the agreement between blood pressure obtained by this method and direct measurement of arterial pressure was much stronger than the agreement between direct and oscillometric measurements, this technique is not commonly used in the NICU. A discussion of basic principles of noninvasive blood pressure measurement in infants is available.[17]

The measurement of blood pressure by oscillometry was first described by Marey in 1876, and Ramsey reported the use of an automated instrument based on the oscillometric technique (Dinamap, Critikon, Tampa, FL) in 1979.[8,23] This device is able to measure cuff oscillations at given pressures as sensed by a pressure transducer; systolic pressure is the pressure at which cuff oscillation begins to increase as the cuff is deflated. Mean pressure is the lowest cuff pressure at which oscillometric amplitude is maximal, and diastolic pressure is the pressure at which the amplitude of cuff oscillations stops decreasing.[7]

The agreement between blood pressure values obtained directly and by oscillometry has generally been good.[24] However, some investigators have found that the agreement is poor, and suggested that noninvasive techniques are not sufficiently accurate for routine use.[25] Of course, when comparing direct and noninvasive methods, it is important to ensure accuracy of the reference method by performing dynamic calibration (frequency response and damping coefficient) for each infant.[17] However, this exercise is not always noted.[16]

One well-documented reason for lack of agreement with intra-arterial blood pressure may be use of an inappropriate cuff size when performing oscillometric measurements. Sonesson and Broberger reported that mean blood pressure was overestimated with a cuff width to arm circumference ratio of 0.33-0.42.[26] Accuracy improved with a ratio of 0.44-0.55. In the study by Kimble and colleagues, the appropriate cuff width to arm circumference ratio was 0.45-0.70 (Fig. 3-2).[27] It is of concern that several investigators have found that blood pressure determined by oscillometry overestimates directly obtained blood pressure, since this relationship might lead to failure to treat hypotensive neonates. As noted earlier, this overestimation might be due to a cuff that is too small.[26] In a study of 12 VLBW neonates, Diprose and colleagues reported that the oscillometric method overestimated blood pressure in hypotensive infants.[28] Cuff width to arm circumference ratios were not reported in this study (although the authors commented that the cuffs actually may have been too large because of the relatively small size of the patients), and data regarding mean blood pressure were not included. Fanaroff and Wright reported that mean blood pressure during the first 48 postnatal hours, determined by the oscillometric technique, exceeded direct readings by about 3 mm Hg; however, cuff size was not reported.[29] Others also have reported a tendency for oscillometric determinations to exceed direct measurements.[30] Wareham and colleagues noted that diastolic blood pressure was overestimated by the oscillometric method, but systolic and mean blood pressures were underestimated.[31]

Studies comparing blood pressure measurements from upper versus lower limbs have produced conflicting results.[24] In term neonates, Park and Lee observed

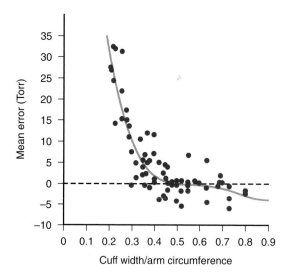

Figure 3-2 A nonlinear regression analysis comparing error (Dinamap minus intra-arterial) with cuff width to arm circumference ratio. Each point represents the average of 10 determinations with the same cuff in a given patient. (From Kimble KJ, Darnall RA Jr, Yelderman M, et al. An automated oscillometric technique for estimating mean arterial pressure in critically ill newborns. Anesthesiology. 1981;54:423-425 1. Used with permission from Lippincott Williams & Wilkins.)

no difference in blood pressure between arm and calf.[32] Piazza and colleagues compared upper and lower limb systolic blood pressure in term neonates in the first 24 hours and found that higher readings in the upper versus lower limb were more common than vice versa.[33] However, higher readings in the lower limb were sufficiently common (28%) for these investigators to conclude that either possibility should be considered normal. In subsequent follow-up of 25 of the study neonates up to three years of age, systolic blood pressure was higher in the lower extremities in 24/25.

More recently, Cowan and colleagues determined arm and calf blood pressure in term neonates in active and quiet sleep during the first five postnatal days.[34] The increase in blood pressure during this period was greater in the arm than in the calf, and calf blood pressure appeared to be more dependent on sleep state than did arm blood pressure. Subsequently, Kunk and McCain studied 65 preterm neonates with mean birth weight of 1629 g.[35] During days 1-5, there were no significant differences in systolic, diastolic, and mean blood pressures between arm and calf, although arm blood pressures consistently were slightly higher. On day 7, there was a significant difference with arm greater than calf for systolic blood pressure by an average of 2.7 mm Hg.

Papadopoulos and colleagues compared three oscillometric devices [Dinamap 8100 (Critikon), SpaceLabs M90426 (SpaceLabs Medical), and the Module HP M1008B (Hewlett-Packard; HP)] to a simulator.[36] The Dinamap and SpaceLabs readings were in good agreement with the reference method, whereas mean errors for systolic and diastolic blood pressure with the HP device were 21 and 15 mm Hg, respectively.

Pichler and colleagues[37] compared two commonly used oscillometric systems, the HP-Monitor CMS Model 68 S with Module HP M1008B and the Dinamap 8100. By Bland-Altman analysis, it was shown that mean blood pressure determined by the Dinamap was significantly higher than with the HP. This study is difficult to interpret since direct determination of blood pressure was not made for comparison. However, it does point out that results in noninvasive determination of blood pressure may be dependent on the system used by a particular NICU.

More recently, Dannevig and colleagues compared blood pressure obtained with three different monitors (Dinamap Compact, Criticare Model 506 DXN2, and Hewlett-Packard Monitor with the HP MI008B Module) with determinations made with an invasive system (Hewlett-Packard).[38] Twenty neonates (birth weight 531-4660 g) were studied during the first postnatal week. Difference between oscillometric and invasive pressures (measurement deviance) was related to two factors:

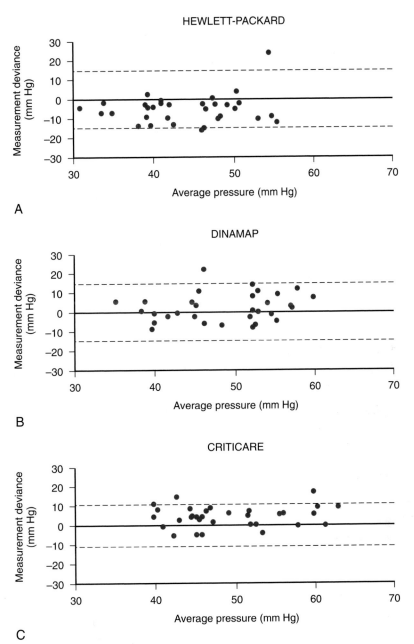

Figure 3-3   Bland-Altman plots comparing invasively measured arterial blood pressure and measurements obtained with three oscillometric devices (Dinamap, Criticare, Hewlett-Packard). (From Dannevig I, Dale HC, Liestol K, Lindemann R. Blood pressure in the neonate: three noninvasive oscillometric pressure monitors compared with invasively measured blood pressure. Acta Paediatr. 2005;94:191-196, Fig. 1. Used with permission from Taylor & Francis.)

(1) size of infant and (2) monitoring system. In smaller infants, the noninvasively measured value tended to be too high, and as arm circumference increased, measurement deviance decreased with all monitors. The Hewlett-Packard gave lower pressure readings than either the Criticare or Dinamap (Fig. 3-3); Criticare and Dinamap tended to show too high a value in the smallest infants, while Hewlett-Packard tended to give too low a value in the larger infants. These investigators concluded that blood pressure should preferably be measured invasively in severely ill neonates and preterm infants.

While caution in the interpretation of indirectly obtained blood pressure measurements is prudent, the clinical usefulness of this technique has been demonstrated. In many instances, the trend in blood pressure in a particular infant is of critical importance, and the exact absolute value may be of less relevance. Fortunately, those critically ill neonates in whom decisions regarding treatment of possible hypotension need to be made are the patients most likely to have arterial access. When the most frequently used site for direct access (umbilical artery) is not available, as in the case presented at the beginning of this chapter, direct access via a peripheral artery should be considered.

In summary, the best method for routine noninvasive blood pressure measurement is the oscillometric method, and the sophisticated bedside cardiorespiratory monitoring systems in current use allow the clinician to monitor blood pressure at set intervals and display the results on the same screen that shows heart rate, oxygen saturation, and so forth. As noted earlier, use of the proper cuff size is critical. Although differences among various oscillometric monitors have been demonstrated, at this time there does not seem to be conclusive evidence to favor a particular monitor system over all others.

Normative Data for Blood Pressure in Neonates

The establishment of normal values for blood pressure in newborn infants has been attempted by numerous investigators, and there is fairly good agreement in the results reported from various institutions.[39] However, studies that have sought to determine normal ranges for blood pressure often have weaknesses, such as retrospective data collection, small numbers, and use of both invasive and noninvasive blood pressure values.[40] Laughon and colleagues noted that physicians' preferences rather infant well-being determined "normal" blood pressure reported in previous studies of untreated infants, and considered the large variation in treatment of hypotension that they observed among centers (29-98%) to be supportive of this concept.[41] Of course, it is highly likely that improved data regarding what constitutes unsafe and unacceptable blood pressure in high-risk neonates would reduce the current striking center variability in percentage of neonates treated. The Cardiology Group on Cardiovascular Instability in Preterm Infants concluded recently that there is no consensus regarding the definition of hypotension in the neonate.[42]

In most studies, blood pressure is higher in larger, more mature infants, and there is an increase in blood pressure with increasing postnatal age.[7,15,24] Small for gestational age (SGA) infants may have lower blood pressure than larger babies of comparable gestational age, although comparable blood pressure values also have been reported.[24,43] As suggested earlier, "normative values" may be influenced by management protocols within a given institution. Also, most studies have not determined that the "physiologic range" for blood pressure is occurring simultaneously with normal organ blood flow.[44,45] Kluckow and Evans reported a weak correlation between mean blood pressure and superior vena cava (SVC) blood flow used for the assessment of systemic blood flow in preterm infants less than 32 weeks' gestation.[45,46] Studies were performed during the first two postnatal days when shunting across the fetal channels prevents the use of the left ventricular output as the measure of systemic blood flow. Conversely, Munro and colleagues reported that ELBW neonates who were hypotensive during the first postnatal days had lower cerebral blood flow than normotensive neonates.[47]

The report by Kitterman and colleagues in 1969 was one of the earliest studies of blood pressure in neonates, and these results were used widely in neonatal intensive care units.[48] However, this study included only nine patients with birth weights ≤ 1500 g. Versmold and colleagues studied 16 stable neonates with birth weights 610 to 980 g (eight infants were small for gestational age); blood pressure during the first 12 postnatal hours was measured directly through an umbilical artery catheter.[49] Despite this report, which demonstrated that the 95% confidence limits for mean blood pressure ranged from 24 to 44 mm Hg, the value of 30 mm Hg has been widely adopted as a critical lower limit for acceptable blood pressure in preterm

Table 3-1 VARIATION OF MEAN BLOOD PRESSURE* WITH BIRTH WEIGHT AT 3 TO 96 HOURS
OF POSTNATAL AGE

Birth Weight (g)	Time (h) Postnatal Age								
	3	12	24	36	48	60	72	84	96
500	35/23	36/24	37/25	38/26	39/28	41/29	42/30	43/31	44/33
600	35/24	36.25	37/26	39/27	40/28	41/29	42/31	44/32	45/33
700	36/24	37/25	38/26	39/28	42/29	42/30	43/31	44/32	45/34
800	36/25	37/26	39/27	40/28	41/29	42/31	44/32	45/33	46/34
900	37/25	38/26	39/27	40/29	42/30	43/31	44/32	45/34	47/35
1000	38/26	39/27	40/28	41/29	42/31	43/32	45/33	46/34	47/35
1100	38/27	39/27	40/29	42/30	43/31	44/32	45/34	46/35	48/36
1200	39/27	40/28	41/29	42/30	43/32	45/33	46/34	47/35	48/37
1300	39/28	40/29	41/30	43/31	44/32	45/33	46/35	48/36	49/37
1400	40/28	41/29	42/30	43/32	44/33	46/34	47/35	48/36	49/38
1500	40/29	42/30	43/31	44/32	45/33	46/35	48/36	49/37	50/38

*Numbers refer to average MBP/tenth percentile for MBP.
From Watkins AMC, West CR, Cooke RWI. Blood pressure and cerebral haemorrhage and ischaemia in very low birthweight
infants. Early Hum Develop 1989;19:103-110. Used with permission from Elsevier Ltd.

neonates. This notion was based on findings suggesting that the lower limit of the
cerebral blood flow autoregulatory curve was around 30 mm Hg, and that neonates
with mean arterial pressures less than 30 mm Hg had a high likelihood of developing central nervous system pathology (see later).[47,50] Subsequently, Watkins and
colleagues reported that the 10th percentile for mean blood pressure for a baby with
a birth weight of 600 g was less than 30 mm Hg until 72 hours postnatal (Table
3-1).[51] Similar low values for extremely preterm neonates were reported by Nuntnarumit and colleagues (Fig. 3-4). This figure demonstrates clearly the striking

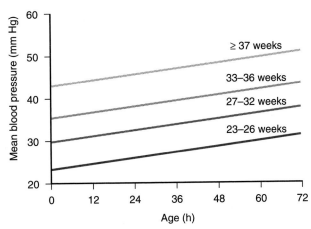

Figure 3-4 Mean blood pressure in neonates with gestational ages of 23 to 43 weeks (n =
103, neonates admitted to NICU). The graph shows the predicted mean blood pressure during
the first 72 h of life. Each line represents the lower limit of 80% confidence interval (two-tail)
of mean blood pressure for each gestational age group; 90% of infants for each gestational
age group will be expected to have a mean blood pressure value equal to or above the value
indicated by the corresponding line, the lower limit of the confidence interval. (Nuntnarumit
P, Yang W, Bada-Ellzey HS. Blood pressure measurements in the newborn. Clin Perinatol.
1999;26:981-996. Used with permission from Elsevier.)

differences in mean blood pressure between term and preterm neonates, but with parallel increases occurring over the first 72 hours postnatal. Interestingly, following an initial decrease during the first 6-12 postnatal hours, cerebral blood flow also increases after delivery in both term and preterm neonates.[7,52] However, the initial decrease is more dramatic in the VLBW patient population, and it is during the ensuing period of rapid improvement in cerebral blood flow (reperfusion) that peri-intraventricular hemorrhage PIVH) occurs.[45]

In 1999, Lee and colleagues demonstrated that the lower 95% confidence interval for mean blood pressure was even lower than reported by Versmold and colleagues, with values of 20 to 23 mm Hg observed in the 500- to 800-g infants.[53,72] These authors cautioned against treatment for a low blood pressure value alone unless there are coexisting signs of hypoperfusion, such as poor capillary return, oliguria, and metabolic acidosis (see later).

Adams and colleagues reported findings of a study of continuously recorded blood pressure in 15 infants with birth weight ≤ 1500 g, utilizing a system capable of measuring and storing 60 data points each minute.[54] When a linear regression analysis of hourly mean blood pressure as a function of postnatal age was calculated, these investigators found significant correlations for gestational age and birth weight with the slopes and intercepts of the linear equations. While these authors noted that the relatively steep rise in mean blood pressure in the less mature infants may be a predisposing factor in the development of intraventricular hemorrhage, it should be noted that birth weight was ≥ 1180 g in 13 of 15 neonates. Subsequently, Cunningham and colleagues performed continuous recordings of blood pressure and noted cyclical variation with hypertensive "waves."[55] They postulated that this blood pressure instability might predispose to intraventricular hemorrhage. Cunningham and colleagues subsequently reported mean blood pressure ranges in 232 VLBW neonates.[56] Intraventricular hemorrhage (IVH) was associated with low blood pressure on the day IVH was noted or on the day before. Periventricular leukomalacia (PVL) was not associated with blood pressure.

In two reports, Hegyi and colleagues described blood pressure ranges in preterm infants in the immediate postnatal period and in the first postnatal week.[57,58] Soon after birth, 20-50% of those neonates with low Apgar scores had blood pressure values below the 5th percentile for healthy infants. Of note, in healthy infants, as well as in those who received mechanical ventilation and in those whose mothers were hypertensive, the limits of systolic and diastolic blood pressure were found to be independent of birth weight and gestational age. In the latter study, blood pressure increased steadily during the first week of life.[58] However, no relationships between blood pressure variables and birth weight, gender, or race were observed.

In a retrospective study, Cordero and colleagues examined mean arterial pressure in 101 neonates with birth weight ≤ 600 g during the first 24 postnatal hours.[59] Mean arterial pressure was similar at birth in stable and unstable neonates, but subsequent increases over the first 24 hours were less in the unstable group, despite a greater incidence of therapy for hypotension. These authors considered failure of mean arterial pressure to increase between 3 and 6 hours postnatal and a mean arterial pressure of ≤ 28 mm Hg at 3 hours postnatal to be a reasonable predictor of the need for therapy for hypotension. It should be noted that mean gestational age was 27 versus 25 weeks in the stable and unstable groups, respectively.

Zubrow and colleagues reported the findings of a large multicenter study conducted by the Philadelphia Neonatal Blood Pressure Study Group.[60] In this investigation, systolic and diastolic blood pressure was significantly correlated with birth weight gestational age, and postconceptional age. In each of four gestational age groups, systolic and diastolic blood pressure was significantly correlated with postnatal age over the first five days of life. LeFlore and colleagues studied 116 VLBW neonates during the first 72 postnatal hours.[61] Mean blood pressure increased 38% during this period (r = .96). Increases in blood pressure in infants with birth weight ≤ 1000 g are shown in Figure 3-5. There was a similar increase in blood pressure

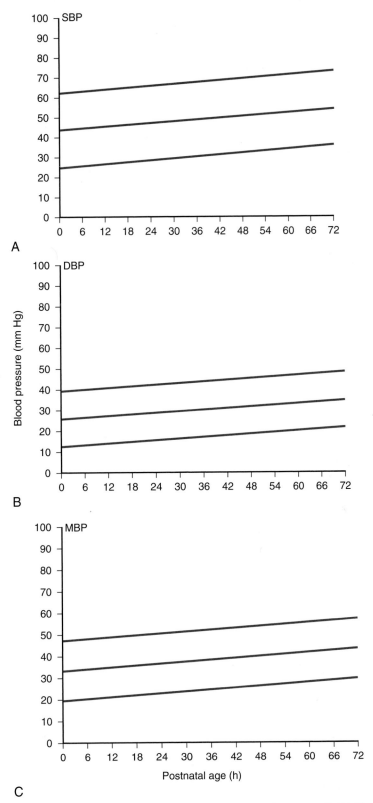

Figure 3-5 Change in systolic blood pressure (SBP) **(A),** diastolic blood pressure (DBP) **(B),** and mean blood pressure (MBP) **(C)** in neonates ≤ 1000 g birth weight (n = 36) during the initial 72 hours postnatal. Lines represent means and 95% confidence intervals ($P < .0001$). Equations for lines of best fit were SBP = 0.17x + 43.2; DBP = 0.13x + 25.8; MBP = 0.14x + 32.9. In each instance, the y-intercept was significantly lower ($P < .001$) than the value for comparable lines of best fit in infants with birth weights 1001–1500 g; however, no significant differences in slopes for the lines of best fit were observed between the two birth weight groups. (From LeFlore JL, Engle WD, Rosenfeld CR. Determinants of blood pressure in very low birth weight neonates: lack of effect of antenatal steroids. Early Hum Dev. 2000;59:37-50. Used with permission from Elsevier.)

Table 3-2   95TH, 50TH, AND 5TH PERCENTILE VALUES OF THE SYSTOLIC, DIASTOLIC, AND MEAN BLOOD PRESSURES FOR 86 HEMODYNAMICALLY STABLE INFANTS DURING THE FIRST POSTNATAL WEEK

	Age (hr)							
BP	1	6	12	18	24	48	72	168
Systolic BP (mm Hg)								
95th percentile	44	50	52	54	55	57	58	61
50th percentile	32	38	40	42	43	45	46	49
5th percentile	20	26	28	30	30	33	34	37
Diastolic BP (mm Hg)								
95th percentile	32	35	36	37	38	39	39	41
50th percentile	23	26	27	27	28	29	30	31
5th percentile	13	16	17	18	18	19	20	21
Mean BP (mm Hg)								
95th percentile	36	41	42	43	44	45	46	48
50th percentile	27	31	33	34	34	36	37	39
5th percentile	17	21	23	24	25	26	27	29

From Batton B, Batton D, Riggs T. Blood pressure during the first 7 days in premature infants born at postmenstrual age 23 to 25 weeks. Am J Perinatol 2007;24:107-116. Used with permission from Thieme Medical Publishers, Inc.

in the neonates with birth weight 1001 to 1500 g. However, mean blood pressure in the smaller infants was approximately 20% less than in the larger infants throughout the study.

More recently, Batton and colleagues reported blood pressure values for 86 neonates with gestational age 23-25 weeks who did not receive treatment for hypotension.[62] Results from birth to 168 hours for the 95th, 50th and 5th percentiles are shown in Table 3-2. Mean arterial pressures ≤25 mm Hg were not uncommon and were not associated with apparent consequences. In comparing the untreated neonates to a group of infants with similar gestational age who did receive treatment for hypotension, it was noted that the treated infants had much lower survival and survival without major morbidity. The authors noted that it was not apparent from their data that the treatment had any beneficial effects. Conversely, Pellicer and colleagues, using the normative data noted earlier (see Fig. 3-4) as criteria for treatment, concluded that cautious use of cardiovascular support to treat early systemic hypotension was safe.[63]

Kent and colleagues reported normative blood pressure data in non-ventilated neonates with gestational age 28-36 weeks.[64] Blood pressure in preterm neonates was similar to that of term infants after two weeks.

The Joint Working Group of the British Association of Perinatal Medicine has recommended that mean arterial blood pressure, in mm Hg, should be maintained at or above the gestational age of the infant in weeks during the immediate postnatal period.[65] In light of the aforementioned studies, this approach seems to have some merit, but further investigation will be required to establish its safety and efficacy; as noted by Dempsey and Barrington, the recommendation by the Joint Working Group was made without supporting data.[40,66] Nevertheless, these guidelines are used very frequently in clinical care, perhaps because of the ease of use. Of course, whether one considers the acceptable blood pressure to be the gestational age in weeks or a value higher than the 10th percentile for gestational age or birth weight, it is important to remember that being born at a very early gestation represents an abnormal situation, and that having a blood pressure in the "normal" range relative to one's peers does not guarantee that this is a safe situation. Using a value for mean blood pressure that was below gestational age as criteria for hypotension, Pellicer and colleagues observed that with the increase in blood pressure, cerebral intravascular oxygenation increased as well following treatment with dopamine or epinephrine in VLBW neonates during the first postnatal day.[67] These findings suggest that mean arterial blood pressures at or below gestational age in VLBW neonates during the first postnatal day are below the autoregulatory blood pressure range for cerebral blood flow. Indeed, the recent findings of Munro and colleagues suggest that a mean blood pressure of <30 mm Hg remains a potentially useful clinical benchmark.[50,68] Conversely, normal cerebral electrical function may be observed in VLBW neonates when the blood pressure is quite low, and a lack of correlation between mean blood pressure and cerebral fractional oxygen extraction has been reported during the first postnatal day.[69,70] Interestingly, recent findings from the same group also suggest that electrical brain activity may be affected at mean arterial blood pressures at or below 23 to 24 mm Hg in VLBW neonates during the first postnatal day.[71] However, one should remember that a likely temporally functional impairment does not necessarily equate to a negative impact on brain development or damage to brain structure just as fainting does not indicate that brain damage has necessarily occurred. In support of this concept, Lightburn and colleagues reported that cerebral blood flow velocity was similar in hypotensive and normotensive extremely low birth weight neonates.[72]

Clearly, more studies relating blood pressure, organ flow, and subsequent outcome are needed especially in the VLBW patient population during the first postnatal days when most of the severe central nervous system pathology may develop. With regard to the case described at the beginning of the chapter, if this infant's mean blood pressure had been stable in the low-to-mid 30s, it would seem reasonable to continue with frequent oscillometric determinations.

The mechanism for the gradual rise in blood pressure during the first postnatal week is unknown, although hemodynamic adjustment of the immature myocardium to the relatively high resistance imposed suddenly at the time of birth certainly plays a role.[4] Urinary prostaglandin E_2 and plasma 6-keto-prostaglandin $F_{1\alpha}$ (stable metabolite of prostacyclin) decrease during the first three postnatal days in preterm neonates.[73] This could result in a rise in vascular tone and increased vascular reactivity.[74] However, the hormonal mechanisms of the postnatal cardiovascular adaptation are more complex than could be explained by changes in one hormone or paracrine system alone as, for instance, the concomitant decrease in catecholamine and vasopressin levels would favor lower blood pressures. Ezaki and colleagues measured plasma levels of vasoactive substances in extremely low birth weight neonates in the first 24 hours after birth.[75] In infants with severe hypotension, dopamine levels were elevated and the norepinephrine/dopamine ratio was decreased, suggesting a role for decreased conversion of dopamine to norepinephrine in the development of severe hypotension. van Bel and colleagues reported that levels of the vasodilator cyclic guanosine monophosphate (cGMP) were increased in neonates with respiratory distress syndrome (RDS) and suggested that lung inflammation resulted in increased heme oxygenase and increased carbon monoxide resulting in increased cGMP (Fig. 3-6).[76] Nitric oxide was similar between the groups, but the incidence of hypotension was higher in the RDS group (Fig. 3-7). Presumably this process would be self-limited with a subsequent increase in BP. It has been reported that vascular smooth muscle protein expression and contractility demonstrate functional maturation during development.[77,78] Thus the rise in blood pressure during the fetal-neonatal transition may reflect decreases in the activity and synthesis of vasodilators, which are critical to fetal survival or related to a disease process such as RDS, as well as intrinsic changes in vascular smooth muscle function occurring prior to and following birth, both of which appear to be developmentally regulated. Finally, maturation of autonomic nervous system function may also play a role in the blood pressure increase during the first postnatal week. In summary, blood pressure is lower in preterm versus term neonates on the first postnatal day, and there is a direct relationship between blood

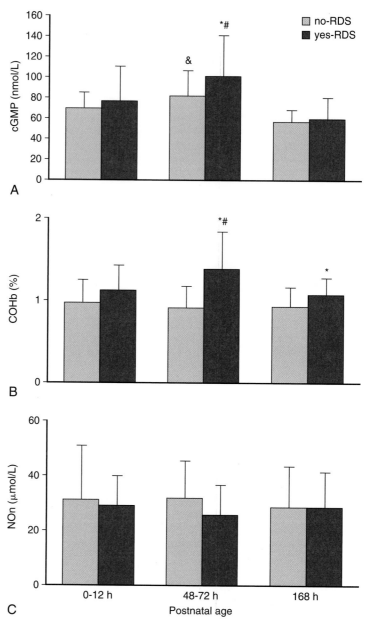

Figure 3-6 **A,** cGMP (nmol/L). **B,** Carboxyhemoglobin (COHb; %). **C,** Plasma levels of nitric oxide (NO) production (NOx; μmol/L) in plasma of infants without respiratory distress syndrome (no-RDS, n = 21) or with RDS (yes-RDS, n = 31), respectively, as a function of postnatal age. *P < .05 vs no-RDS; #P < .05 vs. 0-12 hr and 168 hr yes-RDS; &P < .05 vs. 168 hr no-RDS. (From van Bel F, Latour V, Vreman HJ, et al. Is carbon monoxide-mediated cyclic guanosine monophosphate production responsible for low blood pressure in neonatal respiratory distress syndrome? J Appl Physiol. 2005;98:1044-1049. Used with permission from the American Physiological Society.)

pressure and gestational age over a broad range of maturity at birth. This difference persists through the first postnatal week, as relatively parallel increases in blood pressure are observed in all gestational age groups. Blood pressure continues to increase in preterm and term infants during the first four postnatal months, and when systolic and diastolic blood pressure are plotted against weight, the slopes for VLBW neonates are greater than those observed in low birth weight neonates or those with normal birth weight.[79]

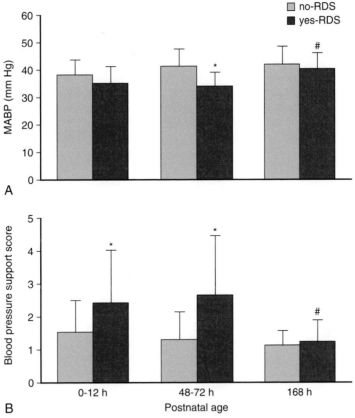

Figure 3-7 Mean arterial blood pressure values (MABP; mmHg) **(A)** and blood pressure support score **(B)** [means (SD)] of no-RDS infants (n = 21) or yes-RDS infants (n = 31), respectively, as a function of postnatal age. *P .05 vs. no-RDS; #P < 0.05 vs 0–12 h (only B) and 48 = 72 hr (A and B) yes-RDS. (From van Bel F, Latour V, Vreman HJ, et al. Is carbon monoxide-mediated cyclic guanosine monophosphate production responsible for low blood pressure in neonatal respiratory distress syndrome? J Appl Physiol. 2005;98:1044-1049. Used with permission from the American Physiological Society.)

Adjuncts to Blood Pressure Measurement in the Diagnosis of Compromised Circulatory Function

Perkin and Levin have described three stages of shock, and it is important to remember that in the initial or compensated stage there may be no or minimal derangement in blood pressure.[80,81] Indirect evidence of changes in nonvital organ perfusion during the compensated phase of shock include oliguria, prolonged capillary refill (greater than 3 s), excessive temperature gradient between surface and core, tachypnea, tachycardia, and pallor.[82] In the uncompensated phase, blood pressure and vital (brain, heart, and adrenal glands) organ perfusion also decrease. Clinical observations of the indirect signs of organ perfusion are important, but can be misleading when used in isolation, especially during the immediate postnatal transition of the VLBW neonate. These signs are most helpful when used together and in conjunction with continuous or frequent blood pressure determinations. Dempsey and colleagues recently reported their experience using such a combination (capillary refill, skin color, heart rate, urine output, level of activity and biochemical findings, in particular the degree of acidosis) and found that withholding therapy in infants whose BP was <gestational age (GA), but whose perfusion indices were reassuring, was associated with an outcome that was as good as that observed in normotensive infants.[83] Wardle et al. studied peripheral tissue oxygenation using near-infrared spectroscopy (NIRS), and oxygen delivery, oxygen consumption, and fractional

oxygen extraction were determined.[84] Although hypotension was associated with lower oxygen delivery and consumption, fractional oxygen extraction and blood lactate concentration were similar to those observed in normotensive infants.

Urine Output

The presence of normal urine output is considered to be an indicator of adequate circulatory function, and might suggest that a blood pressure that appears to be marginal is, in fact, physiologic for that neonate. Conversely, decreased urine output is often cited as evidence that there is circulatory inadequacy and that blood pressure may be too low. These assessments assume, of course, that fluid administration is sufficient, intrinsic renal function is normal, and the impact of the normally high levels of vasopressin and catecholamines on renal function immediately after delivery have been taken into consideration. In addition, there are pathologic situations in which concern regarding hypotension is high, for example, neonates with a hypoxic-ischemic insult, but in whom the kidneys often have sustained significant damage.[85] In this case, the ability to assess urine output as an indicator of cardiovascular function is lost.

As referred to earlier, the other significant problem with quantification of urine output in the clinical decision-making process regarding possible hypotension is that low urine output is physiologic in the first day or so following birth. Accordingly, in some normal term and mostly late preterm infants, the first void may not occur until 24 h after delivery.[86] Unfortunately, this period coincides with a time of great concern, particularly in preterm neonates, for hypotension and possible organ hypoperfusion, particularly of the central nervous system.[4]

Despite these concerns, low urine output (assuming accurate assessment and/or collection) may be an important clinical indicator of circulatory compromise, particularly if there has been previous normal and stable output. If intake has not changed, and the environment is the same (e.g., the patient has not been moved from an incubator to a radiant warmer), then a significant decrease in urine output probably indicates a circulatory problem that needs to be addressed. It is important to remember that at this stage (compensated shock), the blood pressure may be normal because of distribution of organ blood flow to the vital organs, with decreased blood flow to the kidneys as well as other nonvital vascular beds.[80] Conversely, the presence of normal urine output is evidence in favor of adequate circulation.

Metabolic Acidosis

Metabolic acidosis often is considered in a somewhat similar light as oliguria; that is, in its absence there is a tendency to assume that the circulatory status is normal. With inadequate tissue perfusion, tissue hypoxia ensues, and lactic acid is produced. Although sometimes subtle, most clinicians regard development of metabolic acidosis (in a patient whose pulmonary gas exchange is adequate) as an ominous finding that supports the presence of circulatory inadequacy.

Occasionally, peripheral perfusion is so poor that lactate is formed but not "mobilized" to the general circulation and the site of blood gas determination. When this is the case, the clinician often has findings other than metabolic acidosis (e.g., very low blood pressure) to help with the diagnosis of circulatory insufficiency.

Finally, the clinician must differentiate anion-gap (lactic) acidosis from non-anion-gap (bicarbonate wasting) acidosis in the neonate. This is of particular importance in the VLBW patient population where renal bicarbonate wasting due to renal tubular immaturity is the rule rather than the exception. Therefore only following the changes in base deficit may not be sufficient for the indirect assessment of the hemodynamic status, and measurement of serum lactate levels may be indicated when the status of tissue perfusion is unclear.[87]

Hyperkalemia

Kluckow and Evans examined the relationship between low systemic blood flow (as estimated by SVC blood flow) and early changes in serum potassium in preterm neonates.[88] The mean minimum blood flow was significantly lower in those neonates who became hyperkalemic versus those with normokalemia, and a rate of rise of serum potassium greater than 0.12 mmol/L/hr in the first 12 h predicted a low flow state with 93% accuracy. This interesting observation deserves further study, but it may provide the clinician with another tool for overall assessment of cardiovascular stability. However, the complexity of the regulation of the distribution of total body potassium between the intra- and extracellular compartments (primarily determined by the functional maturity and activity of the sodium-potassium ATPase) and that of the function of the immature kidneys warrants cautiousness when using the changes in serum potassium levels as supporting or refuting evidence of poor systemic perfusion in the neonate, especially during the period of immediate postnatal adaptation.

Heart Rate

The association of tachycardia with shock is a classic observation frequently made in combat situations and in civilians with severe trauma and blood loss. For the neonate, an increase in heart rate is the most effective way to increase cardiac output, since the ability to increase stroke volume is somewhat limited. Thus one might assume that tachycardia is a reliable sign of hypotension and circulatory inadequacy; however it is important to note that most hypotensive neonates are not hypovolemic, particularly in the early postnatal period.[89]

Problems with the use of heart rate to indicate hypotension are many, however. Firstly, there is a wide range of normal for heart rate.[90] Secondly, there are many factors other than hypotension that cause a neonate to be tachycardic, such as hunger, pain, agitation, elevated body temperature, excessive noise levels, and pharmacologic agents. Heart rate was lower in lambs whose mothers received betamethasone.[91] Thirdly, a neonate with hypotension also may be hypoxic, and the typical response of the fetus and, to a certain extent, of the neonate (unlike the older child or adult) to hypoxia is a vagally mediated decrease in the heart rate. Also, if myocardial damage has occurred and is responsible for the observed hypotension, the heart may not be able to maintain a sustained increase in rate. In a recent study of preterm neonates, systemic blood flow and heart rate were not significantly correlated.[45]

Despite these issues, assessment of heart rate may be useful and should be considered in the neonate with suspected hypotension. A clear increase from a previously stable baseline, in the absence of others factors causing tachycardia, should suggest that a measured blood pressure that seems to be marginal may truly represent significant circulatory compromise.

Capillary Refill Time and Central-Peripheral Temperature Difference

Capillary refill time (CRT) has been studied extensively in neonates, children, and adults, and is an assessment that tends to provoke strong emotions among those who either do or do not consider it useful clinically.[24] The CRT is determined by blanching an area of skin and measuring the elapsed time until baseline color returns. The test was described originally by Beecher and colleagues in 1947, was part of the Trauma Score, and is used as a tool in life support programs, including Pediatric Advanced Life Support.[24,92] Numerous studies of CRT have determined that age, ambient and skin temperature, anatomic site of measurement, and duration of pressure influence the value obtained.[93,94]

Wodey and colleagues studied 100 neonates who required intensive care and found no correlation between CRT and shortening fraction, left atrial diameter/aortic diameter ratio, blood pressure, or heart rate.[95] However, a significant correlation between CRT and cardiac index was observed. LeFlore and Engle studied healthy term newborns at 1-4 hours after delivery.[96] Brief (1-2 sec) and extended (3-4 sec) pressure was applied at various anatomic sites. Although an inverse relationship between CRT and blood pressure would be expected, this was not observed. In several instances, a highly significant direct relationship was observed, suggesting

Table 3-3   RELATIONSHIP BETWEEN CPTD AND CRT AND OTHER PARAMETERS AT 3 AND 10 H POSTNATAL AGE

CPTd or CRT	Sn	Sp	PPV	NPV	LR+	LR–
CPTd ≥ 2°C						
3 hr	29 (15-42)	78 (65-90)	20 (8-32)	85 (74-96)	1.29	0.92
10 hr	41 (27-55)	66 (52-79)	41 (27-55)	66 (52-79)	1.19	0.90
All observations	40 (32-48)	69 (61-77)	23 (16-30)	83 (77-90)	1.30	0.87
CRT ≥ 3 sec						
3 hr	54 (45-63)	79 (72-86)	23 (16-31)	93 (89-98)	2.55	0.58
10 hr	59 (50-68)	75 (67-82)	51 (42-60)	80 (73-87)	2.33	0.55
All observations	55 (50-60)	80 (76-84)	33 (29-38)	91 (88-94)	2.78	0.56
CRT ≥ 4 sec						
3 hr	38 (30-47)	93 (88-97)	38 (30-47)	93 (88-97)	5.24	0.66
10 hr	26 (18-33)	97 (93-100)	77 (70-84)	74 (67-82)	7.44	0.77
All observations	29 (24-33)	96 (94-98)	55 (50-60)	88 (85-91)	6.84	0.75

Values in parentheses are 95% confidence intervals: LR+, positive likelihood ratio; LR–, negative likelihood ratio; NPV, negative predictive value; PPV, positive predictive value; Sn, sensitivity; Sp, specificity.
Data from: Osborn DA, Evans N, Kluckow M. Clinical detection of low upper body blood flow in very premature infants using blood pressure, capillary refill time, and central-peripheral temperature difference. Arch Dis Child Fetal Neonatal Ed 2004;89:F168-F173. Used with permission from BMJ Publishing Group.

that vasoactive substances present in the early post-delivery period caused increased vascular resistance, increased blood pressure, and prolonged CRT.

Osborn and colleagues studied the ability of CRT, central-peripheral temperature difference (CPTd) ≥ 2°C and blood pressure to detect low SVC flow in neonates less than 30 weeks' gestation. Results for CPTd and CRT are listed in Table 3-3.[97] Sensitivity improved to 78% when mean blood pressure less than 30 mm Hg and central CRT ≥ 3 sec were used in combination. Tibby and colleagues found that neither CRT nor CPTd correlated well with any hemodynamic variables in postcardiac surgery children.[98]

Measurement of CRT has become a routine part of physical examination. Its use should be accompanied by an appreciation of its limitations. The use of CPTd, a test not performed as frequently as CRT, has similar limitations.

Clinical Factors that May Affect Blood Pressure

As discussed earlier, it appears that birth weight, gestational age, and postnatal age are significant determinants of blood pressure in the VLBW neonate. Additional demographic and clinical variables that may influence blood pressure in this high-risk population are reviewed later. Clinical situations associated with severe alterations in blood pressure, such as blood loss, asphyxia, and sepsis, are discussed elsewhere in this book.

Maternal Age and Blood Pressure

In a large study (Project Viva, Harvard Vanguard Medical Associates), Gillman and colleagues observed a direct relationship between maternal age and newborn systolic blood pressure.[99] In 96% of neonates, blood pressure was measured before 72 hours of postnatal age. In a mixed linear regression model, systolic blood pressure in newborns (mean gestational age 39.7 weeks) increased by 0.8 mm Hg for each increase of 5 years in maternal age, even after controlling for potentially confounding factors. Maternal blood pressure was also a strong independent predictor of newborn blood pressure. For every 10 mm Hg rise in third trimester maternal systolic blood pressure, newborn systolic blood pressure increased by 0.9 mm Hg.[99]

Route of Delivery

Faxelius and colleagues compared sympathoadrenal activity and peripheral blood flow in term infants delivered vaginally and by cesarean section.[100] Peripheral vascular resistance was higher both at birth and at 2 hours' postnatal in the vaginally delivered infants, corresponding to higher catecholamine concentrations. However, in this relatively small study (n = 24) mean blood pressures were similar between the groups. More recently, Agata and colleagues reported significantly higher catecholamine concentrations in vaginally delivered infants versus those delivered by cesarean section; left ventricular output and its regional distribution showed a similar pattern in the two groups.[101] Pohjavuori and Fyhrquist found an association between cord blood arginine vasopressin (AVP) and adrenocorticotropic hormone (ACTH) levels, route of delivery, and blood pressures.[102] Vaginally delivered infants had the highest blood pressures and AVP and ACTH levels, followed by those delivered by cesarean section with labor and then those delivered by elective cesarean section. These studies were performed in term neonates; in VLBW infants blood pressures were similar in infants delivered vaginally versus those delivered by cesarean section.[61,100-102] Likewise in the study by Zubrow and colleagues, stepwise multiple linear regression analysis did not identify route of delivery as a significant determinant of blood pressure variation in preterm neonates.[60] Breech delivery has been associated with blood pressure in the lower range of normal.[103]

Time of Umbilical Cord Clamping

Interest in delayed cord clamping has been primarily due to the possibility of reduced need for transfusion in preterm neonates. Mercer and colleagues reported that initial mean blood pressure was higher in neonates with delayed cord clamping (approximately 30-45 seconds versus 5-10 seconds in the immediate clamping group), and infants in the delayed cord clamping group were three to four times more likely to have mean BP > 30 mm Hg.[104] More recently, Baenzigar and colleagues reported significantly higher MBP at 4 hours but not at 24 or 72 hours in infants with cord clamping delayed 60-90 seconds.[105] Hosono and colleagues found that umbilical cord milking resulted in higher blood pressure in the first 12 hours postnatal and a reduced need for blood pressure support during the first 120 hours.[106]

Patent Ductus Arteriosus

Cardiovascular effects of patent ductus arteriosus (PDA) in preterm lambs were studied by Clyman and colleagues in a model in which ductal size could be regulated. Highly significant decreases in diastolic blood pressure were observed with any size left-to-right ductal shunt, while systolic blood pressure did not change with a small shunt and changed only slightly with either moderate or large shunt.[107]

Ratner and colleagues studied 34 preterm infants of whom 17 developed clinically significant PDA.[108] These investigators noted that diastolic blood pressure less than 28 mm Hg was suggestive of the presence of PDA. While diastolic blood pressure was significantly decreased in the PDA group from the first postnatal day, of note, systolic blood pressure was lower after the second day only. Following ligation of the PDA, blood pressures were similar to those in the non-PDA group.

Evans and Moorcraft found similar blood pressures with or without PDA in infants with birth weight 1000 to 1500 g.[109] However, in those with birth weight less than 1000 g, mean, systolic, and diastolic blood pressures were lower in infants with PDA versus those without PDA. Furthermore, these hemodynamic effects could be demonstrated well before the PDA became clinically apparent. These authors cautioned against the use of volume expanders and/or inotropic agents in this population, since these treatments might be counterproductive if the etiology of the hypotension were a hemodynamically significant but clinically silent PDA.

Furthermore, volume expansion appears to be a risk factor for development of a symptomatic PDA in VLBW neonates.[110,111] It is apparent that problems with low blood pressure related to PDA, especially diastolic blood pressure, may result in inadequate perfusion of many organs secondary to the "vascular steal" phenomenon.[112] Although there was considerable variability in their results, Freeman-Ladd and colleagues reported a significant negative correlation ($r = -.48$, $P<.002$) between superior mesenteric pulsatility index (PI) and the ratio of the PI of the left pulmonary artery and the PI of the descending aorta.[113] Management of this clinical problem is, of course, best directed at closure of the PDA rather than at increasing the blood pressure by other means. Of note, significant elevation of systemic blood pressure associated with clinical deterioration has been observed following PDA ligation.[114,115] This may be secondary to increased afterload, and there is limited evidence that milrinone may be beneficial in this situation.[116]

Apnea

Circulatory changes resulting from apnea in the neonate have been summarized by Miller and Martin.[117] The initial decrease in heart rate is accompanied by a rise in pulse pressure, usually secondary to an increase in systolic pressure, occasionally accompanied by a fall in diastolic pressure.[118] These events presumably are secondary to increased filling volume associated with bradycardia, which leads to enhanced stroke volume in accordance with Starling's law. As the severity of apnea and bradycardia increases, blood pressure may decrease, along with a fall in cerebral blood flow velocity.[119] Thus during prolonged apnea, cerebral perfusion may decrease significantly, placing the infant at risk for brain injury.

Respiratory Support

Infants with severe respiratory distress syndrome (RDS) may have lower blood pressure than that observed in premature neonates without RDS or in infants with less severe RDS.[76,120,121] An association in infants with RDS between marked fluctuations in arterial blood pressure and fluctuating cerebral blood-flow velocity has been demonstrated; the association between this pattern and intraventricular hemorrhage (IVH) may be mediated as much by alterations on the venous side of the cerebral circulation as by alterations on the arterial side.[122,123] In a study in which a lower coefficient of variation of systolic blood pressure was observed, blood pressure fluctuation actually was lower in infants who developed IVH.[124] Also, an association between acute hypocarbia and marked systemic hypotension has been reported.[125] This association places infants at very high risk for central nervous system injury (see Chapters 2 and 16).

Three aspects of respiratory management in preterm neonates might be expected to most likely have an effect on blood pressure: (1) use of increased airway pressures, given either by constant positive airway pressure (CPAP) or conventional or high frequency ventilation, (2) suctioning of the airway, and (3) instillation of an exogenous surfactant preparation into the airway. Holzman and Scarpelli reported no effect of positive end-expiratory pressure (PEEP) on mean arterial pressure in normal dogs.[126] More recently, de Waal and colleagues studied the effects of changes in PEEP from 5 to 8 cm H_2O.[127] Systolic and diastolic blood pressures were unchanged, but there was a significant decrease in right ventricular output. In neonates, Yu and Rolfe observed no change in mean arterial pressure with or without CPAP.[128] In some studies in which systemic blood pressure did not fall despite high airway pressures, it was shown that an increase in systemic vascular resistance occurred.[129,130] Kluckow and Evans and Evans and Kluckow observed a highly significant negative influence of mean airway pressure on mean blood pressure in preterm neonates requiring mechanical ventilation.[46,131] Similarly, Skinner and colleagues reported a negative correlation between systemic blood pressure and mean airway pressure in 33 preterm neonates with RDS.[132] Decreases in blood pressure fluctuations during mechanical ventilation may be achieved through use of various methods of synchronized mechanical ventilation as shown by Hummler and colleagues.[133]

Perlman and Volpe studied 35 intubated preterm neonates undergoing routine suctioning.[134] Mean blood pressure increased during suctioning in all but one patient, and these investigators concluded that the observed increases in cerebral blood flow velocity and intracranial pressure were directly related to the increased blood pressure. Perry and colleagues reported that blood pressure elevations were temporally related to suctioning and other procedures, and they associated systolic blood pressure above a "stability boundary" with increased risk for PIVH.[135] Omar and colleagues studied blood pressure responses to care procedures (suctioning, chest auscultation and physiotherapy, mouth rinsing, diaper changing, and nasogastric feeding) in 22 ventilated, preterm infants.[136] In general, blood pressure responses were biphasic, with a decrease in blood pressure followed by a greater and longer-lasting increase. Kalyn and colleagues found that use of a closed suction technique (infant not disconnected from ventilator) was associated with enhanced physiologic stability, and that elevations in systolic blood pressure were greater with open suctioning.[137]

Numerous investigators have studied physiologic effects of surfactant instillation in neonates, and differences in these reports may be secondary to dosing, technique of administration, adjustments in ventilator settings to avoid significant changes in PCO_2 levels, or other factors.[7,24] In most studies, any effects on blood pressure were transient. There may be greater hemodynamic effects associated with natural surfactant preparations, perhaps related to their generally more rapid pulmonary effects and greater ability to release local vasoactive mediators when compared with artificial surfactant preparations.

Antenatal Steroids

Infusion of cortisol into the sheep fetus results in increased arterial pressure and decreased blood volume.[138] Stein and colleagues observed that neonatal sheep that received hydrocortisone prenatally had increased cardiovascular function despite a marked attenuation in the anticipated surge of plasma catecholamine concentrations and a decrease in epinephrine secretion rate.[139] In addition, adenylyl cyclase activity in the myocardial tissue was increased.[139]

Several reports have suggested that neonatal blood pressure is higher in preterm infants whose mothers received antenatal steroids to hasten fetal lung maturity.[140,141] This finding would not be unexpected, since previous studies have suggested that sick preterm neonates may have relative adrenocorticosteroid insufficiency, and successful treatment with hydrocortisone or dexamethasone of hypotension refractory to conventional therapies has been documented.[24,142]

Kari and colleagues performed a randomized, controlled trial to study whether prenatal dexamethasone improves the outcome of preterm neonates who receive exogenous surfactant.[140] While neonates whose mothers received dexamethasone tended to have higher mean arterial blood pressure during the first three postnatal days, this relationship was less clear when adjustment for birth weight was made, in which case a significant difference in blood pressure was noted only 2 hours following the initial dose of surfactant. Subsequently, Moise and colleagues studied the amount of blood pressure support received by extremely preterm infants (23-27 weeks' gestation) whose mothers did or did not receive antenatal steroids.[141] Infants not exposed to antenatal steroids had lower mean blood pressures from 16 to 48 h postnatally. Furthermore, the use of dopamine was increased in the infants not exposed to antenatal steroids. Garland and colleagues linked the reduction in severe IVH observed in infants whose mothers received antenatal steroids to normal blood pressures in those infants.[143] Demarini and colleagues reported that mean blood pressures during the first 24 hours postnatal were increased in VLBW infants whose mothers received antenatal steroids, and that volume expansion and vasopressor support were decreased in those infants.[144] Mildenhall and colleagues found that exposure to multiple courses of antenatal glucocorticoids was associated with increased blood pressure and myocardial thickness after birth.[145] In a subsequent randomized trial of single versus repeat antenatal steroid courses, the same investigators found similar blood pressure and myocardial wall thickness between the two

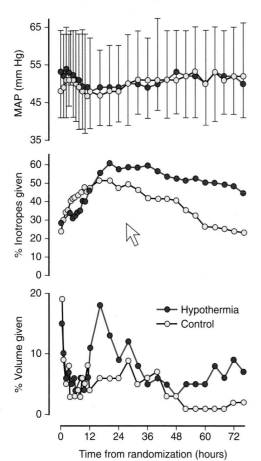

Figure 3-8 Time sequence of changes in mean arterial blood pressure (MAP) (**A**, mm Hg) and the percentage of infants receiving either inotropes (**B**, % inotropes given) or volume for cardiovascular support (**C**, % volume given). MAP data are median (10th, 90th percentile). (From Battin MR, Thoresen M, Robinson E, et al. Does head cooling with mild systemic hypothermia affect requirement for blood pressure support? Pediatr. 2009;123:1031-1036. Used with permission from the American Academy of Pediatrics.)

groups.[146] The aforementioned findings in human neonates have been supported by studies in animals.[24,91]

Conversely, LeFlore and colleagues reported no differences in blood pressures in 116 VLBW neonates whose mothers did or did not receive antenatal steroids.[61] Similar results were obtained by Omar and colleagues and Cordero and colleagues.[59,147] Mantaring and Ostrea reported a tendency for higher mean blood pressure in infants of ≥ 1000 g whose mothers received antenatal steroids but a tendency for lower mean blood pressure in infants <1000 g who were exposed to antenatal steroids.[148] Leviton and colleagues found no difference in the incidence of lowest mean blood pressure less than 30 mm Hg in infants whose mothers did or did not receive a complete course of antenatal glucocorticoid prophylaxis.[149] Recently, Dalziel and colleagues reported that blood pressure at 6 years of age did not differ between children exposed prenatally to betamethasone and those not exposed.[150]

Therapeutic Hypothermia

The use of head or systemic cooling in infants with hypoxic-ischemic encephalopathy has become a common practice. Battin and colleagues recently reported an analysis of cardiovascular data from the Cool Cap Trial.[151] Despite similar mean arterial blood pressures in cooled and control neonates, cardiovascular support was significantly greater in the cooled neonates from 24 to 76 hours (Fig. 3-8). The investigators suggested that this might reflect changes in physician behavior, with more cautious withdrawal of therapy for hypotension in the intervention group versus the controls. However, a decreased cardiovascular responsiveness to catechol-amines at lower body temperatures might have played a role as well.

Other Indicators of Changes in Circulatory Function

Maternal smoking may be associated with increased diastolic blood pressure in the neonate.[152] Beratis and colleagues reported that both systolic and diastolic blood pressure were increased in infants of mothers who smoked, that there was a direct relationship between neonatal blood pressure and the number of cigarettes smoked, and that the effect could persist for at least 12 months.[153] Although maternal hyper-tension may be a factor associated with higher neonatal blood pressure, this is not consistently reported.[24,57,58,61,99,148] In discordant twins, blood pressure is higher in the larger versus the smaller twin; with twin-twin transfusion, blood pressure decreases over the first 24 hours postnatal in the recipient twin.[154] Cocaine exposure in utero has been shown to be associated with increased blood pressure on the first day of life in term neonates, and increased circulating catecholamine concentrations have been demonstrated.[24] The use of antenatal magnesium sulfate therapy intended to decrease the incidence of brain damage in preterm neonates has increased, and Shokry and colleagues described decreased cerebral blood flow with decreases in peak systolic velocity, end-diastolic velocity and mean velocity in cerebral arteries in neonates exposed to antenatal magnesium sulfate.[155]

Mean arterial pressure was unchanged, but arterial pressure variability was decreased with both pancuronium and pethidine (meperidine) while fentanyl and midazolam may cause hypotension in neonates.[156] There is recent concern that use of the induction agent propofol in neonates may be associated with significant hypotension.[157] Sammartino and colleagues recently reported a case of propofol overdose associated with propofol infusion syndrome (PRIS).[158] PRIS often is fatal, and the clinical picture includes metabolic acidosis, bradycardia, lipemic plasma, rhabdomyolysis, and renal failure. The infant described was born at 24 weeks, and moderate hypotension was part of the initial clinical presentation. Simons and col-leagues concluded that blood pressure, blood pressure variability and use of inotro-pes were not influenced by morphine infusion.[159] Others have found decreased blood pressure with the use of diamorphine or morphine, and similar findings were observed in the NEOPAIN trial.[160-162] A secondary analysis of the NEOPAIN data, while confirming the association with hypotension, found that preemptive morphine analgesia was not significant in regression models tested for the outcomes of severe IVH, any IVH or death.[163]

Noise exposure, a major concern in a busy NICU, was associated with elevated BP as well as increased heart rate.[164] Numerous studies have demonstrated that blood pressure may increase as well as decrease with pneumothorax.[123,165] Seizure activity may have variable effects on blood pressure.[123] Increased neonatal blood pressure has been documented in infants with chronic lung disease who receive dexametha-sone therapy and in infants whose formula is diluted with water that has an elevated sodium concentration.[24,166] Finally, a condition referred to as late-onset circulatory dysfunction (LCD) has been reported frequently in Japan.[167] LCD occurs in preterm neonates who were previously stable and is characterized by sudden hypotension and oliguria; it is associated with development of periventricular leukomalacia.

Conclusion

Recent studies have broadened our knowledge of the complex processes controlling fetal and neonatal blood pressure. Clinical studies in VLBW neonates have provided normative data for blood pressure, especially in the first few postnatal days, and have demonstrated that many of the more immature preterm infants have mean blood pressures in the 20-25 mm Hg range especially during the first postnatal day. On the other hand, as noted earlier, having a blood pressure in the "normal range" does not necessarily guarantee that it is safe. Adjunctive assessments such as urine output and CRT may be helpful, particularly when considered together, but the clinician at the bedside often faces a difficult dilemma in weighing the risks and benefits of therapy for presumed low blood pressure. Further outcome-based studies are needed to address the issue of confirmation of acceptable cardiovascular status in preterm and term neonates adjusted for gestational and postnatal age.

References

1. Lou HC, Skv H, Psych C, et al. Low cerebral blood flow: a risk factor in the neonate. J Pediatr. 1979;95:606-609.
2. Kopelman AE. Blood pressure and cerebral ischemia in very low birth weight infants. J Pediatr. 1990;116:1000-1002.
3. Guyton AC, Hall JE. Textbook of medical physiology, 9th ed. Philadelphia: WB Saunders; 1996.
4. Kluckow M. Low systemic blood flow and pathophysiology of the preterm transitional circulation. Early Hum Dev. 2005;81:429-437.
5. Soleymani S, Borzage M, Seri I. Hemodynamic monitoring in neonates. Advances and challenges. J Perinatol. 2010;30:S38-S45.
6. Emery EF, Greenough A. Assessment of non-invasive techniques for measuring blood pressure in preterm infants of birthweight less than or equal to 750 grams. Early Hum Dev. 1993;33: 217-222.
7. Nuntnarumit P, Yang W, Bada-Ellzey HS. Blood pressure measurements in the newborn. Clin Perinatol. 1999;26:981-996.
8. Darnall RA. Blood-pressure monitoring. In: Brans Y, Hay WJ, eds. Physiological monitoring and instrument diagnosis in perinatal and neonatal medicine. Cambridge: University Press; 1995:246-266.
9. O'Rourke MF. What is blood pressure? Am J Hypertens. 1990;3:803-810.
10. Gardner RM. Direct blood pressure measurement—dynamic response requirements. Anesthesiology. 1981;54:227-236.
11. Park MK, Robotham JL, German VF. Systolic pressure amplification in pedal arteries in children. Crit Care Med. 1983;211:286-289.
12. Lotze A, Rivera O, Walton DM. Blood pressure monitoring. In: MacDonald MG, Ramasethu J, eds. Atlas of procedures in neonatology, 3rd ed. Philadelphia: Lippincott Williams and Wilkins; 2002: 51-59.
13. Weindling AM. Blood pressure monitoring in the newborn. Arch Dis Child. 1989;64:444-447.
14. Cunningham S, Symon AG, McIntosh N. Changes in mean blood pressure caused by damping of the arterial pressure waveform. Early Hum Devel. 1994;36:36:27-30.
15. Butt WW, Whyte H. Blood pressure monitoring in neonates: comparison of umbilical and peripheral artery catheter measurements. J Pediatr. 1984;105:630-632.
16. Darnall RA. Noninvasive blood pressure measurement in the neonate. Clin Perinatol. 1985;12: 31-49.
17. Stebor AD. Basic principles of noninvasive blood pressure measurement in infants. Adv Neonatal Care. 2005;5:252-261.
18. Association for the Advancement of Medical Instrumentation. American National Standard. Manual, Electronic, or Automated Sphygmomanometers, ANSI/AAMI SP10. Arlington, VA: ANSI; 2002.
19. Nelson RM, Stebor AD, Groh CM, et al. Determination of accuracy in neonates for non-invasive blood pressure device using an improved algorithm. Blood Press Monit. 2002;7:123-129.
20. Nwankwo MU, Lorenz JM, Gardiner JC. A standard protocol for blood pressure measurement in the newborn, Pediatrics. 1997;99:E10.
21. Andriessen P, van den Bosch-Ruis W, Jan Ten Harkel D, et al. Feasibility of noninvasive continuous finger arterial blood pressure measurements in very young children, aged 0-4 years. Pediatr Res. 2008;63:691-696.
22. Langbaum M, Eyal FG. A practical and reliable method of measuring blood pressure in the neonate by pulse oximetry. J Pediatrics. 1994;125:591-595.
23. Ramsey M. Noninvasive automatic determination of mean arterial pressure. Med Biol Eng Comput. 1979;17:11-18.
24. Engle WD. Definition of normal blood pressure range. The elusive target. In: Kleinman CS, Seri I, Polin RA, eds. Hemodynamics and cardiology. Neonatology questions and controversies. Philadelphia: Saunders Elsevier; 2008:39-65.
25. Pellegrini-Caliumi G, Agostino R, Nodari S, et al. Evaluation of an automatic oscillometric method and of various cuffs for the measurement of arterial pressure in the neonate. Acta Paediatr Scand. 1982;71:791-797.
26. Sonesson S-E, Broberger U. Arterial blood pressure in the very low birthweight neonate. Acta Paediatr Scand. 1976;87:338-341.
27. Kimble KJ, Darnall RA, Yelderman M, et al. An automated oscillometric technique for estimating mean arterial pressure in critically ill newborns. Anesthesiology. 1981;54:423-425.
28. Diprose GK, Evans DH, Archer LNJ, et al. Dinamap fails to detect hypotension in very low birthweight infants. Arch Dis Child. 1986;61:771-773.
29. Fanaroff AA, Wright E. Profiles of mean arterial blood pressure (MAP) for infants weighing 501-1500 grams. Pediatr Res. 1990;27:205A.
30. Chia F, Ang AT, Wong TW, et al. Reliability of the Dinamap non-invasive monitor in the measurement of blood pressure of ill Asian newborns. Clin Pediatr (Philadelphia). 1990;29:262-267.
31. Wareham JA, Haugh LD, Yeager SB, et al. Prediction of arterial blood pressure in the premature neonate using the oscillometric method. Am J Dis Child. 1987;141:1108-1110.

32. Park MK, Lee DH. Normative arm and calf blood pressure values in the newborn. Pediatrics. 1989;83:240-243.
33. Piazza SF, Chandra M, Harper RG, et al. Upper- vs lower-limb systolic blood pressure in full-term normal newborns. Am J Dis Child. 1985;139:797-799.
34. Cowan F, Thoresen M, Walloe L. Arm and leg blood pressures—are they really so different in newborns? Early Hum Dev. 1991;26:203-211.
35. Kunk R, McCain GC. Comparison of upper arm and calf oscillometric blood pressure measurement in preterm infants. J Perinatol. 1996;16:89-92.
36. Papadopoulos G, Mieke S, Elisaf M. Assessment of the performances of three oscillometric blood pressure monitors for neonates using a simulator. Blood Press Monit. 1999;4:27-33.
37. Pichler G, Urlesberger B, Reiterer F, et al. Non-invasive oscillometric blood pressure measurement in very-low-birthweight infants. a comparison of two different monitor systems. Acta Paediatr. 1999;88:1044-1045.
38. Dannevig I, Dale HC, Liestol K, et al. Blood pressure in the neonate. three non-invasive oscillometric pressure monitors compared with invasively measured blood pressure. Acta Paediatr. 2005;94:191-196.
39. Engle WD. Blood pressure in the very low birth weight neonate. Early Hum Dev. 2001;62:97-130.
40. Dempsey EM, Barrington KJ. Treating hypotension in the preterm infant: when and with what. a critical and systematic review. J Perinatol. 2007;27:469-478.
41. Laughon M, Bose C, Allred E, et al. Factors associated with treatment for hypotension in extremely low gestational age newborns during the first postnatal week. Pediatrics. 2007;119:273-280.
42. Short BL, van Meurs K, Evans JR, et al. Summary proceedings from the cardiology group on cardiovascular instability in preterm infants. Pediatrics. 2006;117:S34-S39.
43. Strambi M, Vezzosi P, Buoni S, et al. Blood pressure in the small-for-gestational age newborn. Minerva Pediatr. 2004;56:603-610.
44. Seri I, Evans J. Controversies in the diagnosis and management of hypotension in the newborn infant. Curr Opin Pediatr. 2001;13:116-123.
45. Kluckow M, Evans N. Low superior vena cava flow and intraventricular haemorrhage in preterm infants. Arch Dis Child Fetal Neonatal Ed. 2000;82:F188-F194.
46. Kluckow M, Evans N. Relationship between blood pressure and cardiac output in preterm infants requiring mechanical ventilation. J Pediatr. 1996;129:506-512.
47. Munro MJ, Walker AM, Barfield CP. Hypotensive extremely low birth weight infants have reduced cerebral blood flow. Pediatrics. 2004;114:1591-1596.
48. Kitterman JA, Phibbs RH, Tooley WH. Aortic blood pressure in normal newborn infants during the first 12 hours of life. Pediatrics. 1969;44:959-968.
49. Versmold HT, Kitterman JA, Phibs RH, et al. Aortic blood pressure during the first 12 hours of life in infants with birth weight 610 to 4,220 grams. Pediatrics. 1981;67:607-613.
50. Miall-Allen VM, de Vries LS, Whitelaw AGL. Mean arterial blood pressure and neonatal cerebral lesions. Arch Dis Child. 1987;62:1068-1069.
51. Watkins AMC, West CR, Cooke RWI. Blood pressure and cerebral haemorrhage and ischaemia in very low birthweight infants. Early Hum Develop. 1989;19:103-110.
52. Kehrer M, Blumenstock G, Ehehalt S, et al. Development of cerebral blood flow volume in preterm neonates during the first two weeks of life. Pediatr Res. 2005;58:927-930.
53. Lee J, Rajadurai VS, Tan KW. Blood pressure standards for very low birthweight infants during the first day of life. Arch Dis Child Fetal Neonatal Ed. 1999;81:F168-F170.
54. Adams MA, Pasternak JF, Kupfer BM, et al. A computerized system for continuous physiologic data collection and analysis; initial report on mean arterial blood pressure in very low-birth-weight infants. Pediatrics. 1983;71:23-30.
55. Cunningham S, Deere S, McIntosh N. Cyclical variation of blood pressure and heart rate in neonates. Arch Dis Child. 1993;69:64-67.
56. Cunningham S, Symon AG, Elton RA, et al. Intra-arterial blood pressure reference ranges, death and morbidity in very low birthweight infants during the first seven days of life. Early Hum Dev. 1999;56:151-165.
57. Hegyi T, Carbone MT, Anwar M, et al. Blood pressure ranges in premature infants. I. The first hours of life. J Pediatr. 1994;124:627-633.
58. Hegyi T, Anwar M, Carbone MT, et al. Blood pressure ranges in premature infants. II. The first week of life. Pediatrics. 1996;97:336-342.
59. Cordero L, Timan CJ, Waters HH, et al. Mean arterial pressures during the first 24 hours of life in ≤600-gram birth weight infants. J Perinatol. 2002;22:348-353.
60. Zubrow AB, Hulman S, Kushner H, et al. Determinants of blood pressure in infants admitted to neonatal intensive care units. a prospective multicenter study. J Perinatol. 1995;15:470-479.
61. LeFlore JL, Engle WD, Rosenfeld CR. Determinants of blood pressure in very low birth weight neonates: lack of effect of antenatal steroids. Early Hum Dev. 2000;59:37-50.
62. Batton B, Batton D, Riggs T. Blood pressure during the first 7 days in premature infants born at postmenstrual age 23 to 25 weeks. Am J Perinatol. 2007;24:107-116.
63. Pellicer A, del Carmen Bravo M, Madero R, et al. Early systemic hypotension and vasopressor support in low birth weight infants. Impact on neurodevelopment. Pediatrics. 2009;123:1369-1376.
64. Kent AL, Meskell S, Falk FC, et al. Normative blood pressure data in non-ventilated premature neonates from 28-36 weeks gestation. Pediatr Nephrol. 2009;24:141-146.

65. Report of a Joint Working Group of the British Association of Perinatal Medicine and the Research Unit of the Royal College of Physicians. Development of audit measures and guidelines for good practice in the management of neonatal respiratory distress syndrome. Arch Dis Child. 1992;67:1221-1227.

66. Seri I, Noori S. Diagnosis and treatment of neonatal hypotension outside the transitional period. Early Hum Dev. 2005;81:405-411.

67. Pellicer A, Valverde E, Elorza MD, et al. Cardiovascular support for low birth weight infants and cerebral hemodynamics; a randomized, blinded, clinical trial. Pediatrics. 2005;115:1501-1512.

68. Munro MJ, Walker AM, Barfield CP. Preterm circulatory support is more complex than just blood pressure; in reply. Pediatrics. 2005;115:1115-1116.

69. Weindling AM, Bentham J. Blood pressure in the neonate. Acta Paediatr. 2005;94:138-140.

70. Kissack CM, Garr R, Wardle SP, et al. Cerebral fractional oxygen extraction in very low birth weight infants is high when there is low left ventricular output and hypocarbia but is unaffected by hypotension. Pediatr Res. 2004;55:400-405.

71. Victor S, Marson AG, Appleton RE, et al. Relationship between blood pressure, cerebral electrical activity, cerebral fractional oxygen extraction, and peripheral blood flow in very low birth weight newborn infants. Pediatr Res. 2006;59:314-319.

72. Lightburn MH, Gauss CH, Williams DK, et al. Cerebral blood flow velocities in extremely low birth weight infants with hypotension and infants with normal blood pressure. J Pediatr. 2009;154:824-828.

73. Engle WD, Arant BS, Wiriyathian S, et al. Diuresis and respiratory distress syndrome: physiologic mechanisms and therapeutic implications. J Pediatr. 1983;102:912-917.

74. Joppich R, Hauser I. Urinary prostacyclin and thromboxane A_2 metabolites in preterm and full-term infants in relation to plasma renin activity and blood pressure. Biol Neonate. 1982;42:179-184.

75. Ezaki S, Suzuki K, Kurishima C, et al. Levels of catecholamines, arginine vasopressin and atrial natriuretic peptide in hypotensive extremely low birth weight infants in the first 24 hours after birth. Neonatology. 2009;95:248-253.

76. van Bel F, Latour V, Vreman HJ, et al. Is carbon monoxide-mediated cyclic guanosine monophosphate production responsible for low blood pressure in neonatal respiratory distress syndrome? J Appl Physiol. 2005;98:1044-1049.

77. Chern J, Kamm KE, Rosenfeld CR. Smooth muscle myosin heavy chain isoforms are developmentally regulated in male fetal and neonatal sheep. Pediatr Res. 1995;38:697-703.

78. Arens Y, Chapados RA, Cox BE, et al. Differential development of umbilical and systemic arteries. II. Contractile proteins. Am J Physiol, Regul Integr Comp Physiol. 1998;274:R1815-R1823.

79. Georgieff MK, Mills MM, Gomez-Marin O, et al. Rate of change of blood pressure in premature and full term infants from birth to 4 months. Pediatr Nephrol. 1996;10:152-155.

80. Perkin RM, Levin DL. Shock in the pediatric patient, Part I. J Pediatr. 1982;101:163-169.

81. Noori S, Seri I. Pathophysiology of newborn hypotension outside the transitional period. Early Hum Dev. 2005;81:399-404.

82. Faix RG, Pryce CJE. Shock and hypotension. In: Donn SM, Faix RG, eds. Neonatal emergencies. Mount Kisco, NY: Futura Publishing; 1991:371-385.

83. Dempsey EM, Hazzani FA, Barrington KJ. Permissive hypotension in the extremely low birthweight infant with signs of good perfusion. Arch Dis Child Fetal Neonatal Ed. 2009;94:F241-F244.

84. Wardle SP, Yoxall CW, Weindling AM. Peripheral oxygenation in hypotensive preterm babies. Pediatr Res. 1999;45:343-349.

85. Myers BD, Moran SM. Hemodynamically mediated acute renal failure. N Engl J Med. 1986;314:97-105.

86. Clark DA. Times of first void and first stool in 500 newborns. Pediatrics. 1977;60:457-459.

87. Deshpande SA, Platt MPW. Association between blood lactate and acid-base status and mortality in ventilated babies. Arch Dis Child. 1997;76:F15-F20.

88. Kluckow M, Evans N. Low systemic blood flow and hyperkalemia in preterm infants. J Pediatr. 2001;139:227-232.

89. Seri I. Inotrope, lusitrope, and pressor use in neonates. J Perinatol. 2005;25(Suppl 2):S28-S30.

90. Garson AJ, Smith RJ, Moak J. Tachyarrhythmias. In: Long W, ed. Fetal and neonatal cardiology. Philadelphia: WB Saunders; 1990:511-518.

91. Smith LM, Ervin MG, Wada N, et al. Antenatal glucocorticoids alter postnatal preterm lamb renal and cardiovascular responses to intravascular volume expansion. Pediatr Res. 2000;47:622-627.

92. Beecher HK, Simeone FA, Burnett, et al. The internal state of the severely wounded man on entry to the most forward hospital. Recent Adv Surg. 1947;22:672-681.

93. Gorelick MH, Shaw KN, Baker MD. Effect of ambient temperature on capillary refill in healthy children. Pediatrics. 1993;92:699-702.

94. Schriger DL, Baraff L. Defining normal capillary refill. variation with age, sex, and temperature. Ann Emerg Med. 1988;17:932-935.

95. Wodey E, Pladys P, Betremieux P, et al. Capillary refilling time and hemodynamics in neonates. A Doppler echocardiographic evaluation. Crit Care Med. 1998;26:1437-1440.

96. LeFlore JL, Engle WD. Capillary refill time is an unreliable indicator of cardiovascular status in term neonates. Adv Neonatal Care. 2005;5:147-154.

97. Osborn DA, Evans N, Kluckow M. Clinical detection of low upper body blood flow in very premature infants using blood pressure, capillary refill time, and central-peripheral temperature difference. Arch Dis Child Fetal Neonatal Ed. 2004;89:F168-F173.

98. Tibby SM, Hatherill M, Murdoch IA. Capillary refill and core-peripheral temperature gap as indicators of haemodynamic status in paediatric intensive care patients. Arch Dis Child. 1999;80: 163-166.
99. Gillman MW, Rich-Edwards JW, Rifas-Shiman SL, et al. Maternal age and other predictors of newborn blood pressure. J Pediatr. 2004;144:240-245.
100. Faxelius G, Lagercrantz H, Yao A. Sympathoadrenal activity and peripheral blood flow after birth. Comparison in infants delivered vaginally and by cesarean section. J Pediatr. 1984;105:144-148.
101. Agata Y, Hiraishi S, Misawa H, et al. Hemodynamic adaptations at birth and neonates delivered vaginally and by cesarean section. Biol Neonate. 1995;68:404-411.
102. Pohjavuori M, Fyhrquist F. Vasopressin, ACTH and neonatal haemodynamics. Acta Paediatr Scand Suppl. 1983;305:79-83.
103. Holland WW, Young IM. Neonatal blood pressure in relation to maturity, mode of delivery, and condition at birth. Br Med J. 1956;2:1331-1333.
104. Mercer JS, McGrath MM, Hensman A, et al. Immediate and delayed cord clamping in infants born between 24 and 32 weeks. A pilot randomized controlled trial. J Perinatol. 2003;23:466-472.
105. Baenziger O, Stolkin F, Keel M, et al. The influence of the timing of cord clamping on postnatal cerebral oxygenation in preterm neonates. A randomized, controlled trial. Pediatrics. 2007;119: 455-459.
106. Hosono S, Mugishima H, Fujita H, et al. Blood pressure and urine output during the first 120 h of life in infants born at less than 29 weeks' gestation related to umbilical cord milking. Arch Dis Child Fetal Neonatal Ed. 2009;94:F328-F331.
107. Clyman RI, Mauray F, Heymann MA, et al. Cardiovascular effects of patent ductus arteriosus in preterm lambs with respiratory distress. J Pediatr. 1987;111:579-587.
108. Ratner I, Perelmuter B, Toews W, et al. Association of low systolic and diastolic blood pressure with significant patent ductus arteriosus in the very low birth weight infant. Crit Care Med. 1985; 13:497-500.
109. Evans N, Moorcraft J. Effect of patency of the ductus arteriosus on blood pressure in very preterm infants. Arch Dis Child. 1992;67:1169-1173.
110. Furzan JA, Reisch J, Tyson JE, et al. Incidence and risk factors for symptomatic patent ductus arteriosus among inborn very-low-birth-weight infants. Early Hum Dev. 1985;12:39-48.
111. Mouzinho AI, Rosenfeld CR, Risser R. Symptomatic patent ductus arteriosus in very-low-birth-weight infants. 1987-1989. Early Hum Dev. 1991;27:65-77.
112. Alverson DC, Eldridge MW, Johnson JD, et al. Effect of patent ductus arteriosus on left ventricular output in premature infants. J Pediatr. 1983;102:754-757.
113. Freeman-Ladd M, Cohen JB, Carver JD, et al. The hemodynamic effects of neonatal patent ductus arteriosus shunting on superior mesenteric artery blood flow. J Perinatol. 2005;25:459-462.
114. McNamara PJ, Stewart L, Shivananda SP, et al. Patent ductus arteriosus ligation is associated with impaired left ventricular systolic performance in premature infants weighing less than 1000 g. J Thorac Cardiovasc Surg. 2010;140:150-157.
115. Noori A, Friedlich P, Seri I, et al. Changes in myocardial function and hemodynamics after ligation of the ductus arteriosus in preterm infants. J Pediatr. 2007;150:597-602.
116. Sehgal A, Francis JV, Lewis AI. Use of milrinone in the management of haemodynamic instability following duct ligation. Eur J Pediatr. 2011;170:115-119.
117. Miller MJ, Martin RJ. Pathophysiology of apnea of prematurity. In: Polin RA, Fox WW, eds. Fetal and neonatal physiology, 2nd ed. Philadelphia: WB Saunders; 1998:1129-1143.
118. Girling DJ. Changes in heart rate, blood pressure, and pulse pressure during apnoeic attacks in newborn babies. Arch Dis Child. 1972;47:405-410.
119. Perlman JM, Volpe JJ. Episodes of apnea and bradycardia in the preterm newborn. Impact on cerebral circulation. Pediatrics. 1985;76:333-338.
120. Cabal LA, Larrazabal C, Siassi B. Hemodynamic variables in infants weighing less than 1000 grams. Clin Perinatol. 1986;13:327-338.
121. Korvenranta H, Kero P, Valimaki I. Cardiovascular monitoring in infants with respiratory distress syndrome. Biol Neonate. 1983;44:138-145.
122. Perlman JM, McMenamin JB, Volpe JJ. Fluctuating cerebral blood-flow velocity in respiratory-distress syndrome. N Engl J Med. 1983;309:204-209.
123. Volpe JJ. Neurology of the newborn, 3rd ed. Philadelphia: WB Saunders; 1995:172-207.
124. Miall-Allen VM, de Vries LS, Dubowitz LM, et al. Blood pressure fluctuation and intraventricular hemorrhage in the preterm infant of less than 31 weeks' gestation. Pediatrics. 1989;83:657-661.
125. Jacobs MM, Phibbs RH. Prevention, recognition, and treatment of perinatal asphyxia. Clin Perinatol. 1989;16:785-807.
126. Holzman BH, Scarpelli EM. Cardiopulmonary consequences of positive end-expiratory pressure. Pediatr Res. 1979;13:1112-1120.
127. de Waal KA, Evans N, Osborn DA, et al. Cardiorespiratory effects of changes in end expiratory pressure in ventilated newborns. Arch Dis Child Fetal Neonatal Ed. 2007;92:F444-F448.
128. Yu VYH, Rolfe P. Effect of continuous positive airway pressure breathing on cardiorespiratory function in infants with respiratory distress syndrome. Acta Paediatr. 1977;66:59-64.
129. Maayan C, Eyal F, Mandelberg A, et al. Effect of mechanical ventilation and volume loading on left ventricular performance in premature infants with respiratory distress syndrome. Crit Care Med. 1986;14:858-860.
130. Hausdorf G, Hellwege H-H. Influence of positive end-expiratory pressure on cardiac performance in premature infants. A Doppler-echocardiographic study. Crit Care Med. 1987;15:661-664.

131. Evans N, Kluckow M. Early determinants of right and left ventricular output in ventilated preterm infants. Arch Dis Child. 1996;74:F88-F94.
132. Skinner JR, Boys RJ, Hunter S, et al. Pulmonary and systemic arterial pressure in hyaline membrane disease. Arch Dis Child. 1992;67:366-373.
133. Hummler H, Gerhardt T, Gonzalez A, et al. Influence of different methods of synchronized mechanical ventilation on ventilation, gas exchange, patient effort, and blood pressure fluctuations in premature neonates. Pediatr Pulmonol. 1996;22:305-313.
134. Perlman JM, Volpe JJ. Suctioning in the preterm infant. Effects on cerebral blood flow velocity, intracranial pressure, and arterial blood pressure. Pediatrics. 1983;72:329-334.
135. Perry EH, Bada HS, Ray JD, et al. Blood pressure increases, birth weight-dependent stability boundary, and intraventricular hemorrhage. Pediatrics. 1990;85:727-732.
136. Omar SY, Greisen G, Ibrahim MM, et al. Blood pressure responses to care procedures in ventilated preterm infants. Acta Paediatr Scand. 1985;74:920-924.
137. Kalyn A, Blatz S, Feuerstake S, et al. Closed suctioning of intubated neonates maintains better physiologic stability. A randomized trial. J Perinatol. 2003;23:218-222.
138. Wood CE, Cheung CY, Brace RA. Fetal heart rate, arterial pressure, and blood volume responses to cortisol infusion. Am J Physiol, Regul Integ Comp Physiol. 1987;253:R904-R909.
139. Stein HM, Oyama K, Martinez A, et al. Effects of corticosteroids in preterm sheep on adaptation and sympathoadrenal mechanisms at birth. Am J Physiol Endocrinol Metab. 1993;264: E763-E769.
140. Kari MA, Hallman M, Eronen M, et al. Prenatal dexamethasone treatment in conjunction with rescue therapy of human surfactant. A randomized placebo-controlled multicenter study. Pediatrics. 1994;93:730-736.
141. Moise AA, Wearden ME, Kozinetz CA, et al. Antenatal steroids are associated with less need for blood pressure support in extremely premature infants. Pediatrics. 1995;95:845-850.
142. Watterberg KL, Scott SM. Evidence of early adrenal insufficiency in babies who develop bronchopulmonary dysplasia. Pediatrics. 1995;95:120-125.
143. Garland JS, Buck R, Leviton A. Effect of maternal glucocorticoid exposure on risk of severe intraventricular hemorrhage in surfactant-treated preterm infants. J Pediatr. 1995;126:272-279.
144. Demarini S, Dollberg S, Hoath SB, et al. Effects of antenatal corticosteroids on blood pressure in very low birth weight infants during the first 24 hours of life. J Perinatol. 1999;19:419-425.
145. Mildenhall LFJ, Battin MR, Morton SMB, et al. Exposure to repeat doses of antenatal glucocorticoids is associated with altered cardiovascular status after birth. Arch Dis Child Fetal Neonatal Ed. 2006;91:F56-F60.
146. Mildenhall L, Battin M, Bevan C, et al. Repeat prenatal corticosteroid doses do not alter neonatal blood pressure or myocardial thickness. Randomized, controlled trial. Pediatrics. 2009;123: e646-e652.
147. Omar SA, DeCristofaro JD, Agarwal BI, et al. Effects of prenatal steroids on water and sodium homeostasis in extremely low birth weight neonates. Pediatrics. 1999;104:482-488.
148. Mantaring JV, Ostrea EM. Effect of perinatal factors on blood pressure in preterm neonates. Pediatr Res. 1996;39:228A.
149. Leviton A, Kuban KC, Pagano M, et al. Antenatal corticosteroids appear to reduce the risk of postnatal germinal matrix hemorrhage in intubated low birth weight newborns. Pediatrics. 1993; 91:1083-1088.
150. Dalziel SR, Liang A, Parag V, et al. Blood pressure at 6 years of age after prenatal exposure to betamethasone. Follow-up results of a randomized, controlled trial. Pediatrics. 2004;114:e373-e377.
151. Battin MR, Thoresen M, Robinson E, et al. Does head cooling with mild systemic hypothermia affect requirement for blood pressure support? Pediatrics. 2009;123:1031-1036.
152. O'Sullivan MJ, Kearney PJ, Crowley MJ. The influence of some perinatal variables on neonatal blood pressure. Acta Paediatr. 1996;85:849-853.
153. Beratis NG, Panagoulias D, Varvarigou A. Increased blood pressure in neonates and infants whose mothers smoked during pregnancy. J Pediatr. 1996;128:806-812.
154. Cordero L, Giannone PJ, Rich JT. Mean arterial pressure in very low birth weight (801 to 1500 g) concordant and discordant twins during the first day of life. J Perinatol. 2003;23:545-551.
155. Shokry M, Elsedfy GO, Bassiouny M, et al. Effects of antenatal magnesium sulfate therapy on cerebral and systemic hemodynamics in preterm newborns. Acta Obstetrica et Gynecologica. 2010;89:801-806.
156. Miall-Allen VM, Whitelaw AGL. Effect of pancuronium and pethidine on heart rate and blood pressure in ventilated infants. Arch Dis Child. 1987;62:1179-1180.
157. Welzing L, Kribs A, Eifinger F, et al. Propofol as an induction agent for endotracheal intubation can cause significant arterial hypotension in preterm neonates. Pediatric Anesthesia. 2010;20: 605-611.
158. Sammartino M, Garra R, Sbaraglia F, et al. Propofol overdose in a preterm baby. May propofol infusion syndrome arise in two hours? Pediatric Anesthesia. 2010;20:958-976.
159. Simons SHP, van Dijk M, van Lingen RA, et al. Randomized controlled trial evaluating effects of morphine on plasma adrenaline/noradrenaline concentrations in newborns. Arch Dis Child, Fetal Neonatal Ed. 2005;90:F36-F40.
160. Barker DP, Simpson J, Pawula M, et al. Randomized, double blind trial of two loading dose regimens of diamorphine in ventilated newborn infants. Arch Dis Child. 1995;73:F22-F26.
161. Sabatino G, Quartulli L, Di Fabio S, et al. Hemodynamic effects of intravenous morphine infusion in ventilated preterm babies. Early Hum Dev. 1997;47:263-270.

A

162. Anand KJS, Hall RW, Desai N, et al. Effects of morphine analgesia in ventilated preterm neonates. Primary outcomes from the NEOPAIN trial. Lancet. 2001;363:1673-1682.
163. Hall RQ, Kronsberg SS, Barton BA, et al. Morphine, hypotension, and adverse outcomes among preterm neonates. Who's to blame? Secondary results from the NEOPAIN trial. Pediatrics. 2005;115:1351-1359.
164. Williams AL, Sanderson M, Lai D, et al. Intensive care noise and mean arterial blood pressure in extremely low-birth-weight neonates. Am J Perinatol. 2009;26:323-329.
165. Zak LK, Donn SM. Thoracic air leaks. In: Donn SM, Faix RG, eds. Neonatal emergencies. Mount Kisco, NY: Futura; 1991:311-325.
166. Pomeranz A, Dolfin T, Korzets Z, et al. Increased sodium concentrations in drinking water increase blood pressure in neonates. J Hypertens. 2002;20:203-207.
167. Kobayashi S, Fujimoto S, Fukuda S, et al. Periventricular leukomalacia with late-onset circulatory dysfunction of premature infants. Correlation with severity of magnetic resonance imaging findings and neurological outcome. Tohoku J Exp Med. 2006;210:333-339.

3

Diagnosis of Neonatal Shock: Methods and Their Clinical Applications

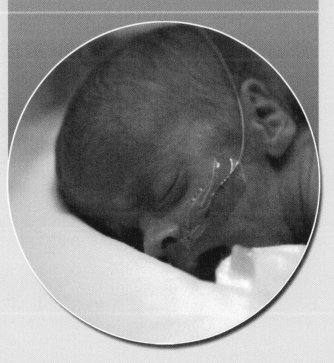

CHAPTER 4

Methods to Assess Systemic and Organ Blood Flow in the Neonate

Gorm Greisen, MD, PhD

This chapter describes the methods available to assess organ blood flow in the neonate, and discusses their strengths, weaknesses, and sources of errors. Most detail is given on Doppler ultrasound and near-infrared (NIR) spectroscopy, since these are the most practical methods, they have been used at the bedside, and are likely to produce new research data in the near future. The measurement of blood flow to the brain (cerebral blood flow, CBF) is described first and in most detail, since this is where most of the experience is. A brief section at the end addresses the experience with assessment of blood flow to other organs.

Organ blood flow is usually expressed in mL/min, as this is the most descriptive unit when an organ is supplied from a single artery and/or drained via a single vein. Indeed, in animal experimentation the simplest method to measure blood flow to an organ is to drain the venous outflow into a calibrated container. The description of blood flow in mL/min has been used to judge the flow to an organ expressed as a fraction of cardiac output. Whether this fraction changes during development or under pathologic conditions such as hypoxia, arterial hypotension, and/or low cardiac output states are important and clinically relevant questions in the field of developmental physiology and pathophysiology. Finally, to allow comparison among groups of infants of different gestational age and thus body weight, it is useful to normalize blood flow for body weight and express it as mL/min/kg.

However, organ blood flow can also be expressed in mL/100 g tissue/min. This measure may refer to an organ as a whole or to a specific region or compartment in a given organ, depending on the method of measurement. The simplest methods to assess organ blood flow use Fick's principle for inert tracers: "Flow equals the rate of change in tissue concentration of tracer divided by the arteriovenous concentration difference of the tracer." This measure is especially useful to assess the flow in relation to metabolism and organ function.

B

It is important to emphasize that blood flow is a complex and dynamic variable. Aside from physiologic fluctuations in organ blood flow governed by the changes in functional activity and thus the metabolic demand of a given organ, blood flow may significantly change within seconds under pathologic conditions such as with abrupt changes in blood pressure or the onset of hypoxia. In addition, blood flow may vary from one part of an organ to the other as during functional activation, or during stress, the distribution may change markedly.

For several decades authors studying the management of circulation during provision of intensive care to the neonate have been pointing out the need to consider blood flow, rather than only arterial blood pressure. Therefore thoughtful neonatal practice would include the use of indirect measures of blood flow, such as skin color, peripheral–core temperature difference, capillary refill time, urine output, and lactic acidosis. Unfortunately, these indirect signs of tissue perfusion either lack sensitivity and specificity (i.e., peripheral–core temperature difference, capillary refill time) or do not represent the changes in the hemodynamic status in a timely manner (i.e., urine output and lactic acidosis).

As for the methods available for the more direct assessment of organ blood flow in neonates, very few units routinely utilize these tools. Why is this so?

There are three main reasons why assessment of organ blood flow has not become routine in the clinical practice. First, none of the many methods used for research has achieved broader application because none satisfies the requirements in terms of ease of use, precision, accuracy, noninvasiveness, and cost. In reality, therefore, no method is truly available to clinicians who want to upgrade their clinical practice. Methods using standard equipment (e.g., ultrasound) require much skill, while the ones, which in principle are "push-button" methods, require special instruments. Second, no method has truly sufficient enough precision. From this standpoint, for research purposes, a method of measurement is appropriate if it is unbiased even if it lacks high precision. Accordingly, although the finding in an individual infant may be imprecise (i.e., uncertain), it is still possible to achieve meaningful and statistically significant results by analysis of the findings from groups of infants. For clinical use, however, it is absolutely necessary that a single measurement is sufficiently precise. Third, research on organ blood flow in neonates has focused on physiology and pathophysiology and done little in the way of defining the clinical benefit of having measures of blood flow in ill infants. This means that there is only little incentive for the clinician to overcome the difficulties presented earlier.

Doppler Ultrasound

Doppler ultrasound to assess changes in CBF was first used in neonates in 1979.[1] As clinical and research interest focused on CBF during this time, several methods, including Doppler ultrasound, were introduced to assess blood flow to the brain of the neonate. The use of Doppler ultrasound for functional echocardiography in the neonate is described in Chapter 5 in detail.

Doppler Principle

According to the Doppler principle, the frequency shift of the reflected sound (the "echo") is proportional to the velocity of the reflector. Since erythrocytes in blood reflect ultrasound, blood flow velocity can be measured based on simple physics. The equation states that the frequency shift equals the flow velocity multiplied by the emitted frequency divided by the speed of sound in the tissue. However, there are several factors that need to be taken into consideration and corrected for with the use of the Doppler principle. First, the apparent velocity has to be corrected for the angle between the blood vessel and the ultrasound beam. Second, it should be kept in mind that multiple frequencies are detected when performing an ultrasound study of a vessel, since the flow velocity decreases from the center of the blood stream toward the vessel wall. In addition, even the vessel wall itself contributes to

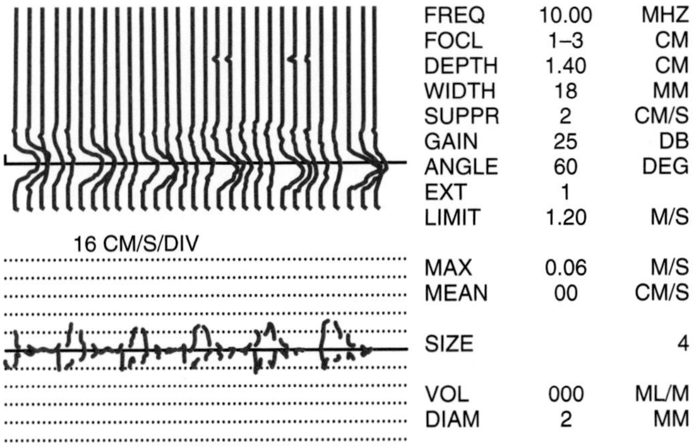

FREQ	10.00	MHZ
FOCL	1–3	CM
DEPTH	1.40	CM
WIDTH	18	MM
SUPPR	2	CM/S
GAIN	25	DB
ANGLE	60	DEG
EXT	1	
LIMIT	1.20	M/S
MAX	0.06	M/S
MEAN	00	CM/S
SIZE		4
VOL	000	ML/M
DIAM	2	MM

16 CM/S/DIV

Figure 4-1 Output from a prototype Doppler instrument with multiple gates built in the late 1980s. The vertical lines represent the mean velocity detected in each of the 128 gates every 50 ms. Together the 128 gates span 18 mm; that is, approximately 0.15 mm is covered by each. The probe was placed on the neck of a newborn infant to measure flow in the common carotid artery. The vertical line is 1.4 cm under the skin. The flow profile is parabolic as expected and steeper during systole. From the flow profile, the diameter can be estimated to be approximately 3 mm at 60° angle of insonation. This is the principle behind color-coded Doppler ultrasound. As a result of the speed of data processing, new instruments have the Doppler information as part of the 2-D ultrasound image. The vessel diameter is then read from the color image by the investigator using electronic calipers. Two principles can be used to estimate mean flow velocity for volumetric Doppler. The sample volume is set so that the entire vessel is covered. The machine can weigh the received mixture of frequency shifts (i.e., velocities) by their intensity (i.e., by the mass of erythrocytes flowing at each velocity). However, intensity is not a perfect measure of mass and not all ultrasound transducers produce homogeneous sonification of the entire vessel. Alternatively, the maximum velocity can be used and divided by a factor of 2. This corresponds to equality of the volume of a parabola with a cylinder of half the height. Maximum frequency is normally well measured, but the method will fail if the flow profile is not parabolic.

the signal. Finally, the velocity is pulsating in nature, as it is faster in systole than in diastole (Fig. 4-1).

First Instruments

The instruments of the 1970s and early 1980s were continuous wave (with no resolution of depth, with no image, and a crude mean frequency shift estimator). Finding an arterial signal was done blindly, using general anatomic knowledge and an audible signal with the frequency shift in the 50-500 Hz range while searching for the loudest pulsating signal with the highest pitch. This left the angle and the true spatial average undetermined, and therefore the scale of measurement uncertain. Indices of pulsatility (resistance index: [(peak systolic flow velocity – end diastolic flow velocity)/end diastolic flow velocity] and pulsatility index: [(peak systolic flow velocity – end diastolic flow velocity)/mean flow velocity]) were often used since these indices are independent of the angle of insonation.

Indices of Pulsatility

Indices of pulsatility reflect downstream resistance to flow and pulsatility in the umbilical artery has achieved great clinical importance in fetal monitoring.[2] In newborn infants, however, the resistance index in the anterior cerebral artery was only weakly associated with cerebral blood flow as measured by ^{133}Xe clearance.[3] In addition, more sophisticated modeling revealed that arterial blood pressure pulsatility and arterial wall compliance are as important determinants of the indices of pulsatility as is the downstream resistance.[4] In summary, Doppler data on resistance indices may be valid and have often been corroborated by other methods, but could be imprecise and heavily biased. In a seminal clinical study, however, the pulsatility index was shown to carry independent prognostic ability in term infants with neonatal hypoxic-ischemic encephalopathy.[5]

Blood Flow Velocity

With the technical advances in the 1980s, duplex scanning combining imaging and Doppler, range-gating limiting flow detection to a small sample volume, and frequency analysis allowing proper maximum and mean frequency shift estimation became available and contributed to more reliable measurement of blood flow velocity. However, this still left the question of accurate determination of the arterial caliber unanswered. This is an important point, as the calculation of absolute organ blood flow in mL/min equals flow velocity (cm/s) multiplied by arterial cross-sectional area (cm^2). The inability to accurately measure the arterial cross-sectional area precludes comparison from one infant to another, one organ to another and, in essence, from one state to another, since arterial caliber varies dynamically in the immature individual.[6,7] In summary, although improved techniques now allow more accurate and precise measurement of flow velocity, it is still uncertain if this has really improved the value of this modality.

Volumetric Measurements

This last hurdle to absolute, volumetric measurement of flow has been addressed using ultrasound imaging to measure arterial cross-sectional area as part of the method. In large-diameter vessels this can now be used quite accurately. For instance, to measure left and right ventricular output, the diameters of the ascending aorta and the pulmonary trunk, respectively, need to be precisely determined. The diameter of these two major vessels is 6-10 mm, and an error of 0.5 mm on the first generation of duplex scanners translated to a reproducibility of 10-15%. Recently, for measurement of superior vena cava (SVC) flow at the vessel's entry into the right atrium with a diameter of 3-6 mm, reproducibility of SVC flow of 14% was reported using a 7-MHz transducer.[8] With the advent of color-coded imaging and the use of higher ultrasound frequencies, volumetric measurement of distributary arteries have also become possible in the newborn. For instance, measurement of blood flow in the right common carotid artery with a diameter of 2-3 mm was reported to have a reproducibility of 10-15% using a 15-MHz transducer, while that in both internal carotid and both vertebral arteries with diameters of 1-2 mm was found to be 7% for the sum of the blood flows in the four arteries using a 10-MHz transducer.[9,10]

Near-Infrared Spectroscopy

NIR spectroscopy is also discussed in Chapters 7 and 8. Transillumination of the head of small animals is possible using NIR spectroscopy and the first clinical research use of this technology was carried out in newborns.[11] Quantitative spectroscopy was subsequently performed in 1986.[12] Over the following years a large number of papers on NIR spectroscopy in newborns have been published.

Geometry

The newborn infant's head is ideally suited for NIR spectroscopy. The overlying tissues are relatively thin, which ensures that the signal is dominated by brain tissue including both the white and gray matter. NIR spectroscopy recordings can be performed with the light applied to one side of the head and received on the other side (transmission mode) in the low birth weight infant with biparietal diameters from 6 to 8 cm. In this situation a large part of the brain is included in the measurement, and the results may be interpreted as assessment of "global" brain blood flow. Larger babies can only be investigated with the emitting and receiving fibers in an angular arrangement (reflection mode), usually with both optodes on the same side of the head. In this situation a smaller volume of brain tissue between the optodes is investigated. This may be chosen on purpose, also in smaller babies, to obtain "regional" results. With a shorter interoptode distance, blood flow in a narrow and shallow tissue volume is investigated with a relatively larger fraction of extracerebral tissues.

Algorithms and Wavelength

Several different types of NIR spectroscopy instruments have been used. The number of wavelengths used has also varied from two to six. With the use of different wavelengths, the mathematical algorithms used to separate the signals of oxyhemoglobin (O_2Hb), deoxyhemoglobin (HHb), and the cytochrome aa3 oxidase difference signal (Cyt.ox), have differed.[13] This may have had an impact on our ability to appropriately analyze the differences in the findings among the different papers, particularly among those published earlier, as some of the differences may have been due to differences in the NIR spectroscopy methodology applied.

Pathlength

The pathlength of light traversing the tissue must be known to calculate concentrations, that is, to measure quantitatively. The pathlength in tissue exceeds the geometric distance between the optodes by a factor of 3-6 and this factor is named the differential pathlength factor (DPF). Correct estimation of pathlength is one of the basic problems in NIR spectroscopy as it varies up to 20% among infants. Although instruments exist that allow direct measurement of pathlength, these are not commonly used.

Quantification of Cerebral Blood Flow

Measurement of blood flow by NIR spectroscopy is based on Fick's principle and utilizes a rapid change in arterial oxyhemoglobin as the intravascular tracer.[14] By using the change in the oxygenation index (OI) observed after a small sudden change in the arterial concentration of oxygen, CBF (in mL/100 g/min) can be calculated as $CBF = \Delta OI/(k \times \int SaO_2 \times dt)$, where OI is measured in units of μmol/L, and $k = $ Hgb $\times 1.05 \times 100$. Hgb is blood hemoglobin in mmol/L (tetraheme), SaO_2 is given in %, and t is time, in min (Fig. 4-2).

Assumptions

The method of measuring CBF rests on several assumptions. First, during measurement CBF, cerebral blood volume (CBV), and oxygen extraction are assumed to be constant. Second, the period of measurement must be less than the cerebral transit time (approximately 10 s). Finally, this method of CBF measurement also has significant practical limitations For instance, in infants with severe lung disease, SaO_2 may be fixed at a low level despite administration of oxygen, whereas in infants with normal lungs, SaO_2 is near 100% in room air. Although this problem could be overcome by using air-nitrogen mixtures and then switching to room air, results of such experiments have not been reported. In addition, there are significant ethical considerations when using a hypoxic gas mixture in healthy newborns even if for only a brief period of time.

Reproducibility and Validation

Measurements of blood flow with NIR spectroscopy have a reported reproducibility of 17-24% and have been validated against ^{133}Xe clearance in sick newborns. These comparisons constitute important direct external validation of NIR spectroscopy in the brain of human neonates. The agreement between the two methods was found to be acceptable.[15,16]

Indocyanine Green as an Alternative Tracer

A dye, indocyanine green, given by intravenous injection, has been used in place of oxygen utilizing a special fiber optic instrument to measure intra-arterial indocyanine green concentration.[17] The results were similar but the reproducibility of this technique was better (15%) than that of conventional NIR spectroscopy. Recently, an improvement of this method has also been proposed, using a convolution algorithm to account for venous outflow and a noninvasive pulse dye-densitometer for

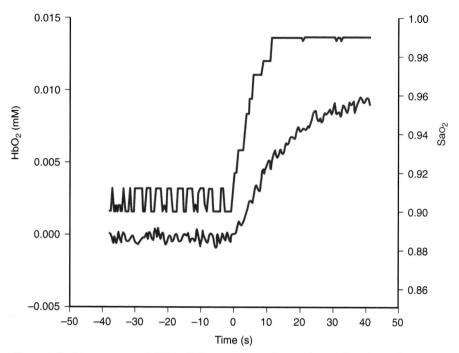

Figure 4-2 Measurement of CBF by NIR spectroscopy in a newborn infant. Arterial saturation (as monitored by a pulse oximeter) is stable at 90-91% until FiO_2 is increased. Within a few seconds the arterial saturation rises to 95% and greater. The rise in cerebral concentration of oxyhemoglobin is slower due to the time it takes for the more highly oxygenated arterial blood to fill the vascular bed of the brain. By restricting the analysis to the first 6 to 8 s as it is assumed that the venous saturation is still unchanged, a simplified version of the Fick's principle can be used. NIR spectroscopy using an intravascular tracer and measuring over a few seconds gives results of "global" cerebral blood flow similar to the result obtained with the use of ^{133}Xe clearance. Xenon is a diffusible tracer equilibrating between blood and tissue. Wash-out is much slower and measurements are made over 8-15 min.

measurement of arterial indocyanine green concentration. The findings were encouraging in piglets, and the method has been utilized in newborn infants.[18,19] Similarly to the conventional NIR spectroscopy methodology, where the sensitivity of the pulse oximeter presents one of the technical problems, the pulse dye-densitometer is the major technical limitation of the NIR spectroscopy method using indocyanine green as the tracer molecule. Therefore, as an alternative, a *blood flow index* has been proposed using the rise-time in cerebral iodocyanine green (ICG) concentration after a rapid intravenous injection.[20] This has a satisfactory coefficient of variability of 10%, and has recently been used to study cerebral auto-regulation directly during epinephrine injection.[21]

Trend Monitoring of Hemoglobin Signals

In principle, NIR spectroscopy allows on-line trending of changes in O_2Hb and HHb, and hence those of total hemoglobin (tHb). Total hemoglobin, the sum of $[O_2Hb]$ and $[HHb]$, is proportional to changes in cerebral blood volume (CBV), which in turn can be used as a surrogate measure of CBF. The appropriateness of this assumption, however, has only been established for reactions to changes in arterial CO_2 tension.[22] Furthermore, constant optode distance is crucial in trend monitoring and if the head circumference changes even by a fraction of a millimeter as a result of change in CBV or brain water content, the trends are significantly biased. In addition, minor changes in the optode-skin contact induce large transients in the signal and/or baseline shifts. Despite these limitations, several investigators have successfully accomplished trend monitoring.

The Hemoglobin Difference, or Oxygenation Index

The difference between [O_2Hb] and [HHb] is called Hbdiff and, when divided by a factor of two, it is known as the oxygenation index (OI). The Hbdiff is an indicator of the mean oxygen saturation of the hemoglobin in all types of blood vessels in the tissue. This measure has been shown to change appropriately in many experimental models and clinical studies, but has important limitations. First, in terms of interpretation, it is not known how much of the signal originates from blood in the arteries, capillaries, or veins. Data in piglets suggest that the arterial-to-venous ratio is about $1:2$.[23] The signal can also be seriously confounded by concomitant changes in tHb, as tHb affects the amount of blood distributed in the arterial, capillary or venous compartments. Finally, the lack of a fixed zero-point makes it impossible to specify a threshold for intervention or even an alarm level for clinical use.

Coherence of the Spontaneous Variability of Cerebral Hemoglobin Oxygenation and Variability of Arterial Blood Pressure as an Indication of Cerebral Autoregulation

Coherence is a statistical measure of correlation between two parameters in the frequency domain; that is, the finding of high coherence shows that cerebral oxygenation varies at the same rate as does arterial blood pressure. This has been proposed as a useful indicator of impaired autoregulation and suggested to be associated with brain injury.[24] In stable infants, however, it may take several hours of signal recording to obtain a statistically stable estimate of coherence and hence, the coherence method is not likely to become clinically useful.[25]

Diffuse Correlation Spectroscopy

NIR equipment based on lasers emits highly coherent light waves. When reflected from stationary reflectors in tissue, the coherence tends to decay slowly over 1 to 100 μs, whereas when the light is reflected from moving particles (in tissue this means red blood cells) the coherence decays more rapidly. The autocorrelation as a function of time therefore can be used as *blood flow index*. Although the blood flow index has been correlated to Doppler ultrasound in preterm infants, and to arterial spin labeling by magnetic resonance imaging (MRI) in neonates with congenital heart disease, the correlations have been relatively weak.[26,27]

Quantification of Hemoglobin-Oxygen Saturation

Three different principles are being used in second-generation instruments to measure hemoglobin-oxygen saturation in absolute terms without manipulation of FiO_2 or using another tracer like a dye. With spatially resolved spectroscopy, the detection of the transmitted light at two or more different distances from the light-emitting optode allows monitoring of the ratio of absolute [O_2Hb] to [tHb], that is, the hemoglobin saturation. The hemoglobin saturation measured by this method is called the tissue oxygenation index (TOI) or tissue oxygen saturation (StO_2).[28] This measure is the weighted average of arterial, capillary, and venous blood oxygenation, and hence cannot easily be validated. The measurement depends on the tissue being optically homogeneous, which is unlikely to be the case. Nevertheless, TOI values close to cerebrovenous values have been found, and appropriate changes in TOI have been documented with changes in arterial oxygen saturation and arterial Pco_2. As the signal-to-noise ratio is not as good as that of OI, TOI is less useful for quantifying the response to rapid therapeutic interventions. The other two principles are time-resolved spectroscopy, which detects the time-of-flight of very short light pulses, and phase shift spectroscopy, which detects the phase shift and phase modulation of a continuous frequency-modulated source of light.[29,30] With the use of these two methods, it is also possible to estimate the absolute concentrations of O_2Hb and HHb, and from these to calculate StO_2.

Bias of Tissue Oxygen Saturation

StO_2, similar to OI (see earlier), cannot be compared directly with any other measurement because it represents the findings in a mixture of blood in the arteries, capillaries, and veins. Interestingly, though, StO_2 has recently been validated on the head of young infants with heart disease during cardiac catheterization.[24] In this study, across an StO_2 range of 40-80%, the mean value was almost identical to oxygen saturation in jugular venous blood as measured by co-oximetry. This suggests a significant negative bias as, in addition to venous blood, the StO_2 also represents arterial and capillary blood. This bias is likely to differ between different types of instruments. In addition, StO_2 has not been compared to any other measures of venous saturation in preterm or term neonates; not even internal consistency of StO_2 with SvO_2 measured by NIRS during obstruction of venous outflow has been reported.

Precision of the Tissue Oxygen Saturation

In the study in young infants with heart disease, while the mean difference was negligible, limits of agreement of individual measurements were as wide as -12 to $+11\%$. Since co-oximetry is very precise, this variation represents an estimate of the error of StO_2.[31] Using the same commercial instrument in newborns and young infants, the limits of agreement after optode replacement were found to be -17 to $+17\%$.[32] In preterm or term neonates, the variation associated with replacement of the optodes could fully account for this poor precision.[33] Therefore it is conceivable that the main reason for the significant variability of StO_2 lies in the small anatomic differences between the different positions of the optodes causing the assumption of scatter isotropy to fail. For comparison, arterial hemoglobin oxygen saturation can be measured by pulse oximetry with limits of agreement of $\pm6\%$.

Importance of the Low Precision of the Tissue Oxygen Saturation

StO_2 is a surrogate measure of cerebrovenous saturation. This important physiologic variable is tightly regulated with the normal values being between 60% and 70%. During hypoxemia, or cerebral ischemia, when CBF decreases without a change in cerebral oxygen consumption, cerebrovenous saturation falls. Hence, cerebrovenous saturation is a useful measure of the sufficiency of cerebral perfusion. However, the major technical problem is that for instance a 30% decrease in the CBF will only lead to a drop from 70% to 60% in the cerebrovenous oxygen saturation, which is well within the limits of the error of measurement.

Magnetic Resonance Imaging

Although MRI is discussed in detail in Chapters 9 and 10, this chapter reviews the basics of methodology. The nucleus hydrogen is stable but magnetically asymmetric and hence behaves like a magnetic dipole. Subjected to a strong magnetic field (0.2-3 T), it will tend to align with the field (longitudinal magnetization), in the sense that it rotates around the direction of the magnetic field. This rotation (called *precession*, like a spinning top) occurs at a frequency proportional to the strength of the magnetic field. Exposed to a pulse of electromagnetic energy of proportional frequency at a 90° angle of the field, the rotation may be synchronized resulting in transverse magnetization and a decrease in the longitudinal magnetization. After the pulse, the synchrony continues and re-emits electromagnetic energy for some time. Imaging depends on the gradients in the magnetic field, which makes a particular frequency specific to a specific plane. By the use of gradients in the X, Y, and Z plane, a 3-D reconstruction is possible. Image contrast comes from the fact that tissues differ according to the chemical and physical constitution of their hydrogen nuclei.

Measurement of Blood Flow

Blood flow is essentially moving water, that is, moving hydrogen nuclei, which tend to cause loss of signal. In the simplest way, global CBF may be estimated by imaging

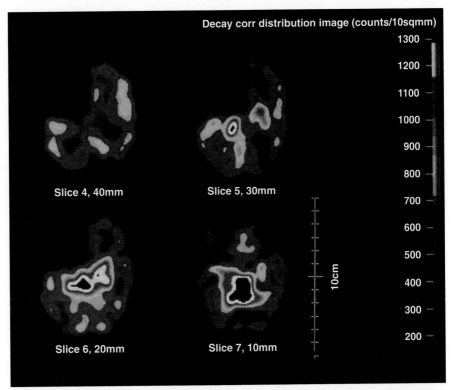

Figure 4-3 Flow images in a near-term newborn infant with a large right frontal subdural hematoma. The four slices are axial at 10, 20, 30, and 40 mm above the orbitomeatal line. The images show no measurable flow to the entire right frontal lobe. Furthermore, flow is high in the central parts of the brain and also appears to be higher in cortex compared to the white matter. However, the latter is not well illustrated due to limited spatial resolution (nominally 8 mm full width at half maximum (FWHM) for this image). The image was made by hexamethylpropyleneamine oxime (HMPAO), a "chemical microsphere" labeled with ^{99m}Tc given intravenously as detected by single photon emission tomography (see later). The HMPAO fixes in tissue during the first pass. The image really is just the distribution of the tracer, that is, of bolus distribution. To translate such an image to flow, in addition to linearization, an estimate of arterial input is required. The latter is very difficult to achieve for HMPAO, but it is easier for some other tracers.

the four arteries on the neck and multiplying their cross-sectional area with the blood flow velocity, estimated by the loss of magnetization caused by fresh blood (water) flowing into the plane of imaging, also called *phase contrast imaging*. This has been successful in newborns, but is more complex than the use of ultrasound and may be less precise.[34] The results are given in mL/s, and should be related to body weight, or more precisely, to brain weight.

Qualitative Flow Imaging (Fig. 4-3)

For qualitative flow imaging, tracer is being used. The tracer usually is gadolinium bound to ethylenediamine tetraacetic acid (EDTA) so that it stays in the vascular compartment.[35] Gadolinium is paramagnetic, that is, it affects the nearby hydrogen nuclei by reducing their relaxation time and hence strongly influences the image. When given intravenously, it accumulates in brain blood vessels and clears in the same way as an intravascular dye for NIR spectroscopy. In adults, gadolinium concentration has been measured near the middle cerebral arteries in order to obtain an arterial input function for the quantification of CBF.

Quantitative Flow Imaging

Arterial spin labeling is performed by applying the radio-frequency pulse to a thick slice (slab) at the base of the skull. This labels the blood in segments of the large arteries supplying the brain. After allowing for the arterial transit time (a little less than a second) to pass, imaging of as many slices as technically possible commences. Regions with higher flow will contain more labeled blood (the bolus distribution principle) and hence a higher signal. Flow is quantified by measuring the relative difference in signal intensity divided by the duration of the labeling pulse. This method also requires correcting for the blood-brain water partition coefficient, any incomplete arterial labeling, and the imaging delay compared to the relaxation time in the blood.[36] This method was recently used in 25 neonates with congenital heart disease during normal ventilation and during inhalation of added CO_2.[37] All babies were mechanically ventilated and sedated. Mean slice CBF was 19.7 ± 9.2 mL/100 g/min and 40.1 ± 20.3 before and during CO_2 inhalation, respectively, giving an overall CBF-CO_2 reactivity of 1 mL/Torr or 35% change per kPa. Although these values appear plausible, the potential for underestimation of CBF has to be recognized. This may be because the arterial transit time at low blood flow is prolonged causing the overestimation of the arterial input. Indeed, Doppler studies have demonstrated that arterial flow velocity in the brain may go as low as 5 cm/s.

Kety-Schmidt Method

Fick's principle for metabolically inert tracers states that the change of the mean tracer concentration in a tissue equals the perfusion rate (flow) multiplied by the arteriovenous concentration difference of the tracer and can be expressed as $dC_t/dt = F \times (C_a - C_v)$. The Kety-Schmidt method was developed specifically to measure blood flow to the brain. Fifteen percent nitrous oxide, a freely diffusible inert gas, is administered by inhalation and tracer concentration in arterial and jugular venous blood is determined by taking six to eight precisely timed blood samples over 10 min after the start of the inhalation. The concentration of nitrous oxide in the brain is estimated by multiplying its venous concentration by the tissue-blood partition coefficient with an equilibrium assumed. By integration of the equation earlier, blood flow is calculated as the nitrous oxide concentration in the brain at 10 min divided by the area under the curve of the arteriovenous concentration difference in time points between 0 and 10 min.

However, the assumption of equilibration may not be correct even after 10 min, if parts of the brain are perfused at low rates and therefore remain unsaturated. This may frequently be the case in infants.[30] In this situation, the wash-in must be followed for at least 15 min. Obviously, regions of the brain that are not perfused will not be represented. Since a counter-current exchange of nitrous oxide from artery to vein may also take place, the difference between venous concentration and tissue concentration will be even greater. The result is an overestimation of the CBF.

The value of CBF obtained by the Kety-Schmidt method is the mean flow over the wash-in period and relates to the part of the brain drained by the jugular vein at the sampling site. Of note is that even at the jugular bulb there may be a small admixture of extracerebral blood.

The Kety-Schmidt method has been used in newborn infants.[38-40] There are several limitations of this method, including a relatively large 2 to 3 mL blood volume requirement for sampling and an unknown reproducibility. However, its main drawback is the need for arterial and jugular venous blood sampling. Catheterization of the jugular bulb in a newborn is technically difficult, and carries a greater risk than catheterization in larger infants and children. In special cases, however, when such a catheter is in place for clinical use, the method can be applied without significant additional risks and it has a great advantage, as it makes it possible to measure global cerebral metabolic rate of oxygen (CMR_{O2}) or glucose (CMR_{glu}) by multiplying the CBF by the cross-brain extraction of oxygen or glucose.

^{133}Xe Clearance

^{133}Xe is a radioactive isotope and also inert. Measurement of CBF by ^{133}Xe clearance is based on a modification of the Kety-Schmidt method. If instantaneous equilibration between brain and venous blood is assumed, the venous concentrations can be derived from tissue concentrations as measured by external detection of the gamma radiation emitted by the ^{133}Xe in the brain. Thus, the need for jugular vein catheterization can be circumvented. When xenon is given intravenously dissolved in saline, the arterial concentration can be estimated by external detection over the chest, assuming equilibrium between alveolar air and arterial blood. In the small neonatal brain, ^{133}Xe clearance provides a measure of global CBF since the detector samples from a brain volume of about 200 mL. The clearance curve analysis allows separate estimates of blood flow to gray and white matter, but the most stable estimate is the mean blood flow (CBF$_\infty$). This is identical to the estimate obtained by the Kety-Schmidt method and is determined over 5 to 10 min and has a reproducibility of 10-15%.[41,42]

Single Photon Emission Computed Tomography

Tomographic images of radiotracer localization may be obtained by methods similar to computed x-ray tomography. Gamma emitting decays (photons) across the brain are detected by a number of collimated detectors from a large number of angles around the head circumference. The image is constructed by back-projection and usually subjected to various smoothing procedures (filters). There is no theoretical limit to the spatial resolution, but the narrow collimation required for high resolution reduces the sensitivity and requires more counts to fill the larger number of pixels (image elements). Furthermore, Compton scatter tends to mask "cold" areas, whereas small high flow structures will be underestimated due to partial volume effects. Spatial resolution is 6 to 12 mm full width at half-maximum (FWHM). The distribution of the radioactive tracers is fixed in the brain tissue during the first passage. Slowly rotating gamma cameras may image the distribution of radioactively labeled substances, such as ^{131}I-iodoamphetamine or ^{99m}Tc-HMPAO (hexamethylpropylene amine oxime).[43,44] The advantage of these compounds is that they may be injected intravenously at any time, whereas the imaging may take place several hours later. Their disadvantage is that only the distribution of flow can be obtained without the ability to calculate absolute flows. Finally, equipment rotating in 5-10 s may follow the local uptake and clearance of ^{133}Xe.[45]

Stable Xenon-Enhanced Computed Tomography

This method is also a variant of the Kety-Schmidt method. Detection of the tracer (stable or nonradioactive xenon) in the brain is based on the high density of xenon to x-rays. By performing repeated x-ray computed tomography (CT) scans during inhalation of 35% xenon, brain saturation can be followed. In principle, the spatial resolution is as good as it is for conventional CT scanning. However, the low brain-blood partition coefficient of xenon in newborn brain results in a low signal-to-noise ratio. Despite these limitations, very low levels of CBF have been documented in young, brain-dead infants.[46] With the advent of Xenon-inhalation for neuroprotection, this technique may be used more frequently again.

Positron Emission Tomography

Positron emission tomography (PET) is similar to single photon emission tomography (SPECT) in image reconstruction, but differs in that PET utilizes the fact that positron annihilation results in two photons emitted always at an angle of 180°. Therefore localization is achieved by only accepting the counts that occur simultaneously at two oppositely positioned detectors and collimation is not needed. Hence the sensitivity is better at high resolution compared to SPECT and the resolution now approaches the theoretical maximum of 3-5 mm representing the average positron movement before annihilation. Biologically relevant positron-emitting isotopes exist (e.g., ^{11}C, ^{13}N, and ^{15}O) and many biochemical substances can also be labeled. PET is ideally suited for receptor studies using specific ligands, since imaging and quantification can be done with picomoles of tracer. As the positron emitting iso-topes are very short-lived (2 min to 2 h), PET requires a nearby cyclotron facility.

Finally, CBF, CBV, cerebral oxygen extraction fraction, CMR_{O2}, and CMR_{glu} may all be measured by PET.[47-50] As the newest PET scanners are very sensitive, the dose of isotope can be reduced, perhaps to a level where nontherapeutic research in newborn infants may become acceptable.

Other Methods

Venous occlusion plethysmography is a standard method for measurement of limb blood flow and has been used to estimate jugular blood flow.[51] In spite of its virtues of technical simplicity and low risk in healthy infants, the method has fallen into disuse, mostly because of concern that low skull compliance yields falsely low values of cranial blood flow.

The slightly pulsatile transcephalic impedance may be measured by applying a small alternating electrical current. The pulsatility correlates with CBF, although the precise basis of the impedance pulsatility remains unclear.[52] This method only has theoretical risks, but only gives qualitative information and is sensitive to movement. Although it appears well suited for long-term monitoring, it has rarely been used.

Measurement of Flow to Other Organs

Doppler ultrasound has been used in newborns for measuring indices of resistance and/or flow velocity in the renal, celiac, superior mesenteric, carotid, and vertebral arteries. A few volumetric studies have been published: whereas recent studies have given plausible values the earlier studies appear to have overestimated flow, most likely caused by overestimation of arterial cross-sectional area due to insufficient resolution at 5 MHz (see Chapter 2).

Flow to the forearm or lower leg can easily be measured by venous occlusion and NIR spectroscopy. Recently, it was shown that the modulation (amplitude) of the plethysmographic signal of a pulse oximeter correlates well with flow.[53]

Conclusion

This chapter describes a number of methods, nearly all tried in newborns because they had worked in adults and because of the need to gather more information about normal brain function and blood supply, brain injury, and long-term neurodevelop-mental sequelae of prematurity, perinatal insult, or critical neonatal illness. Some of the methods have been discarded by the authors themselves. Others have just been tried a few times and characterized as "promising." However, quite a few methods, such as ultrasonography, NIR spectoscopy, PET, and more recently MRI, have been workhorses for individual researchers or groups of researchers. Yet, none of these methods has really been established as a reference. This is a concern because the results obtained by using these more favored yet not cross-validated methods have less credence and usefulness.

Blood flow is probably too complex a physiologic variable for it to be meaning-ful to even think of a "true" value or a "gold standard" in any given organ. Quoting the late Niels Lassen, my mentor in the measurement of CBF, "A method [measuring CBF] must have acceptable precision with a reproducibility of about 10%, and be able to demonstrate a plausible $CBF-CO_2$ reactivity and a reasonable CBF-MABP (mean arterial blood pressure) autoregulation in patients with a normal brain." For use in newborns, it must furthermore be feasible and safe in the intensive care unit and be able to determine absolute CBF and continuously monitor the changes. Unfortunately, none of the methods developed and available has so far lived up to these requirements.

References

1. Bada HS, Hajjar W, Chua C, et al. Noninvasive diagnosis of neonatal asphyxia and intraventricular hemorrhage by Doppler ultrasound. J Pediatr. 1979;95:775-779.

2. Neilson JP, Alfirevic Z. Doppler ultrasound for fetal assessment in high risk pregnancies. The Cochrane Database of Systematic Reviews. 2006;2.
3. Greisen G, Johansen K, Ellison PH, et al. Cerebral blood flow in the newborn infant: comparison of Doppler ultrasound and 133-Xenon clearance. J Pediatr. 1984;104:411-418.
4. Greisen G. Analysis of cerebroarterial Doppler flow velocity waveforms in newborn infants: towards an index of cerebrovascular resistance. J Perinat Med. 1986;4:181-187.
5. Levene MI, Sands C, Grindulis H, et al. Comparison of two methods of predicting outcome in peri-natal asphyxia. Lancet. 1985;67-69.
6. Drayton MR, Skidmore R. Vasoactivity of the major intracranial arteries in newborn infants. Arch Dis Child. 1987;62:236-240.
7. Malcus P, Kjellmer I, Lingman G, et al. Diameters of the common carotid artery and aorta change in different directions during acute asphyxia in the fetal lamb. J Perinat Med. 1991;19:259-267.
8. Kluckow M, Evans N. Superior vena cava flow in newborn infants: a novel marker of systemic blood flow. Arch Dis Child. 2000;82:F182-F187.
9. Sinha AK, Cane C, Kempley ST. Blood flow in the common carotid artery in term and preterm infants: reproducibility and relation to cardiac output. Arch Dis Child. 2006;91:31-35.
10. Ehehalt S, Kehrer M, Goelz R, et al. Cerebral blood flow volume measurement with ultrasound: interobserver reproducibility in preterm and term neonates. Ultrasound Med Biol. 2005;31:191-196.
11. Brazy JE, Lewis DV, Mitnisk MH, et al. Noninvasive monitoring of cerebral oxygenation in preterm infants: preliminary observation. Pediatrics. 1985;75: 217-225.
12. Wyatt JS, Cope M, Delpy DT, et al. Quantification of cerebral oxygenation and haemodynamics in sick newborn infants by near infrared spectrophotometry. Lancet. 1986;2:1063-1066.
13. Matcher SJ, Elwell CE, Cooper CE, et al. Performance of several published tissue near infrared spectroscopy algorithms. Anal Biochem. 1995;227:54-68.
14. Edwards AD, Wyatt JS, Richardson CE, et al. Cotside measurement of cerebral blood flow in ill newborn infants by near-infrared spectroscopy. Lancet. 1988;2:770-771.
15. Skov L, Pryds O, Greisen G. Estimation cerebral blood flow in newborn infants: comparison of near infrared spectroscopy and ^{133}Xe clearance. Pediatr Res. 1991;30:570-573.
16. Bucher HU, Edwards AD, Lipp AE, et al. Comparison between near infrared spectroscopy and 133Xenon clearance for estimation of cerebral blood flow in critically ill preterm infants. Pediatr Res. 1993;33:56-60.
17. Patel J, Marks K, Roberts I, et al. Measurement of cerebral blood flow in newborn infants using near infrared spectroscopy with indocyanine green. Pediatr Res. 1998;643:34-39.
18. Brown DW, Picot PA, Naeini JG, et al. Quantitative near infrared spectroscopy measurement of cerebral hemodynamics in newborn piglets. Pediatr Res. 2002;51:564-570.
19. Kusaka T, Okubo K, Nagano K, et al. Cerebral distribution of cardiac output in newborn infants. Arch Dis Child Fetal Neonatal Ed. 2005;90:F77-F78.
20. Wagner BP, Gertsch S, Ammann RA, et al. Reproducibility of the blood flow index as noninvasive, bedside estimation of cerebral blood flow. Intensive Care Med. 2003;29(2):196-200.
21. Wagner BP, Ammann RA, Bachmann DC, et al. Rapid assessment of cerebral autoregulation by near-infrared spectroscopy and a single dose of phenylephrine. Pediatr Res. 2011 Jan 20. [Epub ahead of print].
22. Pryds O, Greisen G, Skov L, et al. The effect of PaCO2 induced increase in cerebral blood volume and cerebral blood flow in mechanically ventilated, preterm infants. Comparison of near infra-red spectrophotometry and 133Xenon clearance. Pediatr Res. 1990;27:445-449.
23. Brun NC, Moen A, Borch K, et al. Near-infrared monitoring of cerebral tissue oxygen saturation and blood volume in newborn piglets. Am J Physiol. 1997;273:H682-H686.
24. Tsuji M, Saul JP, du Plessis A, et al. Cerebral intravascular oxygenation correlates with mean arterial pressure in critically ill premature infants. Pediatrics. 2000;106;625-632.
25. Hahn GH, Christensen KB, Leung TS, et al. Precision of coherence analysis to detect cerebral auto-regulation by near-infrared spectroscopy in preterm infants. J Biomed Opt. 2010;15:037002.
26. Buckley EM, Cook NM, Durduran T, et al. Cerebral hemodynamics in preterm infants during posi-tional intervention measured with diffuse correlation spectroscopy and transcranial Doppler ultra-sound. Opt Express. 2009;17:12571-12581.
27. Durduran T, Zhou C, Buckley EM, et al. Optical measurement of cerebral hemodynamics and oxygen metabolism in neonates with congenital heart defects. J Biomed Opt. 2010;15:037004.
28. Suzuki S, Takasaki S, Ozaki T, et al. A tissue oxygenation monitor using NIR spatially resolved spectroscopy. SPIE. 1999;3597:582-592.
29. Ijichi S, Kusaka T, Isobe K, et al. Quantification of cerebral hemoglobin as a function of oxygenation using near-infrared time-resolved spectroscopy in a piglet model of hypoxia. J Biomed Optics. 2005;10:024-026.
30. Zhao J, Ding HS, Hou XL, et al. In vivo determination of the optical properties of infant brain using frequency-domain near-infrared spectroscopy. J Biomed Opt. 2005;10:024-028.
31. Nagdyman N, Fleck T, Schubert S, et al. Comparison between cerebral tissue oxygenation index measured by near-infrared spectroscopy and venous jugular bulb saturation in children. Intensive Care Med. 2005;31:846-850.
32. Dullenkopf A, Kolarova A, Schulz G, et al. Reproducibility of cerebral oxygenation measurement in neonates and infants in the clinical setting using the NIRO 300 oximeter. Pediatr Crit Care Med. 2005;6:344-347.

4

B

33. Sorensen LC, Greisen G. Precision of measurement of cerebral tissue oxygenation index using near infrared spectroscopy in term and preterm infants. J Biomed Op. 2006;11:05400.
34. Benders MJ, Hendrikse J, de Vries LS, et al. Phase contrast magnetic resonance angiography measurements of global cerebral blood flow in the neonate. Pediatr Res. 2011 Feb 28. [Epub ahead of print].
35. Tanner SF, Cornette L, Ramenghi LA, et al. Cerebral perfusion in infants and neonates: preliminary results obtained using dynamic susceptibility contrast enhanced magnetic resonance imaging. Arch Dis Child. 2003;88:525-530.
36. Wang J, Licht DJ, Jahng GH, et al. Pediatric perfusion imaging using arterial spin labelling. J Magn Res Imag. 2003;18:404-413.
37. Licht DJ, Wang J, Silvestre DW, et al. Preoperative cerebral blood flow is diminished in neonates with severe congenital heart defects. J Thorac Cardiovasc Surg. 2004;128:841-849.
38. Sharples PM, Stuart AG, Aynsley-Green A, et al. A practical method of serial bedside measurement of cerebral blood flow and metabolism during neurointensive care. Arch Dis Child. 1991;66:1326-1332.
39. Garfunkel JM, Baird HW, Siegler J. The relationship of oxygen consumption to cerebral functional activity. J Pediatr. 1954;44:64-72.
40. Frewen TC, Kissoon N, Kronick J, et al. Cerebral blood flow, cross-brain oxygen extraction, and fontanelle pressure after hypoxic-ischemic injury in newborn infants. J Pediatr. 1991;118:265-271.
41. Greisen G, Pryds O. Intravenous ^{133}Xe clearance in preterm neonates with respiratory distress. Internal validation of CBF-infinity as a measure of global cerebral blood flow. Scand J Clin Lab Invest. 1988;48:673-678.
42. Greisen G, Trojaborg W. Cerebral blood flow, PaCO2 changes, and visual evoked potentials in mechanically ventilated, preterm infants. Acta Paediatr Scand. 1987;76:394-400.
43. Rubinstein M, Denays R, Ham HR, et al. Functional imaging of brain maturation in humans using iodine ^{123}I-iodoamphetamine and SPECT. J Nucl Med. 1989;30:1982-1985.
44. Denays R, Ham H, Tondear M, et al: Detection of bilateral and symmetrical anomalies in technecium-99 HMPAO brain SPECT studies. J Nucl Med. 1992;33:485-490.
45. Chiron C, Raynaud C, Maziere B, et al. Changes in regional cerebral blood flow during brain maturation in children and adolescents. J Nucl Med. 1992;33:696-703.
46. Ashwal S, Schneider S, Thompson J. Xenon computed tomography measuring blood flow in the determination of brain death in children. Ann Neurol. 1989;25:539-546.
47. Volpe JJ, Herscovitch P, Perlman JM, et al. Positron emission tomography in the newborn. Extensive impairment of regional cerebral blood flow with intraventricular hemorrhage and hemorrhagic cerebral involvement. Pediatrics. 1983;72:589-601.
48. Powers WJ, Raichle ME. Positron emission tomography and its application to the study of cerebrovascular disease in man. Stroke. 1985;16:361-376.
49. Chugani HT, Phelps ME, Mazziotta JC. Positron emission tomography study of human brain functional development. Ann Neurol. 1987;22:487-497.
50. Altman DI, Perlman JM, Volpe JJ, et al. Cerebral oxygen metabolism in newborns. Pediatrics. 1993;92:99-104.
51. Cross KW, Dear PRF, Hathorn MKS, et al. An estimation of intracranial blood flow in the newborn infant. J Physiol. 1979;289:329-345.
52. Colditz P, Greisen G, Pryds O. Comparison of electrical impedance and ^{133}Xe clearance for the assessment of cerebral blood flow in the newborn infant. Pediatr Res. 1988;24:461-464.
53. Zaramella P, Freato F, Quaresima V, et al. Foot pulse oximeter perfusion index correlates with calf muscle perfusion measured by near-infrared spectroscopy in healthy neonates. J Perinatol. 2005;25:417-422.

CHAPTER 5

Functional Echocardiography in the Neonatal Intensive Care Unit

Nicholas J. Evans, DM, MRCPCH

A continuing unresolved issue in the intensive care of the newborn infant is the lack of tools with which to monitor cardiovascular and hemodynamic function. In most neonatal intensive care units (NICUs), there is the ability to continuously monitor invasive blood pressure and heart rate and that is all. Beyond that, heavy reliance is often placed on poorly validated and probably inaccurate measures of hemodynamic well-being such as acid-base status, skin capillary refill time, and urine output. In the intensive care of the older subject, there is a range of tools for monitoring cardiac output such as thermodilution, continuous Doppler methodologies, and derivations from blood pressure waveforms (Chapter 6).[1] None of these are available for the neonate, partly because of the need to miniaturize, partly because of commercial conceptions of the NICU as a limited market, and partly because of the complexities of the transitional circulation. The only available, noninvasive method to continuously monitor cardiac output in neonates is based on a novel approach to electrical impedance monitoring (see Chapter 6). However, this method has not yet been validated in neonates.

Doppler echocardiography provides a noninvasive technique from which it is possible to derive estimates of a wide range of hemodynamic parameters. Traditionally, it has been specialists who work predominantly outside the NICU (mainly cardiologists) who have had the skills to derive these measures. This resulted in a predominantly snapshot picture of neonatal hemodynamics. Increasingly, neonatal intensivists are developing echocardiographic skills themselves.[2] The fact that they are in the NICU all the time has allowed more systematic serial studies, which, in turn, is allowing the research and clinical monitoring potential of these methodologies to develop further. This chapter describes the functional Doppler echocardiographic measures that can be used in the assessment of the sick newborn infant and how they can be used in common clinical scenarios. Other chapters in this book provide more details on findings using some of these methods and how the information derived might be used to guide clinical management.

Doppler Ultrasound

In the simplest terms, ultrasounds reflect off solid or liquid interfaces of different densities to allow definition of structure. In the heart, this is the interface between muscle, fiber, and blood. Projection of these structures against time allows definition of movement, both of the structures themselves but also relative to other structures. This is the essence of M-mode and two-dimensional (2-D) imaging.

The Doppler principle can be applied to ultrasounds because they change frequency as they reflect off moving objects. The direction of change in frequency depends on the direction of movement of the object. Movement toward the transmission source increases frequency while movement away decreases the frequency. This frequency shift is directly proportional to the velocity of the moving object as long as the direction of movement, or angle of insonation, is within 20° of straight toward or straight away from the transmission source. So when this is applied to blood moving in the heart and blood vessels, the various types of Doppler allow determination of both direction and velocity of blood flow.

Accurate determination of velocity allows two further factors to be derived. Firstly, the pressure gradient can be determined via the modified Bernoulli equation. This describes the relationship between pressure gradient and velocity in a fluid stream (pressure gradient = $4 \times$ velocity^2). Secondly, because flow of a fluid in streamline is the product of mean velocity and cross-sectional area of the stream, if we can estimate the diameter of a blood vessel and measure the mean velocity of the blood, we can estimate blood flow. In the neonate, these flow measures can really only be made in major vessels, as smaller peripheral vessels are too small to measure size accurately.

Two-Dimensional Imaging and Normal Cardiac Structure

The prerequisite to developing skills in functional echocardiography is a good understanding of cardiac anatomy and the ability to obtain and understand 2-D images from each of the four main ultrasound windows. A common starting point for people wanting to learn echocardiography has been to look over the shoulder of an experienced operator. Many an ultrasound ambition has fallen fallow in this wasteland of a learning approach. You will never learn this way; your understanding will always be one step behind the operator. As ultrasound is essentially a process of converting a 3-D structure into a series of 2-D cuts, if you understand the anatomy in spatial terms, the 2-D images will explain themselves. If you do not understand the anatomy, the 2-D images will remain a mystery. The heart is more difficult to conceptualize in 3-D space than other organs because it is not symmetrical but with application this understanding is possible.

It is beyond the scope of this chapter to describe normal 2-D imaging in detail; other resources are available.[3,4] However, to illustrate the points made here, the reader is taken through one view that is particularly useful for hemodynamic assessment: the low parasternal long axis view of the pulmonary artery. The four images in Figure 5-1 represent the chambers of the heart being progressively built up from back to front. On each image, the white line represents where the ultrasound beam will cut in the image. By examining how the line transects each of the structures, you should be able to build up in your own mind how the image will look. This is shown (with more detailed explanation in the legend) for both the heart model and an ultrasound image in Figure 5-2. The pulmonary artery is particularly good for

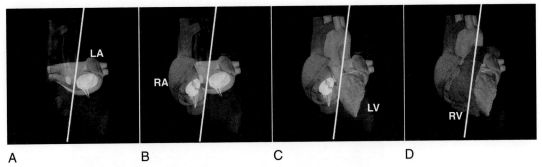

A   B   C   D

Figure 5-1   These four frames show the chambers of the heart being progressively added from back to front. The white line shows where the ultrasound beam will transect the heart. **A,** The left atrium (LA) at the back of heart with two pulmonary veins coming in each side posteriorly. **B,** The right atrium (RA), which is to the right and slightly in front of the LA. **C,** The endocardial surface of the left ventricle (LV), which receives blood toward the apex through the mitral valve and ejects it into the ascending aorta, which runs toward the right shoulder in front of the LA. **D,** The anterior nature of the right ventricle, which wraps in front of the LV outflow tract before ejecting blood posteriorly into the pulmonary artery. (See Expert Consult site for color image.)

Doppler studies because its posterior direction takes the blood directly away from the transducer at a minimal angle of insonation. A basic understanding of 2-D imaging can be derived from learning three to four images like this for each of the four ultrasound windows, subcostal, apical, and low and high parasternal.

M-mode ultrasound was the precursor to 2-D imaging and is where ultrasounds down one transmission line are plotted against time (Fig. 5-3). It remains a useful modality for assessing movement of structures and the higher resolution and edge definition allow for more accurate measurement of dimensions at defined time points in the cardiac cycle.

Types of Doppler

There are three main types of Doppler in common usage: pulsed wave, continuous wave, and color Doppler. Pulsed wave Doppler is most commonly used because it allows you to focus your velocity assessment at a particular site through an operator guided "range gate" (Fig. 5-4). The limitation of pulsed wave is that it cannot assess higher velocities, usually those greater than about 2 m/s. Continuous wave Doppler allows assessment of higher velocities but is less focused, receiving signals from the whole path of transmission. Typically both pulsed and continuous wave Doppler are

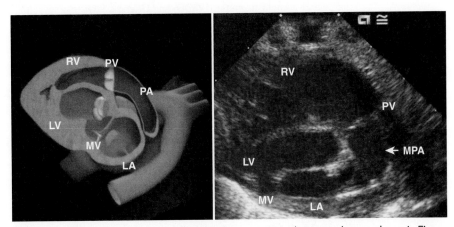

Figure 5-2   A heart model and an ultrasound picture cut in the same plane as shown in Figure 5-1. The RV is seen at the front connecting with the posteriorly directed pulmonary artery. Behind the RV is the LV outflow tract and the LA and mitral valve. (See Expert Consult site for color image.)

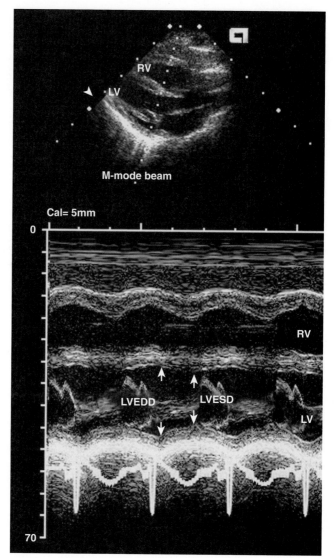

Figure 5-3 M-mode plots the ultrasound signals from the single beam (shown on a 2-D image) against time. This allows movement and dimensions to be more accurately measured. The LV end-diastolic diameter (LVEDD) and LV end-systolic diameter (LVESD) are shown. (See Expert Consult site for color image.)

displayed as a velocity time plot, with flow toward the transducer shown as a positive plot and away as a negative plot (see Fig. 5-4).

Color Doppler is a development of pulsed wave Doppler where the frequency shift is mapped onto the 2-D image, with flow toward and away from the transducer plotted as different colors. Conventionally, flow away is mapped as blue and toward is mapped as red. Color Doppler has a range of uses but is particularly useful in functional echocardiography to guide pulsed Doppler study and to assess patency of the ductus arteriosus (see Fig. 5-4).

What Can Be Measured with Functional Echocardiography in the Neonatal Intensive Care Units?

There are a range of parameters that can be assessed using functional echocardiography, including ductal and atrial shunting (presence, direction, and degree),

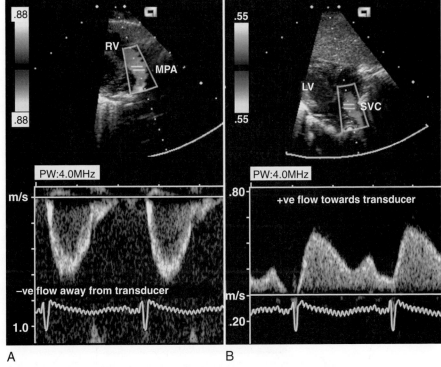

Figure 5-4 Pulsed Doppler assesses flow velocity at a defined location (= sign on 2-D image). Flow away from the transducer is negative **(A)** and toward the transducer positive **(B)**. Color Doppler maps those signals onto the 2-D image with flow away coded blue **(A)** and toward coded red **(B)**. (See Expert Consult site for color image.)

pulmonary artery pressure, flow measures (right and left ventricular output and superior vena cava flow), and myocardial function measures. One factor to emphasize is the close interrelationship of many of these measures. It is a basic rule of fluid mechanics that measurement at a single point in a streamline can be influenced by factors both upstream and downstream of that point. So it is in the heart where, if you take a single measurement, you will often not be able to interpret that measure unless you know what is happening both upstream and downstream from that measure. A commonly encountered example of this in neonatology is a left-to-right ductal shunt, which will increase the volume load (preload) on the left ventricle and reduce the afterload. So measures of left ventricular input and output in the presence of a significant ductal shunt will be high and measures of function very good, but neither will give you any information about the well-being of the systemic circulation. For this reason, studies, whether for research or clinical reasons, need to be as complete as possible.

It also needs to be emphasized that, in common with all noninvasive measures, there are limitations to the accuracy of Doppler ultrasound measurements. Most will have intraobserver variability of about 10% and interobserver variability of about 20%. The findings need to be interpreted with these limitations to accuracy in mind. These limitations will be minimized if you use more than one method to measure a parameter as a cross-check, take averages from repeated measures, and limit the number of different observers taking a measurement in the same baby.

We now start by discussing the factors that define the complexity of the transitional circulation relative to the mature circulation, the shunts through the fetal channels, and the potential lability of pulmonary vascular resistance and hence pulmonary arterial pressure.

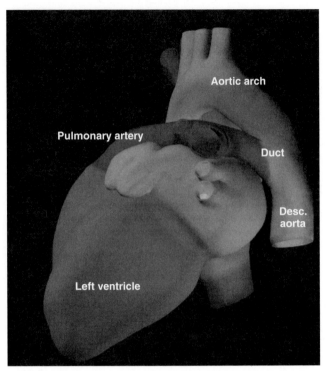

Figure 5-5 A model of the heart viewed from the left-hand side. It can be seen that the ductus arteriosus is a continuation of the pulmonary artery and describes an arch into the descending aorta. It is slightly offset to the left reflecting the need to connect with the left-sided descending aorta. (See Expert Consult site for color image.)

Ductal Shunting

Ductal Patency and Direction of Shunting

Many neonatologists have a conception of the ductus arteriosus as a dichotomous variable, that is, it is either open or closed. Nothing could be further from the truth and, when viewing the duct with ultrasound, there is great variability both in size (or degree of constriction) and the direction of shunting. The duct can be directly imaged with 2-D ultrasound. Anatomically, it is a continuation of the main pulmonary artery that is slightly offset to the left reflecting the arch it describes into the descending aorta (Fig. 5-5). Thus with the ultrasound transducer placed at the left upper sternal edge and the beam in a true sagittal plane (straight up and down the body), the duct can be seen leaving the main pulmonary artery close to the junction with the left pulmonary artery and describing an arch into the descending aorta. Patent ducts that are minimally constricted are readily apparent on 2-D imaging (Fig. 5-6), but differentiating a functionally closed from a well-constricted duct needs color Doppler. Figure 5-7A shows the predominantly blue color Doppler of flow in the main and left pulmonary artery with no flow apparent through the duct. Two-dimensional imaging with color Doppler allows assessment not only of ductal patency but also the degree of ductal constriction. The contrast between the well-constricted duct in Fig. 5-7B and the unconstricted one in Fig. 5-7C is apparent. With a well-optimized color Doppler study, it is possible to derive a semi-quantitative assessment of the degree of constriction by measuring the minimum diameter of the shunt within the course of the ductus.[5]

Color Doppler also allows some assessment of the direction of shunting but accurate assessment of direction of shunting requires pulsed Doppler. The direction of blood flow through the duct is determined by the continuum of the relative

5

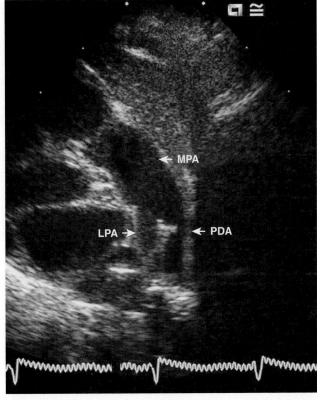

Figure 5-6 A 2-D image of a patent duct adjacent to the root of the left pulmonary artery, which is seen in this section as a diverticulum inferior to the duct. The duct describes an arch that is in continuity with the anterior wall of the main pulmonary artery. (See Expert Consult site for color image.)

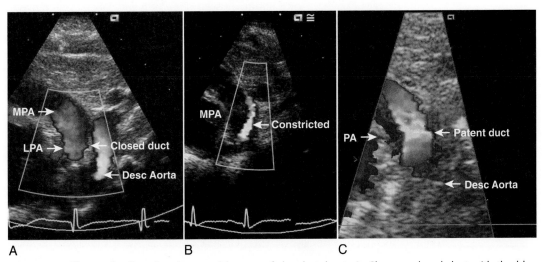

A   B   C

Figure 5-7 Three-color Doppler ultrasound images of the ductal cut. **A,** Shows a closed duct with the blue streams of the pulmonary artery and descending aorta. The absence of color in the line of the duct shows that it is functionally closed. **B,** Shows the red stream of a left-to-right shunt through a constricted duct, streaming back up the anterior wall of the pulmonary artery. **C,** Shows a left-to-right shunt though an unconstricted duct. (See Expert Consult site for color image.)

B

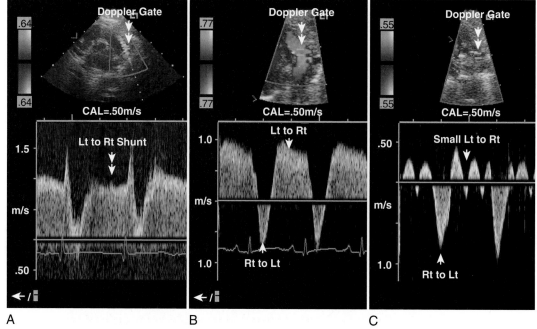

A   B   C

Figure 5-8   The range of pattern of ductal shunt on pulsed Doppler. **A,** Shows the positive (toward the transducer) trace of a pure left-to-right shunt. **B,** Shows a bidirectional shunt with both left-to-right (positive) and right-to-left (negative) components. **C,** Shows a predominantly right-to-left (negative) shunt but with some left-to-right shunt in diastole. Pure right-to-left ductal shunts are uncommon. (See Expert Consult site for color image.)

pressure at each end. When pulmonary pressures are clearly below systemic the shunt will be left to right (Fig. 5-8A); when they are well above systemic pressures, the shunt will be right to left (Fig. 5-8C). When pulmonary pressures are close to but are not clearly above or below systemic pressures throughout the cardiac cycle, varying degrees of bidirectional shunt are seen (Fig. 5-8B and 5-8C). This range of shunt pattern allows assessment of pulmonary artery pressure (described later).

Determination of Hemodynamic Significance

Echocardiographic determination of patency and shunt direction is relatively straightforward; more controversial are the criteria that should be applied to determine hemodynamic significance. In cardiology, the size of a left-to-right shunt is often expressed as the ratio of pulmonary to systemic blood flow (Qp:Qs); this, in turn, can be derived by measuring both ventricular outputs with Doppler. With a ductal shunt, the left ventricular output measures the pulmonary blood flow and the right ventricular output, the systemic blood flow. Unfortunately, you cannot use this routinely in the transitional circulation because of the interatrial shunts, discussed later, which confound right ventricular output as a measure of systemic blood flow.[6] We were able to measure Qp:Qs in a cohort of preterm babies with a patent ductus arteriosus (PDA) in whom there was minimal atrial shunting and compare it to a variety of suggested criteria of ductus arteriosus hemodynamic significance.[7] The criteria that had the closest correlation with Qp:Qs was the diameter as measured from the color Doppler as shown in Fig. 5-7. In babies born before 30 weeks during the postnatal week, if the ductal diameter was less than 1.5 mm, the shunt was usually insignificant; if greater than 1.5 mm, the shunt was usually significant. If the diameter was over 2 mm, the Qp:Qs was usually more than 2:1 (i.e., pulmonary blood flow twice as high as systemic). The other measure that was useful was the pattern of diastolic flow in the postductal descending aorta. Normally this flow is forward but, in the presence of an increasing shunt back through a duct, this flow direction becomes progressively absent and then retrograde (Fig. 5-9). In the

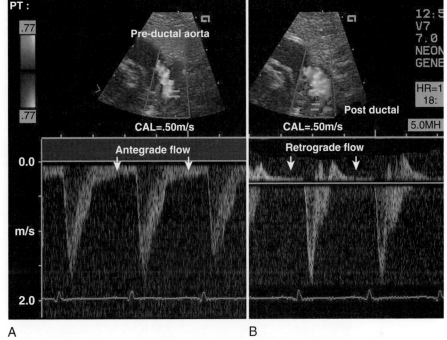

Figure 5-9 Compares the normal forward diastolic flow **(A)**, which is also seen with a patent ductus arteriosus (PDA) in the preductal aorta with the retrograde diastolic flow seen in the postductal aorta in the presence of a significant PDA. (See Expert Consult site for color image.)

aforementioned studies, retrograde diastolic flow was associated with a mean Qp:Qs of 1.6 (i.e., pulmonary blood flow is 60% more than systemic).[7] The same phenomenon that reduces diastolic flow in the postductal aorta also increases diastolic flow in the branch pulmonary arteries. So increased diastolic and/or mean velocities in the left pulmonary artery (LPA) has been described as a marker of significance.[8] This measure does have the advantage of being technically easier than Doppler in the postductal aorta, just requiring a small adjustment of the Doppler range gate from the ductus into the left pulmonary artery (Fig. 5-10).

El Hajjar and colleagues performed a similar validation but used superior vena cava (SVC) flow (see later) as a surrogate for Qs to avoid the confounding effect of any atrial shunt.[9] They studied a cohort of 23 babies born before 31 weeks and found that ductal diameter over 1.4 mm/kg, left atrial to aortic root ratio (LA:Ao) over 1.4, LPA mean velocity over 0.42 m/s or LPA diastolic velocity over 0.2 m/s, all predicted an left ventricular output (LVO):SVC ratio greater than 4 (approx Qp:Qs > 2) with more than 90% specificity and sensitivity. In clinical practice having determined that the predominant direction of shunting was left to right, we would use the diameter of the duct as the primary determinant of significance and the direction of diastolic flow in the descending aorta and LPA diastolic velocities as confirmatory adjunct measures.

Natural History of Postnatal Constriction

In healthy term babies, the ductus constricts quickly after birth but some shunting is commonly apparent on color Doppler during the first 12-24 hours.[10,11] In term babies with high oxygen requirements, the ductus also usually constricts quickly, particularly when the problem is primarily in the pulmonary parenchyma. A minority of such babies will have a patent ductus after postnatal day 1.[12] In term babies with primary persistent pulmonary hypertension of the newborn (PPHN), the ductus is more likely to remain patent but is still often well constricted.[12]

In the preterm population, the constriction of the ductus in the early hours after birth varies widely from those where the constriction would be equivalent to

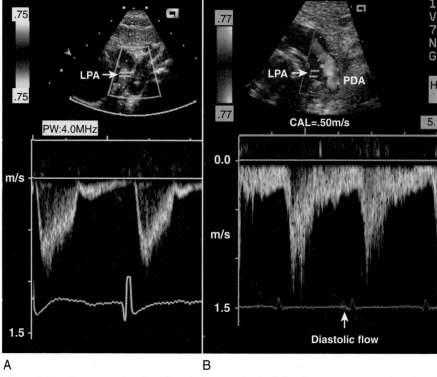

Figure 5-10 Compares the diastolic velocity seen in the left pulmonary artery with a closed duct with the increased diastolic velocity (in this case 0.5 m/s) seen with a significant PDA. (See Expert Consult site for color image.)

a term baby to those where there is no constriction.[13,14] Contrary to popular belief, even at this early time, the dominant direction of shunting is left to right. In those babies where constriction fails, large systemic to pulmonary shunts can result. So the hemodynamic impact of a ductal shunt in reducing systemic blood flow and increasing pulmonary blood flow can be present from very early after birth.[14] These shunts are invariably clinically silent in the first 2 days, so will only be detected if looked for echocardiographically.[15,16] The degree of early ductal constriction also predicts persisting patency, so early echocardiography may offer a way of targeting early treatment of the duct.[5,13,14,17]

Atrial Shunting

The incompetent foramen ovale is commonly considered as a site for right-to-left shunting but not for the much more common left-to-right shunting (Fig. 5-11).[6,7] The atrial septum is best imaged from the subcostal four-chamber view. From this window, it can be imaged in its full length with the foramen ovale easily distinguishable as the loose foraminal flap tissue moves both ways during the cardiac cycle. Some assessment of the relative pressures in the two atria can be derived from this movement but assessment of shunting needs color Doppler. The color Doppler scale needs to be optimized for the usual low velocity of interatrial shunts and, when placed over the foramen ovale, the stream of any shunt should be apparent (see Fig. 5-11). Some assessment of the degree of atrial shunting can be derived from the size of the color stream and the ease with which it is imaged.[6,7] Like in the ductus, color Doppler gives a good impression of shunt direction but accurate assessment requires pulsed Doppler. The shunt patterns between the atria are complex reflecting a complex pressure relationship. Some shunting through the foramen ovale is commonly apparent even in normal healthy babies and although the dominant direction

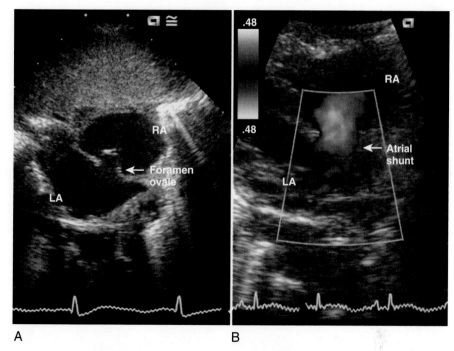

Figure 5-11 A, The 2-D appearance of the atrial septum and foramen ovale in the subcostal four-chamber view. **B,** The color Doppler of a left-to-right shunt through an incompetent foramen ovale. (See Expert Consult site for color image.)

of shunting is left to right, it is very common to detect a short period of right-to-left shunt in diastole (Fig. 5-12). Thus some degree of bidirectional shunting is a normal finding in the newborn. Indeed, Hiraishi and colleagues demonstrated that right-to-left atrial shunting for up to 30% of the cardiac cycle was normal in the neonate.[18] As right heart pressures rise, the duration of right-to-left shunting within the cardiac cycle will increase. A pure right-to-left atrial shunt is surprisingly uncommon in babies with pulmonary hypertension although you do see it in extreme cases. A pure right-to-left atrial shunt should always raise the possibility of congenital heart disease such as total anomalous pulmonary venous drainage.

In the term baby, left-to-right atrial shunting is usually trivial and transient but, in the preterm baby, it can be both significant and quite persistent.[6] The foramen ovale becomes smaller relative to the rest of the heart during the last trimester, so some of this may relate to structural immaturity. However, it is also related to ductal shunting, which will volume load the left atrium increasing the pressure and driving the left-to-right atrial shunt. It is not uncommon in babies with quite significant ductal shunts to find there is even more blood moving left to right at the atrial level than at the ductal level, and thus both shunts will contribute to a high pulmonary blood flow.[6,7]

Ductal and atrial shunts may not necessarily be in the same direction. This reflects the fact that atrial shunting is determined predominantly by filling (or diastolic pressures) while ductal shunting is determined by pressure throughout the cardiac cycle. Thus it is not uncommon to have a predominantly right-to-left but bidirectional ductal shunt together with a predominantly left-to-right atrial shunt.

Pulmonary Artery Pressure

There are three main methods for estimating pulmonary artery pressure, each of which has strengths and weaknesses. The best methods, because you get a number, involve application of the modified Bernoulli equation to a ductal shunt or a tricuspid incompetence jet.

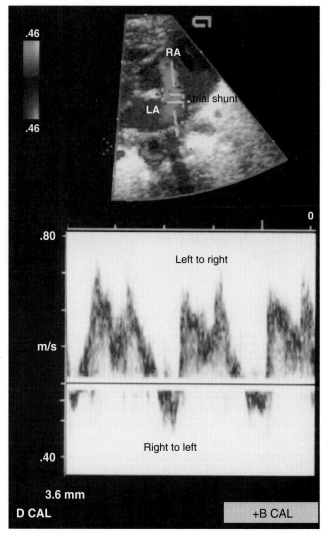

Figure 5-12 Pulsed Doppler of a normal bidirectional atrial shunt with a short period of right-to-left shunting followed by left-to-right shunting. (See Expert Consult site for color image.)

Pulmonary Artery Pressure from a Ductal Shunt

The modified Bernoulli equation states that the pressure gradient down which a fluid stream is traveling will be $4 \times velocity^2$. Thus if we know the pressure in the systemic circulation and we know velocity of a ductal shunt, we can calculate the pressure gradient across the ductus and so derive the pulmonary artery pressure. For example, if a baby has a left-to-right ductal shunt with a maximum velocity of 2 m/s then the pulmonary artery pressure must be $4 \times 2^2 = 16$ mm Hg *less* than the systemic pressure. If the shunt were right to left at 2 m/s then the pulmonary artery pressure must be 16 mm Hg *more* than systemic pressure.

This is not so straightforward with the common bidirectional ductal shunt pattern that appears as pulmonary pressures start to rise. This bidirectional pattern results from the fact that the pressure wave at each end of the duct is not synchronous (Fig. 5-13). The pressure wave from the right heart arrives before that from the left. This means that there is some right-to-left shunting in early systole well before pulmonary pressures exceed systemic. It can be seen from Fig. 5-13 that, as pulmonary artery pressure rises relative to systemic, so the velocity and duration of right-to-left shunting will increase. Musewe and colleagues estimated that, when the

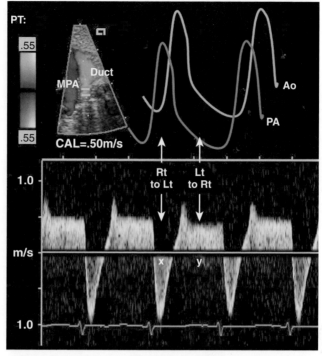

Figure 5-13 The two waveforms represent the simultaneous pressure wave at the pulmonary (blue) and aortic (red) end of the duct. The pressure wave at the pulmonary end rises before that at the aortic end. As pulmonary pressure rises (but remains sub-systemic) some right-to-left shunting occurs in early systole. As pulmonary pressure rises further so the duration of this right-to-left shunt (x) increases. When the duration of right-to-left shunt is more than about 30% of the cardiac cycle, pulmonary pressure is usually suprasystemic. (See Expert Consult site for color image.)

duration of right-to-left shunt was more than about 30% of the cardiac cycle, pulmonary artery pressure was usually suprasystemic.[19] Less than 30% of the cardiac cycle suggests pulmonary artery pressure is less than systemic. So our approach with bidirectional shunting is to measure the duration of right-to-left shunting; then, if it is more than 30%, use the right-to-left velocity to estimate the pulmonary artery pressure (PAP). On the other hand, if it is less than 30%, we use the left-to-right velocity. Apart from this complication, the ductal shunt is very useful for estimating PAP. The main limitation is that the duct will often close, particularly in more mature babies.

Pulmonary Artery Pressure from Tricuspid Incompetence

Incompetence of the tricuspid valve in systole is common in the neonate during the transitional period. It is also more likely to be present with pulmonary hypertension, probably because of the tendency for a dilated right ventricle to dilate the tricuspid valve ring. The velocity of this incompetent jet can be measured with Doppler and, again using the modified Bernoulli equation, the pressure gradient across the tricuspid valve between the right ventricle and right atrium can be assessed. Because we know that right atrial pressure is usually low (5-10 mm Hg), this gradient will approximate to the right ventricular systolic pressure. As long as the pulmonary valve is normal, right ventricular systolic pressure will be the same as pulmonary artery pressure. So if the maximum velocity of a tricuspid incompetence jet is 3 m/s, then the pressure gradient is $4 \times 3^2 = 36$ mm Hg. Conventionally, 5 mm Hg is added to this gradient to reflect right atrial pressure. So the estimated systolic pulmonary artery pressure in this case would be 41 mm Hg (Fig. 5-14).

The accuracy of this method is dependent on minimizing the angle of insonation. Tricuspid incompetence jets can vary in direction, so this is an important potential

B

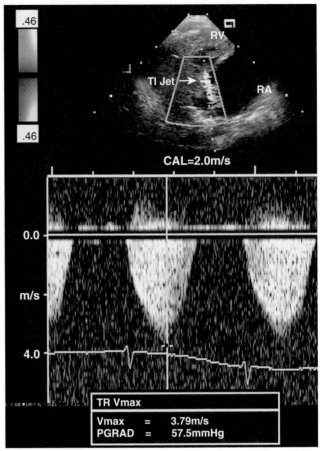

Figure 5-14 An example of tricuspid incompetence. The maximum velocity (Vmax) is 3.79 m/s. This means that the pressure gradient (PGRAD) across the valve is $4 \times 3.79^2 = 57.5$ mm Hg. Adding 5 mm Hg for right atrial pressure, this means that the RV systolic pressure is about 63 mm Hg; this will be the same as pulmonary artery systolic pressure. (See Expert Consult site for color image.)

source of error. When present, this is probably the most accurate of the indirect methods.[20,21] However, the main limitation is that many babies in whom you want to measure pulmonary artery pressure will not have a tricuspid incompetence jet. It was present in only 50% of a cohort of term babies with high oxygen requirements that we studied. Further when pulmonary artery pressure drops, the tricuspid incompetence often disappears, so it is not a very good method for serially monitoring change in pulmonary artery pressure.

Pulmonary Artery Doppler Time to Peak Velocity

This method relies on the observation that as the pulmonary artery pressure rises so the time taken for systolic blood flow to reach its peak velocity in the main pulmonary artery will get shorter.[22] This time to peak velocity (TPV) can be measured and is usually expressed as a ratio to the total right ventricular ejection time (RVET). This method has important limitations to its accuracy and is vulnerable to a range of confounders such as right ventricular dysfunction or position of the Doppler range gate. It has also been shown to be of limited accuracy when PAP is raised due to left-to-right shunting.[23]

Pressure is the product of flow and resistance and may be raised if either or both are raised. Considering the physics of this phenomenon, it is probably more a measure of resistance or compliance of the pulmonary circulation. Hence it may be more accurate when pressure is high due to high resistance rather than high flow. It is probably best regarded as a "ballpark" measure when neither of the other two methods discussed earlier are available. Using this approximation approach, TPV:RVET ratios greater than 0.3 are normal, 0.2-0.3 suggest moderately raised pulmonary artery pressure, and less than 0.2 suggest significantly raised pulmonary artery pressure.[24,25]

Measurement of Blood Flow and Cardiac Output

The physics of fluid dynamics dictate that blood flow within a vessel is the product of the mean velocity of flow and the cross-sectional area of that vessel. With Doppler, it is possible to measure velocity as long as there is a minimal angle of insonation and, with the major vessels around the heart, it is possible to derive cross-sectional area, either directly or by estimating from a measured diameter. These two measures have different methodological requirements, in that velocity measurement requires the blood to be flowing at 0° or 180° to the direction of the ultrasound beam and the best measurement of edges with ultrasound is achieved when the ultrasound beam hits the vessel at 90°. These issues mean that there is a significant intrinsic error associated with these measurements. This is particularly true when cross-sectional area is derived from a diameter where the conversion will magnify the error. Notwithstanding these problems, we do not have any better method for measuring blood flow in major vessels around the heart in neonatology. The most commonly used measures of blood flow in the heart have been the ventricular outputs, particularly left ventricular output.

Left Ventricular Output

Left ventricular (LV) output is derived by measuring blood flow in the ascending aorta. The ascending aorta leaves the heart more horizontally than in an adult, heading initially in the direction of the right shoulder. This direction makes it a great vessel for measuring diameter but an awkward vessel for minimizing angle of insonation to measure velocity. Diameter is usually derived by imaging the ascending aorta in the long axis from the low parasternal window (Fig. 5-15). There is some argument in the literature about the best site for diameter measurement. We have always used the end-systolic internal diameter just beyond the coronary sinus (Fig. 5-15). Others argue that the diameter of the aortic valve ring or of systolic leaflet separation is more accurate. Probably, where you measure is less important than measuring at a consistent site, in a consistent way, and at a consistent time in the cardiac cycle. Cross-sectional area is derived from πr^2. Velocity is best measured from the apical or the suprasternal window but from either view it is difficult to minimize the angle of insonation. Our preference is the apical long axis view because it is better tolerated by the babies.[26] The Doppler range gate is placed just beyond the aortic valve and the velocity time trace is recorded. Mean velocity is usually measured as the area under the systolic envelope called the velocity time integral (VTI) and we would usually average this from five cardiac cycles. Using these measures:

$$\text{stroke volume} = \text{VTI} \times \text{cross-sectional area (mL)}$$

and

$$\text{cardiac output} = \text{stroke volume} \times \text{heart rate (mL/min)}$$

usually also divided by body weight to give mL/kg/min.

This method of measuring LV output has been validated against other more invasive methods.[27,28] In general, the correlation against a range of "gold standards" is good although there is significant interobserver and intraobserver variability. Intraobserver variability is estimated at about 10% and interobserver at about 20%, so ideally serial studies should be made by the same person.[29] The main problem with LV output as a measure of systemic blood flow in the neonate, particularly the premature neonate, is the extent to which it is confounded by a left-to-right ductal

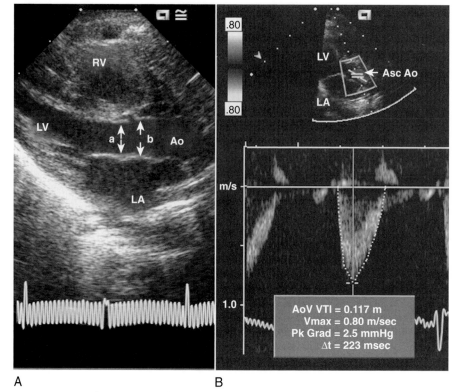

Figure 5-15   A, Shows the site of measurement of aortic diameter. Some authors recommend measurement of valve ring or leaflet separation (a); we usually use the internal diameter beyond the coronary sinus (b). **B,** Shows pulsed Doppler assessment of ascending aortic velocity from the apical long axis view. Velocity time integral (VTI) is derived by tracing around the systolic spectral envelope (VTI = 0.117 m in this case). (See Expert Consult site for color image.)

shunt. If you consider Fig. 5-16, you can see that, in the presence of a ductal shunt, LV output is the sum of systemic blood flow and the shunt across the duct and so it will overestimate systemic blood flow. In fact within this hemodynamic situation, LV output is actually measuring pulmonary blood flow and it is the right ventricular (RV) output that is measuring systemic blood flow. For this reason, RV output is a better measure of systemic blood flow than LV output.

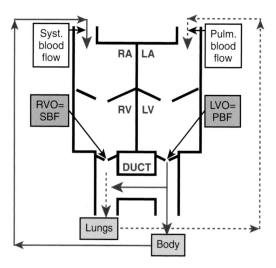

Figure 5-16 This schematic diagram of the heart highlights how, in the presence of a left-to-right ductal shunt, LV output (LVO) is measuring the sum of systemic blood flow and the ductal shunt. This is actually pulmonary blood flow (PBF) and it is RV output (RVO) that is measuring systemic blood flow (SBF).

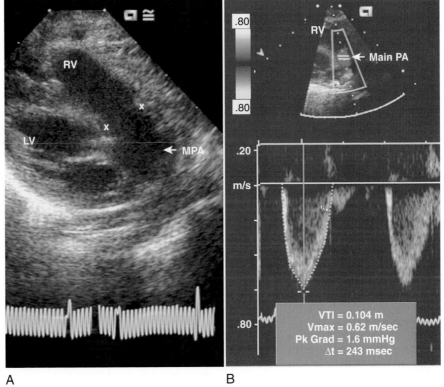

Figure 5-17   A, Shows the site of measurement of pulmonary artery diameter, in end-systole at the valve hinge points. **B,** Shows pulsed Doppler assessment of main pulmonary artery velocity with the range gate just beyond the valve. Velocity time integral (VTI) is derived by tracing around the systolic spectral envelope (VTI = 0.104 m in this case). (See Expert Consult site for color image.)

Right Ventricular Output

This is derived by measuring blood flow in the main pulmonary artery. The main pulmonary artery (MPA) heads in a predominantly posterior direction before bifurcating into the two main branches. This direction makes the MPA a great vessel on which to perform Doppler from the low parasternal window with a minimal angle of insonation but not such a good vessel in which to derive diameter. The pulmonary artery is imaged in the long axis as described under the earlier section on "Two-Dimensional Imaging and Normal Cardiac Structure." We measure diameter from the 2-D image at the insertion of the pulmonary valve leaflets, advancing frame by frame until end-systole, just before the valve closes (Fig. 5-17). The anterior wall is often the most difficult to get a clear view of and there is often a need to experiment with different transducer positions. Doppler is performed from the same window with the range gate just beyond the valve leaflets (see Fig. 5-17). This minimizes any disturbance to the flow pattern from ductal shunting. The measures are then used to calculate RV output in the same way as described for the LV output. Normal values for both right and left ventricular output would be in the range of 150-300 mL/kg/min.

There has been no direct validation of RV output measured in this way. In a group of babies with no atrial shunting and a closed ductus, we found a close correlation between RV output and the directly validated LV output.[7] Just as LV output can be confounded by a left-to-right ductal shunt, RV output can be confounded by a left-to-right atrial shunt.[6,7] While large ductal shunts can develop quite quickly after birth, atrial shunts often take longer to develop, so RV output is a reasonably accurate means of assessing systemic blood flow during the first 24 postnatal hours.

However, this variable and unpredictable confounding of both ventricular outputs as measures of systemic blood flow limits their use for studying the natural history of systemic blood flow in babies. Because of this, we developed the concept of measuring cardiac input rather than output, specifically measuring flow returning to the heart via the superior vena cava (SVC).

Superior Vena Cava Flow

Any pump within a closed fluid circuit can only pump out what returns to it and will only return to it what it pumps out. As input to the pump has to be the same as the output, so it is with the heart. The SVC is a good vessel for Doppler as the angle of insonation on flow is small from the low subcostal window and good images for diameter can be obtained from the parasternal window. From a physiologic point of view, SVC flow is not confounded by shunts through the fetal channels and it represents the portion of systemic blood flow that we are most interested in, that from the upper body and brain.[15,30] It is difficult to find firm data in the literature as to what proportion of upper body blood flow is cerebral blood flow (CBF), although estimates of 70-80% have been suggested for the neonate.[31]

Doppler velocity in the SVC is measured from the subcostal window with the transducer as low as possible to minimize the angle of insonation.[30] The range gate is placed in the mouth of the SVC just as it enters the right atrium. The velocity traces in the SVC can be quite pleomorphic particularly in babies that are breathing spontaneously and there is often some retrograde flow associated with atrial systole. So we would usually average from 10 cardiac cycles and would include any negative trace (Fig. 5-18). For diameter measurement, the SVC is imaged in the long axis from a low to mid-parasternal position and the SVC can be seen entering the right atrium, often deviating anteriorly just before entry.[30] This can be technically the most challenging part of this technique as, with postnatal age, the right lung often inflates over the window. The SVC also varies more in size than the great arteries during the cardiac cycle. To allow for this, we average a maximum and minimum diameter. Whether this is the physiologically correct way to compensate for the variation in diameter is open to question but we adopted this approach because it is simple and easy to apply. These maximum and minimum diameter measurements are much easier from an M-mode trace (see Fig. 5-18). However, as with all M-mode diameter measurement it is important to make sure the ultrasound beam is transecting the vessel at right angles. The calculation for SVC flow is then the same as for LV output. Mean SVC flows increase over the first 48 postnatal hours from about 70 mL/kg/min at 5 hours of age to 90 mL/kg/min at 48 hours. The normal range during the time frame would be between 40 and 120 mL/kg/min and, in babies with minimal shunting, SVC flow is usually between 30% and 50% of total ventricular output.[15,30]

Like RV output, SVC flow has not been directly validated against invasive measures but has been validated against Doppler measured LV output in babies with no shunts.[30] It is a more difficult technique to master than the ventricular outputs and is similarly vulnerable to error, probably more so when the SVC is difficult to image for diameter measurement. Its role is probably more as a research tool than a routine clinical tool and it has given us a consistent means with which to study the natural systemic blood flow in the very premature baby. The findings of these studies are discussed later and are covered in detail in Chapter 12.

Left Pulmonary Artery Velocities: Pulmonary Blood Flow

Just as the shunts through the fetal channels confound ventricular outputs as measures of systemic blood so they also confound them as measures of pulmonary blood flow (PBF). The impact of left-to-right atrial shunting on RV output has been mentioned earlier. A right-to-left ductal shunt will also confound RV output as a measure of PBF, as some of the blood leaving the right ventricle will shunt directly into the systemic circulation. In light of this, velocity of blood flow in the left pulmonary

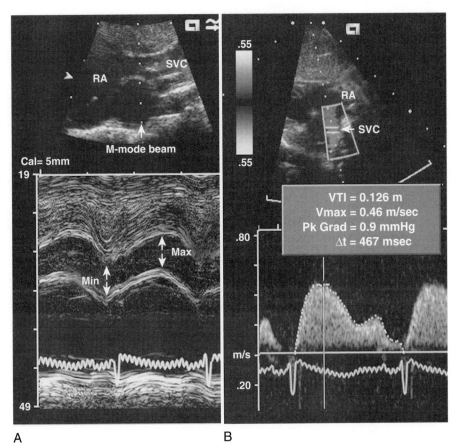

Figure 5-18 A, Measurement of superior vena cava (SVC) diameter from a mid-parasternal sagittal view. The M-mode beam is dropped through the SVC at the point that it starts to funnel out into the RA. Diameter is averaged from a maximum (max) and minimum (min) diameter. **B,** Pulsed Doppler assessment of SVC velocity from a low subcostal view. Velocity time integral (VTI) is derived by tracing around the systolic spectral envelope including any negative trace if present (VTI = 0.126 m in this case). (See Expert Consult site for color image.)

artery (LPA) has been suggested as a method of assessing PBF, which is protected from the confounding effects of the shunts.

LPA velocities are measured from the same view as the ductus arteriosus but moving the transducer slightly to the right and then angling back to the left can open up more of the LPA to view and so minimize the angle of insonation. Normal values for this have been derived in term babies where mean LPA velocities were usually greater than 0.2 m/sec.[32] The study of El Hajjar and colleagues suggested that mean LPA velocity of greater than 0.43 suggests a large ductal shunt.[9] Low velocities have been demonstrated in some babies with PPHN and data suggest that low LPA mean velocity is a good predictor of response to inhaled nitric oxide. In other words, babies with pulmonary hypertension and low pulmonary blood flow are most likely to respond to a vasodilator; indeed, dramatic improvement in LPA velocities can be seen with nitric oxide in such babies (Fig. 5-19).[33]

The problem with this measure is that some babies have a physiologic narrowing at the LPA root and hence acceleration of blood into the LPA. This is a common cause of innocent flow murmurs in all babies but particularly in the preterm baby. The cause of this physiologic narrowing is not known but it is hypothesized that it may be a consequence of the proximity of the LPA to the ductus, so the LPA can be slightly "gathered up" as the ductus constricts. Experientially I would suggest that narrowing at the root of the LPA is uncommon in the

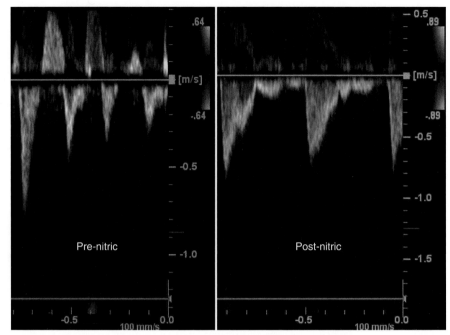

Figure 5-19 Shows velocity in the root of the left pulmonary artery (LPA) before and after commencing inhaled nitric oxide. The pre-nitric velocities are low with ventilator induced variation while the velocities have increased and stabilized with nitric oxide. (See Expert Consult site for color image.)

early postnatal period, particularly when the ductus is still widely patent. Regardless, LPA mean velocities should be interpreted with this potential confounder in mind.

Myocardial Function Measures

Neonatologists often place great importance on the traditional LV myocardial function measures of ejection fraction and fractional shortening, possibly because these can be the only hemodynamic measures given in routine echocardiography reports. They are not very useful measures in the study of neonatal hemodynamics unless the myocardial dysfunction is severe, in which case you do not need to measure anything to know there is a myocardial problem.

Ejection fraction and fractional shortening are essentially derivations of the same measures, which is the difference between the diastolic and systolic dimensions of the left ventricle. They are most commonly derived from an M-mode study of the left ventricle with the M-mode beam transecting the left ventricle at the tips of the mitral valve (Fig. 5-3). The anteroposterior diameter of the left ventricle is measured in end-systole (LVESD) and end-diastole (LVEDD; Fig. 5-3). The fractional shortening (%) is derived as [(LVEDD − LVESD)/LVEDD] × 100. The ejection fraction is really the same measure but the diameter measurements are cubed to convert to an assumed ventricular volume: [(LVEDD^3 − LVESD^3)/LVEDD^3] × 100.

There are several problems with these measures in the neonate; most importantly, M-mode only reflects the movement of the anterior and posterior wall of the left ventricle. In preterm babies, because of the complexities of the transitional circulation, the anterior wall of the neonatal LV moves relatively little during contraction compared to the posterior and lateral walls, so anteroposterior M-mode derivations of these measures underestimate LV function. In light of this observation, Lee and colleagues proposed a method of deriving circumferential shortening by imaging the LV in short axis and tracing the LV endocardial circumference in end-diastole and end-systole and converting to circumferential shortening using the same equation as fractional shortening.[34] The advantage of this method is that it reflects the movement of the entire circumference of the left ventricle not just two walls.

The velocity of fractional (or circumferential) fiber shortening (VCF) is another way to derive a function measure from both these measures by using the LV ejection time (LVET). VCF is derived from following equation VCF = Circumferential shortening / LVET. As VCF is also influenced by the heart rate, some investigators recommend correcting for the heart rate using the following equation: $VCF_c = VCF/\sqrt{RR}$ interval where VCF_c is the velocity of circumferential fiber shortening corrected for heart rate. In essence, VCF measures how fast the myocardium is contracting rather than how far.

Mean fractional shortening in healthy newborns is about 35% with a range from 26% to 40%, although values lower than this were found by Lee and colleagues in healthy preterm babies for the reasons cited earlier.[3,33] Normal velocity of VCF in a group of preterm babies ranged from 0.8 circ/s (±0.15) shortly after birth to 1.0 circ/s (± 0.18) on postnatal day 5. In term babies, the average was 0.9 circ/s (±0.15) at both times.[35]

The overriding problem of all these measures in the neonate is the extent to which they are affected by the load conditions on the left ventricle. Myocardial contractility has three major determinants: the health of the myocardium (which is what we want to assess), the preload on the ventricle (more will improve contractility up to a certain point), and the afterload (more will eventually reduce contractility as the myocardium goes off the top of the Starling curve). So anything that affects the load conditions also affects these contractility measures. Again ductal shunting is the biggest confounder. It increases the preload and reduces the afterload on the left ventricle and so results in excellent measures of contractility in a situation in which hemodynamic health may not be good. Other important confounders include hypovolemia, which reduces contractility, and very high pulmonary vascular resistance in PPHN. PPHN can have interesting effects on myocardial function because the high resistance may compromise RV function but the resulting low pulmonary blood flow will also cause low LV preload and hence apparently poor LV function. None of this is possible to work out if you only have a single measure of LV function and do not know what is happening in the rest of the heart.

The aforementioned scenario highlights that RV function is probably just as important as LV but the shape of the RV does not lend itself as well to reproducible function measures. However, some investigators have started to look at this by deriving normal values for right ventricular volume measures, although it is probably too early to say whether these will develop into clinically useful measures.[36]

One development of these measures, which is argued to be more load independent, is the relationship between VCF and LV wall stress (WS). WS is essentially a calculation of afterload and is derived from an equation that included measures of end-systolic blood pressure (ESP), end-systolic LV posterior wall thickness (h) and end-systolic diameter (D_{es}). The latter is calculated by dividing the end-systolic circumference by π to reduce error from irregularity of the LV shape. The formula is:

$$VWS = 0.34(Des)(ESP)/h[1 + (h/Des)]$$

Generally, as LV WS increases so VCFs will slow down, so a plot of the two will produce a negative correlation slope. The steepness of this slope reflects myocardial function; in other words, the more VCF slows in response to an increase in afterload, the worse the myocardial function. The need to derive a slope means that this needs repeated measures at different wall stress. This limits its use in an individual but it may give useful information in cross sectional data in populations of babies. Figure 5-20 compares the VCF versus WS slopes at 3 hours of age in preterm infants who did and did not develop low systemic blood flow. The steeper slope suggesting worse myocardial function in the babies with low systemic blood flow is apparent.[37]

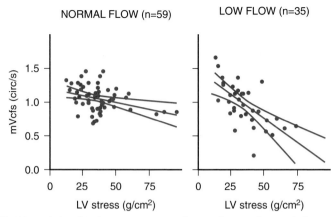

Figure 5-20 The relationship between mean velocity of circumferential shortening (mVCF) and LV wall stress in babies who maintained normal systemic blood flow (SBF) and those who developed low SBF. The low SBF babies have a steeper slope suggesting more limited myocardial response to increased LV wall stress.

Myocardial Function: Future Developments

Data are beginning to emerge in the newborn on two further methodologies for assessing myocardial function, namely measures of diastolic function and tissue Doppler measures. At the moment these data are mainly normal values, so the role of these methods in clinical or research assessment of hemodynamic pathophysiology is not yet clear. I will describe both briefly here.

Diastolic Function

Diastolic relaxation is an active process in the heart and a compromise of this relaxation can have just as marked effects on cardiac output as compromised systolic function. In essence, these measures are all derived from the Doppler waveform of the ventricular inflow (Fig. 5-21). This flow pattern reflects the two phases of diastole with an early peak in flow velocity reflecting early ventricular filling (the E wave) with ventricular relaxation and a later peak reflecting active filling as a result of atrial systole (the A wave). A variety of measures of diastolic function can be derived from this flow pattern, most of which are reflections of either velocities of the two phases (maximum, mean, and relative E and A wave ratios) or the acceleration and deceleration times of the two phases. The latter measures need correcting for heart rate and, at faster heart rates in the newborn, the A wave can be difficult to distinguish from the E wave. Velocity measures taken in isolation will also be as much a reflection of the load conditions as the diastolic function; again the duct will be a big confounder especially in neonates during the immediate postnatal transition.

In the mature healthy heart, 80% of filling occurs in early diastole, so relative dominance of the A wave is a marker of impaired diastolic function. However, in healthy term and preterm neonates, the mean ratio is 1.1 : 1 and 1 : 1, respectively, suggesting that reduced diastolic function is normal in the neonate.[3] In both term and preterm babies, diastolic function measures improve over the first few months after birth.[38] Like most myocardial function measures, there are more data available for the left than right side of the heart. While these measures give interesting physiological insight into the precarious state of the preterm circulation, their relationship to clinical outcome and their role in the assessment of an individual infant have not been clarified.

Tissue Doppler

This methodology uses the low Doppler shift frequencies of high energy generated by the ventricular wall motion, frequencies that are purposely filtered out in standard Doppler blood flow studies.[39] There are essentially three variables in ventricular wall

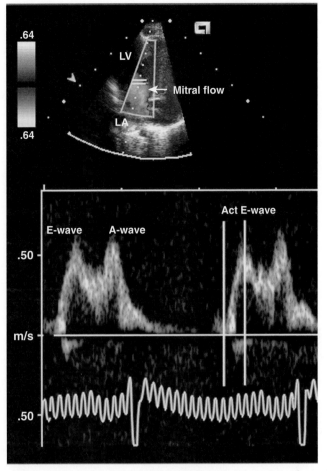

Figure 5-21   Shows the normal neonatal pulsed Doppler velocity trace of mitral valve flow that is used to measure diastolic function. The E-wave represents early filling due to active ventricular relaxation while the A-wave represents filling due to atrial systole. Act E-wave shows the acceleration time of early diastolic filling. (See Expert Consult site for color image.)

motion: velocity, acceleration, and displacement. We tend to think of ventricular function in terms of circumferentially orientated fibers but longitudinally orientated contraction is just as important. The M-mode myocardial function measures discussed earlier give information on displacement and circumferential contraction, but tissue Doppler allows much better assessment of velocity, acceleration, and longitudinal contraction. Longitudinal contraction is mainly due to contraction of subendocardial fibers and there is evidence from older subjects that abnormalities of wall motion may initially appear in the longitudinal axis. Because the apex of the heart stays relatively stationary during the cardiac cycle, longitudinal motion is assessed best from a four-chamber apical view with the Doppler range gate at the base of the heart (Fig. 5-22). From this view, motion of ventricular septal base and tricuspid and mitral annulus can be assessed. The velocity spectral trace has waves that reflect wall velocity in systole and the two phases of diastole.

In older subjects, where much of the tissue Doppler research has been done, there is some evidence that this methodology has significant advantages over more traditional measures of myocardial function.[39] Mori and colleagues have established some normal data in term newborns in comparison to older children.[40] Nestaas and colleagues studied healthy term babies over the first 3 days and found that there were large inter individual variations in these measures depending on the location of measurement and the quality of the ultrasound window and images.[41] They

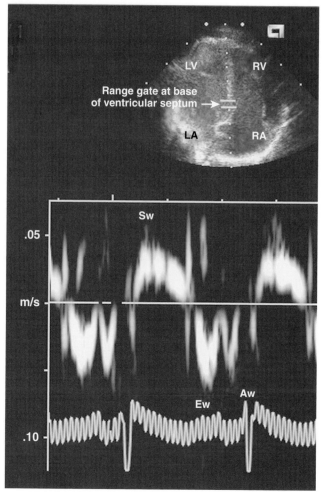

Figure 5-22 Shows the tissue Doppler velocity spectrum of longitudinal wall motion at the base of the ventricular septum. Sw shows peak systolic motion velocity, Ew is peak early diastolic filling motion velocity and Aw is peak atrial systolic motion velocity. (See Expert Consult site for color image.)

concluded that they may be more useful for summary data between groups of babies than make assessments in an individual baby. So, like diastolic function measures, the clinical usefulness of these measures in the assessment of an individual infant remains to be established.

Functional Echocardiography in the Neonatal Intensive Care Units in Specific Clinical Situations

Like almost all other diagnostic modalities, there is no evidence that functional echocardiography improves neonatal outcomes. However it can provide useful hemodynamic information in almost any sick baby. While many newborn services will have access to consultative echocardiography services, to fulfill its potential functional echocardiography needs to be integrated into care in a way that is difficult to achieve unless neonatologists develop these skills themselves.[42,43] Introduction of such clinician-performed ultrasound (CPU) at the point of care encounters varying degrees of resistance in different clinical settings.[44] From the neonatal clinician's perspective, there is the benefit of immediate diagnostic information, from the perspective of the specialties that have traditionally provided these diagnostic services, there are concerns about quality and competence and the risk of diagnostic error.

The experience of most services that have successfully incorporated CPU, including functional echocardiography, is that CPU does not replace the need for consultative ultrasound services. Indeed if true collaboration exists, they often complement each other.

Probably the greatest risk is that of important congenital heart disease being missed. Because clinician-performed functional echocardiography in a NICU mainly examines structurally normal hearts, the ability to recognize the abnormal patterns of congenital heart disease (CHD) comes early in the learning process. Indeed some training in recognizing common congenital heart abnormalities should be part of that learning process. However, this should not be relied on to exclude CHD. In any situation where the primary question is "Does this baby have a structurally normal heart?" it is *vital* that an echocardiogram be performed early in the clinical course by someone skilled in establishing structural normality, usually a pediatric cardiologist. In most babies for whom the primary question is "What are the hemodynamics in this sick baby?" the heart will be structurally normal. But there are babies in whom both questions must be answered. Hence, if a neonatologist is going to undertake functional echocardiography, the importance of working in close collaboration with a pediatric cardiologist cannot be emphasized strongly enough. Questions remain about the training and accreditation of neonatologists to perform ultrasound including echocardiography, and several countries are beginning to progress these issues. In Australia and New Zealand, there is now a certificate of clinician-performed ultrasound specifically for neonatologists.[44]

There are four common scenarios in which functional echocardiography plays an important role: (1) the very preterm baby during the transitional period; (2) the baby with suspected PDA; (3) the baby with clinically suspected circulatory compromise (usually hypotensive); and (4) the baby with suspected PPHN. In all these situations, the echocardiogram should be as complete as possible; later, measures that are particularly important in each situation are outlined.

Very Preterm Baby During the Transitional Period

The hemodynamic pathology of the first 12 hours of life of the very preterm infant is described in more detail in Chapter 12. It is a period of exquisite vulnerability to low systemic blood flow and, in our studies, this low systemic blood flow has been associated with a range of adverse preterm outcomes.[14,45] We try to perform an echocardiogram between 3 and 9 hours of age in all babies born before 28 weeks and babies born after 27 weeks with significant respiratory compromise. This echocardiogram includes a measure of systemic blood flow and an assessment of early ductal constriction and shunt direction.

Measurement of Systemic Blood Flow

We recommend measuring both RV output and SVC flow as a cross-check against each other. SVC flow will usually be between 30% and 50% of total systemic blood flow (SBF). For clinical purposes, RV output is a reasonably accurate marker of low SBF because atrial shunts are not usually large early after birth (see earlier). Full flow measures are time-consuming to derive and, because velocity in the MPA is the dominant determinant of RV output, measuring the maximum velocity in the MPA (PA V_{max}) provides a simple way to screen for low SBF (Fig. 5-23). In our studies, if the PA V_{max} is greater than 0.45 m/s, low SBF is unlikely and, if the PA V_{max} is less than 0.35 m/s, most babies will have low SBF. Between 0.35 and 0.45 m/s is a gray zone where discriminatory accuracy is less good. In practice, I would recommend screening with PA V_{max} and then doing full RV output and/or SVC flow measures in those with a PA V_{max} less than 0.45 m/s.[46]

Assessment of Early Ductal Constriction and Shunt Direction

We would assess the degree of ductal constriction by measuring minimum diameter from the color Doppler and the pattern of shunting. The latter is usually predominantly left to right but often has a bidirectional component at this stage. We do this

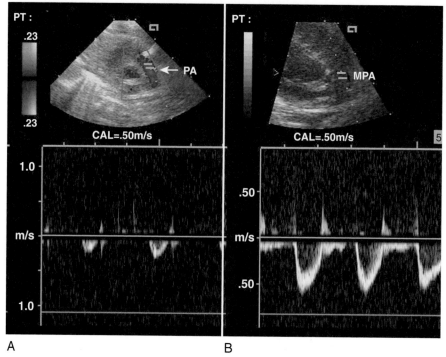

Figure 5-23   Doppler velocity in the pulmonary artery in two babies. **A,** The low V_{max} of about 0.2 m/s in a baby with low systemic blood flow (SBF) compared with **(B)**, a normal V_{max} of about 0.6 m/s. (See Expert Consult site for color image.)

because it has been shown that constriction at this stage predicts subsequent persisting patency.[5,13,14,17]

Preterm Infant with Suspected PDA

This will usually be a baby beyond the first 24 h with signs and/or symptoms suggestive of a PDA. In our hands, an echocardiogram on such a baby includes:

- Color Doppler confirmation of patency and minimum diameter from the color Doppler, as a means of assessing likely significance.
- Pulsed Doppler assessment of shunt direction.
- Pulsed Doppler assessment of direction of diastolic flow in the postductal descending aorta.
- Pulsed Doppler assessment of velocity of mean and diastolic flow in the left pulmonary artery.

In babies born before 30 weeks with a PDA with a predominantly left-to-right shunt, a minimum diameter between 1.5 and 2 mm will usually mark a significant shunt and, when greater than 2 mm, the shunt will almost always be significant. Retrograde diastolic flow in the postductal descending aorta and increased velocity flow (diastolic > 0.2 m/sec or mean > 0.43 m/sec) in the LPA support the observation that the shunt is likely to be significant.

Baby with Clinically Suspected Circulatory Compromise

The approach here will vary depending on the presentation. The term baby presenting at birth with low Apgar scores and persisting pallor will usually be due to post-hypoxic acidosis. But an acute fetal bleed with hypovolemia can present this way and the characteristic poorly filled ventricles seen on echocardiography can be helpful in making this diagnosis quickly. In an acute postnatal circulatory collapse in a term baby, then, the need to exclude a ductal dependent systemic circulation is paramount. In the preterm baby undergoing intensive care, such acute collapses will usually have a respiratory origin but it may be cardiac, such as cardiac tamponade from a long line extravasating into the pericardium or a ductal dependent systemic circulation. In such situations, prompt diagnosis with echocardiography will be lifesaving. The more common situation for the neonatologist will be the preterm baby with persisting hypotension. These babies usually have a structurally normal heart and functional echocardiography in our practice includes the following:

- A full assessment of ductal patency and significance. PDA causes a global reduction in systolic and diastolic blood pressure during the first postnatal week.[47]
- A measure of systemic blood flow, RV output, and/or SVC flow. As the baby grows older, more caution is needed in using pulmonary artery velocities to screen for low flow because significant atrial shunts become more common. In fact, low systemic blood flow is uncommon after the first 24 h. Most hypotensive babies after day 1 will have normal or sometimes high systemic blood flow suggesting loss of vascular tone is more important than low cardiac output after the transitional period.[14,48,49]
- A visual assessment of myocardial contractility is important in these babies. If it looks poor, I would measure LV fractional shortening.

Baby with Suspected Primary Persistent Pulmonary Hypertension of the Newborn

This is usually the term or near term baby with high oxygen and ventilator requirements. Congenital heart disease can present this way, so these babies must have this possibility excluded early on in their course. Once structural abnormality has been excluded, functional echocardiography in our practice includes the following:

- An assessment of pulmonary artery pressure, ideally from a tricuspid incompetence jet or a ductal shunt. Measure both, if they are present, as a cross-check against each other. Pulmonary artery pressure is surprisingly difficult to predict from a baby's clinical condition.[12] The highest pulmonary pressure is found in babies with primary idiopathic PPHN (who may not have very high FiO_2 requirements) and babies with severe lung disease.
- An assessment of systemic blood flow, RV output and or SVC flow. These measured are commonly low in such babies, particularly in the first 24 h.[12]
- An assessment of ductal constriction and direction of shunting. The ductus usually constricts early and closes in these babies; often well before the oxygen requirement falls.[12]
- An assessment of degree and direction of atrial shunting.
- Measurement of mean velocity in the root of the left pulmonary artery.

Conclusion

There is a wealth of hemodynamic information that can be derived by functional echocardiography in the sick neonate. A common theme to many of the research findings in this area is how different actual hemodynamic findings are from what one might expect from conventional thinking in particular clinical scenarios. Further, it is striking how variable hemodynamics are between individual babies and also within the same baby with time. Without echocardiography, you will be guessing the hemodynamics and much of the data would suggest that you will be wrong a fair amount of the time. For functional echocardiography to fulfill its clinical potential, it needs to be available at any time and at short notice in the NICU. Some NICUs will have external diagnostic services that can provide this sort of service but many do not have this sort of access. In these situations, there is much to be said for the neonatologists themselves developing echocardiographic skills in close collaboration with their cardiologists.

References

1. Hoffman GM, Ghanayem NS, Tweddell JS. Noninvasive assessment of cardiac output. Semin Thoracic Cardiovas Surg: Ped Cardiac Surg Annual. 2005:12-21.
2. Evans N. Echocardiography on neonatal intensive care units in Australia and New Zealand. J Paediatr Child Health. 2000;36:169-171.

B

3. Skinner J, Hunter S, Alverson D, eds. Echocardiography for the neonatologist. London: Churchill Livingstone; 2000.

4. Evans N, Malcolm G. Practical echocardiography for the neonatologist. Two multimedia CD-ROMs, Royal Prince Alfred Hospital, 2000 and 2002. www.cs.nsw.gov.au/rpa/neonatal.

5. Evans N, Malcolm G, Osborn DA, et al. Diagnosis of patent ductus arteriosus in preterm infants. Neoreviews. 2004;5:e86-e97.

6. Evans N, Iyer P. Incompetence of the foramen ovale in preterm infants requiring ventilation. J Pediatr. 1994;125:786-792.

7. Evans N, Iyer P. Assessment of ductus arteriosus shunting in preterm infants requiring ventilation: effect of inter-atrial shunting. J Pediatr. 1994;125:778-785.

8. Suzumura H, Nitta A, Tanaka G, et al. Diastolic flow velocity of the left pulmonary artery of patent ductus arteriosus in preterm infants. Pediatr Int. 2001;43:146-151.

9. El Hajjar M, Vaksmann G, Rakza T, et al. Severity of the ductal shunt: a comparison of different markers. Arch Dis Child Fetal Neonatal Edition. 2005;90(5):F419-FF22.

10. Evans N, Archer LNJ. Postnatal circulatory adaptation in term and healthy preterm neonates. Arch Dis Child. 1990;65:24-26.

11. Lim MK, Hanretty K, Houston AB, et al. Intermittent ductal patency in healthy newborn infants: demonstration by colour Doppler flow mapping. Arch Dis Child. 1992;67:1217-1218.

12. Evans N, Kluckow M, Currie A. The range of echocardiographic findings in term and near term babies with high oxygen requirements. Arch Dis Child. 1998;78:105-111.

13. Kluckow M, Evans N. High pulmonary blood flow, the duct, and pulmonary hemorrhage. J Pediatr. 2000;137:68-72.

14. Kluckow M, Evans N. Low superior vena cava flow and intraventricular haemorrhage in preterm infants. Arch Dis Child. 2000;82:F188-F194.

15. Skelton R, Evans N, Smythe J. A blinded comparison of clinical and echocardiographic evaluation of the preterm infant for patent ductus arteriosus. J Paediat Child Health. 1994;30:406-411.

16. Davis P, Turner-Gomes S, Cunningham K, et al. Precision and accuracy of clinical and radiological signs in premature infants at risk of patent ductus arteriosus. Arch Pediatr Adolesc Med. 1995;149: 1136-1141.

17. Kluckow M, Evans N. Early echocardiographic prediction of symptomatic patent ductus arteriosus in preterm infants undergoing mechanical ventilation. J Pediatr. 1995;127:774-779.

18. Hiraishi S, Agata Y, Saito K, et al. Interatrial shunt flow profiles in newborn infants: a colour flow and pulsed Doppler echocardiographic study. Br Heart J. 1991;65:41-45.

19. Musewe NN, Poppe D, Smallhorn JF, et al. Doppler echocardiographic measurement of pulmonary artery pressure from ductal Doppler velocities in the newborn. JACC. 1990;15:446-456.

20. Yock PG, Popp RL. Non invasive estimation of right ventricular systolic pressure by Doppler ultrasound in patients with tricuspid regurgitation. Circulation. 1984;70:657-662.

21. Chan KL, Currie PJ, Seward JB, et al. Comparison of three Doppler ultrasound methods in the prediction of pulmonary artery pressure. JACC. 1987;9:549-554.

22. Kosturakis D, Goldberg SJ, Allen HD, et al. Doppler echocardiographic prediction of pulmonary arterial hypertension in congenital heart disease. Am J Cardiol. 1984;53:1110-1115.

23. Matsuda M, Sekiguchi T, Sugishita Y, et al. Reliability of non-invasive estimates of pulmonary hypertension by pulsed Doppler echocardiography. Br Heart J. 1986;56:158-164.

24. Evans N, Archer LNJ. Postnatal circulatory adaptation in term and healthy preterm newborns. Arch Dis Child. 1990;65:24-26.

25. Evans N, Archer LNJ. Doppler assessment of pulmonary artery pressure and extrapulmonary shunting in the acute phase of hyaline membrane disease. Arch Dis Child. 1991;66:6-11.

26. Mandelbaum-Isken VH, Linderkamp O. Cardiac output by pulsed Doppler in neonates using the apical window. Pediatr Cardiol. 1991;12:13-16.

27. Alverson DC, Eldridge M, Dillon T, et al. Non invasive pulsed Doppler determination of cardiac output in neonates and children. J Pediatr. 1982;101:46-50.

28. Mellander M, Sabel KG, Caidahl K, et al. Doppler determination of cardiac output in infants and children: comparison with simultaneous thermodilution. Pediatr Cardiol. 1987;8:241-246.

29. Hudson I, Houston A, Aitchison T, et al. Reproducibility of measurements of cardiac output in newborn infants by Doppler ultrasound. Arch Dis Child. 1990;65:15-19.

30. Kluckow M, Evans N. Superior vena cava flow. A novel marker of systemic blood flow. Arch Dis Child. 2000;82:F182-F187.

31. Drayton MR, Skidmore R. Vasoactivity of the major intracranial arteries in newborn infants. Arch Dis Child. 1987;62:236-240.

32. Gournay V, Cambonie G, Rozé JC. Doppler echocardiographic assessment of pulmonary blood flow in healthy newborns. Acta Paediatrica. 1998;87(4):419-423.

33. Rozé JC, Storme L, Zupan V, et al. Echocardiographic investigation of inhaled nitric oxide in newborn babies with severe hypoxaemia. Lancet. 1994;344(8918):303-305.

34. Lee LA, Kimball TR, Daniels SR, et al. Left ventricular mechanics in the preterm infant and their effect on measurement of cardiac performance. J Pediatr. 1992;120:114-119.

35. Takahashi Y, Harada K, Kishkumo S, et al. Postnatal left ventricular contractility in very low birth weight infant. Pediatr Cardiol. 1997;18:112-117.

36. Clark SJ, Yoxall CW, Subhedar NV. Measurement of right ventricular volume in healthy term and preterm neonates. Arch Dis Child, Fetal Neonatal Ed. 2002;87:F89-F93.

37. Osborn D, Evans N, Kluckow M. Left ventricular contractility and wall stress in very preterm infants in the first day of life. Pediatr Res. 2007;61:335-340.

38. Schmitz L, Stiller B, Pees C, et al. Doppler-derived parameters of diastolic left ventricular function in preterm infants with a birth weight <1500 g: reference values and differences to term infants. Early Human Develop. 2004;76:101-114.

39. Isaaz K. Tissue Doppler imaging for the assessment of left ventricular systolic and diastolic function. Curr Opin Cardiol. 2002;17:431-442.

40. Mori K, Nakagawa R, Nii M, et al. Pulsed wave Doppler tissue echocardiography assessment of the long axis function of the right and left ventricles during the neonatal period. Heart. 2004;90: 175-180.

41. Nestaas E, Stoylen A, Brunvand L, et al. Tissue Doppler derived strain and strain rate during the first 3 days of life in healthy term neonates. Pediatr Res. 2009;65:357-362.

42. Kluckow M, Seri I, Evans N. Functional echocardiography: an emerging clinical tool for the neonatologist. J Pediatr. 2007;150:125-130.

43. Kluckow M, Seri I, Evans N. Echocardiography and the neonatologist. Pediatr Cardiol. 2008;29(6): 1043-1047.

44. Evans N, Gournay V, Cabanas F, et al. Point-of-care ultrasound in the neonatal intensive care unit: international perspectives. Semin Fetal Neonatal Medicine 2011;16:61-68.

45. Osborn DA, Evans N, Kluckow M. Hemodynamic and antecedent risk factors of early and late periventricular/intraventricular hemorrhage in premature infants. Pediatrics. 2003;112:33-39.

46. Evans N. Which inotrope in which baby? Arch Dis Child. 2006;91:F213-F220.

47. Evans N, Moorcraft J. Effect of patency of the ductus arteriosus on blood pressure in very preterm infants. Arch Dis Child. 1992;67:1169-1173.

48. Noori S, Friedlich P, Wong P, et al. Haemodynamic changes after low-dosage hydrocortisone administration in vasopressor-treated preterm and term neonates. Pediatrics. 2006;118(4):1456-1466.

49. Lopez SL, Leighton JO, Walther FJ. Supranormal cardiac output in the dopamine and dobutamine dependent preterm infant. Pediatr Cardiol. 1997;18:292-296.

5

CHAPTER 6

Assessment of Cardiac Output in Neonates: Techniques Using the Fick Principle, Pulse Wave Form Analysis, and Electrical Impedance

Markus Osypka, PhD, Sadaf Soleymani, MS,
Istvan Seri, MD, PhD, HonD, Shahab Noori, MD, RDCS

- Fick Principle
- Echocardiography
- Electrical Cardiometry
- Pulse Contour Method
- Conclusion
- References

As discussed in Chapter 1 in detail, assessment of the cardiovascular system and thus treatment of critically ill neonates with cardiovascular compromise hinge on the ability to monitor at least two of the three interdependent cardiovascular parameters (blood pressure, cardiac output, and systemic vascular resistance), determining systemic and organ blood flow and thus oxygen delivery to the tissues. In the following equation, Ohm's law is applied to systemic blood flow:

$$CO = k \cdot \frac{(MAP - CVP)}{SVR} \qquad (6.1)$$

where CO = cardiac output (i.e., systemic blood flow), (MAP − CVP) = pressure difference between mean arterial pressure (MAP) and central venous pressure (CVP), SVR = systemic vascular resistance, k = constant, and

$$DO_2 = CO \cdot CaO_2 \qquad (6.2)$$

where DO_2 = oxygen delivery to the tissues, CO = cardiac output, and CaO_2 = arterial oxygen content.

At present, only blood pressure can be monitored continuously in absolute numbers in real time albeit only invasively (Chapter 3). Since monitoring SVR is currently not possible, continuous noninvasive real-time assessment of beat-to-beat cardiac output has become the "holy grail" of modern-day neonatal intensive care. With the ability to continuously monitor both blood pressure and cardiac output in real time, the neonatologist would likely be able to more accurately diagnose and treat neonatal shock (Chapters 1 and 12).

Expectations for an ideal method for the assessment of cardiac output include appropriate validation, accuracy in real time, absolute numbers, a method that is reliable, practical, affordable, and easy to use, and data that are easily stored and retrieved. Usefulness for assessing systemic blood flow in neonates with extracardiac and intracardiac shunting would be an additional but important requirement. None of the presently available and routinely used methods fulfill all off these requirements (Fig. 6-1).

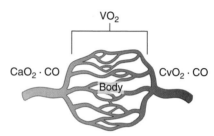

Figure 6-1 The Fick principle utilizing oxygen concentration in arterial and pulmonary artery blood. See text for details.

This chapter discusses the most important techniques with the potential to assess cardiac output, since some novel techniques for monitoring cardiac output in the neonate have been introduced.

The hemodynamic monitoring methods discussed in this chapter have been established and used in adult patients (Table 6-1). They differ in their applicability to neonates with respect to invasiveness, spot check versus continuous measurements, and the requirements to be met by the patient. The size a of neonate, which can be less than 500 g, and corresponding stroke volume and cardiac output values usually around 1-2 mL/kg and 150-250 mL/min/kg, respectively, construct a significant limitation to the applicability of any cardiac output method especially to the preterm neonatal patient population.

Fick Principle

Methods using the Fick principle might utilize the direct Fick method or one of its modifications to render the technique more clinically applicable. However, the modifications often come at the expense of accuracy.

In 1870, German physiologist Adolf Eugen Fick stated that the volume of blood flow in a given period (cardiac output) equals the amount of a substance entering the bloodstream in the same period divided by the difference in concentrations of the substance upstream and downstream, respectively.[1]

Table 6-1 MAJOR METHODS OF CARDIAC OUTPUT MEASUREMENT

Method	Characteristics	Type of Measurement	Requirements from Patient
Direct Fick principle	Invasive	Noncontinuous, requires blood samples and analysis to obtain CO	Acceptance of face mask, central vascular access, absence of shunts between venous and arterial system
Echocardiography (Doppler velocimetry)	Noninvasive	Noncontinuous, requires analysis to obtain SV/CO results	Specific body position, patient needs to be at rest
Thoracic electrical bio-impedance and electrical cardiometry	Noninvasive	Continuous or spot check, real-time display of results	Patient needs to be at rest, no/minimal movement of skin areas close to surface sensors
Pulse contour analysis	Invasive	Continuous, real-time display of results	Arterial blood pressure line

CO, cardiac output; SV, stroke volume.
See text for details.

Oxygen Fick (O$_2$-Fick) Method

Determination of cardiac output according to the direct Fick method requires application of a face mask (or some means of assessing oxygen consumption) and consideration of arterial and venous oxygen saturation, which is usually obtained by taking blood samples for laboratory analysis.

The direct Fick method employing a measurement of pulmonary oxygen uptake (see later) is considered the "gold standard" for assessing cardiac output. It is of note though that recent advances in magnetic resonance imaging (MRI) technology have initiated a shift in our thinking and cardiac output measurement by MRI is now considered by many as the "gold standard" for measurement of cardiac output (see Chapter 10). According to the direct Fick principle, cardiac output is calculated by dividing oxygen consumption (VO$_2$) by the difference in the oxygen content of the aortic blood (CaO$_2$) and the mixed venous blood (CvO$_2$) (see Fig. 6-1). The applicability in its original form, that is, measuring VO$_2$ instead of assuming it, is limited to the fact that a face mask must be used. With respect to the application in neonates, further limitation includes that multiple blood sampling is required.

With oxygen being the substance for this method, Fick's principle states that during steady-state, the oxygen taken up in the pulmonary system (pulmonary oxygen uptake) equals the oxygen consumption in the tissues.

Cardiac output (pulmonary blood flow) can be calculated by dividing the pulmonary oxygen uptake by the oxygen concentration gradient (difference) between arterial blood (CaO$_2$) and venous blood (CvO$_2$). Under steady-state condition, tissue oxygen consumption is equal to pulmonary oxygen uptake (VO$_2$).

Hence,

$$CO = \frac{VO_2}{CaO_2 - CvO_2} \tag{6.3}$$

where CO = cardiac output in L /min, VO$_2$ = pulmonary oxygen uptake in mL O$_2$/min, CaO$_2$ = oxygen concentration of arterial blood in mL O$_2$/L, CvO$_2$ = oxygen concentration of venous blood (preferably determined in the pulmonary artery) in mL O$_2$/L.

Pediatric and adult patients differ significantly in oxygen consumption. The cardiac index is higher by 30-60% in neonates and infants to help meet their increased oxygen consumption.[2] Fetal hemoglobin, present in fetal life and, in decreasing concentration, up to 3-6 months following birth, has higher oxygen affinity and thus does not deliver oxygen to the tissues as effectively as adult hemoglobin does after delivery when arterial oxygen saturation increases from the fetal levels of 75% to 98-100%. In neonates, the combination of a higher hemoglobin concentration (17-19 g/dL compared with 13.5-17.5 g/dL in men and 12-16 g/dL in women), higher blood volume per kg body weight, and increased cardiac output compensate for the decreased release of oxygen from hemoglobin to the tissues.

Pulmonary Oxygen Uptake (VO$_2$)

Pulmonary oxygen uptake (VO$_2$), or oxygen consumption, can be obtained via a Douglas bag, using indirect calorimetry by spirometry or metabolic monitors, such as the Datex-Ohmeda Deltatrac II metabolic monitor as well as by mass spectrometry using the direct Fick method.[3] Table 6-2 depicts VO$_2$ measurements obtained in different patient populations and under different clinical conditions.[4-6]

Alternatively, for the adult population, VO$_2$ can be estimated following a regression equation suggested by Krovetz and Goldbloom based on height and weight.[7]

$$VO_{2EST} = \frac{((1.39 \cdot height) + (0.84 \cdot weight) - 3.56)}{BSA} \tag{6.4}$$

where VO$_{2EST}$ = estimated pulmonary oxygen uptake (indexed by body surface area [BSA]) in mL O$_2$/min/m^2, height measured in cm, and weight measured in kg.

Table 6-2 PULMONARY OXYGEN UPTAKE (VO2) (OXYGEN CONSUMPTION) IN DIFFERENT PATIENT POPULATIONS

Group	VO$_2$ (Mean ± SD)	Notes
Adults	$125 \ \dfrac{mL \ O_2}{min \ m^2}$	Indexed for body surface area (BSA)
Healthy newborns [Bauer et al, 2002][4]	$6.7 \pm 0.6 \ \dfrac{mL \ O_2}{min \ kg} - 7.1 \pm 0.4 \ \dfrac{mL \ O_2}{min \ kg}$	Indexed for weight n = 7
Neonates with Sepsis [Bauer et al, 2002][4]	$7.0 \pm 0.3 \ \dfrac{mL \ O_2}{min \ kg} - 8.2 \pm 0.4 \ \dfrac{mL \ O_2}{min \ kg}$	n = 10
Mechanically ventilated preterm infants [Shiao, 2006][5]	$8.0 \pm 3.73 \ \dfrac{mL \ O_2}{min \ kg}$	<8 hours after blood draw (n = 202)
	$11.3 \pm 5.65 \ \dfrac{mL \ O_2}{min \ kg}$	≥ 8 hours after blood draw (n = 65)
Preterm and term infants before and one hour after feeding [Stothers and Warner, 1979][6]	$4\text{-}8 \ \dfrac{mL \ O_2}{min \ kg}$ (estimated from Fig. 6-1)	n = 9 preterm infants n = 9 term infants
Term infants during sleep	$5.97 \ \dfrac{mL \ O_2}{min \ kg}$ during REM sleep	n = 30
	$5.72 \ \dfrac{mL \ O_2}{min \ kg}$ during non-REM sleep	

Pulmonary oxygen uptake in adults, healthy term newborns, neonates with sepsis, mechanically ventilated preterm neonates, and preterm and term neonates before and after feeding.[4-6]
REM, rapid eye movements. See text for details.

In addition, LaFarge and Miettinen developed a regression equation based on age and heart rate, which distinguishes between the genders[8]:

$$VO_{2EST} = 138.1 - (17.04 \cdot \ln(age)) + (0.378 \cdot HR) \text{ for females} \qquad (6.5)$$

$$VO_{2EST} = 138.1 - (11.49 \cdot \ln(age)) + (0.378 \cdot HR) \text{ for males} \qquad (6.6)$$

where VO_{2EST} = estimated pulmonary oxygen uptake (indexed by BSA) in mL O_2/min/m^2, age in years, and heart rate in beats per minute (bpm).

These regression equations determine an estimated VO$_2$ indexed by BSA. However, for neonates it is common to use body mass (weight) as an index.

The estimation of VO$_2$, which is also referred to as the indirect Fick method, is subject to errors for the determination of cardiac output potentially exceeding 50%. Because of the potential errors and its questionable adaptability to neonates, the cardiac output obtained by indirect Fick method may be used in neonates for orientation purposes only.

Oxygen Concentration Gradient (CaO$_2$ – CvO$_2$)

Oxygen concentration (CO$_2$) is calculated by determining hemoglobin (Hb) and oxygen saturation (SO$_2$), which traditionally is obtained by blood gas analysis:

$$CO_2 = \left(Hb \left(\frac{g}{dL} \right) \cdot 1.36 \left(\frac{mL \ O_2}{g} \right) \cdot SO_2 \right) + \left(PO_2 (mmHg) \cdot 0.0032 \left(\frac{mL \ O_2}{dL \ mmHg} \right) \right) \qquad (6.7)$$

where Hb = hemoglobin in g/dL, SO$_2$ = arterial (pulmonary vein) oxygen saturation (normal value ≈ 99%) and venous (pulmonary artery) oxygen saturation (normal value ≈ 75%), and PO$_2$ = partial pressure of oxygen in mm Hg or kPa (1 mmHg ≈ 133 Pa = 0.133 kPa) with normal values between 80 and 100 mm Hg (10.6-13.3 kPa). Values ≤ 40 mmHg (5.3 kPa) are considered extremely low.

Table 6-3 HEMOGLOBIN CONCENTRATIONS IN DIFFERENT AGE GROUPS

Group	Hemoglobin (Hb) g/dL	Notes [References]
Healthy men	13.5-17.5	
Healthy women	12-16	
Healthy newborns	17-19	[2]
Newborns with anemia	<13	Anemia sufficient to jeopardize oxygen-carrying capacity of the blood [2]
Infants < 6 months of age with anemia	<10	Anemia sufficient to jeopardize oxygen-carrying capacity of the blood] [2]

See text for details.

Note that the aforementioned equation obtains oxygen content (CO_2) in mL O_2/dL. To obtain oxygen concentration (CO_2) in mL O_2/L, one needs to multiply the result by 10 (1 L = 10 dL).

Because in the normal range of PaO_2, dissolved oxygen contributes very little to the total oxygen-carrying capacity, oxygen content can be approximated by

$$CO_2 \approx Hb\left(\frac{g}{dL}\right) \cdot 1.36\left(\frac{mL\ O_2}{g}\right) \cdot SO_2 \tag{6.8}$$

and the gradient by

$$CaO_2 - CvO_2 \approx Hb\left(\frac{g}{dL}\right) \cdot 1.36\left(\frac{mL\ O_2}{g}\right) \cdot (SaO_2 - SvO_2) \tag{6.9}$$

Alternative to blood gas analysis, SaO_2 and SvO_2 may be obtained via catheters (e.g., Opticath catheter in combination with Oximetric-3 monitors, Abbott Critical Care Systems, Abbott Laboratories, Abbott Park, IL). Arterial oxygen saturation (SaO_2) may be approximated noninvasively by SpO_2 obtained via pulse oximetry.

Table 6-3 summarizes the hemoglobin levels at different age groups and in different medical conditions. Neonates may show increased levels of carboxyhemoglobin (HbCO) and methemoglobin (MetHb), and these levels have to be accounted for to ensure accurate assessment of the oxygenation status.

Cardiac Index (Calculation Examples)

Assuming an adult with a VO_2 of 125 mL O_2/min/ m^2, Hb of 15 g/dL, SaO_2 of 99%, and SvO_2 of 75%:

$$CaO_2 - CvO_2 \approx Hb\left(\frac{g}{dL}\right) \cdot 1.36\left(\frac{mL\ O_2}{g}\right) \cdot (SaO_2 - SvO_2)$$

$$= 15\frac{g}{dL} \cdot 1.36\frac{mL\ O_2}{g} \cdot (99 - 75)\%$$

$$= 4.90\frac{mL\ O_2}{dL}$$

With VO_2 normalized for BSA, the cardiac index (CI) is

$$CI = \frac{VO_2}{CaO_2 - CvO_2} = \frac{125\left(\frac{mL\ O_2}{min\ m^2}\right)}{4.90\left(\frac{mL\ O_2}{dL}\right)} = 25.5\left(\frac{dL}{min\ m^2}\right) = 2.55\left(\frac{L}{min\ m^2}\right)$$

Unlike in the adult and pediatric patient, where CO is normalized for BSA, cardiac output in neonates is usually normalized by body mass, or weight. Assuming a neonate with VO_2 of 7 mL O_2/min/kg, Hb of 17 g/dL, SaO_2 of 99%, and SvO_2 of 75%:

$$CaO_2 - CvO_2 \approx Hb\left(\frac{g}{dL}\right) \cdot 1.36\left(\frac{mL\ O_2}{g}\right) \cdot (SaO_2 - SvO_2)$$

$$= 17\frac{g}{dL} \cdot 1.36\frac{mL\ O_2}{g} \cdot (99 - 75)\%$$

$$= 5.55\frac{mL\ O_2}{dL}$$

With VO_2 normalized for weight, the cardiac index (CI) is

$$CI = \frac{VO_2}{CaO_2 - CvO_2} = \frac{7.0\left(\frac{mL\ O_2}{min\ kg}\right)}{5.55\left(\frac{mL\ O_2}{dL}\right)} = 1.26\left(\frac{dL}{min\ kg}\right) = 0.126\left(\frac{L}{min\ kg}\right)$$

According to this calculation, cardiac output is 126 mL/kg/min in a neonate under physiologic circumstances. In a study by Tibby and colleagues in five neonates with birth weights $\leq$ 3.2 kg following surgical correction of their congenital heart disease,[9] the median cardiac index (CI) was 138 mL/kg/min. However, CI measured by echocardiography in neonates averages around 200 mL/kg/min. There are several reasons why our calculation suggests lower cardiac output compared with echocardiography-assessed CI. While the Hb concentration assumed in the equation is normal for term neonates in the transitional period, it is likely high for neonates who underwent cardiac catheterization for clinical reasons and had their CI determined using the Fick principle. These patients' oxygen consumption is also likely to be higher than that of a healthy term neonate. In addition, the methods using the direct Fick principle yield a lower CI compared with that assessed by echocardiography because of the approximately 20% physiologic shunting present in the lungs. Indeed, if we change the Hb concentration and the VO_2 to 15 g/dL and 8 mL O_2/min/kg, respectively, and add 20% to compensate for the physiologic shunting in the lungs, we get a CI of 196 mL/kg/min, which is the same as the estimated 200 mL/kg/min of average CI determined by echocardiography.

Carbon Dioxide Fick (CO_2-Fick) Method

With the CO_2-Fick method, instead of using oxygen as a marker, the exchange of carbon dioxide may be used. The following two methodologies use this principle: the modified carbon dioxide Fick method (mCO_2F) and the carbon dioxide rebreathing technology (CO_2R).

Modified Carbon Dioxide Fick Method (mCO_2F)

The modified carbon dioxide Fick method is based on the principle that steady-state carbon dioxide production in the tissue is equal to pulmonary carbon dioxide exchange (VCO_2)

$$CO = \frac{VCO_2}{CvCO_2 - CaCO_2} \tag{6.10}$$

where CO = cardiac output in L/min, VCO_2 = pulmonary carbon dioxide exchange in mL CO_2/min, $CaCO_2$ = carbon dioxide concentration of arterial blood in mL CO_2/min, and $CvCO_2$ = carbon dioxide concentration of venous blood (preferably determined in the pulmonary artery) measured in ml CO_2 /L.

Pulmonary carbon dioxide exchange (VCO_2) may be measured using volumetric capnography. In a ventilated patient, VCO_2 can be determined by analysis of the expiratory airflow (Q_{exp}) and carbon dioxide fraction in the expiratory air ($FeCO_2$):

$$VCO_2 = \left\{ \int_0^T Q_{exp(t)} \cdot FeCO_2(t) \cdot dt \right\} \cdot T^{-1} \qquad (6.11)$$

where Q_{exp} = expiratory airflow in L/min, $FeCO_2$ = carbon dioxide fraction in expiratory air (gradient) in ml CO_2/L, and T= time in minutes.

Carbon dioxide in an arterial or venous blood sample (C_bCO_2) may be measured by the Douglas equation.[10] This method was has been used in a validation study in an animal model.[11]

Carbon Dioxide Rebreathing Technology (CO₂R)

In the rebreathing method, CO_2 concentration may be estimated from exhaled gas. However, this would only yield an estimate of the nonshunted blood flow participating in gas exchange, also referred to as *pulmonary capillary blood flow* (Q_{PCBF}). The blood bypassing the lung (shunted blood flow) may be estimated and added to Q_{PCBF} to determine overall cardiac output as follows[12]:

$$CO = Q_{PCBF} + Q_{SHUNT} \qquad (6.12)$$

where Q_{PCBF} = pulmonary capillary blood flow (estimate also referred to as the *differential Fick partial rebreathing method* [$Q_{PCBF} = \Delta VCO_2/\Delta CaCO_2$]) in L/min, ΔVCO_2 = change in carbon dioxide elimination in mL CO_2/min, $\Delta CaCO_2$ = change in arterial (alveolar) CO_2 content mL CO_2/min, and Q_{shunt} = shunted blood flow in L /min.

The NICO system (Philips Respironics, Pittsburgh, PA) is an example for a monitor incorporating the carbon dioxide rebreathing method. The $\Delta CaCO_2$ is estimated either by considering the alveolar partial pressure of CO_2, that is, $PaCO_2$, and the CO_2 dissociation curve, or by a regression equation, which is a function of hemoglobin and alveolar CO_2:

$$CaCO_2 = 6.957[Hb] + 94.864) * \log(1.0 + 0.1933\, PaCO_2) \qquad (6.13)$$

where Hb = hemoglobin in g/dL and $PaCO_2$ = arterial (alveolar) partial pressure in mm Hg.[12]

The most often used method to compensate for the shunted blood flow (Qs) is to employ venous and arterial blood gases if they are available.[12] Other methods for estimating a shunt employ the use of pulse oximetry (SpO_2) and inspired oxygen concentration.[12,13] When using a noninvasive approach, an adaptation of Nunn's isoshunt plots describing the relationship between PaO_2 and FiO_2 for different levels of intrapulmonary shunting (in percent) may be utilized.[12,14]

Echocardiography

Echocardiography is considered primarily an imaging technique, which obtains images of structures of heart, the valves, and vessels, and of the function of the heart (see Chapter 5). A secondary use of echocardiography is to estimate stroke volume, cardiac output, organ blood flow, and shunting across the fetal channels during transition, to assess shunts under pathologic circumstances, and to evaluate myocardial function and the pulmonary circulation (see Chapter 5). Echocardiography employs ultrasound and relies on the Doppler phenomenon to determine blood velocity. With respect to the estimation of stroke volume, the ultrasound beam is directed preferably toward the direction of the blood flow in the aorta. Based on the difference in ultrasound frequency between the emitted beam and the beam reflected from the moving red blood cells, velocity is obtained. This specific application of echocardiography is also referred to as *Doppler velocimetry*. Ultrasound is also used to determine the diameter of the aorta at the location of the Doppler insonation, and thereof the cross-sectional area (CSA) of the aorta.

The principle underlying ultrasonic measurement of stroke volume (SV) is quite simple: if the distance (d, measured in cm) traversed by a cylindrical column of blood is measured over its ejection interval (t, measured in s) and multiplied by the measured cross-sectional area conduit (CSA, measured in cm²) through which it flows, then SV (measured in mL) can be calculated as:

$$SV = CSA \cdot d \qquad (6.14)$$

where CSA of the aorta is calculated via diameter measurements employing ultrasonic echo imaging. The distance (d) is calculated using Doppler envelope of blood velocity extracted from ultrasonic Doppler velocimetry.

According to the Doppler principle, when an emitted ultrasonic wave of constant magnitude is reflected (backscattered) from a moving object (red blood cell), the frequency of the reflected ultrasound is altered. The frequency difference between the ultrasound emitted (f_0) and that received (f_R) by the Doppler transducer is called frequency shift $\Delta f = f_R - f_0$. This instantaneous frequency shift depends upon the magnitude of the instantaneous velocity of the reflecting targets, their direction with respect to the Doppler transducer, and the cosine of angle at which the emitted ultrasound intersects these targets[15]:

$$\Delta f = \frac{2 f_0 \cdot v_i \cdot \cos\theta}{C} \qquad (6.15)$$

where Δf is the instantaneous frequency shift; f_0 the emitted constant magnitude of ultrasonic frequency; C is the speed (propagation velocity) of ultrasound in tissue (blood) (1540-1570 m/s); θ is the incident angle formed by the axial flow of red blood cells and the emitted ultrasonic signal, and v_i is the instantaneous velocity of red cells within the scope of the interrogating ultrasound perimeter or target volume.

By algebraic rearrangement:

$$v_i = \frac{C}{2 f_0} \cdot \frac{\Delta f}{\cos\theta} \qquad (6.16)$$

Since C and f_0 are constants, then:

$$v_i = K \cdot \frac{\Delta f}{\cos\theta}. \qquad (6.17)$$

If the angle of incidence between the axial flow of blood and the ultrasonic beam is 0°, that is, $\theta = 0°$, then cosine θ equals 1, and thus:

$$v_i = K \cdot \Delta f$$
$$v_i \propto \Delta f \qquad (6.18)$$

Since from the opening of aortic valve, velocity rapidly accelerates from zero to reach a maximum (peak velocity) during the first one third or one half of ejection phase of systole and a more gradual deceleration phase back to zero velocity occurring with the closure of aortic valve, v_i is not constant. Therefore, in order to obtain the distance d traversed by the cylindrical column of blood according to the model described earlier, v_i has to be integrated over time, that is, from the point in time t_0 representing the opening of the aortic valve to t_1 representing the closure of the aortic valve:

$$d(t) = \int_{t_0}^{t_1} v_i(t)\,dt = SVI \qquad (6.19)$$

where this integral is called the systolic velocity integral (SVI) and defines the stroke distance in centimeters.

Stroke volume is then calculated as

$$SV = CSA \cdot SVI \qquad (6.20)$$

Table 6-4 AORTIC RADIUS/DIAMETER AND CORRESPONDING CROSS-SECTIONAL AREA, ASSUMING A CIRCULARLY SHAPED AORTA

Radius (r) mm	Diameter (d) mm	CSA mm^2	Relative change of CSA			
2.5	5.0	19.6				
3.0	6.0	28.3	44%	larger than when r =	2.5	mm
3.5	7.0	38.5	36%	larger than when r =	3.0	mm
4.0	8.0	50.3	31%	larger than when r =	3.5	mm
4.5	9.0	63.6	27%	larger than when r =	4.0	mm

Relatively small errors in determining the true diameter of the aorta result in significant errors when calculating the CSA, and in turn stroke volume and cardiac output.
CSA, cross-sectional area.
See text for details.

A number of assumptions are made when developing the latter equation.[16-19] A first assumption is that the blood flows in the ascending aorta in an undisturbed laminar flow. As under some conditions, the flow can be turbulent, this assumption has questionable validity.

Another important problem is that the assumption of a circular aorta of constant internal diameter is only fulfilled superficially in a largely undetermined patient population. In fact, aortas of patients are oval or have the shape of an irregular circle. Furthermore, the ascending aorta is not rigid, as assumed, since it pulsates during systolic ejection producing 5-17% changes in the cross-sectional area from its diastolic to systolic pressure extremes.[20]

Moreover, even if the aorta were circular, the accuracy of any echocardiographic method is limited by spatial resolution. Indeed, poor correlation has been found between aortic diameters measured intraoperatively with those measured by a commercially available A-mode echo device preoperatively.[21] In addition, errors in echocardiographic diameter (D) are magnified to the second power (CSA = $\pi \cdot D^2/4$). This becomes more of an issue with the smaller diameter of the aorta in the neonate. Table 6-4 presents a range of aortic radiuses/diameters and for each range the corresponding CSA. The last column refers to the relative change of CSA if the diameter of the aorta was assessed larger by 1 mm (at the 5-mm aortic diameter of neonates, especially preterm neonates, the echocardiographically "measured" CSA would indeed be 44% larger than the actual).

Errors in the velocity measurement are increased by interrogating the axial blood flow at an angle greater than 0° by the emitted ultrasonic signal. However, because the cosine of $\theta < 20°$ is close to 1 (Table 6-5), determining velocity with an acceptable accuracy is still possible. With the increase in angle of insonation (θ) beyond 20°, the velocity is progressively underestimated and therefore angle correction is needed.

In order to improve the measurement quality, esophageal Doppler velocimetry has been introduced. As this approach can realistically only be deployed under

Table 6-5 UNDERESTIMATION OF VELOCITY PER ANGLE OF INSONATION

Angle of Insonation (θ)	Cos θ	Underestimation of Velocity
0	1	0
10	0.98	2%
20	0.94	6%
30	0.87	13%
40	0.77	23%

Cos, cosine
See text for details.

anesthesia, it not an option for neonatal monitoring even if probes small enough to fit the esophagus of a neonate were applied.

Echocardiography has its first and foremost use as an imaging technique to evaluate the mechanical function of the neonate's heart. Employing echocardiography for Doppler velocimetry and determination of stroke volume and cardiac output is a readily available and frequently utilized option at the bedside. The accuracy of stroke volume and cardiac output measurements using echocardiography, however, depends highly on the skills of the operator and the various sources of error must be taken into account when utilizing this method.

Electrical Cardiometry

The noninvasive and easy-to-apply Electrical Cardiometry (AESCULON®/ICON®, Cardiotronic–Osypka Medical, La Jolla, CA, USA/Berlin, Germany) and other impedance-based methods for determining cardiac output extract the changes in thoracic impedance caused by the cardiac cycle. Recording these changes over time produces a waveform, also referred to as the *impedance cardiogram*, which looks akin to an invasive pressure waveform. The methods differ in which component of bio-impedance is utilized to create the impedance cardiogram, and in the interpretation of this waveform.

Bio-impedance is a property of the particular biological tissue and is dependent on the frequency of the electrical current applied. Each tissue in the thoracic compartment, such as blood, organ tissue, or bone, has specific bio-impedivity, or bio-impedance. Blood has very low bio-impedance, in contrast to bone tissue or compartments filled with air, such as the lungs at peak inspiration. Accordingly, the embodiment of bio-impedance measurement is to obtain the respiration rate.

Obtaining hemodynamic parameters from bio-impedance measurements is a two-step process. In a first step, signal acquisition and processing has to acquire and record the portion of the change of bio-impedance specifically related to cardiac activity, referred to as the impedance cardiogram. The surface electrocardiogram (ECG), which is usually recorded in parallel, can serve as a reference for specific landmarks occurring in the course of the impedance cardiogram. Most hemodynamic parameters (except blood pressure) are not the result of a direct measurement. Therefore, a model and related assumptions are applied to derive from a measurement a hemodynamic parameter. The same applies to impedance cardiogram, no matter how it was derived and which component of impedance (resistance or reactance, or magnitude or phase) was pursued. Interpretation of the impedance cardiogram is the second step of the process. One of the models developed to obtain stroke volume from the impedance cardiogram is Impedance Cardiography (ICG).[22] Electrical Velocimetry is a more recent model applied to the impedance cardiogram, which overcomes several limitations of ICG, such as the ability to monitor stroke volume in children and neonates.[23,24] Electrical Velocimetry is incorporated into Electrical Cardiometry monitors.

Obtaining the Impedance Cardiogram

The estimation of stroke volume and cardiac output by means of thoracic electrical bio-impedance (TEB) requires the application of a low magnitude (~2 mA), high-frequency (30-100 KHz) alternating current to the thorax. International safety standards refer to this current as a *patient auxiliary current* and define frequency-dependent maximum amplitudes.

Bio-impedance is calculated as the ratio of the measured voltage $U(t)$ and the applied current $I(t)$:

$$Z(t) = \frac{U(t)}{I(t)} \, (\text{Ohm's law}) \qquad (6.21)$$

Electrical Velocimetry (the model) and Electrical Cardiometry (the method) are trademarks of Osypka Medical (La Jolla, CA, USA, and Berlin, Germany).

If the current $I(t)$ is of constant amplitude, the bio-impedance $Z(t)$ is proportional to the measured voltage $U(t)$:

$$Z(t) \approx U(t). \tag{6.22}$$

Upon application of an alternating current (AC), in contrast to a direct current (DC), as provided by a battery, tissue impedance (Z) comprises not only a resistive component but also a reactive component. The reactive component causes a shift in phase between the alternating current applied and the alternating voltage measured. This occurs because biological tissue can be modeled as a network of electrical resistances (e.g., blood plasma) and capacitors (e.g., cell membranes). Accordingly, electrical bio-impedance is defined by two components: bio-resistance and bio-reactance (in a Cartesian coordinate system) or, redundantly, magnitude and phase (polar coordinates). Impedances such as bio-impedance are also referred to as *complex* impedances.

To make matters worse (or better, if one begins to appreciate the wealth of information contained in it), bio-impedance and its components are dependent on the frequency of the current applied. Imagine a cell membrane, which cannot be "crossed" by an alternating current of low frequency but becomes more and more "permeable" to a current with increasing frequency. This applies to electrical impedance and is one of the reasons why bio-impedance-based methods apply an electrical current usually in the range of 30-100 KHz and not much higher or lower.

The various tissue compartments in the human thorax have different electrical properties and thus bio-impedances. Within the thorax, bio-impedances are considered

- Static, such as bone tissue
- Quasistatic, such as the bio-impedance of some edema as it does not change significantly from minute to minute
- Dynamic, changing their bio-impedance in accordance with the respiratory circle, such as the lungs filling with or releasing air
- Dynamic, changing their bio-impedance in accordance with the cardiac circle, such as the heart filling with blood and the aorta and pulmonary artery passing the stroke volume

When measuring the temporal course of bio-impedance of the thorax, $Z(t)$, the result is the sum of the arrangement of tissue impedance in series and in parallel to each other. Most prevalent are the static and quasistatic impedances referred to as Z_0, followed by a fairly significant dynamic change in bio-impedance corresponding to the respiratory circle $[\Delta Z_R(t)]$, and, to a lesser degree, a change in bio-impedance corresponding to the cardiac cycle $[\Delta Z_C(t)]$, all of which are superimposed:

$$Z(t) = Z_0 + \Delta Z_R(t) + \Delta Z_C(t) \tag{6.23}$$

Because the determination of stroke volume and cardiac output is of interest, the respiratory component of thoracic bio-impedance is omitted (practically by applying high-pass filters), and thus reducing bio-impedance to

$$Z(t) = Z_0 + \Delta Z_C(t). \tag{6.24}$$

Measurement of Thoracic Electrical Bio-impedance

TEB is usually measured in the longitudinal direction of the human body, with surface electrodes (or sometimes electrodes on an esophageal catheter) placed in such a way that the electrical field established by the application of an alternating current encompasses the heart and, more preferably, the ascending aorta and a portion of the descending aorta. The reason for the focus on the aorta rather than the heart is that the most significant rapid change (decrease) in bio-impedance related to the blood circulation $[\Delta Z_C(t)]$, occurs shortly (50-70 msec) after aortic valve opening and thus this change is considered to be a phenomenon related to the aorta.

Figure 6-2 illustrates the attachment of an array of four surface ECG electrode-sensors to the left side of the neck and the lower thorax (approximately at the level of the xiphoid process) for measurement of thoracic electrical bio-impedance.

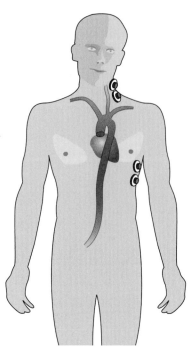

Figure 6-2   Electrode array for measuring thoracic bio-impedance. See text for details.

Typically, an alternating current (AC) of low constant amplitude (up to 5 mA) and high frequency (f_{AC} = 30-100 kHz, also referred to as the *carrier signal*) is applied via the pair of outer electrode sensors to the thorax. The resulting voltage, containing a voltage proportional to $\Delta Z_C(t)$ and the surface ECG vector on top of the carrier signal [f_{AC}] and a surface ECG is obtained via the inner pair of electrode sensors. Electrode sensors may be arranged differently, or electrode sensors added, all for the purpose of obtaining the changes in bio-impedance related to the cardiac cycle.

To obtain the impedance cardiogram, that is, the temporal course of $\Delta Z_C(t)$, the carrier signal, f_{AC} must be removed from $Z(t) = Z_0 + \Delta Z_R(t) + \Delta Z_C(t)$. The technical term for this process is *demodulation*. There are several approaches to demodulation in the analog and digital electronic domain. Furthermore, the demodulation process can be tailored toward the complex bio-impedance, that is, bio-resistance and bio-reactance, or focus on magnitude or phase. Following demodulation, filters separate the surface ECG, Z_0, and $\Delta Z_C(t)$, and possibly other artifacts.

Demodulation reveals a bio-impedance signal, which consists of a significant offset and a relatively small portion of changes. The bigger portion of the changes in bio-impedance is attributed to the respiration cycle. Inspiration causes an increase in thoracic bio-impedance, while expiration corresponding with a decrease in air contents results in a decrease in bio-impedance. The smaller portion of the changes matches the period of the cardiac cycle. Accordingly, devices intended to obtain the respiration rate focus on the bigger changes in bio-impedance, while devices intended to estimate stroke volume and cardiac output focus on the smaller, cardiac-related changes.

Demodulation can be tailored to retrieve the resistive or reactive component of bio-impedance, or magnitude and phase. Magnitude and phase can be calculated from the resistive and reactive part of bio-impedance, and vice versa. The temporal course of any of the bio-impedance components looks very much alike (Fig. 6-3), although signal levels and signal-to-noise ratio may vary.

Bio-impedance and Bio-reactance

Upon application of an alternating current (AC), bio-impedance determines not only the amplitude of applied current and measured voltage but also their phase to each

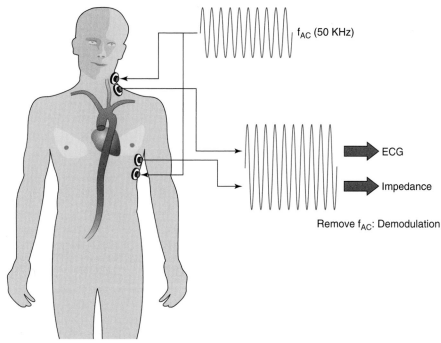

f_{AC} (50 KHz)

ECG

Impedance

Remove f_{AC}: Demodulation

6

Figure 6-3   Demodulation. Application of an alternating current of a certain carrier frequency (f_{AC}; 50 KHz) requires removal of this carrier frequency from the measured voltage signal, a process named *demodulation*. See text for details.

other. If bio-impedance consisted of a resistive component only, the measured sinusoidal signal of the voltage would be in phase with the sinusoidal signal of the applied current. Biological tissues, however, containing compartments and cell membranes, show electrical properties similar to an electrical capacitor, or an array of capacitors. With bio-impedance consisting of both resistive and so-called reactive components, the measured sinusoidal signal of the voltage is subject to a phase shift compared to the sinusoidal signal of the applied current. For biological tissue, bio-impedance is defined as

$$Z(t) = R(t) + j \cdot G(t) \qquad (6.25)$$

where $Z(t)$ = thoracic electrical bio-impedance, R = bio-resistance (also referred as the "real part of impedance") and G = bio-reactance (also referred to as the "imaginary part of impedance"). The letter j indicates that resistance and reactance must be treated as vector components and cannot simply be added algebraically.

Figure 6-4 illustrates the two-dimensional nature of impedance. When, due to respiratory changes or changes related to the cardiac cycle, impedance in the thoracic region changes, both magnitude and phase (or equivalently, resistance and reactance) might contribute to the change as indicated by the continuous line connecting the impedance vectors. Either component can be used to obtain a temporal course of a signal waveform very much akin to an arterial pressure waveform (Fig. 6-5). Albeit signal levels and signal-to-noise ratio may vary. Magnitude and phase can be calculated from the resistive and reactive part of bio-impedance, and vice versa.

Figure 6-6 illustrates the temporal course of the change in bio-impedance along with the corresponding surface ECG. For convenience purposes, the change of bio-impedance signal is shown inverted, revealing not only a striking resemblance with an arterial blood pressure signal waveform but approximating its reciprocal, the change in conductivity.

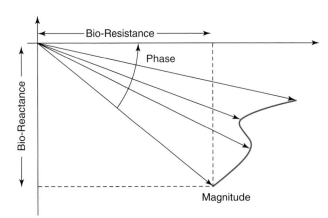

Figure 6-4 Two dimensions of impedance in a Cartesian coordinate system defined by bio-resistance. The two dimensions of impedance in a Cartesian coordinate system defined by bio-resistance are shown on the horizontal axis and bio-reactance on the vertical axis. During the course of a cardiac cycle, thoracic impedance may change along the continuous curve, showing changes in bio-resistance and bio-reactance. Alternatively, impedance is described by its magnitude and phase, with both values changing during the course of a cardiac cycle. See text for details.

It is important to determine the change of impedance, the rate of change. Indeed,

$$dZ(t)/dt$$

is also referred to as the first time-derivative and its temporal course is shown at the bottom of Figure 6-6. Note that from this nonphysiologic, artificial waveform, specific landmarks can be obtained, such as aortic valve opening (marked as B) and aortic valve closure (marked as X). The temporal difference of these landmarks determines left-ventricular ejection time (LVET). Another landmark is the maximum deflection of

$$dZ(t)/dt$$

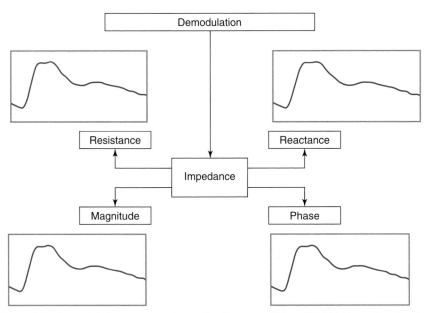

Figure 6-5 Demodulation removes the carrier frequency (30 to 100 KHz) from the signal of interest (the bio-impedance signal) and can be tailored toward obtaining the different components of impedance. Their temporal courses are very much alike and, after filtering out the effects of respiration, the changes resemble an atrial pressure waveform. Of note is that the temporal courses of resistance and magnitude are on top of a significant offset (not shown), like waves in the sea.

Figure 6-6 Temporal course of surface electrocardiogram (ECG), the cardiac-related change of bio-impedance [$-dZ(t)$], and the rate of change of bio-impedance [$-dZ(t)/dt$] are shown. The rate of change of bio-impedance is a calculated (i.e., artificial) signal waveform and used for waveform analysis (such as determination of minima and maxima).

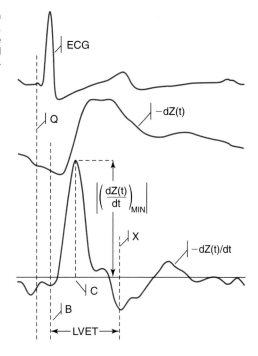

(marked as C) corresponding to the maximum rate of change of bio-impedance (or conductivity) following aortic valve opening (B). Since the inverse of the

$$dZ(t)/dt$$

signal waveform is shown, the amplitude at C is actually the minimum and accordingly labeled as

$$\left| \left(\frac{dZ(t)}{dt} \right)_{MIN} \right|$$

The impedance cardiogram, $\Delta Z_C(t)$, that is, the purely electrical signal waveform akin to an arterial pressure waveform, is of importance for determining stroke volume and cardiac output. Of additional interest is the static thoracic impedance, Z_0, or its reciprocal, as it provides a measure of overall thoracic fluid content (TFC, sometimes referred to as TFI, thoracic fluid index):

$$TFC = \frac{1,000}{Z_0} \tag{6.26}$$

Interpretation of the Impedance Cardiogram

Most hemodynamic parameters cannot be measured directly but require a theoretical model for interpretation of the measurement results. For instance, measurements of electrical voltages on or in the body require the model of the electrocardiogram (ECG) in order to become useful. To estimate oxygen saturation in arterial blood (SpO_2), the absorption of light at different wavelengths is measured, and SpO_2 is determined thereof. Estimating stroke volume from thoracic bio-impedance measurements is no exception. A model must be established to translate the impedance cardiogram $\Delta Z_C(t)$ into a meaningful estimate for stroke volume and cardiac output.

A hemodynamic parameter measured can only be as accurate and reliable as the theoretical model. Thus, knowledge or proper assumption of the origin of the signal measured is the key to modeling. The general formula to determine stroke volume by means of bio-impedance (SV_{TEB}) is

$$SV_{TEB} = C_P \cdot \overline{v}_{FT} \cdot FT; \qquad (6.27)$$

where C_P = a patient constant (volume), usually determined from the patient's body mass (weight) and height; $\overline{v}_{FT}$ = mean velocity during flow time; and FT = flow time.

Impedance Cardiography/Impedance Plethysmography

Kubicek and colleagues modeled the thorax as two parallel conductive cylinders of equal length (L), one representing the aorta and one the remaining thoracic volume, with L being the distance between the sensing electrodes (see Fig. 6-2; inner electrodes).[25] Implicitly, they attributed the systolic portion of $\Delta Z_C(t)$ to the dilation of the aorta following aortic valve opening. According to this model, the first time-derivative of $\Delta Z_C(t)$ corresponds to the velocity of volumetric expansion, and the maximum deflection,

$$\left| \left(\frac{dZ(t)}{dt} \right)_{MIN} \right|$$

or its normalized form,

$$\frac{\left| \left(\frac{dZ(t)}{dt} \right)_{MIN} \right|}{Z_0}$$

becomes an equivalent to *peak* velocity (of volumetric expansion). Accordingly, stroke volume is estimated as

$$SV_{ICG} = V_{ICG} \cdot \frac{\left| \left(\frac{dZ(t)}{dt} \right)_{MIN} \right|}{Z_0} \cdot LVET \qquad (6.28)$$

where V_{ICG} is an estimate of the volume of the thoracic cavity.

Sramek modified the model replacing the cylindrical assumption of thoracic volume by a truncated cone and Bernstein added to the model by correcting actual weight for ideal weight.[22,26] Kubicek's model and its derivations, which attribute the rapid change in thoracic bio-impedance shortly following aortic valve opening to volumetric changes in the aorta, are also referred to as "impedance plethysmography" or "classic" impedance cardiography (ICG).

However, the SV formula and the corresponding model failed to prove its accuracy. First of all, SV and

$$\frac{\left| \left(\frac{dZ(t)}{dt} \right)_{MIN} \right|}{Z_0}$$

are not proportional, which leads to significant discrepancies when patients deviated in body size and composition from normal adults. Indeed, many questions about the model remained only vaguely answered:

1. While the ascending aorta expands (Windkessel phenomenon), a good portion of the stroke volume is already flowing towards the periphery. How does the model account for this portion of the SV?
2. How does the model account for a less or more compliant aorta?
3. The maximum rate of change of bio-impedance usually occurs about 55-60 ms after aortic valve opening, while peak aortic velocity occurs approximately 100 ms after aortic valve opening.

Bernstein and Osypka took a quite different approach and established the model of electrical velocimetry, where not volumetric changes of the aorta but changes in the resistivity of the blood flowing through the aorta cause the rapid change in bio-impedance.[23,24] Electrical velocimetry attributes the rapid change in impedance (or its reciprocal, admittance) following aortic valve opening to the fact that the pulsatile blood flow aligns the previously more randomly oriented red blood cells in the aorta in parallel with the blood flow, allowing the electrical current to traverse the red blood cells much easier. Instead of (complex) impedance, its reciprocal, (complex) admittance can be determined. Complex admittance is defined by conductance and susceptance (Cartesian coordinate system) or magnitude of admittance and phase (polar coordinates).

Alignment of Erythrocytes and Electrical Velocimetry

The method of electrical velocimetry is based on the fact that the conductivity of the blood in the aorta changes during the cardiac cycle.

Prior to opening of the aortic valve, the red blood cells (erythrocytes) assume a random orientation—there is no blood flow in the ascending aorta (Fig. 6-7). The electrical current applied must circumvent the red blood cells for passing through the aorta, which results in a higher voltage measurement and, thus, lower conductivity. Very shortly after aortic valve opening, the pulsatile blood flow forces the red blood cells to align in parallel with the blood flow (mechanical properties of the disc-shaped red blood cells). The electrical current applied bypasses the red blood cells more easily, which results in a lower voltage measurement and thus in a higher conductivity. For technical reasons, impedance rather than conductivity is measured. Impedance is reciprocal to conductivity. The shape of the inverted change-of-impedance waveform, $-dZ(t)$, is akin to the change-of-conductivity waveform. Since the $-dZ(t)$ signal waveform also shows resemblance with an arterial pressure waveform, it has become common use to display the inverted change-of-impedance waveform, $-dZ(t)$, and read it as a change-of-conductivity waveform.

Figure 6-8 illustrates the course of the surface ECG (waveform on top), $-dZ(t)$ (second waveform from top), the calculated, artificial $-dZ(t)/dt$ signal (third waveform from top) and the pulse plethysmogram (obtained by pulse oximetry; bottom waveform). The change from random orientation to alignment of red blood cells

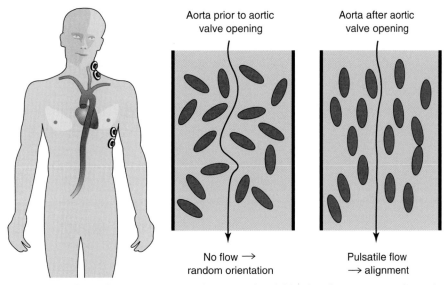

Figure 6-7 Electrode arrangement and proposed red blood cell orientation. Electrode arrangement and proposed orientation of red blood cells in the aorta prior to and shortly after aortic valve opening are shown. See text for details.

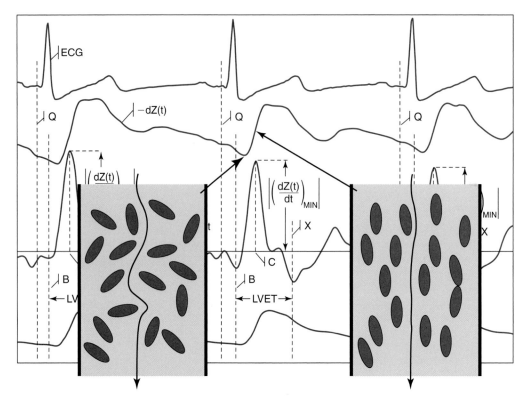

Figure 6-8 Parallel recordings of electrocardiogram (ECG), impedance waveforms, and pulse plethysmogram. Temporal course of parallel recordings of ECG, impedance waveforms, and pulse plethysmogram are shown, along with the proposed orientation of red blood cells in the aorta before and shortly after aortic valve opening. See text for details.

upon opening of the aortic valves generates a characteristic steep, beat-to-beat increase of conductivity (corresponding to a steep decrease of impedance). The red arrows point to the two states shown in the change-of-conductivity signal. The steeper the slope of the $-dZ(t)$ signal, or the higher the peak amplitude of $-dZ(t)/dt$, the quicker the alignment process and, thus, the higher the contractility of the heart.

Doppler velocimetry "interrogates" the erythrocytes in the aorta to determine their velocity. *Electrical velocimetry* also interrogates the erythrocytes but determines their change in orientation to derive blood velocity.

The model of electrical velocimetry considers

$$\frac{\left|\left(\dfrac{dZ(t)}{dt}\right)_{MIN}\right|}{Z_0}$$

as an ohmic equivalent for peak aortic acceleration, and defines an index of contractility (ICON):

$$ICON = \frac{\left|\left(\dfrac{dZ(t)}{dt}\right)_{MIN}\right|}{Z_0} \cdot 1,000. \qquad (6.29)$$

The ohmic equivalent to mean blood velocity ($\overline{v}_{FT}$) is determined by the root mean square transformation:

$$\overline{v}_{FT} = \sqrt{\frac{\left|\left(\dfrac{dZ(t)}{dt}\right)_{MIN}\right|}{Z_0}} \qquad (6.30)$$

The higher the mean blood velocity ($\overline{v}_{FT}$) during flow time, the more SV the left ventricle ejects.

The model of electrical velocimetry corrects the flow time for heart rate, that is, applies a corrected flow time (FT$_C$) to the computation of stroke volume:

$$FT_C = \frac{LVET}{\sqrt{T_{RR}}}; \qquad (6.31)$$

where LVET is the measured left-ventricular ejection time and T_{RR} is the measured R-R interval. The longer FT$_C$ or LVET, the more SV the left ventricle ejects.

Stroke volume is then obtained as

$$SV = V_{EPT} \cdot \sqrt{\frac{\left|\left(\dfrac{dZ(t)}{dt}\right)_{MIN}\right|}{Z_0}} \cdot FT_C \qquad (6.32)$$

where V_{EPT} = volume of electrically participating tissue, a patient constant derived from the patient's body mass (weight) and height.

Pulse Contour Method

The pulse contour method, also referred to as pulse contour analysis, is a technique of estimating and monitoring beat-to-beat stroke volume and cardiac output continuously from an invasively obtained arterial pulse pressure waveform.[27] Cardiac output is derived from waveform analysis and related (proprietary) algorithms considering pulse pressure (the difference between systolic and diastolic pressure), the shape of the waveform or the area under the waveform, or all of the above.

The German physiologist Otto Frank described the circulation in terms of a Windkessel model. *Windkessel* is a German term describing a form of pressure equalization caused by a volume or boundary, which is elastic. Windkessel literally means "air chamber" but it has been used to imply an elastic reservoir. The Windkessel model likens the effect of the elastic arteries in dampening the arterial pulse to that of an air chamber in eighteenth century fire engines.

Accordingly, Frank described the transformation of the pulsatile blood flow ejected by the heart into a more continuous flow that reaches the periphery. Upon aortic valve opening (Fig. 6-9), the pulsatile blood flow though the aorta causes the elastic aorta to expand (akin to the air chamber to be compressed; Fig. 6-10), temporarily storing a portion of the stroke volume with its expansion. Following the peak flow when the pressure created by the contraction of the heart becomes less than the pressure it took to expand the aorta, the aorta begins to regain its normal form by pushing the portion of the stroke volume contained in its expanded size back toward the blood flow.

However, unlike the fire engine, the cardiovascular system is a closed-loop system. Accordingly, the flow generated by the pump and "smoothed" by the Windkessel-effect of the aorta returns to the pump. In the model (Fig. 6-10), the return tube is considered equivalent to the systemic vascular resistance. This somewhat simplistic model of the cardiovascular system, taking into account aortic compliance and systemic vascular resistance, is referred to as the "2-element Windkessel model" and it is of importance for the understanding of the pulse contour method. Table 6-6 compares the Windkessel system and the cardiovascular system based on corresponding properties and functions.

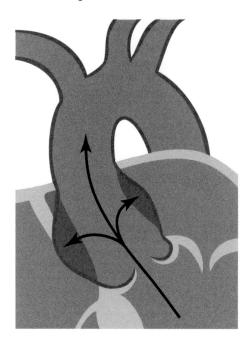

Figure 6-9 Volumetric expansion of the ascending aorta shortly after aortic valve opening. Volumetric expansion of the ascending aorta is depicted shortly after aortic valve opening. The temporary storage of a portion of the stroke volume, followed by its release, attenuates the pulsatile flow leaving the left ventricle, and thus transforms it into a more continuous flow pattern modulated by the compliance of the aorta. See text for details.

According to Ohm's law applied to the systemic blood flow (Equation 6.1)

$$CO = k \cdot \frac{(MAP - CVP)}{SVR}$$

cardiac output is proportional to the pressure difference of $MAP - CVP$ provided that systemic vascular resistance (SVR) is constant. The challenge for any monitoring system employing the pulse contour analysis is to accommodate cardiac output (or stroke volume) for any changes to SVR and for any individual deviation from the normal compliance of the aorta. Furthermore, the location of the pressure measurement within the arterial system must be taken into account as pressure and the shape of the pressure waveform change.

Accordingly, frequent calibration by another trusted cardiac output method, and/or incorporation of algorithms correcting for aortic compliance and changes in

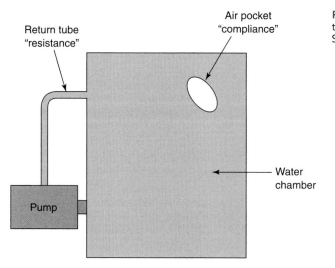

Figure 6-10 Windkessel model adapted to the heart and the systemic arterial system. See text for details.

Table 6-6   WINDKESSEL MODEL AS APPLIED TO THE CARDIOVASCULAR SYSTEM

	Windkessel System	Cardiovascular System
Technique	Pump featuring a handle bar for pumping water first into a water tank with increased compression of the air pocket and from there towards the water hose	Heart (= pump) followed by a compliant aorta (= air pocket), and from there towards the systemic vasculature (= water hose)
Purpose	Transform pulsatile water flow into more continuous water flow	Transform pulsatile blood flow into more continuous blood flow
Means	Elastic air chamber within a sturdy water tank	Compliant (or elastic) aorta and arteries
Pump	Hand-operated pump	Heart
Time when pump builds pressure	Pushing the bar down to pump more water into the water tank	Left-ventricular ejection time
Time when pump lacks building pressure	Pulling the bar up to suck more water	Diastole and the early part of systole prior to aortic valve opening

The Windkessel system is used as a model of the cardiovascular system to illustrate the elastic properties of the aorta and arterial system.

systemic vascular resistance are performed and recommended when using the pulse contour method.

PiCCO Technology

The pulse contour analysis employed by the PiCCO system (Pulsion Medical Systems SE, München, Germany) is calibrated through transpulmonary thermodilution. Once calibrated, the arterial pressure waveform, in particular the area under the systolic part of the arterial pulse curve, is analyzed beat-to-beat (Fig. 6-11). In addition to determining the area under the pressure curve and other factors, calculation of the continuous pulse contour cardiac output also involves aortic compliance measured by transpulmonary thermodilution.

$$PCCO = cal \cdot HR \cdot \int_{Systole} \left(\frac{P(t)}{SVR} + C(p) \cdot \frac{dP}{dt} \right) dt \qquad (6.33)$$

where PCCO = cardiac output by the pulse contour method; cal = patient-specific calibration factor (determined by transpulmonary thermodilution); HR = heart rate; P(t)/SVR = area under the systolic portion of the pressure curve; C(p) = compliance of the aorta; dP/dt = shape of the pressure curve.

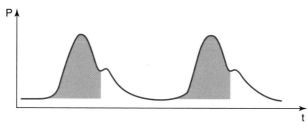

Figure 6-11 Principles of cardiac output assessment by pulse contour analysis. Area under the systolic portion of the pressure waveform and other factors are the basis for calculation of continuous pulse contour cardiac output (PCCO). See text for details (Adapted from Gödje O, Höke K, Goetz AE, et al. Reliability of a new algorithm for continuous cardiac output determination by pulse-contour analysis during hemodynamic instability. Crit Care Med. 2002; 30:52-58.)

LiDCO Technology

The algorithm employed in the LiDCO system (LiDCO Ltd., London, United Kingdom) is based on the assumption that the net power change in a heartbeat is the balance between the input of mass of blood (stroke volume) minus the blood mass lost to the periphery during the beat.[29] Although the arterial pulse waveform is used to determine what is referred to as the *beat period* and the *net power change across the whole beat*, this technique does not rely on the morphology of the waveform and is therefore not considered a true *pulse contour* method.

A proprietary algorithm transforms the arterial pressure waveform into a standardized volume waveform, which undergoes the digital signal process of autocorrelation. This way, both the period of the beat and a power factor assumed to be proportional to a nominal stroke volume are determined. The nominal stroke volume can then be scaled to the actual stroke volume by calibration via an independent indicator (lithium) dilution measurement.

In theory, the main advantage of what LiDCO refers to as the "pulse power algorithm" (essentially determining the autocorrelation) is that it is less sensitive to the site of the arterial pressure measurement. Any arterial site can be used because the morphology of the pressure signal does not contribute to the cardiac output estimate rather the outcome of the autocorrelation process. Furthermore, although the LiDCO system provides for calibration by the lithium dilution technique, other cardiac output methods can be utilized, too. The main limitation of this technology beside the need for calibration, is the use of lithium.

FloTrac System

The FloTrac system (Edwards Lifesciences, Irvine, CA) derives cardiac output from pulse pressure and a factor χ, which accounts for both systemic vascular resistance and aortic compliance (also referred to as the vascular tone) according to the equation:

$$CO_{AP} = HR \cdot \sigma_{AP} \cdot \chi; \tag{6.34}$$

where HR = heart rate (beat/min); σ_{AP} = standard deviation of arterial pulse pressure around the mean arterial pressure (mm Hg); χ = conversion factor accounting for systemic vascular resistance and arterial compliance C(P) with χ being a function of σ_{AP}, C(P), body surface area (BSA), mean arterial pressure (MAP) and the statistical moment μ which is determined by skewness (symmetry) and kurtosis (distinctness of a peak) as well as other mathematical derivatives.

Arterial compliance, $C(P)$ is determined according to the following equation:

$$C(P) = L \cdot \frac{\dfrac{A_{MAX}}{\pi \cdot P_1}}{1 + \left(\dfrac{P - P_0}{P_1}\right)^2} \tag{6.35}$$

where L = estimated length of aorta; A_{MAX} = aortic root cross-sectional area maximum; P = arterial pressure; P_1 = the width of compliance curve at half of maximum compliance; P_0 = pressure at which compliance reaches its maximum.

According to the manufacturer, the FloTrac algorithm requires no calibration because the conversion factor "χ" autocorrects for the patient's changing vascular tone. So far, the FloTrac system has only been tested in adults.

Conclusion

The methods discussed in this chapter rely on different principles to obtain stroke volume and cardiac output (Table 6-7).

Determination of cardiac output using direct Fick principle (oxygen-Fick method) requires application of a face mask or some other means to assess oxygen consumption and measurement of arterial and venous oxygen saturation, which

Table 6-7 OVERVIEW OF UNDERLYING PHYSICAL PRINCIPLES, MEASUREMENTS, DERIVATIONS FROM MEASUREMENTS

Method	Technique	Measurement	Measurement-Derivatives
Echocardiography (Doppler velocimetry)	Ultrasound	Shift of ultrasound frequency (Doppler phenomenon) due to reflection of ultrasound beam at mechanical structures (aortic valve, wall, red blood cells); Heart rate (HR)	Cross-sectional area (CSA) of the aorta (at the interrogation of the ultrasound beam); Aortic flow profile over time (between opening and closure of aortic valve); the area under this flow profile is calculated and referred to as the systolic velocity integral (SVI); $SV = CSA \times SVI$; $CO = SV \times HR$
Direct Fick Principle	Face mask for assessing oxygen consumption, arterial and venous blood sampling	Oxygen consumption (VO_2), arterial oxygen content (CaO_2), venous blood oxygen saturation (CvO_2), hemoglobin (HB)	$C_A \approx HB \times 1.36 \times SaO_2$ $C_V \approx HB \times 1.36 \times SvO_2$ $$CO = \frac{VO_2}{(C_A - C_V)} \cdot 100$$
Thoracic electrical bio-impedance (TEB)/electrical cardiometry (EC)	Application of a low magnitude, high frequency (30-100 KHz) alternating current to thoracic area	Voltage due current application and calculating the temporal course (bio) impedance (usually separated into its two components either magnitude and phase or bio-resistance and bio-reactance); Base impedance (Z_0) or conductivity (Y_0), maximum rate of change of magnitude, phase, resistance or reactance; Heart rate (HR)	Left-ventricular ejection time (LVET), also referred to as flow time (FT) Thoracic fluid content (TFC), also referred to as thoracic fluid index (TFI) Equivalent to peak aortic acceleration, from which mean blood velocity during flow time (v_{FT}) is derived Considers height and/or weight of patient to calculate a patient constant (V_{EPT}) $SV = V_{EPT} \times v_{FT} \times FT$; $CO = SV \times HR$
Pulse contour analysis	Arterial line	Temporal course of arterial pressure	$CO = f$ (e.g., PP, morphology)

See text for abbreviations and details.

requires central vascular access to obtain blood samples for laboratory analysis. Due to the limitations associated with the use of a face mask and the need for blood samples, continuous monitoring is not possible. Furthermore, the need for central vascular access and repeated blood samples and additional methodology-related limitations do not allow for the routine use of this method in the neonatal patient population.

Although the modified CO_2-Fick technique is reliable, the method is complicated and shares many disadvantages of the oxygen-Fick method including the requirement for arterial and venous blood sampling. The CO_2-rebreathing Fick method is noninvasive and can provide a semicontinuous CO measurement. However, it is limited to children weighing less than 15 kg, is only applicable in intubated patients, and is affected by increased CO_2 production, high cardiac output state, and intrapulmonary shunts.

Due to its inherent inaccuracy, echocardiography is not considered the primary method of choice for determining cardiac output in adults but is the most frequently used method in neonates. Obviously, echocardiography can only be employed for spot checks and its error percentage for estimating cardiac output is only about 30%, which is generally borderline acceptable for a method assessing cardiac output.

For many decades, obtaining stroke volume and cardiac output by means of thoracic electrical bio-impedance was restricted to the adult patient population, with application to children being the exception. Electrical Cardiometry, which employs a relatively new approach to the interpretation of the acquired bio-impedance signals, appears to have opened the way for safe and effective monitoring of infants and perhaps neonates. Although Electrical Cardiometry allows for noninvasive and continuous cardiac output monitoring, this technique also has its limitations. As changes of bio-impedance related to the cardiac cycle are of small amplitude compared to, for instance, changes related to respiration, motion artifacts are an important limitation in patients not at rest. Electrical Cardiometry has been validated against invasive methods of cardiac output measurements with excellent correlations in animals, adult humans, and children with congenital heart defects. As for neonates, recent data suggest it has a precision comparable to echocardiography.[30] Further validation and testing of its clinical applicability in the neonatal population are currently underway.

Pulse contour analysis derives stroke volume and cardiac output directly from analysis of the arterial blood pressure waveform. The main limitation of this method is the assumptions that need to be made about systemic vascular resistance, either by considering systemic vascular resistance as constant or estimating it by an algorithm. So far, pulse contour analysis has not been closely studied in neonates.

Finally, it needs to be emphasized that without developing an accurate, noninvasive, continuous, easy-to-use and appropriately validated method to monitor cardiac output in the neonate, further advances in our understanding of transitional cardiovascular physiology and neonatal cardiovascular compromise and its treatment cannot be achieved.

References

1. Shapiro E. Adolf Fick-forgotten genius of cardiology. Am J Cardiol. 1972;30:662-665.
2. Rusy L, Usaleva E. Education resources of the World Federation of Societies of Anaesthesiologists: paediatric anaesthesia review. Practical procedures. Update in Anaesthesia. 1998;8:1-8.
3. de Boode WP. Neonatal hemodynamic monitoring: validation in an experimental animal model. Radboud University Nijmegen: Enschede, The Netherlands; 2010.
4. Bauer J, Hentschel R, Linderkamp O. Effect of sepsis syndrome on neonatal oxygen consumption and energy expenditure. Pediatrics. 2002;110:e69.
5. Shiao SY. Oxygen consumption monitoring by oxygen saturation measurements in mechanically ventilated premature neonates. J Perinat Neonatal Nurs. 2006;20:178-189.
6. Stothers JK, Warner RM. Effect of feeding on neonatal oxygen consumption. Arch Dis Child. 1979;54:415-420.
7. Krovetz LJ, Goldbloom S. Normal standards for cardiovascular data. I. Examination of the validity of cardiac index. Johns Hopkins Med J. 1972;130:174-186.
8. LaFarge CG, Miettinen OS. The estimation of oxygen consumption. Cardiovasc Res. 1970;4:23-30.
9. Tibby SM, Hatherill M, Marsh MJ, et al. Clinical validation of cardiac output measurements using femoral artery thermodilution with direct Fick in ventilated children and infants. Intensive Care Med. 1997;23:987-991.
10. Douglas AR, Jones NL, Reed JW. Calculation of whole blood CO2 content. J Appl Physiol. 1988;65:473-477.
11. de Boode WP, Hopman JC, Daniëls O, et al. Cardiac output measurement using a modified carbon dioxide Fick method: a validation study in ventilated lambs. Pediatr Res. 2007;61:279-283.
12. Jaffe MB. Partial CO2 rebreathing cardiac output—operating principles of the NICO system. J Clin Monit Comput. 1999;15:387-401.
13. Sapsford DJ, Jones JG. The PIO2 vs. SpO2 diagram: a non-invasive measure of pulmonary oxygen exchange. Eur J Anaesthesiol. 1995;12:375-386.
14. Nunn JF. Applied respiratory physiology, 4th ed. Oxford, England: Butterworth; 1993.
15. Milnor W. Methods of measurement. In: Milnor W, ed. Hemodynamics. Baltimore: Williams & Wilkins; 1982:272.
16. Gardin JM, Tobis JM, Dabestani A, et al. Superiority of two-dimensional measurement of aortic vessel diameter in Doppler echocardiographic estimates of left ventricular stroke volume. J Am Coll Cardiol. 1985;6:66-74.

17. Donovan KD, Dobb GJ, Newman MA, et al. Comparison of pulsed Doppler and thermodilution methods for measuring cardiac output in critically ill patients. Crit Care Med. 1987;15:853-857.
18. Waters JS, Kwan O, Kerns G. Limitations of Doppler echocardiography in the calculation of cardiac output. Circulation. 1982;66(Suppl II):122 (abstract).
19. Waters JS, Kwan OL, DeMaria AN. Sources of error in the measurements of cardiac output by Doppler techniques. Circulation. 1983;68(Suppl II):229 (abstract).
20. Greenfield JC Jr, Patel DJ. Relation between pressure and diameter in the ascending aorta of man. Circ Res. 1962;10:778-781.
21. Mark JB, Steinbrook RA, Gugino LD, et al. Continuous noninvasive monitoring of cardiac output with esophageal Doppler ultrasound during cardiac surgery. Anesth Analg. 1986;65:1013-1020.
22. Bernstein DP: Noninvasive cardiac output measurement. In: Shoemaker WC, ed. Textbook of critical care, 2nd ed. WB Saunders Company, Philadelphia; 1989:159-185.
23. Bernstein DP, Osypka MJ. Apparatus and method for determining an approximation of the stroke volume and the cardiac output of the heart. US Patent No. 6,511,438. 2001.
24. Bernstein DP. Impedance cardiography: pulsatile blood flow and the biophysical and electrodynamic basis for the stroke volume equations. J Electr Bioimp. 2010;1:2-17.
25. Kubicek WG, Karnegis JN, Patterson RP, et al. Development and evaluation of an impedance cardiac output system. Aerosp Med. 1966;37:1208-1212.
26. Bernstein DP. A new stroke volume equation for thoracic electrical bio-impedance: theory and rationale. Crit Care Med. 1986;14:904-909.
27. Hofer CK, Ganter MT, Zollinger A. What technique should I use to measure cardiac output? Curr Opin Crit Care. 2007;13:308-317.
28. Gödje O, Höke K, Goetz AE, et al. Reliability of a new algorithm for continuous cardiac output determination by pulse-contour analysis during hemodynamic instability. Crit Care Med. 2002;30:52-58.
29. Rhodes A, Sunderland R. Arterial pulse power analysis: the LiDCO Plus System. In: Pinsky MR, Payen D, eds. Update in intensive care and emergency medicine. Springer-Verlag: Berlin Heidelberg; 2005:183-192.
30. Noori S, Drabu B, Soleymani S, Seri I. Continuous non-invasive cardiac output measurements in the neonate by electrical velocimetry: a comparison with echocardiography. Arch Dis Child Fetal-Neonatal Ed, in press; 2012.

CHAPTER 7

Near-Infrared Spectroscopy and Its Use for the Assessment of Tissue Perfusion in the Neonate

Suresh Victor, PhD, MRCPCH, and Michael Weindling, MD, FRCP, FRCPCH, Hon FRCA

Light-based approaches to the assessment of a tissue's oxygen status are attractive to the clinician because they provide the possibility of continuous noninvasive measurements. For example, pulse oximetry, which relies on emission and absorption of light in red and infrared frequencies (660 and 940 nm, respectively), has become widely used in clinical practice. However, this technology only measures hemoglobin oxygen saturation, which is variably related to the partial pressure of oxygen in arterial blood and not oxygen delivery. The arterial oxygen saturation is estimated by measuring the transmission of light through the pulsatile tissue bed; the microprocessor analyses the changes in light absorption due to pulsatile arterial flow and ignores the component of the signal which is non-pulsatile and which results from blood in the veins and tissues. Near-infrared (NIR) spectroscopy technology takes this further and utilizes light in the near-infrared range (700 to 1000 nm).

Using one NIR spectroscopy technique (the continuous wave method with partial venous occlusion, described in more detail later), venous oxygen saturation can be determined, and, from this, oxygen delivery and consumption can be measured. Blood flow can also be measured by continuous wave NIR spectroscopy and the Fick approach, either with a bolus of oxygen or with dye.[1,2] However, these methods only allow for intermittent measurements and, more recently, another NIR spectroscopy technique (the time-of-flight method, also described in more detail later) has been used to measure an index of tissue oxygenation continuously.[3] Cytochrome activity can also be assessed, but this has not been utilized in any regular clinical or even research application.[4,5]

NIR spectroscopy instrumentation consists of fiber optic bundles or optodes placed either on opposite sides of the tissue being interrogated (usually a limb or the head of a young baby) to measure transmitted light, or close together to measure reflected light. Light enters through one optode and a fraction of the photons are captured by a second optode and conveyed to a measuring device. Multiple light emitters and detectors can also be placed in a headband to provide tomographic imaging of the brain.

This chapter reviews the principles of NIR spectroscopy, quantifies physiologic variables, and gives clinically relevant observations that have been made using this technology. Clinical aspects of the use of NIR spectroscopy in neonatology are discussed in Chapter 8.

Principles of Near-Infrared Spectroscopy

NIR spectrophotometers are applied in the food industry, geological surveys, and in laboratory analysis. Jöbsis first introduced its use for human tissue in 1977.[6] Since 1985, NIR spectrophotometers have been used in newborn infants.

NIR spectroscopy relies on three important phenomena:

- Human tissue is relatively transparent to light in the NIR region of the spectrum.
- Pigmented compounds known as *chromophores* absorb light as it passes through biological tissue.
- In tissue, there are compounds whose absorption differs depending on their oxygenation status.

Human tissues contain a variety of substances whose absorption spectra at NIR wavelengths are well defined. They are present in sufficient quantities to contribute significant attenuation to measurements of transmitted light. The concentration of some absorbers such as water, melanin, and bilirubin remains virtually constant with time. However, the concentrations of some absorbing compounds, such as oxygenated hemoglobin (HbO_2), deoxyhemoglobin (HbR), and oxidized cytochrome oxidase (Cyt aa3) vary with tissue oxygenation and metabolism. Therefore changes in light absorption can be related to changes in the concentrations of these compounds.

Dominant absorption by water at longer wavelengths limits spectroscopic studies to less than about 1000 nm. The lower limit on wavelength is dictated by the overwhelming absorption of HbR less than 650 nm. However, between 650 and 1000 nm, it is possible with sensitive instrumentation to detect light that has traversed 8 cm of tissue.[7]

The absorption properties of hemoglobin alter when it changes from its oxygenated to its deoxygenated form. In the NIR region of the spectrum, the absorption of the hemoglobin chromophores (HbR and HbO_2) decreases significantly compared to that observed in the visible region. However, the absorption spectra remain significantly different in this region. This allows spectroscopic separation of the compounds using only a few sample wavelengths. HbO_2 has its greatest absorbency at 850 nm. Absorption by HbR is maximum at 775 nm, so measurement at this wavelength enables any shift in hemoglobin oxygenation to be monitored. The isobestic points (the wavelength at which two substances absorb light to the same extent) for HbR and HbO_2 occur at 590 and 805 nm, respectively. These points may be used as reference points where light absorption is independent of the degree of saturation.

The major part of the NIR spectroscopy signal is derived from hemoglobin, but other hemoglobin compounds, such as carboxyhemoglobin, also absorb light in the NIR region.[8] However, the combined error due to ignoring these compounds in the measurement of the total hemoglobin signal is probably less than 1% in normal blood. Nevertheless, when monitoring skeletal muscle using NIR spectroscopy, myoglobin and oxymyoglobin must be considered because their near-infrared absorbance characteristics are similar to hemoglobin.

Near-Infrared Spectrophotometers

Three different methods of using NIR light for monitoring tissue oxygenation are currently used:

- Continuous wave method[9-11]
- Time-of-flight method (also known as time-domain or time-resolved)[12]
- Frequency domain method[11]

The continuous wave method has a very fast response but registers relative change only and it is therefore not possible to make absolute measurements using this technique. Nevertheless, these instruments have been widely used for research studies.[1,2,5,13-25] The time-of-flight method needs extensive data processing but provides more accurate measurements. It enables one to explore different information

Table 7-1 EXTINCTION COEFFICIENTS OF HBO$_2$ AND HB AND
DIFFERENT WAVELENGTHS

Wavelength (nm)	HbO$_2$	Hb
772	0.71	1.36
824	0.983	0.779
844	1.07	0.778
907	1.2520	0.892

provided by the measured signals and has the potential to become a valuable tool in research and clinical environments. The third approach, which uses frequency domain or phase modulation technology, has a lower resolution than that of the time-of-flight method but has the potential to provide estimates of oxygen delivery sufficiently quickly for clinical purposes. This frequency domain or phase modulation technology is potentially the best candidate for the neonatal intensive care setting and for bedside usage. The principles used in the three methods are described later.

Continuous Wave Instruments

In continuous wave spectroscopy, changes in tissue chromophore concentrations from the baseline value can be obtained from the modified Beer-Lambert law.[9] The original Beer-Lambert law describes the absorption of light in a nonscattering medium and states that, for an absorbing compound dissolved in a non-absorbing medium, the attenuation is proportional to the concentration of the compound in the solution and the optical pathlength. Therefore, $A = E \times C \times P$, where A = absorbance (no units), E = extinction coefficient or molar absorbtivity (measured in L/mol/cm), P = pathlength of the sample (measured in cm), and C = concentration of the compound (measured in mol/L). Wray and colleagues characterized the extinction coefficient of hemoglobin and oxygenated hemoglobin between the wavelengths of 650 and 1000 nm.[26] The extinction coefficients determined by them at four specific wavelengths are as shown in Table 7-1. Mendelson and colleagues showed that the absorption coefficients of fetal and adult hemoglobin are virtually identical.[27]

However, the application of the Beer-Lambert law in its original form has limitations. Its linearity is limited by:

- Deviation in the absorption coefficient at high concentrations (>0.01 M) due to electrostatic interaction between molecules in close proximity; fortunately such concentrations are not met in biological media
- Scattering of light due to particulate matter in the sample
- Ambient light

When light passes through tissue, it is scattered because of differences in the refractive indices of various tissue components. The effect of scattering is to increase the pathlength traveled by photons and the absorption of light within the tissue. Cell membranes are the most important source of scattering. In neonates, skin and bone tissue become important when the optodes are placed less than 2.5 cm apart.[28]

Thus for light passing through a highly scattering medium, the Beer-Lambert law has been modified to include an additive term, K, due to scattering losses, and a multiplier to account for the increased optical pathlength due to scattering.

Where the true optical distance is known as the differential pathlength (DP), P is the pathlength of the sample, and the scaling factor is the differential pathlength factor (L): thus DP = $P \times L$. The modified Beer-Lambert law, which incorporates these two additions, is then expressed as $A = P \times L \times E \times C + K$, where A is absorbance, P is the pathlength, E is the extinction coefficient, C is the concentration of the compound, and K is a constant. Unfortunately, K is unknown and is dependent on the measurement geometry and the scattering coefficient of the tissue investigated. Hence this equation cannot be solved to provide a measure of the absolute

Table 7-2 DIFFERENTIAL PATHLENGTH FACTORS

	Van der Zee et al.[28]	Duncan et al.[29]
Preterm head	3.8 ± 0.57	—
Term head	—	4.99 ± 0.45
Adult forearm	3.59 ± 0.78	4.16 ± 0.78

B

concentration of the chromophore in the medium. However, if K is constant during the measurement period, it is possible to determine a change in concentration (ΔC) of the chromophore from a measured change in attenuation (ΔA). Therefore, $\Delta A = P \times L \times E \times \Delta C$, or

$$\Delta C = \Delta A / P \times L \times E$$

The differential pathlength factor describes the actual distance traveled by light. As it is dependent on the amount of scattering in the medium, its measurement is not straightforward. The differential pathlength factor has been calculated on human subjects of different ages and in various tissues. Van der Zee and colleagues and Duncan and colleagues conducted optical pathlength measurements on human tissue and their results are as shown in Table 7-2.[28,29]

There is a small change in optical pathlength with gestation, but this is negligible and a constant relationship is assumed.[30] Despite gross changes in oxygenation and perfusion before and after death in experimental animals, the optical pathlength at NIR wavelengths was found to be nearly constant (maximum difference <9%).[31]

In a medium containing several chromophores (C_1, C_2, and C_3) the overall absorbance is simply the sum of the contributions of each chromophore.

Therefore

$$A = (E_1C_1 + E_2C_2 + E_3C_3)P \times L$$

For a medium containing several chromophores C_1, C_2, C_3

$$\Delta C_1 = Q_1\Delta A_1 + R_1\Delta A_2 + S_1\Delta A_3 + T_1\Delta A_4$$

$$\Delta C_2 = Q_2\Delta A_1 + R_2\Delta A_2 + S_2\Delta A_3 + T_2\Delta A_4$$

$$\Delta C_3 = Q_3\Delta A_1 + R_3\Delta A_2 + S_3\Delta A_3 + T_3\Delta A_4$$

where ΔA_1, ΔA_2, ΔA_3, and ΔA_4 represent changes in absorption at wavelengths such as 774 nm, 825 nm, 843 nm, and 908 nm. ΔC_1, ΔC_2, and ΔC_3 represent changes in the concentrations of C_1, C_2, and C_3 (such as HbR, HbO_2, and Cyt aa3). The 12 values of Q, R, S, and T are functions of the absorption coefficients of HbR, HbO_2, and Cyt aa3. They are termed *near-infrared coefficients*. Since the pathlength is wavelength dependent, a modification of these inverse matrix coefficients is listed in Table 7-3.[32]

Examples of instruments using continuous wave technology are the NIRO 500 and NIRO 100, made by Hamamatsu Photonic, Japan.

Table 7-3 INVERSE MATRIX COEFFICIENTS FOR HB, HBO_2, AND CYTOCHROME AA3 AT DIFFERENT WAVELENGTHS

	774 nm	825 nm	843 nm	908 nm
Hb	1.363	−0.9298	−0.7538	0.6747
HbO_2	−0.7501	−0.5183	−0.0002	1.8881
Cyt aa3	−0.1136	0.7975	0.4691	−1.0945

Spatially Resolved Spectroscopy

The continuous wave method, which measures only the intensity of light, is very reliable, but allows only relative or trend measurements due to the lack of information available about pathlength.[9] To address this problem using current continuous wave instruments, multiple optodes operating simultaneously are placed around the head. This allows for a pathlength correction, but only when the tissue being interrogated is assumed to be homogeneous. This modification is called spatially resolved spectroscopy. It has reasonable signal-to-noise ratio and the depth of brain tissue, which can be measured from the surface, varies typically between 1 and 3 cm.

Spatially resolved spectroscopy is a method that measures hemoglobin oxygen saturation. In contrast to standard continuous wave NIR spectroscopy, this technique gives absolute values. A light detector measures tissue oxygenation index with three sensors at different distances from the light source. Scatter and absorption attenuate light passing into tissue. If the distance between the light source and the sensor is large enough (>3 cm), the isotropy of scatter distribution becomes so homogeneous that the loss due to scatter is the same at the three sensors. Tissue oxygenation index (TOI) is calculated according to the diffusion equation as follows:

$$TOI(\%) = \frac{K_{HbO_2}}{K_{HbO_2} + K_{HbR}}$$

where K is the constant scattering contribution. A similar concept is used in calculating regional oxygen saturation (rSO$_2$).

The NIRO 300 (Hamamatsu Inc., Hamamatsu, Japan) was used to determine the cerebral TOI in 15 preterm infants between 26 and 29 weeks' gestation during the first three days after birth. The median TOI increased progressively during the days after birth. It was 57% (95% CI, 54-65.7%) on the first day, 66.1% on the second day (95% CI, 61.9-82.3%), and 76.1% on the third day (95% CI, 67.8 to 80.1%).[33] In a group of eight preterm infants with hypothermia (body temperature < 35°C), the TOI was found to increase on warming four infants with perinatal asphyxia.[34] Naulaers and colleagues have suggested that by using TOI as a measure of venous oxygen saturation, it is possible to measure an equivalent of the fractional extraction of oxygen continuously.[34] Recently, Dullenkopf and associates examined the reproducibility of cerebral TOI.[35] There was good agreement for sensor-exchange experiments (removing the sensor and reapplying another sensor at the same position) and simultaneous left-to-right forehead measurements revealed only small differences (<5%) and no significant differences between corresponding values.[35] The same group also showed that much of the variability of cerebral TOI was due to cerebral venous oxygen saturation.[36] A point about methodology for assessing the reliability of such tests was made by Sorensen and Greisen, who showed that optodes needed to be reapplied and measured at least five times before the precision of the mean value can be assumed to be comparable to pulse oximetry.[37] A mean difference of 8.5% (95% CI, 5.4-11.6%) was shown when two probes were placed on the same patient's head at different positions.[38]

Quaresima and colleagues concluded that TOI reflected mainly the saturation of the intracranial venous compartment of circulation.[39] There has been variability in the results of studies aimed at correlating TOI with jugular venous bulb oximetry, possibly because of assumptions made about the distribution of cerebral blood between the arterial and venous compartments. Several studies used a fixed ratio of 25:75,[40-42] but Watzman and colleagues described an arterial-to-venous ratio of 16:84 in normoxia, hypoxia and hypocapnia and also observed considerable biological individual variability.[40-43]

The mean ±SD of cerebral rSO$_2$ of 223 normal full-term neonates was 62 ± 2 %, higher than the cerebral rSO2 of term babies with hypoxic ischemic encephalopathy, which was 53 ± 3%.[44,45]

Time-of-flight Instruments

This time-resolved technique consists of emitting a very short laser pulse into an absorbing tissue and recording the temporal response (time-of-flight) of the photons at some distance from the laser source.[12] This method uses a mathematical approximation that is based on diffusion theory to allow for the separation of effects due to light absorbance from those due to light scattering. Thus the time-of-flight method permits differentiation of one tissue from another. In addition, the scattering component provides further useful information, which may be used for imaging. Functional imaging is an exciting application of the time-of-flight method because, in conjunction with hemoglobin status, scattering changes, which can be mapped optically, may provide information about the electrical and vascular interaction, which determines the functional status of the brain. Disadvantages of this technique, which still need to be addressed, are the large amount of data, which means that data are collected and analyzed relatively slowly (minutes), and information obtained at bedside is not displayed instantaneously but rather a few minutes later.

There have only been a few reports on the use of time of flight instruments in neonates.[3] Measurements in neonates at the bedside have not been possible because of the size and the cost of typical laboratory equipment needed for these measurements. However, a new portable time resolved spectroscopy (TRS) device (TRS-10, Hamamatsu Photonics K.K., Hamamatsu, Japan), which has a high data acquisition rate, was recently used clinically. This TRS system can be used (1) for continuous absolute quantification of hemodynamic variables, and (2) for better estimation of light-scattering properties by measurement of differential pathlength factors.

Frequency Domain Instruments

The frequency domain method is based on the modulation of a laser light at given frequencies.[11] The frequency domain instrument determines the absorption coefficient and reduces scattering coefficient of the tissue by measuring the AC, DC, and phase change as functions of distance through the tissue. This method allows for correction of the detected signal for the different scattering effects of the fluid and tissue components of the brain using data-processing algorithms. Moreover, the phase and amplitude shifts can be used for localization of the signal. Since pathlength is measured directly, the hemoglobin saturation can be measured to ±5% in in vitro models and ±10% in piglets. Problems include noise and leakage associated with the high frequency signal, but the devices are very compact and appropriate for bedside/incubator use. Further refinement of the technology will be needed to improve accuracy in the clinical setting.

Examples of instruments using this frequency domain technology are manufactured by ISS, Inc., Champaign, IL.

Measurements of Physiologic Variables

As previously stated, continuous wave NIR spectroscopy does not give absolute quantitative measurements. In order to derive quantitative values for physiologic variables, it is necessary to produce changes in the concentrations of the measured chromophore. This has been done by changing the volume of the cerebral venous compartment, either by tilting the subject head-down or, as we have done, by partial venous occlusion, or by using changes in cerebral blood volume induced by ventilation.[20,46,47] By observing the ratio of the changes in chromophores or the change in chromophore concentration in comparison to another measured variable, it is possible to calculate different physiologic variables.

Some assumptions are made. It is assumed that the receiving and transmitting fiber optodes do not move in position and that the distance between the optodes and the scattering characteristics of the tissue remain constant during a measurement. Also, for cerebral measurements it is assumed that there is no contribution to the NIR spectroscopy signal from extra-cerebral hemoglobin.[48]

Continuous wave NIR spectroscopy has been used in a number of ways to make measurements relevant to neonatal cerebral and peripheral hemodynamics. The technique has been used to measure peripheral and cerebral venous oxygen saturation, and cerebral and peripheral blood flow.

Venous Oxygen Saturation

Intermittent measurements of both cerebral and peripheral venous oxygen saturation (SvO_2) have been made using this technology.[16,20,46,47,49] The assumption is made that in a steady state, arterial and venous blood flows are equal. The approach for measuring both cerebral and peripheral SvO_2 is similar, namely to induce a brief increase in the venous compartment (and hence in the concentration of venous hemoglobin) and then to measure that change.

Cerebral Venous Oxygen Saturation

Three techniques have been described for the measurement of cerebral SvO_2 using NIR spectroscopy.[20,46,47] Each involves the calculation of cerebral SvO_2 from the relative changes in HbO_2 and total hemoglobin (the sum of oxygenated and deoxygenated hemoglobin or HbT) that occur when there is an increase in the venous blood volume of the brain. As mentioned earlier, this is achieved either by gravity using a tilt technique, or by partial jugular venous occlusion or by using changes in cerebral blood volume induced by ventilation.[20,46,47]

The partial jugular venous occlusion technique for the measurement of cerebral SvO_2 was developed by our group in Liverpool, UK, and validated by Yoxall and colleagues.[20] In this technique, the monitoring optodes were positioned on the infant's head in the temporal or frontal regions of the same side. The optodes were held firmly in place without any movement using a Velcro band (Ohmeda). A minimum interoptode distance of 2.5 cm was ensured. In order to establish a baseline, the NIR spectroscopic data were monitored for a short period when no changes were made. Then a brief jugular venous occlusion was made using gentle pressure on the side of the neck over the jugular vein. The compression lasted for about 5-10 s, after which the pressure was released. The brief compression of the jugular vein led to an increase in the blood volume in the head. Since there was no arterial occlusion and because the occlusion was brief, all the increase in hemoglobin concentration monitored using NIR spectroscopy may be assumed to be due to venous blood within the head. The relative changes in HbO_2 concentration and HbT concentration monitored could then be used to calculate the saturation of venous blood within the tissue studied.

Data were recorded every 0.5 s on to a laptop computer using the Onmain program developed at University College London. The differential pathlength factor was set according to Table 7-2. The interoptode spacing was measured accurately using calipers.

Using a spreadsheet, the HbR and HbO_2 data were visually inspected to determine the point at which both started to rise. The 10 data points (5 s) preceding this were averaged to give a baseline (Fig. 7-1). The increase from this baseline was calculated at each point for the next 5 s (10 data points). The venous saturation every 0.5 s for 5 s following the occlusion was calculated from the change in the concentration of HbO_2 (ΔHbO_2) as a proportion of the change in total hemoglobin concentration (ΔHbT). Therefore

$$\text{Cerebral } SvO_2 = \frac{\Delta HbO_2}{\Delta HbT}$$

The SvO_2 was then calculated as the mean of the 10 values thus obtained. Before calculating the value of cerebral SvO_2, the data obtained during each occlusion were observed to check for a steady baseline and a smooth increase after the occlusion.

Five consecutive occlusions were made over a period of approximately 1 to 2 min and the value of cerebral SvO_2 was obtained from the mean of these five occlusions. Using this technique, cerebral SvO_2 was measured noninvasively with minimal disturbance of the subject and repeated measurements could be made.

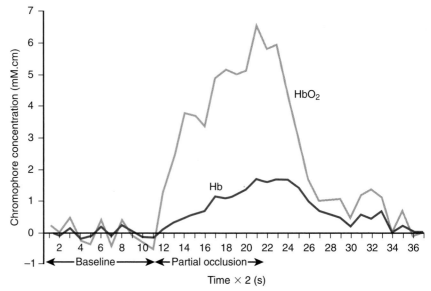

Figure 7-1 Changes in hemoglobin (Hb) and oxygenated hemoglobin (HbO$_2$) following a partial jugular venous occlusion. A 5 s baseline is initially recorded. The partial occlusion lasts for 5 to 10 s. Data are acquired by the NIRO every 0.5 s.

This partial jugular venous occlusion technique was validated by comparison with SvO_2 measured by co-oximetry from blood obtained from the jugular bulb during cardiac catheterization.[20] Fifteen children were studied, aged three months to 14 years (median, 2 years).[20] Cerebral SvO_2 by co-oximetry ranged from 36% to 80% (median, 60%).[20] The mean difference (co-oximeter–NIR spectroscopy) was 1.5%.[20] Limits of agreement were −12.8% to 15.9%.[20] Using partial jugular venous occlusion, measurements were possible in almost all the children studied, including those who were awake and not ventilated and those who were sick and unstable. By contrast, measurements were only possible in 10 of 15 patients studied using the technique described by Wolf and colleagues and results were only obtained in nine of the 22 patients studied using the tilt technique.[46,47] However, the values obtained using the different techniques are reasonably comparable, considering the different populations studied.

Peripheral Venous Oxygen Saturation

Peripheral SvO_2 can be measured by two methods using NIR spectroscopy.[16,50] One approach, which is described in more detail later, involves measuring changes following venous occlusion. It is similar to that used for cerebral SvO_2 and was developed by Wardle and colleagues for preterm infants by adapting a method described and validated by De Blasi and colleagues in adult patients.[16,51] Another approach is a method involving the use of oxygen as an intravascular tracer and it can be used in the same way that measurements of cerebral blood flow are made (see later).[50]

In the venous occlusion method, the optodes were positioned on the upper arm and the interoptode distance was measured using calipers. The optodes were held in place using a small Velcro band (Ohmeda). A brief venous occlusion with a blood pressure cuff around the upper arm was achieved by manually inflating the cuff to 30 mm Hg for approximately 5-10 s. This compression of the arm resulted in a rise in the blood volume within the forearm. Since the venous occlusion was brief and there was no arterial occlusion, all the measured increase in hemoglobin within the tissues monitored was assumed to be due to an increase in the venous blood. During the initial part of a venous occlusion, hemoglobin accumulated in the tissues owing to cessation of venous flow and the rate of hemoglobin flow was equal

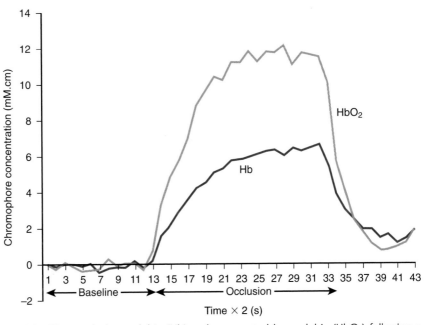

Figure 7-2 Changes in hemoglobin (Hb) and oxygenated hemoglobin (HbO₂) following a forearm venous occlusion. A 5 s baseline is initially recorded. The partial occlusion lasts for 5 to 10 s. Data are acquired by the NIRO every 0.5 s.

to the rate of tissue hemoglobin accumulation during the initial part of the occlusion.

Changes in HbR and HbO_2 concentration were used to calculate the saturation of venous blood within the forearm tissues.

Data were recorded and analyzed as for NIR spectroscopic measurements of cerebral SvO_2 using partial jugular venous occlusion.

$$\text{Peripheral } SvO_2 = \frac{\Delta HbO_2}{\Delta HbT}$$

NIR spectroscopy measures ΔHbT every 0.5 s (Fig. 7-2). Using a similar approach to that for cerebral venous saturation, the HbT data were visually inspected to determine the point at which it started to rise, the ten data points (5 s) preceding this were averaged to give a baseline and the increase from this baseline was calculated at each point for the next 2 s (four data points). As with cerebral SvO_2 measurements, before calculating the value of the peripheral SvO_2 the data from each occlusion were observed to check for a steady baseline and a smooth increase following the occlusion. Five consecutive occlusions over a period of approximately 1-2 min were made and the value of peripheral SvO_2 was obtained from the mean of these five occlusions.

The SvO_2 measurements using the venous occlusion technique made both from the forearms of adults and babies have been compared with co-oximetry measurements. The agreement between the methods was close.[21,22] In 19 adult volunteers, there was a significant correlation between forearm SvO_2 measured by NIR spectroscopy and SvO_2 of superficial venous blood measured by co-oximetry ($r = .7$, $P < .0001$).[22] When the study was repeated in 16 newborn infants there was again a significant correlation between the two measurements ($r = .85$, $P < .0001$).[21] The mean difference between the two techniques was 6% and the limits of agreement were −5.1%-17.1%.[21]

Once venous saturation (using partial venous occlusion and continuous wave NIR spectroscopy) and arterial saturation (using pulse oximetry) are known, fractional oxygen extraction can be measured (see later).

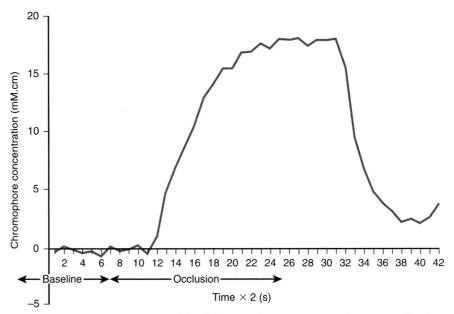

Figure 7-3 Changes in total hemoglobin following a forearm venous occlusion. A 5 s baseline is initially recorded. The partial occlusion lasts for 5 to 10 s. Data are acquired by the NIRO every 0.5 s.

Blood Flow

NIR spectroscopy has also been used as a research tool for measuring cerebral and peripheral blood flow. The methods are described later.

From the measurements made using partial venous occlusion, hemoglobin flow (Hb flow) can also be calculated from the slope of a line through the ΔHbT values during the first 2 s of an occlusion using a least squares method, that is, the rate of increase of HbT within the forearm is used to calculate Hb flow:

$$Hb\ flow = \int \Delta HbT\ dt$$

as shown in Fig. 7-3; and

$$Blood\ flow = \frac{Hb\ flow}{[Hb]}$$

where [Hb] is hemoglobin concentration.

Blood flow (mL/100 mL/min) is calculated by dividing Hb flow (μmol/100 mL/min) by venous [Hb] in μmol/mL. Since the molecular weight of hemoglobin is 64,500 g/mol, blood flow is

$$\frac{Hb\ flow \times 6.45}{[Hb]}$$

where blood flow is in mL/100 mL/min, Hb flow is in μmol/100 mL/min, and [Hb] is in g/dL.

An alternative approach to measure flow by NIR spectroscopy is to use a bolus of oxidized hemoglobin as a non-diffusible intravascular tracer.[1,2,25] In this technique, the monitoring optodes were positioned on the infant's head in the temporal or frontal regions of the same side. The optodes were held firmly in place without any movement using a Velcro band (Ohmeda). A minimum interoptode distance of 2.5 cm was used. In order to establish a baseline, the NIR spectroscopy data were monitored for a short period where no changes were made. The measurement is based on the Fick principle, which states that the amount of a nondiffusible intra-vascular tracer accumulated in a tissue over a time t is equal to the amount delivered in the arterial blood minus the amount removed in the venous blood. If the blood transit time for the brain (t) is less than 6 s, then the amount removed by venous flow will be zero and so increase in tissue tracer content is equal to the amount of tracer delivered by arterial blood flow. Hence, the amount of HbO_2 delivered by arterial flow is arterial Hb flow $\times \int_0^t \Delta SaO_2$, where $\int_0^t \Delta SaO_2$ is the rate of increase in arterial oxygen saturation (SaO_2) and is measured by pulse oximetry. The equation can be rearranged as

$$\text{Hb flow} = \frac{\Delta HbO_2}{\int_0^t \Delta Sao_2 \, dt}$$

Total hemoglobin content [HbT] must remain constant through the measurement. The rise in HbO_2 must therefore be accompanied by an equal fall in HbR. To increase the signal-to-noise ratio ΔHbO_2 is substituted by $\Delta HbD/2$ where HbD = HbO_2 − HbR. The equation now reads

$$\text{Hemoglobin flow} = \frac{\Delta HbD}{\int_0^t \Delta Sao_2 \, dt}$$

where the hemoglobin flow is in µmol/L/min. The SaO_2 is increased by about 5% over less than 6 s. As SaO_2 is measured peripherally and the HbD is measured on the forehead, there may be an interval of not more than 2 s between the rises of each.

Since the molecular weight of hemoglobin is 64,500 g/mol and the tissue density of the brain is 1.05, cerebral blood flow (mL/100 g/min) is

$$\frac{Hb \times 6.14}{[Hb]}$$

where Hb flow is in µmol/L/min and [Hb] is in g/dL.

The oxygen tracer technique has a major drawback in that it self-selects infants within a range of oxygen requirement. Infants who are saturating close to 100% in room air or in small amounts of oxygen cannot increase their oxygen saturations any further with an oxygen bolus. In addition, infants who are on or close to 100% oxygen cannot be given an oxygen bolus.

Physiologic Observations Using Near-Infrared Spectroscopy

Oxygen Delivery

Oxygen delivery (DO_2) is the total amount of oxygen delivered to the tissue per minute.[52] Cerebral oxygen delivery is usually measured as mL of oxygen per 100 g of brain tissue per minute (mL/100g/min).[23]

Oxygen delivery can be calculated from the following formula[23]:

DO_2 = cardiac output × arterial oxygen content

= cardiac output × (oxygen bound to hemoglobin + dissolved oxygen)

= cardiac output × [([Hb] × SaO_2 × 1.39) + (dissolved oxygen)]

where 1.39 is the oxygen-carrying capacity of hemoglobin. As dissolved oxygen is negligible, DO_2 = cardiac output × ([Hb] × SaO_2 × 1.39). While this formula gives the oxygen delivery to the entire body, oxygen delivery to the brain = cerebral blood flow × ([Hb] × SaO_2 × 1.39). Similarly, oxygen delivery to the peripheral tissue = peripheral blood flow × ([Hb] × SaO_2 × 1.39).

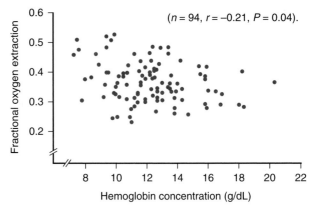

Figure 7-4 Correlation between Hb and peripheral fractional oxygen extraction. (Reproduced with permission from Wardle SP, Yoxall CW, Crawley E, et al. Peripheral oxygenation and anemia in preterm babies. Pediatr Res. 1998;44:125.)

Factors Determining Oxygen Delivery

From the equation DO_2 = cardiac output × ([Hb] × SaO_2 × 1.39) it can be seen that the factors affecting oxygen delivery to the brain are blood flow, hemoglobin concentration, and arterial oxygen saturation. Any one of these measurements alone does not adequately describe oxygen delivery. For example, DO_2 to an organ may be inadequate due to decreased cerebral blood flow despite the presence of normal oxygen saturation and hemoglobin levels.

Effect of Anemia

Despite the importance of hemoglobin in oxygen transport, total hemoglobin concentration is a relatively poor indicator of the adequacy of the provision of oxygen to the tissues and may not accurately reflect tissue oxygen availability.[49] This has been demonstrated in various studies using NIR spectroscopy and is summarized later.

Only a weak but statistically significant negative correlation was demonstrated between blood hemoglobin concentration and cerebral fractional oxygen extraction (FOE) in 91 preterm infants and between blood hemoglobin concentration and peripheral FOE ($n = 94$, $r = -.21$, $P = .04$; Fig. 7-4).[16,18] The authors also compared the cerebral FOE of anemic and nonanemic preterm infants with a relatively small difference in blood hemoglobin concentration between the two groups. There was no significant difference between the cerebral FOE of anemic compared with nonanemic preterm infants.[18] However, cerebral FOE decreased immediately after blood transfusion, suggesting that acute changes may produce an effect.[18]

Peripheral DO_2 increased while peripheral oxygen consumption remained constant after blood transfusion in asymptomatic but not in symptomatic anemic infants.[45] In contrast, observations from animals and adult humans have shown little change in cerebral SvO_2 during anemic hypoxia.[53,54]

Cerebral Oxygen Delivery

Cerebral DO_2 has been calculated using the measurements of cerebral blood flow in preterm infants.[23] The median cerebral DO_2 in infants between 24 and 41 weeks' gestation was 83.2 μmol/100 g/min (range, 33.2-172.3).[23] Cerebral DO_2 overall increases with gestational age ($n = 20$, $\rho = .56$, $P < .012$) and particularly during the first three days after birth (Fig. 7-5).[23,55]

Cerebral Blood Flow (CBF)

Mean global CBF is extremely low in preterm infants and increases with postnatal and gestational age.[51] Using NIR spectroscopy, the median of CBF in preterm infants was 9.3 mL/100 g/min (range, 4.5-28.3).[23] Similar ranges have been reported by

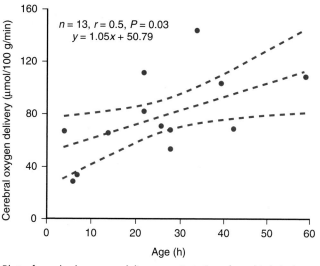

Figure 7-5 Plot of cerebral oxygen delivery against time from birth in hours. There is a significant increase in cerebral oxygen delivery during the measurement, demonstrated by using weighted Pearson correlation coefficient. (Reproduced with permission from Kissack CM, Garr R, Wardle SP, et al. Cerebral fractional oxygen extraction is inversely correlated with oxygen delivery in the sick, newborn, preterm infant. J Cereb Blood Flow Metab. 2005;25:545.)

others using the same technique.[1,25,56] The finding of extremely low CBF in preterm infants using NIR spectroscopy is consistent with measurements of CBF using the xenon clearance technique and using positron emission tomography.[57,58] Cerebral blood flow values of less than 5.0 mL/100 g/min in the normal or near normal brain of the preterm infant are considerably less than the value of 10 mL/100 g/min that is considered to be the threshold for viability in the adult human brain.[59] The very low values of blood flow in the cerebral white matter in the human preterm infant also suggest that there is a small margin of safety between normal and critical cerebral ischemia.[59]

Using the oxygen tracer technique and NIR spectroscopy, CBF was found to increase over the first 3 days after birth in infants between 24 and 31 weeks' gestation.[1] In infants between 24 and 34 weeks' gestation, CBF was independent of mean arterial blood pressure and decreased with decrease in transcutaneous carbon dioxide levels.[25]

NIR spectroscopy was used to investigate the effects of intravenously administered indomethacin (0.1-0.2 mg/kg) on cerebral hemodynamics and DO_2 in 13 very preterm infants treated for patent ductus arteriosus.[55] Seven infants received indomethacin by rapid injection (30 s) and six by slow infusion (20 to 30 min).[60] In all infants CBF, DO_2, blood volume, and the reactivity of blood volume to changes in arterial carbon dioxide tension fell sharply after indomethacin.[55] There were no differences in the effects of rapid and slow infusion.[60]

Peripheral Blood Flow

As described earlier, NIR spectroscopy measures forearm blood flow from the data acquired by the venous occlusion technique.[17,50,51] Using this technique De Blasi and colleagues found that the forearm blood flow in adults at rest was 1.9 ± 0.8 mL/100 mL/min, increasing after exercise to 8.2 ± 2.9 mL/100 mL/min.[51] These values correlated well with those made using forearm plethysmography.[51]

The partial venous occlusion technique was used to study peripheral oxygen delivery in hypotensive preterm infants between 26 and 29 weeks' gestation.[16] In preterm infants, a significant correlation was determined between mean blood pressure and peripheral blood flow (Fig. 7-6).[16,61] Preterm infants with low mean arterial blood pressure of 25 mm Hg (range, 23-27) had median peripheral blood flow of

B

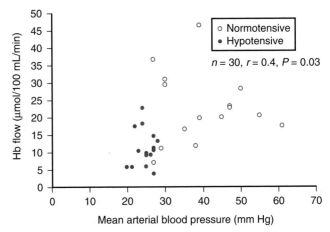

Figure 7-6 Relationship between mean blood pressure and peripheral hemoglobin flow. (Reproduced with permission from Wardle SP, Yoxall CW, Weindling AM. Peripheral oxygenation in hypotensive preterm babies. Pediatr Res. 1999;45:343.)

4.6 mL/100 mL/min (range, 3-5.97). This was significantly lower than the median peripheral blood flow of 8.3 mL/100 mL/min (range, 6.6-10.9) in infants with higher mean arterial blood pressure of 39 mm Hg (range, 30-47).[16] After treatment of hypotension, the median (interquartile range) forearm oxygen delivery increased significantly ($P=.01$) from 37.8 μmol/100 mL/min (25.7-59.5) to 64.2 μmol/100 mL/min (57.1-83.4) (Fig. 7-7).[16] The median (interquartile range) forearm oxygen consumption increased significantly ($P = .02$) from 11.0 μmol/100 mL/min (9.3-2.1.4) to 21.7 μmol/100 mL/min (15.9-26.1) (see Fig. 7-7).[16]

In a study investigating peripheral oxygen delivery and anemia, forearm blood flow did not correlate with the HbF fraction or the red cell volume.[49] Forearm blood flow did not change significantly after transfusion in symptomatic and asymptomatic anemic preterm infants.[49] However, in the same study, there was a significant positive correlation between forearm blood flow and postnatal age.[49]

Oxygen Consumption

Oxygen consumption (VO_2) is defined as the total amount of oxygen consumed by the tissue per minute.[52] The amount of oxygen required by a tissue depends on the

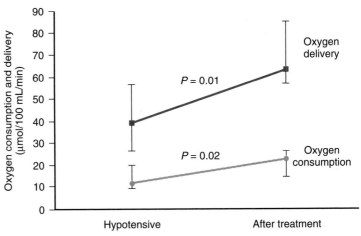

Figure 7-7 Changes in forearm oxygen delivery and oxygen consumption after treatment for hypotension. (Reproduced with permission from Wardle SP, Yoxall CW, Weindling AM. Peripheral oxygenation in hypotensive preterm babies. Pediatr Res. 1999;45:343.)

functional state of the component cells. Some tissues like the brain, the liver, and the renal cortex have persistently high oxygen demands, while tissues like the spleen have low oxygen demands. Other tissues like the skeletal muscle have variable oxygen demands.

The units for cerebral VO_2 are mL of oxygen per 100 g of brain tissue per min.[23] VO_2 can be calculated from the following formula[23]:

$$VO_2 = \text{cardiac output} \times (\text{arterial oxygen content} - \text{venous oxygen content})$$

$$= \text{cardiac output} \times \begin{bmatrix} ([Hb] \times SaO_2 \times 1.39) + (\text{dissolved } O_2) \\ - ([Hb] \times SvO_2 \times 1.39) + (\text{dissolved } O_2) \end{bmatrix}$$

where 1.39 is the oxygen-carrying capacity of hemoglobin. Since VO_2 = cardiac output × [Hb] × (SaO_2 − SvO_2) × 1.39, cerebral or peripheral VO_2 = cerebral or peripheral blood flow × [Hb] × (SaO_2 − SvO_2) × 1.39.

Cerebral Venous Oxygen Saturation and Consumption

By combining measurement of CBF using ^{133}Xe clearance and estimation of cerebral SvO_2 using NIR spectroscopy and head tilt, cerebral VO_2 was calculated as 1.0 mL/100 g/min in nine preterm infants and 1.4 mL/100 g/min in 10 asphyxiated term infants.[46]

We used NIR spectroscopy with partial jugular venous occlusion to determine cerebral SvO_2 and an oxygen bolus to measure CBF in 20 infants (median gestation, 27 weeks; range, 24-41 weeks).[23] The median cerebral VO_2 was 0.52 mL/100 g/min (range, 0.19-1.76) and it increased with maturity in line with cerebral DO_2 (see later) and, presumably, increasing cerebral metabolism.[23]

Peripheral Venous Oxygen Saturation and Consumption

NIR spectroscopy has been used to study SvO_2 and VO_2 in the forearm of preterm infants. Peripheral SvO_2 when measured by co-oximetry was generally slightly higher than that measured by NIR spectroscopy, and this difference was more pronounced at higher levels of SvO_2.[21] This relationship was significant ($r = .528$, $P < .05$, $n = 16$).

In a study comparing forearm VO_2 in anemic preterm infants before and after blood transfusion, no differences were found.[49] This was regardless of whether infants were symptomatic or asymptomatic prior to transfusion.[49]

Peripheral VO_2 increased significantly after treatment of hypotensive preterm infants.[16] In that study, the treatment of hypotension consisted mainly of treatment with dopamine, which is known to stimulate metabolic activity particularly within muscle tissue.[16]

The relationship between the use of dopamine and VO_2 has also been studied using NIR spectroscopy. In a study examining peripheral oxygenation in hypotensive preterm babies, treatment of hypotension using volume and/or dopamine increased forearm DO_2 and VO_2 but did not affect FOE.[16] Low dose dopamine infusion in young rabbits did not alter cerebral hemodynamics and oxygenation.[62]

Fractional Oxygen Extraction

Fractional oxygen extraction (FOE) is the amount of oxygen consumed as fraction of oxygen delivery.[52] It has also been called *oxygen extraction ratio, oxygen extraction,* and *oxygen extraction fraction*.[52,56,63] It is calculated as follows[18,52]:

$$FOE = \frac{VO_2}{DO_2}$$

Since VO_2 = cardiac output × [(Hb × 1.39) × (SaO_2 − SvO_2)] and DO_2 = cardiac output × (Hb × 1.39) × SaO_2, then by simplifying the equation,

$$FOE = \frac{SaO_2 - SvO_2}{SaO_2}$$

Therefore FOE can be calculated if the SaO_2 and SvO_2 are known. SvO_2 is measured using the methods described earlier and peripheral SaO_2 is measured by pulse oximetry. The amount of oxygen dissolved in blood is considered to be negligible.

FOE varies from organ to organ and with levels of activity.[15] Measurements of FOE for the whole body produce a range of approximately 0.15-0.33.[15] That is, the body consumes 15-33% of oxygen transported. The heart and brain are likely to have consistently high values of FOE during active states.[15]

Cerebral FOE can be calculated using the following formula[18]:

$$\text{Cerebral FOE} = \frac{\text{Cerebral } Vo_2}{\text{Cerebral } Do_2}$$

$$= \frac{CBF \times [Hb] \times (SaO_2 - SvO_2) \times 1.39}{CBF \times [Hb] \times SaO_2 \times 1.39}$$

$$= \frac{SaO_2 - SvO_2}{SaO_2}$$

Cerebral SaO_2 is assumed to be equal to peripheral SaO_2 as measured by pulse oximetry. The amount of oxygen dissolved in blood is considered to be negligible.

Using NIR spectroscopy and partial jugular venous occlusion in 41 preterm infants (median gestation, 29 weeks; range, 27-31 weeks), the mean cerebral FOE was 0.292 (SD = 0.06).[18] In that study, there appeared to be no relationship between cerebral FOE and gestational age or postnatal age (median, 9 days; range, 6-19 days).[18] However, when cerebral FOE was measured over the first three days after birth there was a significant decrease in cerebral FOE between days 1 and 2, suggesting an increase in CBF and cerebral oxygen delivery (Fig. 7-8).[14,55,61]

A major determinant of cerebral FOE is arterial carbon dioxide.[18] A negative correlation between arterial carbon dioxide levels and cerebral FOE has been observed in studies on preterm neonates.[18,64] The effect of arterial carbon dioxide on cerebral FOE is related to its effect on cerebral blood flow. The average increase

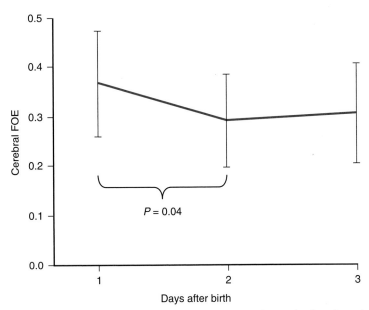

Figure 7-8 Changes in cerebral fractional oxygen extraction during the first three days after birth in sick extremely preterm infants. Data are plotted as means with standard deviations. There is a significant decrease in cerebral fractional oxygen extraction between days 1 and 2. (Reproduced with permission from Kissack CM, Garr R, Wardle SP, et al. Cerebral fractional oxygen extraction is inversely correlated with oxygen delivery in the sick, newborn, preterm infant. J Cereb Blood Flow Metab. 2005;25:545.)

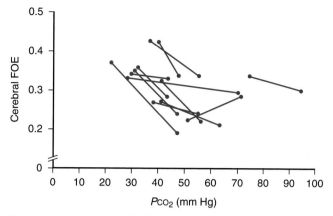

Figure 7-9 Relationship between cerebral fractional oxygen extraction (FOE) and P_{CO_2} within individuals. Measurements within individuals are linked by a line. (Reproduced with permission from Wardle SP, Yoxall CW, Weindling AM. Determinants of cerebral fractional oxygen extraction using near infrared spectroscopy in preterm neonates. J Cereb Blood Flow Metab. 2000;20:272.)

in cerebral FOE with decrease in arterial carbon dioxide was 10.8%/kPa (range, 3.5-29) (Fig. 7-9).[18] This is considerably less than the reported decrease of 67% (range, 13 to 146) in CBF per kPa decrease in arterial carbon dioxide using ^{133}Xe clearance.[65] One possible reason for this may be that cerebral oxygen consumption does not remain constant, but decreases as a protective response to decreased cerebral oxygen delivery induced by hypocarbia.[66,67]

The critical level of blood pressure at which cerebral perfusion becomes compromised has not been clearly determined. Cerebral FOE was not increased in neonates who were considered "hypotensive" when compared with control subjects, and there was no change in cerebral FOE when the blood pressure returned to the normal range after treatment (Figs 7-10 and 7-11).[18] In that study, the median blood pressure was 25 mm Hg (range, 24-27 mm Hg).[18] This was confirmed by other studies examining the relationship between mean blood pressure and cerebral FOE at mean blood pressure levels greater than 20 mm Hg on the first 3 days after birth.[14,61] A study relating CBF to mean blood pressure suggested that the critical level of mean blood pressure was less than 23.7 mm Hg and that CBF at mean blood pressure levels greater than 23.7 mm Hg was independent of mean blood pressure.[25] Since no study was conducted at extremely low levels of mean blood pressure, the

Figure 7-10 Cerebral fractional oxygen extraction was compared between three groups of preterm infants. The bar represents the mean value for each group. (Reproduced with permission from Wardle SP, Yoxall CW, Weindling AM. Determinants of cerebral fractional oxygen extraction using near infrared spectroscopy in preterm neonates. J Cereb Blood Flow Metab. 2000;20:272.)

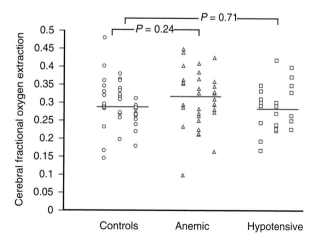

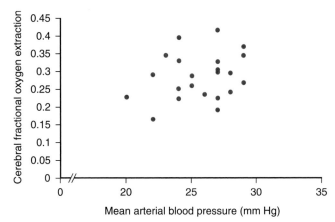

Figure 7-11 Relationship between cerebral fractional oxygen extraction and mean arterial blood pressure in hypotensive group. (Reproduced with permission from Wardle SP, Yoxall CW, Weindling AM. Determinants of cerebral fractional oxygen extraction using near infrared spectroscopy in preterm neonates. J Cereb Blood Flow Metab. 2000;20:272.)

exact nature of the relationships between measures of cerebral oxygenation and mean blood pressure is still unknown.

Left ventricular output was found to have a weak but significant correlation with cerebral FOE.[14] However, much of the relationship was due to two infants with high cerebral FOE. Of the 18 infants with low left ventricular output, cerebral FOE was elevated in only seven. Interestingly, these seven infants were simultaneously hypocarbic.[14] This suggests that left ventricular output, which may be reduced by myocardial hypoxic ischemia as well as hypovolemia, is not an independent determinant of cerebral FOE. Rather, it seems probable that cerebral FOE is only elevated when left ventricular output is low in the presence of hypocarbia. None of these babies developed cerebral white matter injury. Nevertheless, the observation supports other evidence that hypocarbia is a potentially important cause of brain damage. It also adds weight to the proposition that the mechanism of damage when there is hypocarbia is through cerebral vasoconstriction and cerebral hypoperfusion.

Oxygen Delivery–Consumption Coupling

The relationship between cerebral DO_2 and VO_2 has been described using the biphasic model (Fig. 7-12). This model was first described by Cain from animal work using dogs and has subsequently been demonstrated in several other animal models and in critically ill adults and not in preterm babies.[68-71] During the phase B-C, as metabolic demand increases or delivery decreases, FOE (Fig. 7-13) rises to maintain aerobic metabolism and consumption remains independent of delivery.[52] However, at point B—called critical DO_2—the maximum FOE is reached.[52] In phase A-B, when VO_2 is delivery-dependent, any further increase in VO_2 or decline in delivery must lead to tissue hypoxia.[52]

The clinical implication of this model is that tissues, organs, or individuals may be expected to accommodate quite large changes in DO_2 without changes in function or critical damage unless DO_2 is severely curtailed. One mechanism by which the tissues appear to compensate is by increasing FOE. The exact mechanism by which this occurs is unknown. Since oxygen diffusion to the cell is entirely a passive process, it has been suggested that increased oxygen extraction occurs through capillary dilatation and recruitment.[63] However, studies examining this have demonstrated little or no capillary dilatation.[72-74] A theoretical model suggests that alterations in membrane diffusability may be responsible for increasing oxygen extraction.[63] Another possible mechanism is through changing oxygen-hemoglobin dissociation. As arterial oxygen tension decreases, the affinity of oxygen to hemoglobin decreases dramatically due to the sigmoid shaped relationship. Furthermore,

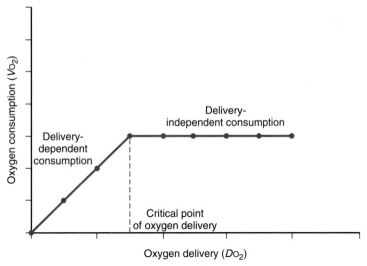

Figure 7-12   Biphasic model for oxygen delivery and oxygen consumption.

the position of the oxygen-hemoglobin dissociation curve changes with changing pH, as may occur if there is local hypoxia and consequent acidosis.

The biphasic model is based on the assumption that VO_2 remains constant during phase B-C. However, the situation in vivo is likely to be different and more complex. VO_2 regulates DO_2 under normal physiologic conditions and DO_2 is likely to vary to ensure balance between delivery and consumption, at least till critical DO_2 is reached. At this time, further decreases in DO_2 result in falling VO_2 with diminished metabolism, although not initially hypoxic tissue damage.

Early Postnatal Adaptation

Serial measurements using NIR spectroscopy have been useful in determining postnatal adaptation in premature infants. There is evidence that cerebral DO_2 increases during the days after birth: cerebral FOE decreases and there are increases in cardiac

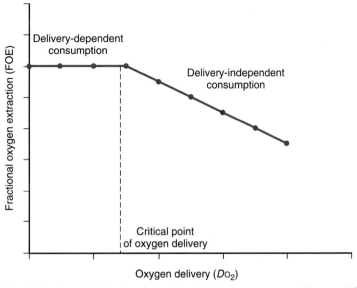

Figure 7-13   Biphasic model showing the relationship between oxygen delivery and fractional oxygen extraction.

output, systemic blood pressure, and CBF.[1,14,75,76] TOI increases during the first three days after birth.[77] These observations suggest that the infant is particularly vulnerable to decreased cerebral DO_2 on the first day after birth and emphasize the importance of careful resuscitation and the need to maintain physiologic stability during the hours after birth.

References

1. Meek JH, Tyszczuk L, Elwell CE, et al. Cerebral blood flow increases over the first three days of life in extremely preterm neonates. Arch Dis Child Fetal Neonatal Ed. 1998;78:F33-F37.
2. Meek JH, Tyszczuk L, Elwell CE, et al. Low cerebral blood flow is a risk factor for severe intraventricular haemorrhage. Arch Dis Child Fetal Neonatal Ed. 1999;81:F15-F18.
3. Ijichi S, Kusaka T, Isobe K, et al. Developmental changes of optical properties in neonates determined by near-infrared time resolved spectroscopy. Pediatr Res. 2005;58:568-573.
4. Dani C, Bertini G, Reali MF, et al. Brain hemodynamic changes in preterm infants after maintenance dose caffeine and aminophylline treatment. Biol Neonate. 2000;78:27-32.
5. Urlesberger B, Pichler G, Gradnitzer E, et al. Changes in cerebral blood volume and cerebral oxygenation during periodic breathing in term infants. Neuropediatrics. 2000;31:75-81.
6. Jöbsis FF, Keizer JH, LaManna JC, et al. Reflectance spectrophotometry of cytochrome aa3 in vivo. J Appl Physiol. 1977;43:858-872.
7. Irwin MS, Thorniley MS, Dore CJ, et al. Near infra-red spectroscopy. a non-invasive monitor of perfusion and oxygenation within the microcirculation of limbs and flaps. Br J Plast Surg. 1995;48:14-22.
8. Mancini DM, Bolinger L, Li H, et al. Validation of near-infrared spectroscopy in humans. J Appl Physiol. 1994;77:2740-2747.
9. Stankovic MR, Maulik D, Rosenfeld W, et al. Role of frequency domain optical spectroscopy in the detection of neonatal brain hemorrhage—a newborn piglet study. J Matern Fetal Med. 2000;9:142-149.
10. Tsuji M, duPlessis A, Taylor G, et al. Near infrared spectroscopy detects cerebral ischemia during hypotension in piglets. Pediatr Res. 1998;44:591-595.
11. Fantini S, Hueber D, Franceschini MA, et al. Non-invasive optical monitoring of the newborn piglet brain using continuous-wave and frequency-domain spectroscopy. Phys Med Biol. 1999;44:1543-1563.
12. Alfano RR, Demos SG, Galland P, et al. Time-resolved and nonlinear optical imaging for medical applications. Ann N Y Acad Sci. 1998;838:14-28.
13. Kissack CM, Garr M, Wardle SP, et al. Postnatal changes in cerebral oxygen extraction in the preterm infant are associated with intraventricular haemorrhage and haemorrhagic parenchymal infarction but not periventricular leukomalacia. Pediatr Res. 2004;56:111-116.
14. Kissack CM, Garr R, Wardle SP, et al. Cerebral fractional oxygen extraction in very low birth weight infants is high when there is low left ventricular output and hypocarbia but is unaffected by hypotension. Pediatr Res. 2004;55:400-405.
15. Wardle SP, Yoxall CW, Weindling AM. Cerebral oxygenation during cardiopulmonary bypass. Arch Dis Child. 1998;78:26-32.
16. Wardle SP, Yoxall CW, Weindling AM. Peripheral oxygenation in hypotensive preterm babies. Pediatr Res. 1999;45:343-349.
17. Wardle SP, Weindling AM. Peripheral oxygenation in preterm infants. Clin Perinatol. 1999;26:947-966.
18. Wardle SP, Yoxall CW, Weindling AM. Determinants of cerebral fractional oxygen extraction using near infrared spectroscopy in preterm neonates. J Cereb Blood Flow Metab. 2000;20:272-279.
19. Wardle SP, Weindling AM. Peripheral fractional oxygen extraction and other measures of tissue oxygenation to guide blood transfusions in preterm infants. Semin Perinatol. 2001;25:60-64.
20. Yoxall CW, Weindling AM, Dawani NH, et al. Measurement of cerebral venous oxyhemoglobin saturation in children by near-infrared spectroscopy and partial jugular venous occlusion. Pediatr Res. 1995;38:319-323.
21. Yoxall CW, Weindling AM. The measurement of peripheral venous oxyhemoglobin saturation in newborn infants by near infrared spectroscopy with venous occlusion. Pediatr Res. 1996;39:1103-1106.
22. Yoxall CW, Weindling AM. Measurement of venous oxyhaemoglobin saturation in the adult human forearm by near infrared spectroscopy with venous occlusion. Med Biol Eng Comput. 1997;35:331-336.
23. Yoxall CW, Weindling AM. Measurement of cerebral oxygen consumption in the human neonate using near infrared spectroscopy: cerebral oxygen consumption increases with advancing gestational age. Pediatr Res. 1998;44:283-290.
24. Meek JH, Elwell CE, McCormick DC, et al. Abnormal cerebral haemodynamics in perinatally asphyxiated neonates related to outcome. Arch Dis Child Fetal Neonatal Ed. 1999;81:F110-F115.
25. Tyszczuk L, Meek J, Elwell C, et al Cerebral blood flow is independent of mean arterial blood pressure in preterm infants undergoing intensive care. Pediatrics. 1998;102(2 Pt 1):337-341.
26. Wray S, Cope M, Delpy DT, et al. Characterization of the near infrared absorption spectra of cytochrome aa3 and haemoglobin for the non-invasive monitoring of cerebral oxygenation. Bioch Biophys Acta. 1988;933:184-192.

27. Mendelson Y, Kent JC, Mendelson Y, et al. Variations in optical absorption spectra of adult and fetal hemoglobins and its effect on pulse oximetry. IEEE Trans Biomed Eng. 1989;36:844-848.
28. van der Zee P, Cope M, Arridge SR, et al. Experimentally measured optical pathlengths for the adult head, calf and forearm and the head of the newborn infant as a function of inter optode spacing. Adv Exp Med Biol. 1992;316:143-153.
29. Duncan A, Meek JH, Clemence M, et al. Optical pathlength measurements on adult head, calf and forearm and the head of the newborn infant using phase resolved optical spectroscopy. Phys Med Biol. 1995;40:295-304.
30. Duncan A, Meek JH, Clemence M, et al. Measurement of cranial optical pathlength as a function of age using phase resolved near infrared spectroscopy. Pediatr Res. 1996;39:889-894.
31. Delpy DT, Arridge SR, Cope M, et al. Quantitation of pathlength in optical spectroscopy. Adv Exp Med Biol. 1989;248:41-46.
32. Essenpreis M, Cope M, Elwell CE, et al. Wavelength dependence of the differential pathlength factor and the log slope in time-resolved tissue spectroscopy. Adv Exp Med Biol. 1993;333:9-20.
33. Naulaers G, Morren G, Van Huffel S, et al. Measurement of tissue oxygenation index during the first three days in premature born infants. Adv Exp Med Biol. 2003;510:379-383.
34. Naulaers G, Cossey V, Morren G, et al. Continuous measurement of cerebral blood volume and oxygenation during rewarming of neonates. Acta Paediatr. 2004;93:1540-1542.
35. Dullenkopf A, Kolarova A, Schulz G, et al. Reproducibility of cerebral oxygenation measurement in neonates and infants in the clinical setting using the NIRO 300 oximeter. Pediatr Crit Care Med. 2005;6:378-379.
36. Weiss M, Dullenkopf A, Kolarova A, et al. Near-infrared spectroscopic cerebral oxygenation reading in neonates and infants is associated with central venous oxygen saturation. Paediatr Anaesth. 2005;15:102-109.
37. Sorensen LC, Greisen G. Precision of measurement of cerebral tissue oxygenation index using near-infrared spectroscopy in preterm neonates. J Biomed Opt. 2006;11:054005.
38. Sorensen LC, Leung TS, Greisen G. Comparison of cerebral oxygen saturation in premature infants by near-infrared spatially resolved spectroscopy: observations on probe-dependent bias. J Biomed Opt. 2008;13:064013.
39. Quaresima V, Sacco S, Totaro R, et al. Noninvasive measurement of cerebral hemoglobin oxygen saturation using two near infrared spectroscopy approaches. J Biomed Opt. 2000;5:201-205.
40. Henson LC, Calalang C, Temp JA, et al. Accuracy of a cerebral oximeter in healthy volunteers under conditions of isocapnic hypoxia. Anesthesiology. 1998;88:58-65.
41. Kurth CD, Levy WJ, McCann J. Near-infrared spectroscopy cerebral oxygen saturation thresholds for hypoxia-ischemia in piglets. J Cereb Blood Flow Metab. 2002;22:335-341.
42. Pollard V, Prough DS, DeMelo AE, et al. Validation in volunteers of a near-infrared spectroscope for monitoring brain oxygenation in vivo. Anesth Analg. 1996;82:269-277.
43. Watzman HM, Kurth CD, Montenegro LM, et al. Arterial and venous contributions to near-infrared cerebral oximetry. Anesthesiology. 2000;93:947-953.
44. Zhou CL, Liu YF, Zhang JJ, et al. [Measurement of birth regional oxygen saturation in neonates in China: a multicentre randomised clinical trial]. Zhonghua Er Ke Za Zhi. 2009;47:517-522.
45. Huang L, Ding H, Hou X, et al. Assessment of the hypoxic-ischemic encephalopathy in neonates using non-invasive near-infrared spectroscopy. Physiol Meas. 2004;25:749-761.
46. Skov L, Pryds O, Greisen G, et al. Estimation of cerebral venous saturation in newborn infants by near infrared spectroscopy. Pediatr Res. 1993;33:52-55.
47. Wolf M, Duc G, Keel M, et al. Continuous noninvasive measurement of cerebral arterial and venous oxygen saturation at the bedside in mechanically ventilated neonates. Crit Care Med. 1997;25:1579-1582.
48. Owen-Reece H, Smith M, Elwell CE, et al. Near infrared spectroscopy. Br J Anaesth. 1999;82:418-426.
49. Wardle SP, Yoxall CW, Crawley E, et al. Peripheral oxygenation and anemia in preterm babies. Pediatr Res. 1998;44:125-131.
50. Edwards AD, Richardson C, van der ZP, et al. Measurement of hemoglobin flow and blood flow by near-infrared spectroscopy. J Appl Physiol. 1993;75:1884-1889.
51. De Blasi RA, Ferrari M, Natali A, et al. Noninvasive measurement of forearm blood flow and oxygen consumption by near-infrared spectroscopy. J Appl Physiol. 1994;76:1388-1393.
52. Leach RM, Treacher DF. The pulmonary physician in critical care ⋅ 2: oxygen delivery and consumption in the critically ill. Thorax. 2002;57:170-177.
53. Borgstrom L, Johannsson H, Siesjo BK. The influence of acute normovolemic anemia on cerebral blood flow and oxygen consumption of anesthetized rats. Acta Physiol Scand. 1975;93:505-514.
54. Paulson OB, Parving HH, Olesen J, et al. Influence of carbon monoxide and of hemodilution on cerebral blood flow and blood gases in man. J Appl Physiol. 1973;35:111-116.
55. Kissack CM, Garr R, Wardle SP, et al. Cerebral fractional oxygen extraction is inversely correlated with oxygen delivery in the sick, newborn, preterm infant. J Cereb Blood Flow Metab. 2005;25:545-553.
56. Greisen G. Cerebral blood flow and energy metabolism in the newborn. Clin Perinatol. 1997;24:531-546.
57. Pryds O, Greisen G, Skov LL, et al. Carbon dioxide-related changes in cerebral blood volume and cerebral blood flow in mechanically ventilated preterm neonates: comparison of near infrared spectrophotometry and [133]xenon clearance. Pediatr Res. 1990;27:445-449.

58. Altman DI, Powers WJ, Perlman JM, et al. Cerebral blood flow requirement for brain viability in newborn infants is lower than in adults. Ann Neurol. 1988;24:218-226.
59. Volpe JJ. Neurobiology of periventricular leukomalacia in the premature infant. Pediatr Res. 2001;50:553-562.
60. Edwards AD, Wyatt JS, Richardson C, et al. Effects of indomethacin on cerebral haemodynamics in very preterm infants. Lancet. 1990;335:1491-1495.
61. Victor S, Weindling AM, Appleton RE, et al. Relationship between blood pressure, electroencephalograms, cerebral fractional oxygen extraction and peripheral blood flow in very low birth weight newborn infants. Pediatr Res. 2006;59:314-319.
62. Koyama K, Mito T, Takashima S, et al. Effects of phenylephrine and dopamine on cerebral blood flow, blood volume, and oxygenation in young rabbits. Pediatr Neurol. 1990;6:87-90.
63. Hayashi T, Watabe H, Kudomi N, et al. A theoretical model of oxygen delivery and metabolism for physiologic interpretation of quantitative cerebral blood flow and metabolic rate of oxygen. J Cereb Blood Flow Metab. 2003;23:1314-1323.
64. Victor S, Appleton RE, Beirne M, et al. Effect of carbon dioxide on background cerebral electrical activity and fractional oxygen extraction in very low birth weight infants just after birth. Pediatr Res. 2005;58:579-585.
65. Greisen G, Trojaborg W. Cerebral blood flow, PaCO2 changes, and visual evoked potentials in mechanically ventilated, preterm infants. Acta Paediatr Scand. 1987;76:394-400.
66. Rosenberg AA. Response of the cerebral circulation to profound hypocarbia in neonatal lambs. Stroke. 1988;19:1365-1370.
67. Rosenberg AA. Response of the cerebral circulation to hypocarbia in postasphyxia newborn lambs. Pediatr Res. 1992;32:537-541.
68. Cain SM. Oxygen supply dependency in the critically ill—a continuing conundrum. Adv Exp Med Biol. 1992;317:35-45.
69. Adams RP, Dieleman LA, Cain SM. A critical value for O_2 transport in the rat. J Appl Physiol. 1982;53:660-664.
70. Mohsenifar Z, Goldbach P, Tashkin DP, et al. Relationship between O_2 delivery and O_2 consumption in the adult respiratory distress syndrome. Chest. 1983;84:267-271.
71. Astiz ME, Rackow EC, Falk JL, et al. Oxygen delivery and consumption in patients with hyperdynamic septic shock. Crit Care Med. 1987;15:26-28.
72. Bereczki D, Wei L, Otsuka T, et al. Hypoxia increases velocity of blood flow through parenchymal microvascular systems in rat brain. J Cereb Blood Flow Metab. 1993;13:475-486.
73. Pinard E, Engrand N, Seylaz J. Dynamic cerebral microcirculatory changes in transient forebrain ischemia in rats: involvement of type I nitric oxide synthase. J Cereb Blood Flow Metab. 2000;20:1648-1658.
74. Seylaz J, Charbonne R, Nanri K, et al. Dynamic in vivo measurement of erythrocyte velocity and flow in capillaries and of microvessel diameter in the rat brain by confocal laser microscopy. J Cereb Blood Flow Metab. 1999;19:863-870.
75. Evans N, Kluckow M. Early determinants of right and left ventricular output in ventilated preterm infants. Arch Dis Child Fetal Neonatal Ed. 1996;74:F88-F94.
76. Cunningham S, Symon AG, Elton RA, et al. Intra-arterial blood pressure reference ranges, death and morbidity in very low birthweight infants during the first seven days of life. Early Hum Dev. 1999;56:151-165.
77. Naulaers G, Morren G, Van Huffel S, et al. Cerebral tissue oxygenation index in very premature infants. Arch Dis Child Fetal Neonatal Ed. 2002;87:F189-F192.

CHAPTER 8

Clinical Applications of Near-Infrared Spectroscopy in Neonates

Petra Lemmers, MD, PhD, Gunnar Naulaers, MD, PhD, and
Frank van Bell, MD, PhD

- ● **Feasibility of NIRS-Monitored rScO$_2$ and cFTOE in Clinical Practice in the NICU**
- ● **Clinical Applications**
- ● **Conclusion**
- ● **References**

Survival of the extremely preterm infant has greatly improved over the last decades. However, perinatal brain damage with adverse neurodevelopmental outcome continues to affect a considerable number of these infants.[1-6] Although the etiology of brain damage is multifactorial and partly unknown (see Chapter 16), hypoxia, hyperoxia, and hemodynamic instability during the first days of postnatal life play an important role.[7-13] It is obvious that further advances in survival and improvements in neurodevelopmental outcomes can only be achieved if we learn more about the underlying pathophysiology so that more effective treatment modalities can be developed. The first step in this direction is to develop the capability to continuously monitor clinically relevant hemodynamic variables and, if possible, treat the underlying condition at an early stage. Continuous monitoring of physiologic parameters such as electrocardiogram (ECG), heart rate, blood pressure, arterial oxygen saturation (SaO$_2$) and temperature are firmly integrated into neonatal intensive care units (NICUs). Recently, amplitude integrated electroencephalography (aEEG) has been introduced in neonatal intensive care as another monitoring technique, to continuously assess cerebral function. Its use, however, is still less common in preterm infants.[14-16] Other novel techniques to continuously monitor additional hemodynamic parameters, such as cardiac output, are discussed in Chapter 6.

Discontinuous techniques to assess cerebral condition, such as cranial ultrasound, Doppler flow velocity measurements, and (advanced) magnetic resonance imaging (MRI) have also been increasingly integrated in the care of infants in the NICU (see Chapters 4, 9, and 10 for details). But these techniques do not provide continuous information on the perfusion and oxygenation of the brain.

What is needed is a reliable clinical tool that monitors oxygenation of the newborn brain noninvasively and continuously to prevent brain damage. A promising method is monitoring cerebral oxygenation by near infrared spectroscopy or NIRS (see Chapter 7).[17-20]

As described in Chapter 7 in detail, the use of NIRS to monitor cerebral perfusion and oxygenation was first described by Jobsis and colleagues in 1977.[21] Since then, many studies have been performed measuring cerebral oxygenation, cerebral blood flow, cerebral blood volume, and fractional oxygen extraction in neonates using the instruments that are mainly based on the Beer-Lambert law. These instruments are well designed for research work; however they remained difficult to use in the clinical setting because of movement artifacts and the fact that no absolute values are provided.[17] The introduction of spatially resolved spectroscopy made it possible to use a new approach to monitoring cerebral oxygenation in the clinical setting. Spatially resolved spectroscopy measures the absorption of light at two or more detectors. By using the diffusion equation, absolute values can be calculated assuming that the scattering for the different distances is constant.[22,23] Another method is to distract the measurement of the closest detector from the measurement of the furthest detector to omit the influence of superficial tissue. However, for instruments using this algorithm, further calibration in vitro or in vivo is still necessary. As discussed in Chapters 4 and 7 in detail, the different instruments used at the moment have different principles of measurement, different wavelengths, different optode distances, and different light emitters (laser or LED). However, they all measure the cerebral oxygenation called the tissue oxygenation index (TOI) or regional cerebral oxygen saturation ($rScO_2$). Despite the different approaches, these measures of cerebral oxygenation reflect the mixed oxygen saturation in the arteries ($\pm25\%$), capillaries ($\pm5\%$), and veins ($\pm70\%$) given as an absolute value that can be measured continuously over prolonged periods of time.

For most of the instruments, a good correlation with the jugular venous saturation has been documented.[24,25] The values are not identical though primarily because $rScO_2$ also reflects the changes in oxygenation in the arterial, capillary, and venous compartments. A comparison in adults between the different monitoring techniques during changes in oxygenation and changes in partial pressure of arterial CO_2 (pCO_2) also yielded a good correlation between the TOI and $rScO_2$.[26,27] In addition, when comparing the left and right side of the brain, the Bland-Altman limits of agreement of $rScO_2$ were -8.5 to $+9.5\%$ with even smaller limits during stable SaO_2 values between 85% and 97%.[28] However, due to the limitations of the technology (see Chapters 4 and 7), it is obvious that these measurements should rather be used for trend measurements instead of precise oxygenation values.

Clinical monitoring cerebral oxygenation by NIRS has already been applied in the intensive care unit for adults and during cardiac surgical procedures.[26,29-31] However, although information concerning cerebral oxygenation may prove to be important in relation to decisions regarding therapy and its impact on outcome, and despite the accumulating but not yet overwhelmingly convincing evidence, the use of NIRS in the daily care of neonates in the NICU is still uncommon.

A second variable of importance when utilizing NIRS to monitor cerebral oxygenation, the cerebral fractional tissue oxygen extraction or cFTOE, is readily derived from $rScO_2$ and SaO_2 based on the following formula: $SaO_2 - rScO_2/SaO_2$. cFTOE is a surrogate indicator of the actual cerebral fractional oxygen extraction, which can be measured with the validated jugular venous occlusion technique (see Chapter 7).[25,32] Naulaers and colleagues reported a positive correlation between NIRS-calculated cFTOE and actual fractional oxygen extraction of the brain in a newborn piglet model.[33] Because cFTOE is a ratio of two variables, an increase might either indicate reduced oxygen delivery to the brain with constant oxygen consumption or increased cerebral oxygen consumption not satisfied by oxygen delivery. The opposite is true in the case of a decrease in cFTOE, reflecting either a decrease of oxygen extraction because of decreased oxygen utilization or an increase of oxygen delivery to the brain while cerebral oxygen consumption has remained unchanged. Obviously, either parameter might change at the same time as well, although relatively rapid changes in cerebral oxygen utilization are less frequently encountered. Although NIRS-derived cFTOE is a less accurate parameter compared to fractional oxygen extraction determined by the jugular occlusion technique, the advantage of its use is that we can now continuously measure an estimate of cerebral oxygen extraction.[34,35]

Feasibility of Near-Infrared Spectroscopy-Monitored $rScO_2$ and cFTOE in Clinical Practice in the NICU

More and more NIRS devices with special neonatal or pediatric sensors and special algorithms have become available. Before interpreting the absolute values though, we have to pay special attention to the differences in the measured values between the different sensors. These values have to be first validated and compared with the values of sensors already in use and with published data on their performance. Indeed, reference values for the neonatal or pediatric sensors in preterm and term neonates should be first established through well-designed studies. These values can then be used for comparison with values obtained during conditions that may affect cerebral oxygenation (see later).

In order to assess the utility of NIRS-monitored $rScO_2$ in clinical practice it is essential to also obtain data on the signal-to-noise ratio and the interpatient and intrapatient variability. When compared with pulse oximetry-measured SaO_2, a reliable and accepted trend monitor for systemic arterial oxygenation, the signal-to-noise ratio is larger for NIRS-measured $rScO_2$.[18] However, when averaging the signal over a longer period, for example, over 30-60 seconds, a rather reliable signal can be obtained with an acceptable signal-to-noise ratio.[18] With respect to intrapatient variability, differences of up to 7% or more have been reported when subsequent measurements are performed with repeated placement of the NIRS sensor. The limits of agreement after sensor replacement are in the −17% to + 17% range.[18,20,36] These values are more than double the limits of agreement for SaO_2.[32] On the other hand, Menke and colleagues described a good reproducibility of NIRS-measured $rScO_2$ with an intermeasurement variance only slightly higher than the physiologic baseline variation.[37] When comparing values during simultaneous monitoring of the left and right frontoparietal regions of the brain, limits of agreement of 7-9% were reported.[28] Moreover, it appears that the experience of the investigator also plays an important role when these issues are being considered.

Reference values of $rScO_2$ or TOI during normal arterial oxygen saturations have been reported in several studies including in preterm neonates, although most studies did not differentiate between postnatal age or the clinical status of the subjects. Mean values (±SD) of $rScO_2$ or TOI ranged between 61% and 75% (±7-±12%), which are comparable to values obtained in adults (Table 8-1).[20,27,36,38-45]

Based on our studies, $rScO_2$ values range between 55% and 85% in stable preterm infants, and these values are being considered "normal" or "expected" for $rScO_2$ in this patient population (Table 8-1). Importantly, an association between $rScO_2$ in neonates with functional or histological compromise of the brain has been documented. Several animal studies in newborn piglets and a human study in neonates with hypoplastic left heart syndrome who underwent open heart surgery have

Table 8-1 REFERENCE VALUES (MEAN [SD]) OF REGIONAL CEREBRAL OXYGEN SATURATION ($rScO_2$)/TISSUE OXYGEN INDEX (TOI) (%) IN ADULTS AND TERM AND PRETERM NEONATES

Adults		67% (± 8)	n = 94[38]
		66% (± 8)	n = 19 ($rScO_2$/TOI)[27]
		68-76%	n = 9 ($rScO_2$)[43]
		61.5 (± 6.1)	n = 14 ($rScO_2$)[44]
Full-term neonates/ infants	Day 12 [0-365]	61% (± 12)	n = 155 (TOI)[39]
	Day 4.5 [0-190]	63% (± 12)	n = 20 (TOI)[36]
	8 min after birth	68% (IQR55-80)	n = 20[45]
Preterm neonates (gestational age < 32 wk)	Day 1	57% [54-66]	n = 15 (TOI)[20]
	Day 2	66% [62-82]	
	Day 3	76% [68-80]	
	NA	75 % (±10.2)	n = 253 (TOI)[40]
	>Day 7	66 % (±8.8)	n = 40($rScO_2$)[41]
	Day 1	70% (±7.4)	n = 38 ($rScO_2$)[42]
	Day 2	71% (±8.8)	
	Day 3	70% (±7.8)	

reported that $rScO_2$ or TOI values lower than 35-45% for more than 30-90 minutes are associated with functional (mitochondrial dysfunction or energy failure) and/or histological damage especially in the hippocampus (a brain region very vulnerable to hypoxia in the perinatal period).[46-48] Moreover, several former studies performed in mostly adult cardiac intensive care units have also reported that a 20% decrease of the baseline value or an absolute rScO2 value of <50% before intervention were associated with hypoxic-ischemic brain lesions.[49,50] In summary, the findings of these studies suggest that $rScO_2$ values below 45-50% for a prolonged period of time should be avoided if possible. We must emphasize though that, at present, we do not have solid evidence that using NIRS monitoring in preterm or term neonates improves outcomes.

Besides its use to detect and thus potentially prevent prolonged low brain tissue oxygen saturation, continuous monitoring of $rScO_2$ can also contribute to the prevention of prolonged hyperoxia of the brain, especially in the extremely preterm infant prone to oxygen toxicity. The importance of avoiding hyperoxia has been increasingly recognized as there is emerging evidence of an association between normal oxygen saturations and improved long-term neurodevelopmental outcome in extremely preterm infants.[13,51,52] With these considerations and presented data in mind, NIRS-monitored $rScO_2$ or TOI and NIRS-derived cFTOE may play an important role in monitoring and improving cerebral oxygenation in the clinical setting in neonates cared for in the NICU.

Clinical Applications

Application of the Sensor and Its Pitfalls

The most important issue regarding the clinical application of noninvasive monitoring of cerebral oxygenation by NIRS is the ability to perform reliable, long-term monitoring of cerebral oxygenation in the most immature and unstable neonates without disturbing the infant. A critical part of initiating the process is the application of the sensor to the head. With appropriate placement, the sensor will allow reliable monitoring of the $rScO_2$ or TOI for a number of days without damaging of the vulnerable skin of the infant. In addition, the sensor in place should not limit access to performing ultrasound studies of the brain, placement of electrodes for aEEG monitoring, or attachment of CPAP devices. Our findings show that application of the NIRS sensor with a soft dark elastic bandage to the frontoparietal part of the head provides protection from ambient light and does not irritate or damage the skin of even the smallest infants while allowing reliable monitoring of $rScO_2$ for extended periods of time. Figure 8-1 shows an example of the application of the NIRS sensor used in all our clinical studies.[17] Alternatively, application of sensors using an adhesive on the skin is possible, and this method is advocated by the manufacturers for most commercially available sensors.

Introduction of the system with structured theoretical and practical courses for nurses and medical staff is an important prerequisite for the successful use of this monitoring method in the clinical practice and to emphasize the potential benefits and risks. In gaining experience, for instance, our nurses have been able to recognize inappropriate transducer placement, improper transducer fixation, or insufficient transducer shielding. In our experience, this resulted in extended periods of uninterrupted and reliable $rScO_2$ monitoring, even in the smallest infants (<600 g) comparable to pulse oximetry-monitored SaO_2. When monitoring and interpreting the values in the daily clinical practice, one has to be aware of several pitfalls. We have already discussed the importance of proper sensor application to prevent movement artifacts and the effect of ambient light. Yet, despite these precautionary measures, phototherapy-induced ambient light sometimes causes disturbances in monitoring $rScO_2$. Therefore covering the sensor with an additional dark piece of material is recommended to restore reliable monitoring. One must also be aware that hematoma or edema of the head and abundant amount of hair or other materials attached to the head, like the plaster of the aEEG electrodes, can cause disturbances in the

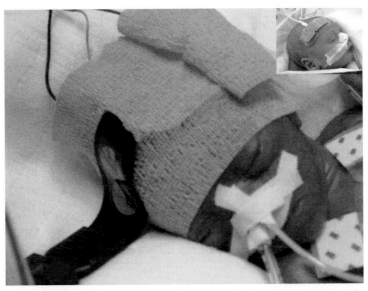

Figure 8-1   Application of the near infrared sensor to the head of a preterm infant in the frontoparietal position using an elastic bandage. The inlay shows the application of the sensor with an adhesive tape (published with permission of the parents). See text for details.

acquisition of the NIRS signal. Finally, movement artifacts and dislocation of the NIRS sensor are additional causes of inappropriate signal and sensor malfunction.

Relation to Other Monitoring Devices

Using the information obtained from NIRS-monitored changes in brain oxygenation, represented by $rScO_2$ or TOI and cFTOE in conjunction with other monitoring devices such as pulse-oximetry-monitored SaO_2, indwelling blood pressure monitoring, heart rate and electrical brain activity generates additional and potentially important information. Following the relation with SaO_2 is mandatory to calculate cerebral oxygen extraction (cFTOE) as described earlier. The relationship between blood pressure and $rScO_2$ may provide information about the presence or absence of cerebral blood flow autoregulation (see later and Chapters 2 and 16).[53-56] As for the use of aEEG in conjunction with NIRS-monitoring of cerebral oxygenation, our group has reported that persistent and unusually high $rScO_2$ values after the first postnatal day in term infants with severe perinatal asphyxia were strongly associated with an abnormal pattern of electrical brain activity by aEEG and adverse neurodevelopmental outcome at 2 years of age.[57] These findings indicate that monitoring cerebral oxygenation and oxygen extraction with NIRS along with other parameters reveals conditions at an early stage that might be associated with poor long-term outcomes. In turn, this type of monitoring will lead to the design of appropriate interventional trials to test the effectiveness of the interventions.

Clinical Conditions Associated with Low rScO2

Perlman and colleagues already reported that the ductal steal phenomenon in cerebral arteries is a risk factor for cerebral damage in the preterm infant.[58] Thus a hemodynamically significant patent ductus arteriosus (PDA) is a condition potentially associated with decreased oxygen delivery to the brain by the impact of the diastolic run-off in the cerebral vessels and the changes in perfusion pressure on cerebral oxygen delivery throughout the entire cardiac cycle. Several recent reports using NIRS-monitored $rScO_2$ found a substantial decrease of cerebral oxygenation to sometimes critically low values in the presence of a hemodynamically significant PDA.[59,60] It appears that infants with a hemodynamically significant PDA unresponsive to pharmacologic closure with cyclooxygenase (COX) inhibitors are especially at risk before and during surgical ligation. Indeed, in a study of 20 infants, we have not infrequently found extremely low $rScO_2$ and high cFTOE values before and during ligation.[61] Moreover, monitoring of these parameters has provided us with early information on the impact of the changes in left-to-right shunting across the duct on cerebral oxygenation and the effectiveness of the treatment initiated to close the PDA. Figure 8-2A provides a representative example of the impact of a hemodynamically significant PDA on cerebral oxygenation and the effect of successful

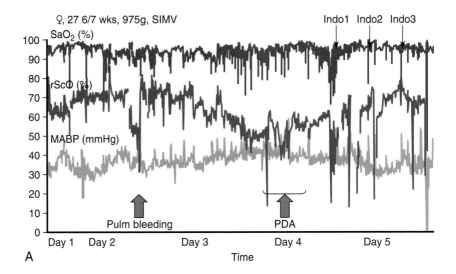

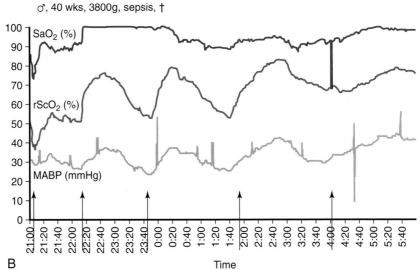

Figure 8-2 A, Representative patterns (including artifacts) of arterial oxygen saturation (SaO_2; red line), regional cerebral oxygen saturation ($rScO_2$; gray line), and mean arterial blood pressure (MABP; pink line) in a male preterm neonate of $27\frac{6}{7}$ weeks' gestation with severe respiratory distress syndrome during the first 5 postnatal days. The infant received exogenous surfactant and was mechanically ventilated. The patient's course was complicated by a pulmonary hemorrhage on day #2 *(arrow)*. Although the pulmonary hemorrhage could have been an early indication of pulmonary overcirculation due to a PDA, the infant developed a hemodynamically significant PDA only on day #4 *(arrow)*, which was successfully treated with indomethacin *(arrows)*. Note the decrease of $rScO_2$ (starting on day #3) to values below 50% at the time of the diagnosis of the hemodynamically significant PDA, and the recovery of $rScO_2$ after the ductus has closed on day #5. See text for details. **B,** Patterns of SaO_2 (red line), $rScO_2$ (gray line), and MABP (pink line) during 8 hours in an infant with a severe sepsis with systemic hypotension. Hypotension was treated with volume expansion and vasopressor-inotropes *(arrows)*. Changes in $rScO_2$ mirrored the changes in blood pressure, suggesting a pressure-passive cerebral circulation with lack of autoregulation of cerebral blood flow. See text for details.

pharmacologic closure of the duct with indomethacin. It should be noted that, unlike ibuprofen, indomethacin decreases and stabilizes cerebral blood flow via mechanisms independent of the drug's effect on the COX enzyme.

Another frequently encountered condition often related to low $rScO_2$ values is systemic hypotension. Hypotension can arise by various conditions including but not restricted to hypovolemia, myocardial dysfunction, the presence of a hemodynamically significant PDA, and sepsis resulting in the inability of the vascular bed to maintain an appropriate peripheral vascular resistance (also see Chapters 1 and 12). Although blood pressure is one of the most frequently measured hemodynamic variables in neonatal intensive care, the lower limits of the gestational- and

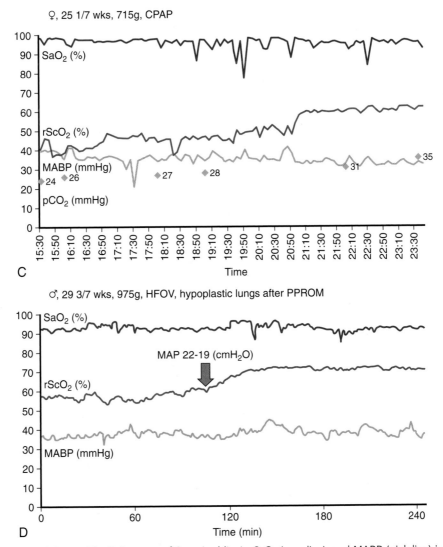

Figure 8-2, cont'd   **C,** Patterns of SaO_2 (red line), $rScO_2$ (gray line), and MABP (pink line) in an extremely preterm infant on CPAP on the first postnatal day. Despite normal blood pressure values and arterial saturations, $rScO_2$ was very low (<50%). Although this infant was breathing spontaneously, she hyperventilated on CPAP to very low pCO_2 values (gray diamonds). Only when pCO_2 increased to > 30 mm Hg, did $rScO_2$ normalize, suggesting the resolution of cerebral hypoperfusion caused by the hypocapnia-induced cerebral vasoconstriction. See text for details. **D,** Patterns of SaO_2 (red line), $rScO_2$ (gray line), and MABP (pink line) in an infant with hypoplastic lungs following prolonged premature rupture of the membranes supported by high-frequency oscillatory ventilation (HFOV) with high mean airway pressures (MAP; 22 cm H_2O). Note the increase of $rScO_2$ after decreasing MAP from 22 to 19 cm H_2O. See text for details. *Continued*

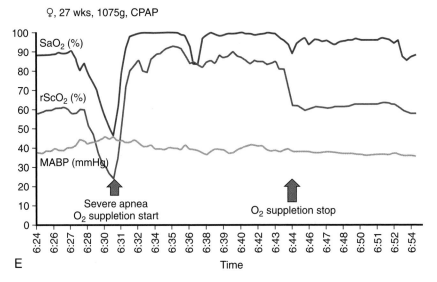

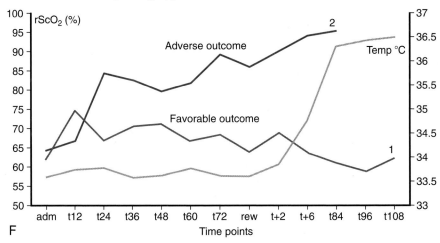

Figure 8-2, cont'd   E, Patterns of SaO$_2$ (red line), rScO$_2$ (gray line), and MABP (pink line) in an infant on CPAP with severe apnea treated with stimulation and supplementary oxygen. The rScO$_2$ increased to very high values and only decreased to baseline after the patient had been weaned off supplemental oxygen. See text for details. **F,** Patterns of rScO$_2$ (gray and red lines) and central temperature (pink line) in two term infants with hypoxic ischemic encephalopathy after severe perinatal asphyxia treated with moderate total body cooling (33.5°C) during the first 72 postnatal hours. Infant #1 had a normal MRI after having been rewarmed on day #5 and subsequently was found to have a favorable neurodevelopmental outcome. Infant #2 had an adverse outcome with severe abnormalities on MRI on day #5. Infant #1 showed normal rScO$_2$ values during hypothermia (time points: admission [adm] until rewarming [rew]) and also during and after rewarming (time points t +2 [2 hours after starting the process of rewarming] until t108 (108 postnatal hours). Infant #2 had normal rScO$_2$ values on admission, increasing to high rScO$_2$ values at 24 hours of age (t24) and beyond. High rScO$_2$ > 24 hours after birth has been shown to be independently associated with adverse neurodevelopmental outcome in infants with hypoxic ischemic encephalopathy after severe perinatal asphyxia. It is thought to be due to decreased utilization of oxygen and the inappropriately high oxygen delivery due to vasodilation. See text for details.

postnatal-age dependent normal blood pressure range is not known (see Chapter 3) and depends on a number of additional factors such as the underlying pathology, the ability of the individual patient to compensate with increasing blood flow to the vital organs and maintain a proper autoregulatory capacity of the cerebrovascular bed (see Chapters 1, 12, and 16). Regional cerebral tissue oxygen saturation in the normal range as well as normal cFTOE values calculated real-time and ranging from 0.10 to 0.46 with a stable hemodynamic and metabolic condition of the infant, might call for consideration of further observation instead of immediately initiating treatment of the apparently low blood pressure values alone (see Chapters 1 and 12). However, clearly more information is needed on this issue before we can identify which hypotensive neonate might benefit from which antihypertensive treatment.

Impaired or absent autoregulatory ability of the cerebral vascular bed has been documented in the critically ill very preterm infant (Chapter 2) and presents a risk for adverse outcomes (see Chapters 2 and 16) and might be one of the causes of insufficient oxygen delivery to the immature brain.[62] Several recent reports have found that NIRS-monitored $rScO_2$ combined with simultaneously monitored mean arterial blood pressure provides information on the status of cerebral autoregulation at a given systemic blood pressure value.[13,54-56,63] This approach assumes that cerebral metabolic rate remains constant and that SaO_2 does not change during the period of the correlation studied. Accordingly, when a change in blood pressure is not associated with changes in cerebral oxygenation (and thus $rScO_2$), cerebral autoregulation is presumed to be present. However, when there is lack of cerebral autoregulation, changes in blood pressure will have an immediate effect on cerebral oxygenation and thus $rScO_2$. Indeed, the findings of Tsuji and colleagues and Wong and colleagues suggest that infants lacking cerebral blood flow autoregulation assessed by NIRS compared with gestational age–matched infants with intact cerebral autoregulation have impaired short- and long-term central nervous system outcomes.[55,64] Several approaches are currently being tested for the continuous and real-time assessment of cerebral blood flow autoregulation.[56,63] Figure 8-2B shows an example of the use of NIRS-monitored $rScO_2$ to assess the autoregulatory ability of the cerebral vascular bed.

Arterial pCO_2 is another important parameter that influences brain perfusion. Actually, changes in pCO_2 cause more robust changes in cerebral blood flow than changes in blood pressure outside the autoregulatory range (Chapter 3). Hypocapnia directly decreases cerebral blood flow and thus cerebral oxygenation (or $rScO_2$) and oxygen delivery (or cFTOE). Therefore monitoring $rScO_2$ and cFTOE can be used as a noninvasive approach to identify changes in pCO_2 again provided that cerebral metabolic rate remains constant and SaO_2 does not change during the period in question.[65] Figure 8-2C shows an example of a preterm infant with low pCO_2 values and low $rScO_2$ values. Only when pCO_2 increased to values greater than 30 mm Hg did $rScO_2$ recover.

Preterm infants with severe respiratory distress syndrome often are mechanically ventilated with high mean inspiratory and/or end-expiratory pressures using conventional high-frequency oscillatory ventilation. The associated increase in intrathoracic pressure might decrease preload and thus cardiac output, resulting in a negative impact on cerebral hemodynamics as reflected in impaired cerebral oxygenation. Indeed, monitoring of the $rScO_2$ has revealed this association in real-time and its use might contribute to early recognition and introduction of corrective measures to prevent such complications (Fig. 8-2D).[16]

Another potential cause of decreased brain oxygenation is severe anemia. Anemia, in neonates with systemic hypotension receiving mechanical ventilation with high mean airway pressures may have an even more profound effect of cerebral oxygen delivery. Van Hoften and colleagues have documented normalization of rScO2 following packed red blood cell transfusions in 33 preterm infants and concluded that cerebral oxygenation in these infants may be at risk at a hemoglobin concentration of less than 6 mmol/L (9.7 g/dL).[66]

Finally, infants with congenital cyanotic heart disease are at particularly high risk of compromised cerebral circulation. Most of these infants with cyanotic heart

Table 8-2   CONDITIONS WITH LOW OR HIGH REGIONAL CEREBRAL OXYGEN SATURATION (RSCO₂)

Low rScO$_2$	High rScO$_2$
Persistent ductus arteriosus (PDA)	Oxygen therapy:
During surgery (PDA)	Pulmonary hypertension (PPHN)
Hypotension	Pneumothorax
Lack of cerebral autoregulation	Apnea
Hypoxia	Perinatal asphyxia
Hypocapnia	Hypercapnia
Anemia	
High mean airway pressure	

disease have baseline rScO$_2$ values below 55% with SaO$_2$ values in the 70-85% range. Of note is that an rScO$_2$ of 55% is below the 2 SD of the "normal" values defined by our data for preterm neonates. Thus neonates with congenital heart disease, even if it is a noncyanotic but duct-dependent lesion, are at risk for cerebral damage especially in combination with the risk factors discussed earlier, including low systemic perfusion, blood pressure, and/or pCO$_2$ values. Importantly, perioperative and postoperative NIRS-measured rScO$_2$ values in this group of infants have been documented to have a predictive value for the occurrence of brain damage in this patient population.[67] Table 8-2 summarizes the clinical conditions associated with low rScO$_2$ values.

Clinical Conditions Associated with High rScO2 Values

NIRS-monitored rScO$_2$ may also be helpful to detect conditions associated with hyperoxemia. Hyperoxemia, especially in the extremely preterm neonate, has been increasingly linked to adverse long-term outcome.[9,12,13] Conditions related to high rScO$_2$ values, thought to be excessive in very preterm neonates, are summarized in Table 8-2.

Oxygen supplementation is the major cause of usually brief periods of hyperoxemia. Brief but repeated episodes of hyperoxemia occur relatively frequently during the recovery of apnea and bradycardia episodes in spontaneously breathing preterm infants treated with additional oxygen supplementation to accelerate normalization of partial arterial oxygen pressure and SaO$_2$ (see Figure 8-2E) and if additional oxygen is provided before routine care or endotracheal intubation. In addition, hyperoxemia occurs unless extreme caution is taken in preterm or term neonates receiving prolonged oxygen therapy for severe respiratory distress syndrome, persistent pulmonary hypertension of the newborn, pneumothorax, or severe bronchopulmonary dysplasia. Despite the increasing awareness that uncontrolled oxygen administration is harmful and oxygen therapy for some of these conditions is obsolete, preventable hyperoxia still occurs. Furthermore, even if oxygen saturation is carefully monitored, oxygen supplementation during episodes of apnea of prematurity often results in hyperoxemia because pulse oximetry-measured SaO$_2$ is not sensitive enough when SaO$_2$ is above 95%. In such cases, provision of concomitant information on cerebral oxygenation may, at least in part, be helpful to minimize the occurrence of these potentially harmful hyperoxia episodes.

Episodes of hypercarbia cause an increase in brain perfusion and thus contribute to a cerebral hyperoxemic state, especially in infants on the ventilator with additional oxygen supplementation. Again, NIRS-monitored rScO$_2$ may be used as an adjunct monitoring technique to aid in appropriately adjusting the oxygen therapy.

In addition to its use as a diagnostic tool to assess cerebral oxygen delivery and extraction, NIRS-monitored rScO$_2$ has been shown to be useful in predicting long-term prognosis in certain patient populations. Our group has reported that, in infants with hypoxic-ischemic encephalopathy following perinatal asphyxia, abnormally high values of NIRS-monitored $rScO_2$ (>85-90%) during the first 24 postnatal hours are strongly and independently associated with adverse neurodevelopmental outcome at 2 years of age.[67] The high values of NIRS-monitored $rScO_2$ are thought to occur because of the low oxygen extraction due to the decreased metabolic activity of the injured brain and as well because of the inappropriately high cerebral oxygen delivery due to the cerebral vasodilatation and vasoparalysis associated with or without the loss of the cerebral autoregulation. Our preliminary data indicate that, even when critically ill neonates with hypoxic-ischemic encephalopathy are treated by therapeutic hypothermia to also ameliorate the secondary injury associated with the ischemia-reperfusion cycle, the pattern of $rScO_2$ changes maintains its prognostic value to assess long-term neurodevelopmental outcome[68] (Figure 8-2F).

Conclusion

At present, NIRS-monitored cerebral oxygenation and oxygen extraction as indicated by $rScO_2$ or TOI and cFTOE, respectively, still lack the precision required for a robust quantitative tool primarily due to high interpatient and intrapatient variability. Moreover, the limits of agreement of this noninvasive bedside method are still beyond what would be considered clinically acceptable. However, when merely used as a trend-monitoring device, substantial changes in NIRS-monitored $rScO_2$, i.e., has the potential to alert the caregiver that potentially harmful changes in brain oxygenation have occurred. Finally, the information provided by the use of this technology has improved our understanding of the limitations of our knowledge and led to the initiation of appropriately designed observational and interventional trials so that the interventions used in the clinical practice can be finally critically tested.

References

1. Anderson PJ, Doyle LW. Cognitive and educational deficits in children born extremely preterm. Semin Perinatol. 2008;32(1):51-58.
2. Wood NS, Costeloe K, Gibson AT, et al. The EPICure study: associations and antecedents of neurological and developmental disability at 30 months of age following extremely preterm birth. Arch Dis Child Fetal Neonatal Ed. 2005;90(2):F134-F140.
3. Wilson-Costello D, Friedman H, Minich N, et al. Improved neurodevelopmental outcomes for extremely low birth weight infants in 2000-2002. Pediatrics. 2007;119(1):37-45.
4. Wilson-Costello D, Friedman H, Minich N, et al. Improved survival rates with increased neurodevelopmental disability for extremely low birth weight infants in the 1990s. Pediatrics. 2005;115(4): 997-1003.
5. Samara M, Marlow N, Wolke D. Pervasive behavior problems at 6 years of age in a total-population sample of children born at </= 25 weeks of gestation. Pediatrics. 2008;122(3):562-573.
6. Wolke D, Samara M, Bracewell M, et al. Specific language difficulties and school achievement in children born at 25 weeks of gestation or less. J Pediatr. 2008;152(2):256-262.
7. Logitharajah P, Rutherford MA, Cowan FM. Hypoxic-ischemic encephalopathy in preterm infants: antecedent factors, brain imaging, and outcome. Pediatr Res. 2009;66(2):222-229.
8. Dammann O, Allred EN, Kuban KC, et al. Systemic hypotension and white-matter damage in preterm infants. Dev Med Child Neurol. 2002;44(2):82-90.
9. Deulofeut R, Critz A, Adams-Chapman I, et al. Avoiding hyperoxia in infants < or = 1250 g is associated with improved short- and long-term outcomes. J Perinatol. 2006;26(11):700-705.
10. Perlman JM, McMenamin JB, Volpe JJ. Fluctuating cerebral blood-flow velocity in respiratory-distress syndrome. Relation to the development of intraventricular hemorrhage. N Engl J Med. 1983;309(4): 204-209.
11. van Bel F, van de BM, Stijnen T, et al. Aetiological role of cerebral blood-flow alterations in development and extension of peri-intraventricular haemorrhage. Dev Med Child Neurol. 1987;29(5): 601-614.
12. Klinger G, Beyene J, Shah P, et al. Do hyperoxaemia and hypocapnia add to the risk of brain injury after intrapartum asphyxia? Arch Dis Child Fetal Neonatal Ed. 2005;90(1):F49-F52.
13. Gerstner B, DeSilva TM, Genz K, et al. Hyperoxia causes maturation-dependent cell death in the developing white matter. J Neurosc. 2008;28(5):1236-1245.
14. Toet MC, Lemmers PM. Brain monitoring in neonates. Early Hum Dev. 2009;85(2):77-84.
15. Hellstrom-Westas L. Continuous electroencephalography monitoring of the preterm infant. Clin Perinatol. 2006 September;33(3):633-647, vi.

16. Hellstrom-Westas L, Rosen I, Svenningsen NW. Cerebral function monitoring during the first week of life in extremely small low birthweight (ESLBW) infants. Neuropediatrics. 1991;22(1):27-32.

17. van Bel F, Lemmers P, Naulaers G. Monitoring neonatal regional cerebral oxygen saturation in clinical practice: value and pitfalls. Neonatology. 2008;94(4):237-244.

18. Greisen G. Is near-infrared spectroscopy living up to its promises? Semin Fetal Neonatal Med. 2006;11(6):498-502.

19. Kissack CM, Garr R, Wardle SP, et al. Cerebral fractional oxygen extraction in very low birth weight infants is high when there is low left ventricular output and hypocarbia but is unaffected by hypotension. Pediatr Res. 2004;55(3):400-405.

20. Naulaers G, Morren G, Van Huffel S, et al. Cerebral tissue oxygenation index in very premature infants. Arch Dis Child Fetal Neonatal Ed. 2002;87(3):F189-F192.

21. Jobsis FF. Noninvasive, infrared monitoring of cerebral and myocardial oxygen sufficiency and circulatory parameters. Science. 1977;23;198(4323):1264-1267.

22. Matcher SJ, Kirkpatrick P, Nahid K, et al. Absolute quantification methods in tissue near infrared spectroscopy. Proc SPIE. 1995;2389:486-495.

23. Suzuki S, Takasaki S, Ozaki T, et al. A tissue oxygenation monitor using NIR spatially resolved spectroscopy. Proc SPIE. 1999;3597:582-592.

24. Nagdyman N, Fleck T, Schubert S, et al. Comparison between cerebral tissue oxygenation index measured by near-infrared spectroscopy and venous jugular bulb saturation in children. Intensive Care Med. 2005;31(6):846-850.

25. Yoxall CW, Weindling AM, Dawani NH, et al. Measurement of cerebral venous oxyhemoglobin saturation in children by near-infrared spectroscopy and partial jugular venous occlusion. Pediatr Res. 1995;38(3):319-323.

26. Thavasothy M, Broadhead M, Elwell C, et al. A comparison of cerebral oxygenation as measured by the NIRO 300 and the INVOS 5100 near-infrared spectrophotometers. Anaesthesia. 2002;57(10):999-1006.

27. Yoshitani K, Kawaguchi M, Tatsumi K, et al. A comparison of the INVOS 4100 and the NIRO 300 near-infrared spectrophotometers. Anesth Analg. 2002;94(3):586-590.

28. Lemmers PM, van Bel F. Left-to-right differences of regional cerebral oxygen saturation and oxygen extraction in preterm infants during the first days of life. Pediatr Res. 2009;65(2):226-230.

29. Murkin JM. NIRS: a standard of care for CPB vs. an evolving standard for selective cerebral perfusion? J Extra Corpor Technol. 2009;41(1):11-14.

30. Hoffman GM. Neurologic monitoring on cardiopulmonary bypass: what are we obligated to do? Ann Thorac Surg. 2006;81(6):S2373-S2380.

31. Williams GD, Ramamoorthy C. Brain monitoring and protection during pediatric cardiac surgery. Semin Cardiothorac Vasc Anesth. 2007;11(1):23-33.

32. Yoxall CW, Weindling AM. The measurement of peripheral venous oxyhemoglobin saturation in newborn infants by near infrared spectroscopy with venous occlusion. Pediatr Res. 1996;39(6):1103-1106.

33. Naulaers G, Meyns B, Miserez M, et al. Use of tissue oxygenation index and fractional tissue oxygen extraction as noninvasive parameters for cerebral oxygenation. A validation study in piglets. Neonatology. 2007;92(2):120-126.

34. Wardle SP, Yoxall CW, Weindling AM. Cerebral oxygenation during cardiopulmonary bypass. Arch Dis Child. 1998;78(1):26-32.

35. Wardle SP, Yoxall CW, Weindling AM. Determinants of cerebral fractional oxygen extraction using near infrared spectroscopy in preterm neonates. J Cereb Blood Flow Metab. 2000;20(2):272-279.

36. Dullenkopf A, Kolarova A, Schulz G, et al. Reproducibility of cerebral oxygenation measurement in neonates and infants in the clinical setting using the NIRO 300 oximeter. Pediatr Crit Care Med. 2005;6(3):344-347.

37. Menke J, Voss U, Moller G, et al. Reproducibility of cerebral near infrared spectroscopy in neonates. Biol Neonate. 2003;83(1):6-11.

38. Misra M, Stark J, Dujovny M, et al. Transcranial cerebral oximetry in random normal subjects. Neurol Res. 1998;20(2):137-141.

39. Weiss M, Dullenkopf A, Kolarova A, et al. Near-infrared spectroscopic cerebral oxygenation reading in neonates and infants is associated with central venous oxygen saturation. Paediatr Anaesth. 2005;15(2):102-109.

40. Sorensen LC, Greisen G. Precision of measurement of cerebral tissue oxygenation index using near-infrared spectroscopy in preterm neonates. J Biomed Opt. 2006;11(5):054005.

41. Petrova A, Mehta R. Near-infrared spectroscopy in the detection of regional tissue oxygenation during hypoxic events in preterm infants undergoing critical care. Pediatr Crit Care Med. 2006;7(5):449-454.

42. Lemmers PM, Toet M, van Schelven LJ, et al. Cerebral oxygenation and cerebral oxygen extraction in the preterm infant: the impact of respiratory distress syndrome. Exp Brain Res. 2006;173(3):458-467.

43. Macleod D, Ikeda K, Vacchiano C. Simultaneous comparison of Fore-sight and INVOS cerebral oximeters to jugular bulb and arterial co-oximetry measurements in heathy volunteers. SCA suppl. 2009;108:101-104.

44. Olopade CO, Mensah E, Gupta R, et al. Noninvasive determination of brain tissue oxygenation during sleep in obstructive sleep apnea: a near-infrared spectroscopic approach. Sleep. 2007;30(12):1747-1755.

45. Fauchere JC, Schulz G, Haensse D, et al. Near-infrared spectroscopy measurements of cerebral oxygenation in newborns during immediate postnatal adaptation. J Pediatr. 2010;156(3):372-376.
46. Hou X, Ding H, Teng Y, et al. Research on the relationship between brain anoxia at different regional oxygen saturations and brain damage using near-infrared spectroscopy. Physiol Meas. 2007;28(10):1251-1265.
47. Kurth CD, McCann JC, Wu J, et al. Cerebral oxygen saturation-time threshold for hypoxic-ischemic injury in piglets. Anesth Analg. 2009;108(4):1268-1277.
48. Dent CL, Spaeth JP, Jones BV, et al. Brain magnetic resonance imaging abnormalities after the Norwood procedure using regional cerebral perfusion. J Thorac Cardiovasc Surg. 2005;130(6):1523-1530.
49. Sakamoto T, Hatsuoka S, Stock UA, et al. Prediction of safe duration of hypothermic circulatory arrest by near-infrared spectroscopy. J Thorac Cardiovasc Surg. 2001;122(2):339-350.
50. Hoffman GM, Ghanayem NS, Stuth EA, et al. NIRS-derived somatic and cerebral saturation difference provides noninvasive real time hemodynamic assessment of cardiogenic shock and anaerobic metabolism. Anesthesiology. 2004;101:A1448.
51. Tin W. Optimal oxygen saturation for preterm babies. Do we really know? Biol Neonate. 2004;85(4):319-325.
52. Chow LC, Wright KW, Sola A. Can changes in clinical practice decrease the incidence of severe retinopathy of prematurity in very low birth weight infants? Pediatrics. 2003;111(2):339-345.
53. De Smet D, Vanderhaegen J, Naulaers G, et al. New measurements for assessment of impaired cerebral autoregulation using near-infrared spectroscopy. Adv Exp Med Biol. 2009;645:273-278.
54. Brady KM, Lee JK, Kibler KK, et al. Continuous time-domain analysis of cerebrovascular autoregulation using near-infrared spectroscopy. Stroke. 2007;38(10):2818-2825.
55. Wong FY, Leung TS, Austin T, et al. Impaired autoregulation in preterm infants identified by using spatially resolved spectroscopy. Pediatrics. 2008;121(3):e604-e611.
56. Brady KM, Mytar JO, Lee JK, et al. Monitoring cerebral blood flow pressure autoregulation in pediatric patients during cardiac surgery. Stroke. 2010;41(9):1957-1962.
57. Toet MC, Lemmers PM, van Schelven LJ, et al. Cerebral oxygenation and electrical activity after birth asphyxia: their relation to outcome. Pediatrics. 2006;117(2):333-339.
58. Perlman JM, Hill A, Volpe JJ. The effect of patent ductus arteriosus on flow velocity in the anterior cerebral arteries: ductal steal in the premature newborn infant. J Pediatr. 1981;99(5):767-771.
59. Lemmers PM, Toet MC, van Bel F. Impact of patent ductus arteriosus and subsequent therapy with indomethacin on cerebral oxygenation in preterm infants. Pediatrics. 2008;121(1):142-147.
60. Underwood MA, Milstein JM, Sherman MP. Near-infrared spectroscopy as a screening tool for patent ductus arteriosus in extremely low birth weight infants. Neonatology. 2007;91(2):134-139.
61. Lemmers PM, Molenschot MC, Evens J, et al. Is cerebral oxygen supply compromised in preterm infants undergoing surgical closure for patent ductus arteriosus? Arch Dis Child Fetal Neonatal Ed. 2010;95(6):F429-F434.
62. Soul JS, Hammer PE, Tsuji M, et al. Fluctuating pressure-passivity is common in the cerebral circulation of sick premature infants. Pediatr Res. 2007;61(4):467-473.
63. Ciacedo A, Naulaers G, Ameye L, et al. Cerebral tissue oxygenation and regional oxygen saturation can be used to study cerebral autoregulation in prematurely born infants. Pediatr Res, in press.
64. Tsuji M, Saul JP, du Plessis A, et al. Cerebral intravascular oxygenation correlates with mean arterial pressure in critically ill premature infants. Pediatrics. 2000;106(4):625-632.
65. Vanderhaegen J, Naulaers G, Vanhole C, et al. The effect of changes in tPCO2 on the fractional tissue oxygen extraction—as measured by near-infrared spectroscopy—in neonates during the first days of life. Eur J Paediatr Neurol. 2009;13(2):128-134.
66. van Hoften JC, Verhagen EA, Keating P, et al. Cerebral tissue oxygen saturation and extraction in preterm infants before and after blood transfusion. Arch Dis Child Fetal Neonatal Ed. 2010;95(5):F352-F358.
67. Toet MC, Flinterman A, Laar I, et al. Cerebral oxygen saturation and electrical brain activity before, during, and up to 36 hours after arterial switch procedure in neonates without pre-existing brain damage: its relationship to neurodevelopmental outcome. Exp Brain Res. 2005;165(3):343-350.
68. Lemmers PMA, Toet MC, Benders MJ, et al. Cerebral oxygenation (RScO2) and aEEG background patterns (BGP) of term neonates during hypothermia after perinatal asphyxia. 2010 SPR/PAS Vancouver (Canada) (A).

CHAPTER 9

Advanced Magnetic Resonance Neuroimaging Techniques in the Neonate with a Focus on Hemodynamic-Related Brain Injury

Matthew Borzage, MS, Ashok Panigrahy, MD,
Stefan Blüml, PhD

- Magnetic Resonance-Compatible Neonatal Incubator
- Magnetic Resonance-Compatible Video Monitoring System
- Neonatal Sized Head Coil
- Diffusion-Weighted Imaging and Diffusion Tensor Imaging of the Neonatal Brain
- Perfusion Imaging of the Neonatal Brain
- Quantitative Proton Magnetic Resonance Spectroscopy of the Neonatal Brain
- References

This chapter discusses the recent advances in magnetic resonance imaging (MRI) with a focus on the evaluation of the neonatal brain. Particularly we will focus on hardware and imaging sequences that are adapted to assess critically ill preterm and term neonates. Hardware developments include systems developed to improve patient safety and image quantity. Examples of these include MR-compatible incubators, MR-compatible video systems, and neonatal-sized head coils. MR sequence development includes sequences useful for assessing hemodynamics and hypoxic ischemic lesions in neonates. Imaging sequences include diffusion-weighted imaging (DWI) and diffusion tensor imaging (DTI). Imaging sequences also include perfusion imaging: blood oxygen level dependent (BOLD), arterial spin labeling (ASL) including continuous ASL (cASL) and pulsed ASL (pASL). Beyond MRI, MR spectroscopy (MRS) provides chemical spectra with clinical utility. These imaging and spectroscopic methods can be used to evaluate acute hypoxic ischemic injury to the neonatal brain.

Magnetic Resonance–Compatible Neonatal Incubator

MR studies of critically ill preterm and term neonates are difficult because of the need to provide consistent, reliable and effective monitoring and support for respiratory and cardiovascular functions and fluid-electrolyte and thermoregulatory homeostasis throughout the examination. Placing an MR scanner adjacent to or within a neonatal intensive care unit (NICU) reduces transport time, and hence reduces the duration for which these must be considered. However addressing these needs during the MR study remains nontrivial. The solution is to develop the ability to provide uninterrupted intensive care including monitoring and full clinical support for critically ill preterm and term neonates while undergoing MR studies. At least two separate MR-compatible incubators have been developed.[1-4] One is commercially available

(Lammers Medical Technology, Lübeck, Germany) and is a system that has been used by the authors.[1]

Design of an MR-compatible incubator requires consideration of certain aspects: air flow, humidity, temperature regulation, physiologic monitoring, integration of respiratory devices, and integration of specialized radiofrequency head and body coils.[2] These are required to provide a safe, controlled environment for imaging critically ill preterm and term newborns (Fig. 9-1). When these aspects are addressed the incubator can reduce the risks of MR and allow it to be more widely employed. Use of the incubator can reduce multiple patient transfers from four to two, eliminates repeated opening and closing of the incubator during normal use, and has shown to be associated with a reduced need for repeated application of anesthesia.[5]

Magnetic Resonance–Compatible Video Monitoring System

Vital sign monitoring and visual observation of the neonate are part of the standard of clinical care in the NICU. While vital sign monitoring during MR studies is common, it is difficult to visually observe the neonate.[5] This is due to a variety of factors including physical distance from the neonate, orientation of the control room, and the presence of visually obstructing objects like an MR-compatible incubator. These factors combine with the small body size of the neonates to make it nearly impossible to appropriately observe the neonate.

One solution is to introduce a video system. A video system can provide real-time color video monitoring of the neonate, thus enabling direct observation of the neonate in the MR scanner. One of the first research MR-compatible incubator systems included an integrated video system for patient monitoring.[2] The video camera was placed into the MR bore to provide a better view than could be obtained otherwise. Commercially available cameras (MRC Systems Gmb, Heidelberg) are approved for use in the MR bore. This particular camera comes in black and white and color versions, but color is useful for secondary monitoring of the perfusion.

Caution is required when installing a video system. Introducing electronic equipment into the MRI suite could precipitate a projectile event in the MR suite, or may result in MR image artifacts.

Neonatal-Sized Head Coil

Because of the small size of a neonatal head, the standard magnetic resonance head coils give suboptimal picture quality in the neonate.[6] The use of radiofrequency coils optimized for newborns improves the quality of MRI.[1] Coils can be tailored to offer superior signal-to-noise ratio (SNR) and image contrast for the neonatal patient population. Improvements in SNR, in turn, can be used to reduce scan time, improve resolution, or do both. Manufacturers are beginning to offer neonatal-sized head coils commercially: Philips, Lammers Medical Technology, and Advanced Imaging Research. The current generation of head coils are "receive" only. The next generation of neonatal head coils will include "receive transmit" coils.

Diffusion-Weighted Imaging and Diffusion Tensor Imaging of the Neonatal Brain

Diffusion-weighted MRI (DWI) is based on the microscopic movement of water molecules in brain tissue.[7] There are two basic imaging sequences that are being used to obtain quantitative information about water diffusion. The two types of images can be combined to calculate the apparent diffusion coefficient (ADC) map. The ADC map is an instrument- and MR sequence-independent parameter.

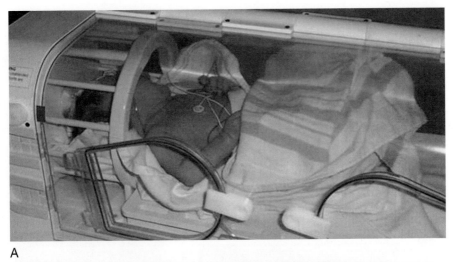

A

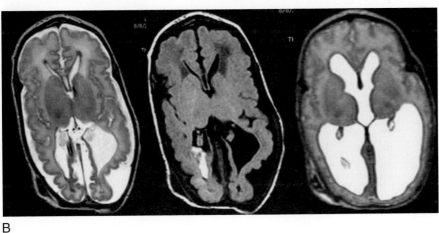

B

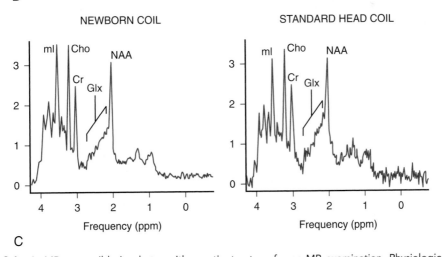

NEWBORN COIL

STANDARD HEAD COIL

C

Figure 9-1 **A,** MR-compatible incubator with a patient set up for an MR examination. Physiologic monitoring is performed using MR-compatible equipment. Note that the specialized newborn head coil is already in place. **B,** T2-weighted FSE MRI (left), FLAIR MRI (middle), and single-shot FSE image (right). **C,** The improvement in signal-to-noise is demonstrated by two MR spectra acquired from 2-month-old babies with the newborn coil (left) and the standard head coil (right). The random noise signal at 0 ppm is approximately three times higher when the standard head coil was used.

B

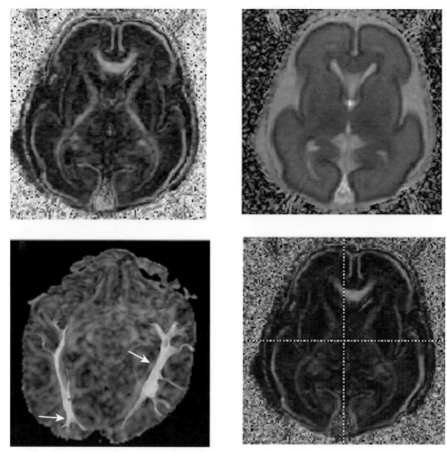

Figure 9-2   Diffusion tensor imaging (DTI) of a preterm neonate (25 weeks' gestation, 1 week old) with fractional anisotropy map (top left), mean diffusivity map (top right), color direction specific (blue: cranial caudal; green: transverse; and red: anterior posterior) fractional anisotropy map (bottom right), and tractography of the optic radiations (bottom left). (See Expert Consult site for color image.)

Diffusion tensor imaging (DTI) uses a set of diffusion-weighted images to obtain a more complete picture of the water diffusion including quantitative parameters.[8-10] These quantitative parameters correlate with sequences of myelination in the developing brain.[10,11] DTI can be used for the evaluation of a neonate with hypoxic-ischemic brain injury and periventricular white matter injury. It can also be used to map white matter tracts because water movement across fibers is hindered by white matter elements, and to generate tractography data to evaluate selected tracts (i.e., optic radiations) in the neonate (Fig. 9-2).[12,13]

Perfusion Imaging of the Neonatal Brain

MRI sequences that measure perfusion in the brain use either exogenous contrast or endogenous contrast methods. The exogenous perfusion contrasts are based on injections that alter either the magnetic relaxation or magnetic susceptibility of tissue.[14] These injections can include manganese, gadolinium, or super-paramagnetic iron oxide. The second class of techniques is based on endogenous contrast. These include BOLD effect, in which changes in blood oxygenation result in change in the magnetic resonance signal. Endogenous contrast methods also include ASL, in which arterial blood is tagged magnetically before it enters the brain tissue and then the amount delivered to the tissue is measured.[15]

Exogenous Contrast Agents

Exogenous contrast agents artificially alter either the magnetic relaxation or magnetic susceptibility so that it contrasts with tissue that would otherwise appear homogeneous. Paramagnetic metal ions are typically used for T1 contrast, and super-paramagnetic particles are typically used for T2 contrast, but both alter other magnetic properties.[16,17]

Manganese can be used as an intravascular contrast agent. Manganese has additional utility due to its ability to replace calcium in functioning neurons. However manganese has not been used clinically due to concerns about its potential toxicity. Indeed, while manganese has an interesting technical ability to image functioning neurons in the neonate, concerns about neurotoxicity preclude general use in humans. However, if the sensitivity of the acquisition can be increased, the concentration of the tracer needed will be less and manganese contrast might prove useful.[18]

Gadolinium has been widely used as an intravascular contrast agent in adult imaging as well as in the neonate, but its application is limited due to concerns about the renal safety of gadolinium given as a bolus.[19,20]

Super-paramagnetic iron oxide (SPIO) has also been used as an intravascular contrast agent. Of particular interest is the use of very small SPIO particles to perform perfusion imaging and to perform SPIO-labeled cell imaging.[16] SPIO imaging can assist in the detection of cerebral ischemia; areas with normal perfusion have signal reduction due to the presence of SPIO, and regions with lower perfusion have higher signal levels. SPIO is ultimately broken down by the body, and animal studies suggest it is a relatively safe MR contrast agent.[16,21]

Using contrast injections, dynamic susceptibility contrast (DSC) images can be acquired. In DSC, intravascular contrast alters the magnetic properties of the body. As the contrast passes through the brain tissue, a magnetic field difference is created between the blood vessel filled with contrast and the surrounding brain tissue. Susceptibility-weighted MR images are then obtained (Fig. 9-3). The perfusion imaging dataset is used to create a signal intensity versus time curve, and this curve can be used to calculate relative cerebral blood volume (CBV), relative cerebral blood flow (CBF), and mean transit time.

One study using dynamic susceptibility contrast-enhanced MRI demonstrated that maps of relative CBF could be acquired in neonates.[19] We have found that depending on the timing of perfusion imaging performed relative to the acute hypoxic injury, there may be a relatively increased flow in the region of acute infarction, which is probably related to luxury perfusion and/or increased metabolism (Fig. 9-4).

Blood Oxygen Level–Dependent Functional Magnetic Resonance Imaging

The BOLD fMRI technique was introduced by Ogawa and colleagues and Kwong and colleagues.[22,23] Using rapid MRI acquisition, these investigators could observe changes in the MR signal caused by transient hemodynamic changes. Functional activation of a neuron increases local oxygen extraction, followed by increased blood flow, which supplies oxygen to tissue in excess of what can be extracted by the cells. The net oxygen content in the venous blood is increased, which reduces the magnetic susceptibility gradient between blood and the surrounding parenchyma. As a result, the MR signal of the affected brain region is increased due to the reduced $T2^*$ spin dephasing.

Task-dependent fMRI using the BOLD effect is an established technique to measure brain activation from passive or active tasks performed during imaging. There have been studies of newborn fMRI, predominantly of the visual system, although the auditory and sensory-motor systems have also been investigated.[24] Since the onset and early postnatal development of hemispheric lateralization in the human brain are unknown, we also studied cortical activation induced by passive extension and flexion of the hand in neonates using fMRI.[25] In contrast to those seen

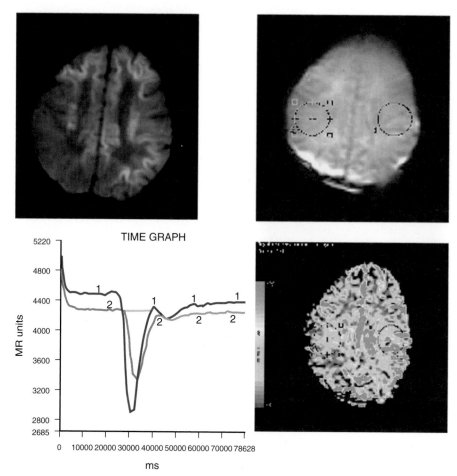

Figure 9-3 Dynamic contrast susceptibility perfusion magnetic resonance imaging (MRI) of hypoxic-ischemic injury in the neonatal brain. Top left: Diffusion map showing abnormal restricted diffusion in the bilateral cerebral cortex, left greater then right, with a "peripheral" pattern of injury. Top right: Gradient echo-echo planar magnetic resonance perfusion raw image obtained at the same level with placement of two ROIs. Bottom left: Time-activity curve showing the signal change over time of the contrast bolus through the region of interest. Bottom right: The generated cerebral blood volume map shows a relatively increased blood flow in the cortex relative to white matter and increased cerebral blood volume in the regions of acute infarction likely representing luxury compensatory reactive perfusion. (See color plate.)

in older age groups, somatosensory areas in the precentral and postcentral gyri of the neonate showed no significant hemispheric lateralization at term. Rather, our findings from independent left- and right-hand experiments suggest the presence of an emerging trend of contralateral lateralization of the somatosensory system at around term gestation (Fig. 9-5). The slight, statistically insignificant advantage of contralateral dominance (9.1% left hand and 12.5% right hand) found in this study suggests a trend toward the lateralization we know in the mature human brain. Findings in infants confirm rapid maturation of lateralization and suggest the presence of a developmental step between birth and about 2-6 months of age. In addition, the symmetry between left- and right-hand findings confirms establishment of unilateral sensorimotor function and validates the methodological approach. In this context, a comprehensive fMRI study of somatosensory genesis in younger premature newborns (24-32 weeks' gestation) and somatosensory pruning in older infants (2-6 months) reported for emerging language lateralization would be intriguing.[26]

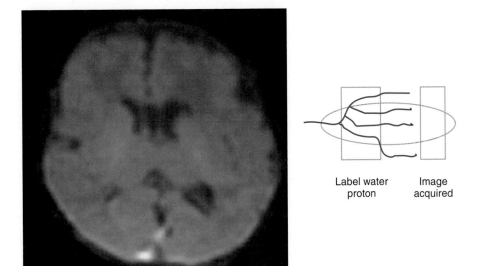

Label water   Image
proton   acquired

9

Figure 9-4 Left panel: Raw unprocessed arterial spin-labeled images acquired using FAIR (flow-sensitive alternating inversion recovery) technique in a full-term newborn signal with a focal area of cavitation seen near the left frontal horn. Note the high signal seen in the straight and the sagittal sinus near the level of the torcula. Also note that the signal intensity of the periventricular and deep white matter in decreased relative to the cortex. Right panel: A diagram showing how arterial blood is tagged by a radiofrequency pulse. The arterial blood then flows into the imaging slice, where its magnetization results in change in signal intensity.

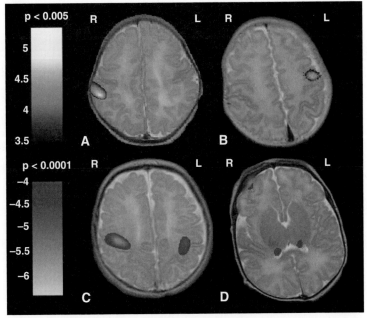

Figure 9-5 Blood oxygen level dependent (BOLD) changes in sensorimotor areas and thalamus from passive extension and flexion stimulation. **A,** Contralateral activation from left-hand stimulation of a 40-week gestation female (at 42 weeks' postmenstrual age) newborn. **B,** Right-hand stimulation of a 26-week gestation female (at 39 weeks' postmenstrual age) newborn. Findings are comparable to adult results for sensorimotor activation. **C,** Bi-hemispheric BOLD changes (36.4% and 31.3% during left and right hand, tasks respectively), which are unique for the newborn population. Bilateral deactivation in a 40-week gestational age male (at 43 weeks' postmenstrual age) newborn from left-hand stimulation. Additional significant BOLD changes were found in frontal lobe and thalamus (41.7% of the population). **D,** Thalamic deactivation in both hemispheres in a 39-week gestational age male (at 42 weeks' postmenstrual age) newborn from left-hand stimulation. (See Expert Consult site for color image.)

Taking these findings together, it appears that the somatosensory system is not specialized between midgestation and early postnatal life, and appears to develop later through postnatal pruning.[26]

Resting BOLD and functional connectivity are emerging alternatives to the task-dependent paradigm. Instead of using a functional event to cause a specific activation, in functional connectivity, low frequency fluctuations in the BOLD signal are compared via mathematical models, which attempt to determine the areas undergoing similar fluctuations.[27] Analysis results in a map indicating areas of the brain that are functionally connected.[27] This method has been demonstrated in the developing brain for neonates, as well young children.[28-30] Studies using these methods have shown that premature infants have different connectivity that is persistent during maturation compared with term birth controls subjects.[31]

Arterial Spin Labeling

The general method of ASL replicates the Fick indicator dilution method. ASL uses a radiofrequency (RF) pulse to label a particular region of tissue containing arteries. Later the regions supplied by these arteries will contrast with the surrounding tissue when the labeled blood from the first region reaches the region to be imaged.[32,33] There are different types of ASL, but more commonly employed methods include continuous ASL (cASL) and pulsed ASL (pASL).[23,34,35] Both allow cerebral perfusion imaging without the use of exogenous contrast agents (Fig. 9-4); further comparison of the methods is found elsewhere.[36]

Continuous Arterial Spin Labeling

In cASL imaging, the RF pulse is active for a longer period and is applied to a labeling region at the base of the head.[33] cASL has shown utility in imaging acute stroke and in quantification of CBF measurements, but its use has been reduced by more advanced varieties of ASL.[37]

Pulsed Arterial Spin Labeling

In pASL, shorter duration RF pulses are used to label the region of tissue, and they are applied just before the blood vessels enter the region of interest.[33] In one study, the pASL technique was used to quantify preoperative CBF in 25 infants with congenital heart disease.[38] The mean CBF value for the cohort was 19.7 ± 9.1 mL/100 g/min. This value is less compared to that found in another study in healthy term infants (50 ± 3.4 mL/100 g/min), which calculated CBF using ^{133}Xe clearance methodology.[39] In this study, periventricular leukomalacia (PVL) occurred in 28% of the cases (7/25) and it was associated with decreased baseline CBF values.[38] However, as there are significant differences in the absolute CBF values among the different methods, one must exercise caution when comparing CBF data from studies using different methods (Chapter 4).

Recently, ASL has been performed with a 3T magnet in neonates for evaluation of regional cerebral perfusion.[40] Interestingly, this study found that perfusion in the basal ganglia (30-39 mL/100 g/min) was higher than in cortical gray matter (16-19 mL/100 g/min) or white matter (10-15 mL/100 g/min).

Of note, with reference to neonates suffering from ischemia-related brain injury, we have found a large incidence of focal white matter necrosis in MRI studies in both preterm and term infants with congenital heart disease.[41] In analyzing the neuropathology of 38 infants dying after cardiac surgery, we tested a set of questions related to the severity and patterns of brain injury, cardiopulmonary bypass (CPB), deep hypothermic circulatory arrest (DHCA), and age of the infants at the time of surgery. In all infants dying after cardiac surgery, irrespective of the modality, cerebral white matter damage (PVL or diffuse white matter gliosis) was the most significant lesion in terms of severity and incidence, followed by a spectrum of gray matter lesions. The patterns of brain injury were not age-related in the limited time-frame analyzed, except that infants who developed acute PVL after both closed and DHCA/CPB surgery (14/38 infants, 34%) were significantly younger at the time of death (median age 13 days) compared with infants without

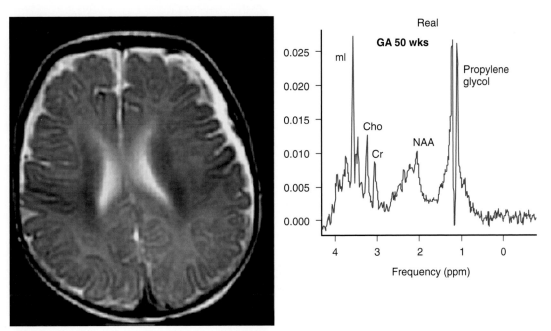

Figure 9-6 Short-echo proton magnetic resonance spectroscopy of occipital gray matter in a full-term neonate showing a propylene glycol (right) peak from a solvent used in medication being administered to the patient.

brain injury (median age at death 42.5 days) (P=.031). This observation suggests that the brain in the neonatal period (during the first 28 postnatal days) might be at higher risk to develop acute PVL even in term neonates, and likely reflects the vulnerability of immature (premyelinating) white matter to hypoxia-ischemia.

Quantitative Proton Magnetic Resonance Spectroscopy of the Neonatal Brain

The signal used by MRI to create anatomical maps is generated primarily by the hydrogen nuclei, also known as protons (^{1}H), of water molecules. In contrast, ^{1}H MRS analyzes signal of protons attached to other molecules. In lieu of an image a chemical spectra can be acquired for a region of interest.

Changes in MRS spectra can be observed in a variety of cases: after ingesting alcohol (there is measurable presence of ethanol); while maintaining specialized diets (e.g., acetone is present after ketogenic diet); and following the administration of medications (e.g., mannitol and propylene glycol solvents for drugs) (Fig. 9-6).[42]

In neonates with hypotensive ischemic brain injury, early acute injury can be detected by ^{1}H MRS when both diffusion imaging and conventional imaging are negative.[43-50] Within the first 24 hours of injury, MRS can detect elevated levels of lactate in the cerebral cortex or basal ganglia depending on the pattern of injury. Reduced levels of N-acetyl-aspartate (NAA) and elevated glutamate and glutamine are then usually detected after 24 hours (Fig. 9-7). The role of MRS in evaluating perinatal white matter injury is similar in the acute phase of injury when initially lactate is elevated, then subsequently NAA is reduced and glutamate and glutamine are elevated. Knowledge of the normal developmental changes in MRS metabolites across development is necessary when interpreting pathologic cases.[43-50] Establishing a database of exams that includes age-matched normal controls and biopsy-proven pathologic cases will assist in interpretation of MRS metabolite spectra; this effort is underway.

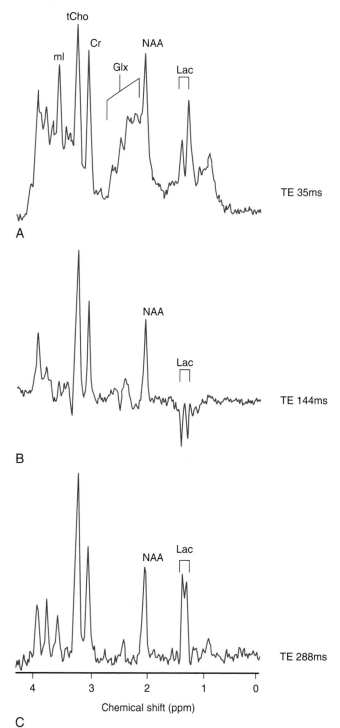

Figure 9-7 Single-voxel proton magnetic resonance spectroscopy (MRS) of the basal ganglia of a term infant with hypoxic-ischemic injury. **A,** A spectrum acquired using short echo time (35 ms), which shows a myoinositol peak (left side of the spectrum), elevated glutamate/glutamine peak next to a reduced NAA peak (middle spectrum), and an elevated lactate doublet next to a lipid peak (right side of the spectrum). **B,** A spectrum acquired using long echo time (144 ms) showing a lactate doublet peak inverted and reduced NAA but with nonvisualization of myoinositol, glutamate, and lipids. **C,** A spectrum acquired using even longer echo time (244 ms); it is similar to Fig. 9-7B except that the lactate doublet has reverted. (See Expert Consult site for color image.)

Acknowledgments

The authors thank Hari Keshava (quantitative diffusion tensor measurements); Stephan Erberich, PhD (neonatal fMRI); Marvin D. Nelson, MD; Istvan Seri, MD, PhD; and Floyd Gilles, MD (support and advice); and the staff of the Newborn and Infant Critical Care Unit and MRI program at CHLA.

Grant support: Radiological Society of North American and Rudi Schulte Research Institute and NIH pediatric research loan repayment grant.

References

1. Blüml S, Friedlich P, Erberich S, et al. MR Imaging of newborns by using an MR-compatible incubator with integrated radiofrequency coils: initial experience. Radiology. 2004;231(2):595-601.
2. Dumoulin C, Rohling K, Piel J, et al. Magnetic resonance imaging compatible neonate incubator. Concepts Magn Reson. 2002;15(2):117-128.
3. Srinivasan R, Loenneker-Lammers T, Shah R. MR compatible incubator for imaging pre- and term neonates. Proc Int Soc Magn Reson Med. 2002;10:799.
4. Srinivasan R, Connolly D, Capener D. Ultrafast magnetic resonance imaging of the neonate in a magnetic resonance-compatible incubator with a built-in coil. Pediatrics. 2004;113(2):150-152.
5. Stokowski L. Ensuring safety for infants undergoing magnetic resonance imaging. Adv Neonatal Care. 2005;5(1):14.
6. Erberich S, Friedlich P, Seri I, et al. Functional MRI in neonates using neonatal head coil and MR compatible incubator. Neuroimage. 2003;20:683-692.
7. Beaulieu C. The basis of anisotropic water diffusion in the nervous system—a technical review. NMR Biomed. 2002;15:435-455.
8. Le Bihan D, Mangin J, Poupon C, et al. Diffusion tensor imaging: concepts and applications. Magn Reson Imag. 2001;13:534-546.
9. Basser P, Pajevic S, Pierpaoli C, et al. In vivo fiber tractography using DT-MRI data. Magn Reson Med. 2000;44:625-632.
10. Wimberger D, Roberts T, Barkovich J, et al. Identification of premyelination by diffusion-weighted MRI. J Comput Assist Tomogr. 1995;19(1):28-33.
11. Evans A. The NIH MRI study of normal brain development i Brain Development Cooperative Group 1. Citeseer. 2006;30:184-202.
12. Mori S, Crain B, Chacko V, et al. Three-dimensional tracking of axonal projections in the brain by magnetic resonance imaging. Ann Neurol. 1999;45(2):247-269.
13. Basser P, Jones DK. Diffusion-tensor MRI: theory, experimental design and data analysis—a technical review. NMR Biomed. 2002;15:456-467.
14. Rosen B, Belliveau J, Veva JM, et al. Perfusion imaging with NMR contrast agents. Magn Reson Med. 1990;14:249-265.
15. Huisman T, Sorrensen AG. Perfusion-weighted magnetic resonance imaging of the brain: techniques and application in children. Eur Radiol. 2004;14:59-72.
16. Krestin G. Superparamagnetic iron oxide contrast agents: physicochemical characteristics and applications in MR imaging. Eur Radiol. 2001;11(2319):2331.
17. Strijkers G, Mulder M, Tilborg GA, et al. MRI contrast agents: current status and future perspectives. Anticancer Agents. 2007;7:291-305.
18. Silva A, Lee J, Aoki I, et al. Manganese-enhanced magnetic resonance imaging (MEMRI): methodological and practical considerations. NMR Biomed. 2004;17:532-543.
19. Tanner S, Cornette L, Ramenghi L, et al. Cerebral perfusion in infants and neonates: preliminary results obtained using dynamic susceptibility contrast enhanced magnetic resonance imaging. Br Med J. 2003;88:525-530.
20. Laswad T, Wintermark P, Alamo L, et al. Method for performing cerebral perfusion-weighted MRI in neonates. Pediatr Radiol. 2009;39:260-264.
21. Weinmann H, Ebert W, Misselwitz B, et al. Tissue-specific MR contrast agents. Eur J Radiol. 2003; 46:33-44.
22. Ogawa S, Lee T, Kay A, et al. Brain magnetic resonance imaging with contrast dependent on blood oxygenation. Proc Natl Acad Sci. 1990;87:9868-9872.
23. Kwong KK, Belliveau JW, Chesler DA, et al. Dynamic magnetic resonance imaging of human brain activity during primary sensory stimulation. Proc Natl Acad Sci. 1992;89(12):5675.
24. Seghier M, Lazeyras F, Huppi P. Functional MRI of the newborn. Semin Fetal Neonatal Med. 2006;6:479-488.
25. Erberich S, Panigrahy A, Friedlich P, et al. Somatosensory lateralization in the newborn brain. Neuroimage. 2006;29:155-161.
26. Dehaene-Lambertz G, Pallier C, Serniclaes W, et al. Neural correlates of switching from auditory to speech perception. Neuroimage. 2005;24:21-33.
27. Biswal B, Yetkin F, Haughton VM, et al. Functional connectivity in the motor cortex of resting human brain using echo-planar MRI. Magn Reson Med. 1995;34:534-541.
28. Fransson P, Skiöld B, Horsch S, et al. Resting-state networks in the infant brain. Proc Natl Acad Sci. 2007;104(39):15531.
29. Liu W, Flax J, Guise K, et al. Functional connectivity of the sensorimotor area in naturally sleeping infants. Brain Res. 2008;1223:42-49.
30. Lin W, Zhu Q, Gao W, et al. Functional connectivity MR imaging reveals cortical functional connectivity in the developing brain. Am J Neuroradiol. 2008;29:1883-1889.
31. Lubsen J, Vohr B, Myers E, et al. Microstructural and functional connectivity in the developing preterm brain. Semin Perinatol. 2011;35(1):34-43.
32. Golay X, Hendrikse J, Lim T. Perfusion imaging using arterial spin labeling. Top Magn Reson Imag. 2004;15(1):10.
33. Wang JJ, Licht DJ. Pediatric perfusion MR imaging using arterial spin labeling. Neuroimag Clin North Am. 2006;16:149-167.
34. Williams D, Detre J, Leigh J, et al. Magnetic resonance imaging of perfusion using spin inversion of arterial water. Proc Natl Acad Sciences. 1992;89:212-216.

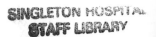

35. Detre JA, Leigh J, Williams D, et al. Perfusion imaging. Magn Reson Med. 1992;23:37-45.
36. Wong EC, Buxton RB, Frank LR. A theoretical and experimental comparison of continuous and pulsed arterial spin labeling techniques for quantitative perfusion imaging. Magn Reson Med. 1998;40(3):348-355.
37. Chalela JA, Alsop DC, Gonzalez-Atavales JB, et al. Magnetic resonance perfusion imaging in acute ischemic stroke using continuous arterial spin labeling. Stroke. 2000;31(3):680.
38. Licht DJ, Wang J, Silvestre D, et al. Preoperative cerebral blood flow is diminished in neonates with severe congenital heart defects. J Thorac Cardiovasc Surg. 2004;128(6):841-849.
39. Greisen G, Børch K. White matter injury in the preterm neonate: the role of perfusion. Develop Neurosci. 2000;23:209-212.
40. Miranda M, Olofsson K, Sidaros K. Noninvasive measurements of regional cerebral perfusion in preterm and term neonates by magnetic resonance arterial spin labeling. Pediatr Res. 2006;60(3): 359-363.
41. Kinney H, Panigrahy A, Newburger J, et al. Hypoxic-ischemic brain injury in infants with congenital heart disease dying after cardiac surgery. Acta Neuropathol. 2005;110:563-578.
42. Seymour K, Blüml S, Sutherling J, et al. Identification of cerebral acetone by 1 H-MRS in patients with epilepsy controlled by ketogenic diet. Magn Reson Material Phys Biol Med. 1999;8:33-42.
43. Kreis R, Hofmann L, Kuhlmann B, et al. Brain metabolite composition during early human brain development as measured by quantitative in vivo 1H magnetic resonance spectroscopy. Magn Reson Med. 2002;48(6):949-958.
44. Ernst T, Kreis R, Ross BD. Absolute quantitation of water and metabolites in the human brain. I. Compartments and water. J Magn Reson. 1993;102:1-8.
45. Shu S, Ashwal S, Holshouser B, et al. Prognostic value of 1H-MRS in perinatal CNS insults. Pediatr Neurol. 1997;14(4):309-318.
46. Hanrahan J, Sargentoni J, Azzopardi D, et al. Cerebral metabolism within 18 hours of birth asphyxia: a proton magnetic resonance spectroscopy study. Pediatr Res. 1996;39(4):584-590.
47. Holshouser B, Ashwal S, Luh G, et al. Proton MR spectroscopy after acute central nervous system injury: outcome prediction in neonates, infants, and children. Radiology. 1997;202:487-496.
48. Hüppi PS, Posse S, Lazeyras F, et al. Magnetic resonance in preterm and term newborns: 1H-spectroscopy in developing human brain. Pediatr Res. 1991;30(6):574-578.
49. Vigneron D, Barkovich A, Noworolski SM, et al. Three-dimensional proton MR spectroscopic imaging of premature and term neonates. Am J Neuroradiol. 2001;22:1424-1433.
50. Hüppi P, Possee S, Lazeyras F, et al. Magnetic resonance in preterm and term newborns: 1H-spectroscopy in developing human brain. Pediatr Res. 1991;30:574-578.

B

CHAPTER 10

Cardiovascular Magnetic Resonance in the Study of Neonatal Hemodynamics

Anthony N. Price, PhD, Alan M. Groves, MD, FRCPCH

10

- ● **Current Understanding of Neonatal Hemodynamics**
- ● **Current Cotside Circulatory Assessment**
- ● **Optimal Circulatory Management**
- ● **Current Cardiovascular Magnetic Resonance Imaging**
- ● **Success of CMR in the Adult Population**
- ● **Performing CMR Imaging in the Newborn**
- ● **Adapting CMR for Use in Newborns**
- ● **Cine CMR**
- ● **Phase contrast CMR**
- ● **Emerging Cardiac Magnetic Resonance Imaging**
- ● **Assessment of Myocardial Motion**
- ● **Potential Role of CMR in the Study of Neonatal Hemodynamics**
- ● **Advantages and Disadvantages of Functional CMR Imaging**
- ● **Conclusion**
- ● **References**

This chapter describes the emerging role of cardiovascular magnetic resonance (CMR) in the study of neonatal hemodynamics. While at the time of publication this approach is very much in its infancy, in our view this is set to change. CMR assessments in adults now have a role in the clinical assessment of ventricular function, cardiomyopathy, myocarditis, and complex congenital heart disease.[1] Similarly the use of brain magnetic resonance imaging (MRI) in the neonate has blossomed since its first reported use in 1982.[2] Brain MRI is now accepted as standard of care for encephalopathic infants, has been used to predict long-term neurodevelopmental outcome in very preterm neonates (Chapter 9), and has led to more than 1000 published research papers in the neonatal population.[3-7]

CMR assessments of neonatal hemodynamic function are neither simple nor inexpensive, but they are entirely noninvasive. This chapter summarizes areas of neonatal hemodynamics where there is significant residual uncertainty over pathophysiology and management, describes the impact of CMR in adult practice, puts forward a safe, effective approach to CMR in the neonate, discusses the current and emerging techniques, and suggests areas for the technique to significantly advance our understanding of developmental cardiovascular physiology and contribute to future changes in the care of critically ill preterm and term neonates with cardiovascular compromise. Our hope is that as the availability of MRI scanners located on or near neonatal intensive care units (NICUs) increases in coming years, CMR will fulfill its significant promise to advance clinical research and thus improve mortality and morbidity in the vulnerable newborn through enhanced hemodynamic monitoring and support.

Current Understanding of Neonatal Hemodynamics

As detailed in Chapters 1, 12, and 16, the most prematurely born infants remain at high risk for death and disability.[8-12] The impact of preterm birth on the population is vast—an estimated annual socioeconomic burden of more than $26 billion in the United States.[13] While in the past respiratory disease was the primary cause of death, high-quality research has improved preterm respiratory care, such that an increasing proportion of deaths occur due to episodes of sepsis or necrotizing enterocolitis.[12,14,15] These systemic inflammatory disorders trigger the release of proinflammatory cytokines, which directly impair myocardial function and drastically alter peripheral vascular control, making circulatory failure the final mechanism of death (Chapters 1, 12 , 14, and 16).[16] Circulatory factors are also linked to key morbidity. Failing cardiac function and abnormal vasoregulation have been shown to cause cerebral hypoperfusion, and episodes of low cerebral blood flow are central to the pathophysiology of preterm brain injury, which causes long-term disability.[17-21]

In our view the pace of research into hemodynamic function has not kept up with that of research into respiratory function, and clinical circulatory care has changed little in the last 20 years. Improving circulatory management has been highlighted as a research priority in preterm infants.[22-24] However, understanding of the pathophysiology, as well as optimal treatment of circulatory failure, is hampered by the limited tools available to monitor circulatory function.[25]

Current Cotside Circulatory Assessment

All circulatory function relies on the interplay of preload, contractility, and afterload (see Chapters 1 and 12). A robust assessment of the newborn circulation therefore needs to quantify preload, contractility, afterload, systemic perfusion, and organ blood flow distribution. Current cotside methods fall short of this ideal, however; in particular, monitoring of circulatory status in the neonatal unit still relies heavily on arterial blood pressure (Chapters 1, 3, and 6). Yet, blood pressure is at best weakly predictive of volume of blood flow, and some studies have suggested no or even an inverse relation between blood pressure and blood flow in certain subpopulations of preterm infants (Chapters 1 and 12).[26-28] Other clinical assessments, such as capillary refill time or volume of urine output also have limited value in indicating circulatory health.[26]

Other chapters in this textbook address the role of many other research and clinical techniques, which have already, or may in the future, enhance our understanding of the transitional circulation. In particular, functional echocardiographic techniques (Chapter 5) have produced significant advances in understanding,[21,29-37] and echocardiography has a role in the assessment of circulatory status at the bedside.[38,39] However, echocardiography has its limitations. For example, current echocardiographic modalities cannot reliably measure cardiac preload, measures of contractility are limited by irregular ventricular contours seen in the newborn period, and measures of cardiac output and systemic perfusion have limited repeatability in the preterm infant.[32,40-44] Other techniques such as near-infrared spectroscopy (NIRS) also have limited repeatability in assessment of perfusion and cannot assess the elements of cardiac preload and contractility, which are necessary to advance understanding of circulatory failure (see Chapters 7 and 8).[45]

Optimal Circulatory Management

Even when the attending clinician is confident that circulatory failure is present, there is very little evidence on how to intervene, what treatment to use, and at what dose.[46-49] The North American ELGAN study and other groups have demonstrated that the rate of vasopressor use in infants of less than 28 weeks' gestation varies between 6% and 64% in different centers (Fig. 10-1), and that this range is not due to differences in illness severity between populations.[50]

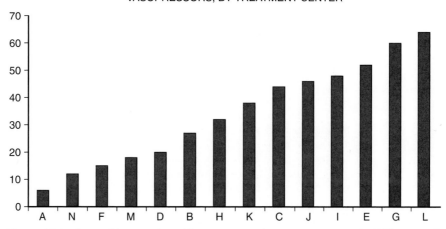

PROPORTION OF INFANTS <28 WEEKS GESTATION TREATED WITH VASOPRESSORS, BY TREATMENT CENTER

Figure 10-1   Rates of intervention with vasopressors by treatment center in 1387 extremely low gestation (<28 week) infants. See text for details. (From Laughon M, Bose C, Allred E, et al. Factors associated with treatment for hypotension in extremely low gestational age newborns during the first postnatal week. Pediatrics. 2007;119:273-280.)

Similar variability has been seen in other studies of vasopressor/inotrope and/or inotrope use and in rates of intervention to close a patent ductus.[51,52] It is clear that clinicians are limited in their understanding of circulatory failure, their ability to detect it, and in their ability to make informed choices on optimal management. Each year thousands of preterm infants are either being exposed to unnecessary, potentially harmful, treatments or are being deprived of potentially beneficial ones.

Current Cardiovascular Magnetic Resonance Imaging

A comprehensive discussion of magnetic resonance (MR) physics is beyond the scope of this textbook, but a few basic principles may be pertinent. For a greater insight, readers are referred to textbooks on the subject as a good starting point.[53] The underlying principle of MR relies upon the fact that certain atomic nuclei exhibit a magnetic moment, which gives rise to a gyromagnetic ratio. This ratio is the rate at which a nucleus can be said to precess in a magnetic field; the product of this and the magnet field strength is called the *Larmor frequency*. Hydrogen atoms, consisting of a single proton, exhibit the highest Larmor frequency and ultimately provide the strongest signal of all MR visible nuclei; coincidently, they are also the most numerous in the human body. When placed into a magnetic field protons will align along the direction of the field, but the measureable signal actually arises from the difference between the number that have aligned parallel versus antiparallel to the magnet field, which typically may be only a few for every million or so protons. This distribution of aligned moments is proportional to the strength of magnet field and thus the main reasons for the drive to use higher field strength magnets in MRI. Collectively the overall net magnetization of the many nuclear magnetic moments that make up a sample can be manipulated by applying radiofrequency (RF) pulses, and allows for the magnetization to be measured using RF receiver coils. Images can be produced that exploit the contrast between different tissue types, which can be due to different concentrations of protons or more powerfully due to differences in their "magnetic" environment. Alternatively, "labeling" protons in a particular way to encode their velocity can also be achieved by applying additional spatially dependent magnetic fields. Further specific issues are discussed with individual methodologies herein.

Success of Cardiovascular Magnetic Resonance in the Adult Population

Cardiac magnetic resonance (CMR) techniques have significantly advanced understanding of cardiovascular physiology and pathophysiology in adults. They are now considered the gold standard functional assessment tool, and their use is supported for a number of routine clinical applications.[1,54,55] These noninvasive assessments of cardiac health are now being gained faster, in more detail, and with greater sophistication than ever before.[54] The range of techniques available has been summarized in a number of recent reviews, but an introduction to some of the primary individual techniques are described herein.[54,56] The key benefits of CMR in the adult population are the ability to quantify the component factors of circulatory function, and in the improved repeatability over echocardiography for assessment of quantitative measures. Critically, improved repeatability can translate into 70-90% reduction in the patient numbers required to prove a hypothesis in research studies.[57]

Performing Cardiovascular Magnetic Resonance Imaging in the Newborn

It is clear that functional CMR will not become a routine clinical assessment tool for the sick newborn infant in the foreseeable future—its applicability is severely restricted by access to an MR scanner which needs to be in close proximity to a neonatal unit. However, the gaps in current knowledge mean that all potential methodologies should be applied to gain the maximum research advance. In particular, if CMR biomarkers of circulatory function can be used as part of the major endpoints in clinical trials of circulatory interventions, it may be possible to perform adequately powered studies on much smaller numbers of infants.[58] Our group therefore began exploring the potential utility of CMR as a research tool in neonatal medicine.[59]

Our group's patient care system for very low birth weight infants undergoing MRI has recently been described.[60] We have demonstrated that MR scans can safely be performed in this population while maintaining respiratory, circulatory and thermal stability. We have now performed cardiac MR examinations in over 180 newborn preterm and term infants without any adverse events. Functional CMR images have been successfully obtained in infants weighing as little as 590 g. All infants are studied purely for research purposes, and all parents have given signed informed consent. The project has been approved by the local regional ethics committee. Scans are carried out using a dedicated neonatal scanner (Philips 3.0 Tesla Achieva system [Best, Netherlands]) installed within the Neonatal Intensive Care Unit at Hammersmith Hospital.

In all cases cardiac MR images are obtained after infants have been allowed to fall into a natural sleep after a feed and careful swaddling. Neither sedative medication nor anesthesia is used. In many cases a vinyl vacuum bag filled with plastic beads is used to augment immobilization (Natus Medical Inc., San Carlos, CA). Infants are scanned with oxygen saturation, heart rate, and continuous temperature monitoring; a pediatrician or trained neonatal nurse is also in attendance throughout each scan. Protection from acoustic noise is achieved by applying moldable dental putty to the ears and covering them with neonatal ear muffs (Natus Minimuffs, Natus Medical Inc., San Carlos, CA).[60]

Scans can be performed free breathing, with the provision of nasal continuous positive airway pressure or low flow oxygen as clinically indicated. In older children, most CMR scans are performed during sedation or anesthesia, and image acquisitions occur either during enforced breath-holds, or by use of a navigator bar to coordinate image acquisition with diaphragmatic movement. However, to date our neonatal cardiac images have been obtained without the need for sedation/anesthesia or respiratory navigation. While this approach improves both the acceptability of the technique and limits scan acquisition times, we are currently investigating newer approaches to cope with respiratory motion. Traditional methods employed in adult CMR, such as breath-holding or respiratory navigators, are not suitable, or reliable

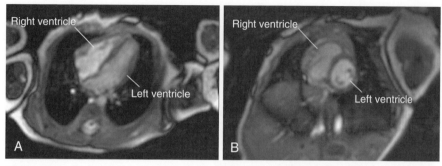

Figure 10-2   Four chamber **(A)** and short axis **(B)** views obtained with steady-state free precession sequences in a newborn. See text for details. (Reproduced with permission from Groves AM, Chiesa G, Durighel G, et al. Functional cardiac MRI in preterm and term newborns. Arch Dis Child Fetal Neonatal Ed. 2011;96:F86-F91.)

10

enough, for use in neonates. Techniques are being investigated that will allow for retrospective handling of data corrupted by respiratory motion, and also the bulk body motions that may occur during scanning of non-sedated infants. This could both allow for improvements in image quality by reducing artifacts and allow further cardiac physiology to be explored; for example, by evaluating the cardiac function during different parts of the respiratory cycle.

Adapting Cardiovascular Magnetic Resonance for Use in Newborns

The majority of adult CMR studies are currently performed at 1.5-Tesla field strength. Discussion on the specific challenges faced when imaging at higher field strengths are outside the scope of this review.[61] However, as mentioned, the main drive to higher field systems comes from the increased signal offered as field strength increases, which may confer a substantial benefit for imaging small neonates. The initial process of image optimization we have undergone to maximize scan quality has previously been described.[58]

The major challenges faced in performing CMR in neonates arise from the need to significantly increase image resolution, both spatially (due to the size of the heart) and temporally (due to the rapid heart rates). These requirements place increased demands on the scanner hardware. In addition, the standard imaging protocols applied to adults may not be directly transferable, and thus require modification to be used for scanning small neonates.

Cine Cardiovascular Magnetic Resonance

Cine CMR plays a central role in any CMR assessment by producing time-resolved images of the heart that can be used to analyze cardiac function.[62] Typically, in adults, an MR acquisition method known as steady-state free precession (SSFP) is used because it provides images with excellent contrast between blood and muscle while also having very high signal-to-noise efficiency.[63] The technique applies rapid repetitive radiofrequency pulses and subsequently acquires data, referenced relative to the electrocardiogram (ECG) trace to allow retrospective reordering, that can produce dynamic images of the beating heart. Applying this technique at higher fields (>1.5 T) does, however, become more of a challenge and requires more careful calibration of the scanner to avoid detrimental image artifacts that can occur with this particular acquisition method.[61] Cine images acquired in the newborn infant typically have a temporal resolution of around 10 ms, a spatial (in-plane) resolution of less than 1 mm, a slice thickness of 3-5 mm, and can be acquired in around 30 seconds per slice.[58,59] Scans can be acquired in any imaging plane (see four chamber and short axis views shown in Fig. 10-2).

Rather than simply describing function in a single plane, a stack of contiguous short axis images are routinely acquired to encompass the entire volume of the left

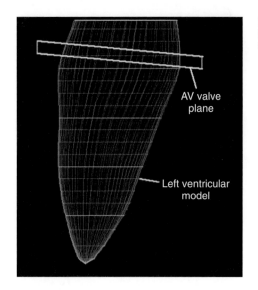

B

Figure 10-3 Three-dimensional model of left ventricular function reconstructed from a stack of short axis images. See text for details.

AV valve
plane

Left ventricular
model

and right ventricles.[62] Endocardial and epicardial borders can be traced at end-diastole and end-systole at each level of the stack of images to reconstruct three-dimensional (3-D) models of ventricular function (Fig. 10-3).

These models are constructed directly from imaging of the whole heart, and without the assumptions on ventricular geometry which weaken the equivalent two-dimensional echocardiographic estimations.[41] Some software packages (e.g., CMR Tools, Cardiovascular Imaging Solutions, London) also produce models incorporating the systolic base-to-apex motion of the heart, which contributes significantly to cardiac output.[64]

Cine CMR techniques can therefore provide data on left ventricular preload (end-diastolic volume), contractility (ejection fraction), and output (stroke volume) from these 3-D models. Our group has constructed a nomogram (Fig. 10-4) for these data from a cohort of 75 infants with median birth weight 1886 g (790-4140 g), birth gestation 33 weeks (25-42 weeks), postnatal age at scan 9 days (1-73 days), weight at scan 2192 g (790-4140 g), and gestation at scan 35 weeks (28-42 weeks). Forty-six infants had been admitted to the neonatal unit; 29 were term or near-term infants on the postnatal ward. While normal range for left ventricular output varied with age this was not the case for end-diastolic volume, end-systolic volume, and ejection fraction. Lower limits of population normal (defined as the 2.5th centile) have therefore been defined for these variables as 1.8 mL/kg, 0.4 mL/kg, and 58% respectively.

In addition to enabling assessments of cardiac preload and ejection fraction, which have not previously been readily assessed by echocardiography, our data demonstrate that these quantitative CMR measures have significantly improved repeatability compared with traditional echocardiographic methods. This improved repeatability will hopefully translate into a significantly decreased subject number for adequately powered clinical trials, as seen in adults.[57]

Phase Contrast Cardiovascular Magnetic Resonance

Phase contrast (PC) techniques are a way in which images can be made sensitive to how far protons have moved during a particular "encoding" time prior to the acquisition of signal.[56,65] This ultimately means that MR can be used to generate images with signal intensity directly (and quantifiably) proportional to the velocity of tissue or more importantly blood. By utilizing this technique with an ECG-synchronized cine (time-resolved) acquisition, the flow of blood can be directly measured

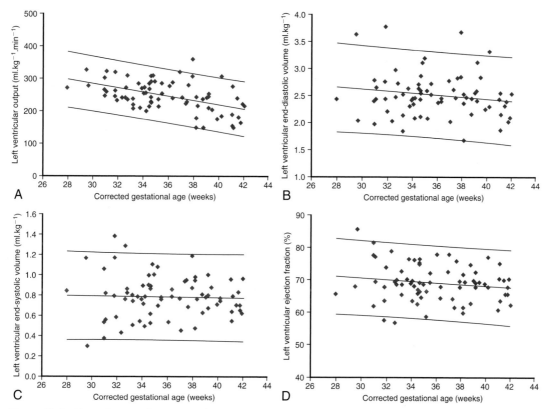

Figure 10-4   Normal ranges by corrected gestational age at scan for steady-state free precession assessment of left ventricular output **(A)**, end-diastolic volume **(B)**, end-systolic volume **(C)**, and ejection fraction **(D)**. (Reproduced with permission from Groves AM, Chiesa G, Durighel G, et al. Functional cardiac MRI in preterm and term newborns. Arch Dis Child Fetal Neonatal Ed. 2011;96:F86-F91.)

throughout the cardiac cycle. Phase contrast imaging planes can be again placed in any orientation, allowing quantification of volume of flow in any large blood vessel.[56,58] Phase contrast images acquired in the newborn infant have a temporal resolution of around 15 ms, and advances in sequence development and receiver coil technology mean that images can now be acquired with a spatial (in-plane) resolution of 0.4-0.6 mm and a slice thickness of 2-4 mm in around 90-180 seconds.[66]

The particular value of PC imaging in the neonate lies in quantification of flow at multiple points in the circulation. The persistence of fetal shunt pathways in the preterm neonate means that neither left nor right ventricular output represent true systemic or pulmonary perfusion.[30] Cardiac MR allows quantification of flow in the superior vena cava (SVC) and descending aorta (DAo), both of which are considered to be acceptable markers of systemic perfusion in the preterm neonate.[32,43,58] Our group has constructed a nomogram (Fig. 10-5) for these data from a cohort of 28 newborn infants with proven ductal closure. These infants had median birth weight 1856 g (965-4140 g), birth gestation 33 weeks (28-41 weeks), postnatal age at scan 10 days (2-22 days), weight at scan 2055 g (1015-4140 g), and gestation at scan 34 weeks (29-41 weeks).[58]

In addition, flow can be assessed in the internal carotid and basilar arteries, the sum of which equals total brain blood flow.[67] By combining PC imaging with assessment of cerebral volume, the cerebral blood flow per unit tissue volume can also be calculated.[66]

PC MRI is a validated technique in the adult.[56] Our data also demonstrate that quantification of SVC and DAo flow with phase contrast CMR has significantly

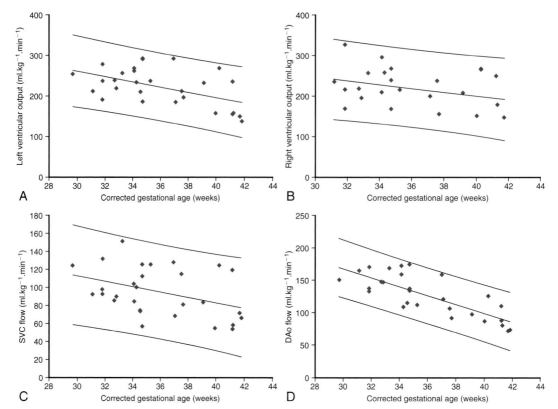

Figure 10-5   Normal ranges by corrected gestational age at scan for phase contrast assessment of left ventricular output **(A)**, right ventricular output **(B)**, superior vena caval flow **(C)**, and descending aortic flow **(D)**. See text for details. (Reproduced with permission from Groves AM, Chiesa G, Durighel G, et al. Functional cardiac MRI in preterm and term newborns. Arch Dis Child Fetal Neonatal Ed. 2011;96:F86-F91.)

improved repeatability compared with prior echocardiographic cohorts.[32,43,44,58] This may be because echocardiographic techniques measure diameter which then has to be squared to estimate area, and then multiplied by the measured velocity of blood flow, producing a potential multiplication of errors.[44] In contrast, PC MRI techniques measure velocity in each voxel across the vessel area and total flow is estimated by summing of signal over all of these voxels, so potentially smoothing out errors. Provisional data also suggest that the sum of SVC and DAo correlates closely with left ventricular output when the ductus is closed, supporting the notion that the sum of SVC and DAo flow is a reasonable surrogate for total systemic perfusion, and giving scope for the volume of ductus arteriosus shunt to be estimated as the difference between left ventricular output and the sum of SVC and DAo flow.[58]

Emerging Cardiac Magnetic Resonance Imaging

3-D Visualization of Flow with Phase Contrast

Whereas 2-D PC techniques allow quantification of flow within a single blood vessel, 3-D techniques allow visualization of flow in entire regions of the body.[68] Specialist postprocessing software allows the user to trace the path of a notional bolus of blood from within any vessel, throughout the cardiac cycle. We have applied these techniques in newborn infants and used Gyrotools software (Gyro-Tools Ltd., Switzerland) to visualize flow in the aortic arch and pulmonary arteries (Fig. 10-6).[69]

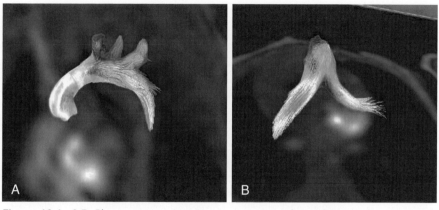

Figure 10-6   3-D Phase contrast imaging in a term newborn showing the aortic arch **(A)** visualized from subject's left side, and the pulmonary bifurcation **(B)** visualized from subject's back. See text for details. (See Expert Consult site for color image.) (Reproduced with permission from Groves AM. Cardiac magnetic resonance in the study of neonatal haemodynamics. Semin Fetal Neonatal Med. 2011;16(1):36-41.)

These techniques also allow quantification of flow in the vessels imaged, providing scope for the techniques to quantify volumes of systemic blood flow in multiple vascular beds, and to assess true volume of pulmonary blood flow, including that derived from shunting through the ductus arteriosus.

In addition to these assessments of flow in the great vessels, 3-D PC techniques have revealed fascinating patterns of intracardiac flow. Healthy adults have exhibited consistent rotational flow patterns within the cardiac atria, which are hypothesized to maintain the momentum of inflowing blood, with the direction of rotational flow allowing blood to "slingshot" into the ventricles following atrioventricular valve opening. While computational modelling studies have not demonstrated a momentum-conserving impact of rotational flow in the adult left ventricle, significant interest in the complexities of intracardiac flow patterns continues. Our initial work suggests that intracardiac flow patterns may be disrupted in newborn infants, potentially impairing diastolic ventricular function.[70]

Assessment of Myocardial Motion

A number of MR techniques give the potential for noninvasive quantification of myocardial motion.[62] Myocardial tagging techniques use "magnetization preparation" pulses to transiently saturate myocardial tissue along set lines or grids, producing low signal areas.[71] These "tags" are then distorted by the motion of the cardiac musculature (Fig. 10-7).

A number of techniques are in use in adults but still require adaptation for use in the preterm neonate. One candidate for development in the newborn is complementary spatial modulation of magnetization (CSPAMM) which has been shown to have improved tag persistence and temporal resolution in adults,[72] and widely available automated analysis packages such as harmonic phase (HARP) can be applied to the images.[73]

Once adapted for use in the newborn infant, tagging techniques may be able to provide quantitative measures of radial, longitudinal and rotational motion of the heart, again providing sensitive biomarkers for assessing the impact of inotropic and lusitropic agents on intrinsic myocardial contractility. These measures may also prove to be valuable tools to support validation of emerging echocardiographic techniques such as tissue Doppler imaging and speckle tracking.[74]

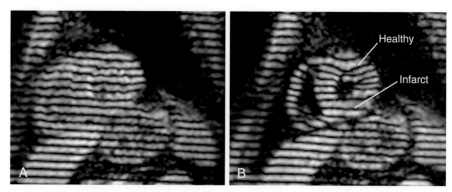

Figure 10-7 Complementary spatial modulation of magnetization (CSPAMM) images taken from an adult with inferior myocardial infarction. End-diastolic short axis image **(A)** shows tag location prior to contraction. End-systolic short axis image **(B)** shows distortion of tags in the anterior myocardium, but nondistortion in the infarcted posterior myocardium. See text for details. (Images courtesy of Dr. Declan O'Regan, Imperial College London. Reproduced with permission from Groves AM. Cardiac magnetic resonance in the study of neonatal haemodynamics. Semin Fetal Neonatal Med. 2011;16[1]:36-41.)

Potential Role of Cardiovascular Magnetic Resonance in the Study of Neonatal Hemodynamics

As acknowledged previously, functional CMR will not become a routine clinical assessment tool for the sick newborn infant in the foreseeable future. However, there is evidence that as a research tool the technique can add significantly to the study of neonatal hemodynamics.

Definition of the Pathophysiology of Circulatory Failure

Significant gaps in the understanding of the pathophysiology of neonatal circulatory failure persist (Chapters 1 and 12). In what circumstances is cardiac preload deficient, such that treatment with fluid volume is indicated?[75] Is intrinsic myocardial contractility impaired in preterm infants, or those with advanced sepsis/necrotizing enterocolitis?[76,77] Does increased systemic vascular resistance in the newborn period specifically impair contractility?[35,76] Does the decreased systemic vascular resistance caused by autonomic central nervous system immaturity and dysregulated cytokine release following preterm birth, oxidant stress, and/or sepsis/necrotizing enterocolitis affect preload and thus contractility, afterload, and perfusion pressure (Chapters 1 and 12)? What is the relationship between systemic blood pressure and systemic (and cerebral) blood flow in the newborn period?[26,28,78]

By providing detailed, repeatable, quantifiable measures of cardiac preload, contractility, afterload, and systemic perfusion, our hope is that by studying a cohort of newborn preterm infants a number of these questions can be answered.

Acting as a Biomarker in Studies Assessing the Cardiovascular Effects of Vasopressor/Inotropes, Inotropes, and Lusitropes

As previously mentioned there is great variability in rates of the use of vasopressor/inotropes and inotropes among different neonatal specialist centers.[50,51] While guidelines suggest that it is advisable to keep systemic arterial blood pressure in a "normal" range, the evidence for this approach is not convincing primarily because blood pressure is the dependent variable among the three major cardiovascular factors determining central cardiovascular function (Chapter 1).[46,47,79,80] Moreover, as all of the factors directly or indirectly affecting cardiac output and systemic vascular resistance as well as the individual's ability to compensate for the decreases in tissue oxygen delivery influence the individual's "normal" blood pressure range, population-based normal blood pressure values do not necessarily apply to a given individual (Chapters 1, 3, and 12). In certain conditions, misguided interventions increasing blood pressure inappropriately in the given hemodynamic scenario may raise systemic vascular resistance to the point where systemic blood flow becomes compromised.[81,82] While multicenter controlled clinical trials are necessary to define whether or not an intervention improves the long-term health of a population of neonates, such trials have significant financial and opportunity costs, and the majority of them have so far produced negative results. This is, at least in part, due to our lack of appropriate understanding of, and ability to appropriately monitor and diagnose, the nature of the underlying hemodynamic compromise (Chapters 1, 6, and 12). Phase 2 trials in small numbers of infants with circulatory compromise could be performed to allow CMR to define the short-term hemodynamic impact of various vasopressor/inotropes and inotropes on cardiac preload, contractility, afterload, and systemic (and cerebral) perfusion.[57] Such trials, having defined the short-term circulatory impact of these agents, could contribute to the chances of success of subsequent larger phase 3 trials. Similarly, phase 2 trials powered by CMR could define the short-term impact of corticosteroid usage and intervention to close a patent ductus arteriosus.[83,84]

Guiding the Development of Emerging Echocardiographic Techniques

The scope for cotside echocardiographic techniques to improve understanding of circulatory function and assist in assessment of individual infants is vast.[38,85] The ready availability of the technique, and its immediate visualization and quantification of function, clearly mean that its clinical applicability outstrips CMR. While echocardiography has significant limitations (Chapter 5), the technology behind the techniques continues to rapidly advance. Real-time 3-D echocardiography could potentially be used to assess cardiac filling and ejection fraction with improved accuracy.[86] Tissue Doppler imaging has already been employed to study a number of cohorts of newborn infants, and can provide key quantification of myocardial contractility.[87-89]

However, both techniques require significant optimization from the approaches currently in use in older subjects. The choice of optimal image settings, views, and analysis is not yet clear, and would be greatly assisted by the ability to compare multiple echocardiography techniques with a validated gold standard. By progressing the development of echocardiography techniques, CMR may eventually enhance the ability of all clinicians to reliably assess circulation at the cotside. This will allow the results of the pathophysiologic and pharmacologic interventional studies described above to be generalized to the majority of neonatal units, allowing advances in care for the greatest number of infants.

Advantages and Disadvantages of Functional Cardiovascular Magnetic Resonance Imaging

The multiple advantages of CMR imaging in terms of the complexity and repeatability of circulatory assessment have been described earlier in this chapter. One of the most important aspects of the advantages of CMR that needs to be emphasized is the possibility to use the technology as the clinical gold standard for central hemodynamic measurements.

However, assessments of cardiac function and blood flow volume using CMR do not take into account tissue oxygen demand or utilization. It is also important to acknowledge other disadvantages of the technique, the most significant being access to the MR scanner. The process of CMR requires physical movement of the patient to an MR scanning suite. While this is an additional handling episode, we have been able to demonstrate that the process can occur without apparent adverse effect.[60] The potential for adverse effects from the imaging modality itself must be considered, although MR imaging is considered extremely safe, provided it is performed within internationally agreed limits.[90] The risk of metallic objects either causing skin burns during the scan, or becoming a projectile as they approach the main magnetic field, are both significant. A thorough metal checking process, to prevent these complications is mandatory.[90] The expense of the technique is significant, and is related to standard MR scan costs, as well as the need for specialist cardiac radiographers to optimize image acquisition, and MR physicists to optimize methodology.

Conclusion

Functional CMR imaging is feasible in the newborn infant, and may contribute significantly to understanding of circulatory function in this population. The detailed assessments provided, and the robust repeatability of the techniques, may allow conclusions to be drawn from interventional studies in relatively small numbers of infants.

Acknowledgments

We are grateful to Prof. David Edwards, Prof. Jo Hajnal, Prof. Reza Razavi, Miss Giuliana Durighel, Miss Kathryn Broadhouse, Dr. Anna Finnemore, Dr. David Cox, and the staff of Queen Charlotte's and Chelsea Hospital Neonatal Unit for their assistance with the project. The MR scanning facilities are supported by the Garfield Weston Foundation, the Medical Research Council, and the Imperial College Comprehensive Biomedical Research Centre. ANP and AMG are supported by an MRC Clinician Scientist Fellowship awarded to AMG. Study sponsors had no involvement in data collection, analysis, or interpretation.

References

1. Hendel RC, Patel MR, Kramer CM, et al. ACCF/ACR/SCCT/SCMR/ASNC/NASCI/SCAI/SIR 2006 appropriateness criteria for cardiac computed tomography and cardiac magnetic resonance imaging: a report of the American College of Cardiology Foundation Quality Strategic Directions Committee Appropriateness Criteria Working Group, American College of Radiology, Society of Cardiovascular Computed Tomography, Society for Cardiovascular Magnetic Resonance, American Society of Nuclear Cardiology, North American Society for Cardiac Imaging, Society for Cardiovascular Angiography and Interventions, and Society of Interventional Radiology. J Am Coll Cardiol. 2006;48:1475-1497.
2. Levene MI, Whitelaw A, Dubowitz V, et al. Nuclear magnetic resonance imaging of the brain in children. Br Med J (Clin Res Ed). 1982;285:774-776.
3. Ment LR, Bada HS, Barnes P, et al. Practice parameter: neuroimaging of the neonate: report of the Quality Standards Subcommittee of the American Academy of Neurology and the Practice Committee of the Child Neurology Society. Neurology. 2002;58:1726-1738.
4. Rutherford M, Biarge MM, Allsop J, et al. MRI of perinatal brain injury. Pediatr Radiol. 2010; 40:819-833.
5. Panigrahy A, Borzage M, Bluml S. Basic principles and concepts underlying recent advances in magnetic resonance imaging of the developing brain. Semin Perinatol. 2010;34:3-19.
6. Lequin MH, Dudink J, Tong KA, et al. Magnetic resonance imaging in neonatal stroke. Semin Fetal Neonatal Med. 2009;14:299-310.
7. Boardman JP, Dyet LE. Recent advances in imaging preterm brain injury. Minerva Pediatr. 2007;59:349-368.
8. Marlow N, Wolke D, Bracewell MA, et al. Neurologic and developmental disability at six years of age after extremely preterm birth. N Engl J Med. 2005;352:9-19.
9. Horbar JD, Badger GJ, Carpenter JH, et al. Trends in mortality and morbidity for very low birth weight infants, 1991-1999. Pediatrics. 2002;110:143-151.
10. Shankaran S, Fanaroff AA, Wright LL, et al. Risk factors for early death among extremely low-birth-weight infants. Am J Obstet Gynecol. 2002;186:796-802.
11. Mangham LJ, Petrou S, Doyle LW, et al. The cost of preterm birth throughout childhood in England and Wales. Pediatrics. 2009;123:e312-e327.
12. Stoll BJ, Hansen NI, Bell EF, et al. Neonatal outcomes of extremely preterm infants from the NICHD Neonatal Research Network. Pediatrics. 2010;126:443-456.
13. Behrman R, Stith Butler A. Preterm birth: causes, consequences, and prevention/Committee on Understanding Premature Birth and Assuring Healthy Outcomes, Board on Health Sciences Policy. Washington, DC: The National Academies Press; 2007.
14. Doyle LW, Gultom E, Chuang SL, et al. Changing mortality and causes of death in infants 23-27 weeks' gestational age. J Paediatr Child Health. 1999;35:255-259.
15. Stoll BJ, Hansen N, Fanaroff AA, et al. Late-onset sepsis in very low birth weight neonates: the experience of the NICHD Neonatal Research Network. Pediatrics. 2002;110:285-291.
16. Ng PC, Li K, Wong RP, et al. Proinflammatory and anti-inflammatory cytokine responses in preterm infants with systemic infections. Arch Dis Child Fetal Neonatal Ed. 2003;88:F209-F213.

17. West CR, Groves AM, Williams CE, et al. Early low cardiac output is associated with compromised electroencephalographic activity in very preterm infants. Pediatr Res. 2006;59:610-615.
18. Kusaka T, Okubo K, Nagano K, et al. Cerebral distribution of cardiac output in newborn infants. Arch Dis Child Fetal Neonatal Ed. 2005;90:F77-F78.
19. Young RS, Hernandez MJ, Yagel SK. Selective reduction of blood flow to white matter during hypotension in newborn dogs: a possible mechanism of periventricular leukomalacia. Ann Neurol. 1982;12:445-448.
20. Volpe JJ. Neurobiology of periventricular leukomalacia in the premature infant. Pediatr Res. 2001;50:553-562.
21. Hunt RW, Evans N, Rieger I, et al. Low superior vena cava flow and neurodevelopment at 3 years in very preterm infants. J Pediatr. 2004;145:588-592.
22. Evans JR, Short BL, Van Meurs K, et al. Cardiovascular support in preterm infants. Clin Ther. 2006;28:1366-1384.
23. Jobe AH. The cardiopulmonary system: research and training opportunities. J Perinatol. 2006;26(suppl 2):S5-S7.
24. Short BL, Van Meurs K, Evans JR. Summary proceedings from the cardiology group on cardiovascular instability in preterm infants. Pediatrics. 2006;117:S34-S39.
25. Kluckow M. Low systemic blood flow and pathophysiology of the preterm transitional circulation. Early Hum Dev. 2005;81:429-437.
26. Osborn DA, Evans N, Kluckow M. Clinical detection of low upper body blood flow in very premature infants using blood pressure, capillary refill time, and central-peripheral temperature difference. Arch Dis Child Fetal Neonatal Ed. 2004;89:F168-F173.
27. Tyszczuk L, Meek J, Elwell C, et al. Cerebral blood flow is independent of mean arterial blood pressure in preterm infants undergoing intensive care. Pediatrics. 1998;102:337-341.
28. Groves AM, Kuschel CA, Knight DB, et al. The relationship between blood pressure and blood flow in newborn preterm infants. Arch Dis Child Fetal Neonatal Ed. 2008;93:F29-F32.
29. Kluckow M, Evans N. Relationship between blood pressure and cardiac output in preterm infants requiring mechanical ventilation. J Pediatr. 1996;129:506-512.
30. Evans N, Kluckow M. Early determinants of right and left ventricular output in ventilated preterm infants. Arch Dis Child Fetal Neonatal Ed. 1996;74:F88-F94.
31. Kluckow M, Evans N. Low superior vena cava flow and intraventricular haemorrhage in preterm infants. Arch Dis Child Fetal Neonatal Ed. 2000;82:F188-F194.
32. Kluckow M, Evans N. Superior vena cava flow in newborn infants: a novel marker of systemic blood flow. Arch Dis Child Fetal Neonatal Ed. 2000;82:F182-F187.
33. Kluckow M, Evans N. Low systemic blood flow and hyperkalemia in preterm infants. J Pediatr. 2001;139:227-232.
34. Evans N, Kluckow M, Simmons M, et al. Which to measure, systemic or organ blood flow? Middle cerebral artery and superior vena cava flow in very preterm infants. Arch Dis Child Fetal Neonatal Ed. 2002;87:F181-F184.
35. Osborn DA, Evans N, Kluckow M. Left ventricular contractility in extremely premature infants in the first day and response to inotropes. Pediatr Res. 2007;61:335-340.
36. Osborn DA, Evans N, Kluckow M, et al. Low superior vena cava flow and effect of inotropes on neurodevelopment to 3 years in preterm infants. Pediatrics. 2007;120:372-380.
37. Paradisis M, Evans N, Kluckow M, et al. Randomized trial of milrinone versus placebo for prevention of low systemic blood flow in very preterm infants. J Pediatr. 2009;154:189-195.
38. Kluckow M, Seri I, Evans N. Functional echocardiography: an emerging clinical tool for the neonatologist. J Pediatr. 2007;150:125-130.
39. Groves AM, Kuschel CA, Skinner JR. International perspectives: the neonatologist as an echocardiographer. Neoreviews. 2006;7:e391-e399.
40. Hruda J, Rothuis EG, van Elburg RM, et al. Echocardiographic assessment of preload conditions does not help at the neonatal intensive care unit. Am J Perinatol. 2003;20:297-303.
41. Lee LA, Kimball TR, Daniels SR, et al. Left ventricular mechanics in the preterm infant and their effect on the measurement of cardiac performance. J Pediatr. 1992;120:114-119.
42. Chew MS, Poelaert J. Accuracy and repeatability of pediatric cardiac output measurement using Doppler: 20-year review of the literature. Intens Care Med. 2003;29:1889-1894.
43. Groves AM, Kuschel CA, Knight DB, et al. Echocardiographic assessment of blood flow volume in the SVC and descending aorta in the newborn infant. Arch Dis Child Fetal Neonatal Ed. 2008;93:F24-F28.
44. Lee A, Liestol K, Nestaas E, et al. Superior vena cava flow: feasibility and reliability of the off-line analyses. Arch Dis Child Fetal Neonatal Ed. 2010;95:F121-F125.
45. Patel J, Marks K, Roberts I, et al. Measurement of cerebral blood flow in newborn infants using near infrared spectroscopy with indocyanine green. Pediatr Res. 1998;43:34-39.
46. Fanaroff JM, Wilson-Costello DE, Newman NS, et al. Treated hypotension is associated with neonatal morbidity and hearing loss in extremely low birth weight infants. Pediatrics. 2006;117:1131-1135.
47. Kuint J, Barak M, Morag I, et al. Early treated hypotension and outcome in very low birth weight infants. Neonatology. 2009;95:311-316.
48. Batton B, Zhu X, Fanaroff J, et al. Blood pressure, anti-hypotensive therapy, and neurodevelopment in extremely preterm infants. J Pediatr. 2009;154:351-357.
49. Dempsey EM, Al Hazzani F, Barrington KJ. Permissive hypotension in the extremely low birthweight infant with signs of good perfusion. Arch Dis Child Fetal Neonatal Ed. 2009;94:F241-F244.

50. Laughon M, Bose C, Allred E, et al. Factors associated with treatment for hypotension in extremely low gestational age newborns during the first postnatal week. Pediatrics. 2007;119:273-280.
51. Al-Aweel I, Pursley DM, Rubin LP, et al. Variations in prevalence of hypotension, hypertension, and vasopressor use in NICUs. J Perinatol. 2001;21:272-278.
52. Laughon M, Bose C, Clark R. Treatment strategies to prevent or close a patent ductus arteriosus in preterm infants and outcomes. J Perinatol. 2007;27:164-170.
53. McRobbie DW. MRI from picture to proton, 2nd ed. Cambridge, UK: Cambridge University Press; 2007:394.
54. Finn JP, Nael K, Deshpande V, et al. Cardiac MR imaging: state of the technology. Radiology. 2006; 241:338-354.
55. Constantine G, Shan K, Flamm SD, et al. Role of MRI in clinical cardiology. Lancet. 2004;363: 2162-2171.
56. Kilner PJ, Gatehouse PD, Firmin DN. Flow measurement by magnetic resonance: a unique asset worth optimising. J Cardiovasc Magn Reson. 2007;9:723-728.
57. Grothues F, Smith GC, Moon JC, et al. Comparison of interstudy reproducibility of cardiovascular magnetic resonance with two-dimensional echocardiography in normal subjects and in patients with heart failure or left ventricular hypertrophy. Am J Cardiol. 2002;90:29-34.
58. Groves AM, Chiesa G, Durighel G, et al. Functional cardiac MRI in preterm and term newborns. Arch Dis Child Fetal Neonatal Ed. 2011;96:F86-F91.
59. Foran AM, Fitzpatrick JA, Allsop J, et al. Three-tesla cardiac magnetic resonance imaging for preterm infants. Pediatrics. 2007;120:78-83.
60. Merchant N, Groves A, Larkman DJ, et al. A patient care system for early 3.0 Tesla magnetic resonance imaging of very low birth weight infants. Early Hum Dev. 2009;85:779-783.
61. Gutberlet M, Noeske R, Schwinge K, et al. Comprehensive cardiac magnetic resonance imaging at 3.0 Tesla: feasibility and implications for clinical applications. Invest Radiol. 2006;41:154-167.
62. Pujadas S, Reddy GP, Weber O, et al. MR imaging assessment of cardiac function. J Magn Reson Imaging. 2004;19:789-799.
63. Thiele H, Nagel E, Paetsch I, et al. Functional cardiac MR imaging with steady-state free precession (SSFP) significantly improves endocardial border delineation without contrast agents. J Magn Reson Imaging. 2001;14:362-367.
64. Odland HH, Brun H, Sejersted Y, et al. Longitudinal myocardial contribution to peak systolic flow and stroke volume in the neonatal heart. Pediatr Res. 2011;70(4):345-351.
65. Fogel MA. Assessment of cardiac function by magnetic resonance imaging. Pediatr Cardiol. 2000;21:59-69.
66. Varela M, Groves AM, Arichi T, et al. Mean cerebral blood flow measurements using phase contrast MRI in the first year of life. NMR Biomed 2011; In Press.
67. Benders MJ, Hendrikse J, De Vries LS, et al. Phase-contrast magnetic resonance angiography measurements of global cerebral blood flow in the neonate. Pediatr Res. 2011;69:544-547.
68. Markl M, Kilner PJ, Ebbers T. Comprehensive 4D velocity mapping of the heart and great vessels by cardiovascular magnetic resonance. J Cardiovasc Magn Reson. 2011;13:7.
69. Groves AM. Cardiac magnetic resonance in the study of neonatal haemodynamics. Semin Fetal Neonatal Med. 2011;16(1):36-41.
70. Groves AM, Durighel G, Tusor N, et al. Disruption of intracardiac flow patterns in the newborn infant. Pediatr Res. 2012; In Press.
71. Moore CC, McVeigh ER, Zerhouni EA. Quantitative tagged magnetic resonance imaging of the normal human left ventricle. Top Magn Reson Imaging. 2000;11:359-371.
72. Ibrahim el SH, Stuber M, Schar M, et al. Improved myocardial tagging contrast in cine balanced SSFP images. J Magn Reson Imaging. 2006;24:1159-1167.
73. Pan L, Prince JL, Lima JA, et al. Fast tracking of cardiac motion using 3D-HARP. IEEE Trans Biomed Eng. 2005;52:1425-1435.
74. Cho GY, Chan J, Leano R, et al. Comparison of two-dimensional speckle and tissue velocity based strain and validation with harmonic phase magnetic resonance imaging. Am J Cardiol. 2006;97:1661-1666.
75. Seri I. Circulatory support of the sick preterm infant. Semin Neonatol. 2001;6:85-95.
76. Toyono M, Harada K, Takahashi Y, et al. Maturational changes in left ventricular contractile state. Int J Cardiol. 1998;64:247-252.
77. Maeder M, Fehr T, Rickli H, et al. Sepsis-associated myocardial dysfunction: diagnostic and prognostic impact of cardiac troponins and natriuretic peptides. Chest. 2006;129:1349-1366.
78. Munro MJ, Walker AM, Barfield CP. Hypotensive extremely low birth weight infants have reduced cerebral blood flow. Pediatrics. 2004;114:1591-1596.
79. Report of the Second Working Group of the British Association of Perinatal Medicine. Guidelines for good practice in the management of neonatal respiratory distress syndrome. British Association of Perinatal Medicine; 1998.
80. Barrington KJ. Hypotension and shock in the preterm infant. Semin Fetal Neonatal Med. 2008;13:16-23.
81. Zhang J, Penny DJ, Kim NS, et al. Mechanisms of blood pressure increase induced by dopamine in hypotensive preterm neonates. Arch Dis Child Fetal Neonatal Ed. 1999;81:F99-F104.
82. Osborn D, Evans N, Kluckow M. Randomized trial of dobutamine versus dopamine in preterm infants with low systemic blood flow. J Pediatr. 2002;140:183-191.
83. Seri I, Tan R, Evans J. Cardiovascular effects of hydrocortisone in preterm infants with pressor-resistant hypotension. Pediatrics. 2001;107:1070-1074.

84. Shimada S, Kasai T, Hoshi A, et al. Cardiocirculatory effects of patent ductus arteriosus in extremely low-birth-weight infants with respiratory distress syndrome. Pediatr Int. 2003;45:255-262.

85. Evans N, Gournay V, Cabanas F, et al. Point-of-care ultrasound in the neonatal intensive care unit: international perspectives. Semin Fetal Neonatal Med. 2011;16:61-68.

86. Simpson JM, Miller O. Three-dimensional echocardiography in congenital heart disease. Arch Cardiovasc Dis. 2011;104:45-56.

87. Negrine RJS, Chikermane A, Wright JGC, et al. Measurement of myocardial velocities in preterm neonates using tissue Doppler imaging. Arch Dis Child Fetal Neonatal Ed. 2010 Oct 30. [Epub ahead of print; PMID: 21037287]

88. Nestaas E, Stoylen A, Sandvik L, et al. Feasibility and reliability of strain and strain rate measurement in neonates by optimizing the analysis parameters settings. Ultrasound Med Biol. 2007;33:270-278.

89. Nestaas E, Stoylen A, Brunvand L, et al. Tissue Doppler derived longitudinal strain and strain rate during the first 3 days of life in healthy term neonates. Pediatr Res. 2009;65:357-362.

90. Shellock FG, Crues JV. MR procedures: biologic effects, safety, and patient care. Radiology. 2004;232:635-652.

10

CHAPTER 11

Assessment of the Microcirculation in the Neonate

Ian M. R. Wright, MBBS, DCH, MRCP(Paeds)UK, FRACP,
Michael J. Stark, PhD, MRCP, and Vicki L. Clifton, PhD

Why Assess the Microcirculation?

The cardiorespiratory system is crucial in the perinatal adaptation of the human fetus to extra-uterine life. Most infants who die do so in the first few days of life and exhibit evidence of cardiovascular compromise. The cardiovascular system, as addressed in the other chapters in this book in detail, has a number of crucial components that affect the overall performance of the system, including the pump, the circulating volume, and the peripheral vasculature (Chapters 1, 5, and 12). It is being increasingly recognized, however, that a component of the latter, the microvasculature, represents a significant controller of the overall function and specifically that the microvasculature, as opposed to the macrovascular conductance vessels, is crucially important in the delivery of oxygen and nutrients to the tissues of the entire body. In addition, the flow within the microcirculation also reflects the combined action of the other, more central, components of the circulation and thus the endpoint of total cardiovascular efficiency.

So, what comprises the microvascular system? Current accepted definitions of the components of the microvasculature include, from proximal to distal, arterioles, capillaries, arteriolar-venular shunts, and venules.[1] In practice, this is all vascular tissue under 100 micrometers in diameter. Although lymphatic function is not discussed here, it can have significant influence on overall microvascular function, is known to be an active process, and has had little study in the neonatal population.[2] The microvasculature has regional and organ-specific specialization but also has global function and responses, thus representing one of the largest virtual "organs" in the body. As nearly all tissue needs to be in close proximity to a blood supply for oxygen and nutrient delivery, even the lens of the eye in the preterm neonate, the microvasculature reaches throughout the body.[3] It has been estimated that in an adult, the capillary component of the microvasculature alone covers in excess of 6000 m^2 in cross-sectional area. It is estimated that 5% of the circulating blood volume is in the capillaries at any time, but the capillary system has the ability to increase its capacity by 4-fold. Similar estimations have not been undertaken in the newborn but the fact that the baby is growing and has a less organized capillary network may mean it has an even greater proportional capacity.

Those involved with the care of the newborn are aware of the growth of the microvasculature in the context of the retina. Retinopathy of prematurity (ROP) remains a significant cause of blindness in the population born preterm, but its study has also allowed us to understand much more about the growth and development of the microvasculature during development. We know more about the role of the oxygenation level on vascular growth, understand that a number of factors, including but not restricted to vascular endothelial growth factor (VEGF) and the prorenin/angiotensin system, are responsible for the angiogenesis and pruning of the growing tree.[4-6] We do not often consider that the process of angiogenesis and vasculogenesis and its refinement are going on throughout the developing preterm infant. Therefore, understanding the effects, process, and outcomes within the microvasculature is important in understanding cardiovascular compromise at different gestational and postnatal ages and thus some of the long-term consequences of prematurity.

Studying and understanding the microcirculatory status are therefore extremely important to achieve a more complete understanding of the circulation in both clinical and experimental work with preterm or sick term newborns. This has led to the development and use of a number of methods for the assessment of the microcirculation, many of which have been applied to neonatal and perinatal subjects. This chapter reviews the sites and techniques that have been used, outlines current findings, and addresses the questions relevant to the understanding of the circulation in general and the microcirculation in particular in the preterm and sick term neonate.

Where to Study the Microcirculation in the Human Newborn?

Clearly, as the microcirculation is virtually ubiquitous throughout the body, the possibilities for observation and measurement are widespread. In the animal model, a number of the techniques have been used to assess flow in a selection of vascular beds, including laser Doppler flowmetry in skin, muscle, brain, liver, gastrointestinal tract, and kidneys, videomicroscopy in the microcirculation of the brain, skin, and gut blood flow measurement, as well as Xenon clearance techniques.[7-16] Techniques such as the use of microspheres or perfusate casts limited to animal work are reviewed elsewhere.[17] The noninvasive requirements for most human investigation, especially in neonates, have lead to more peripheral sites being targeted with different methods including heat conductance, skin temperature changes, laser Doppler, videomicroscopy, Xenon clearance, saturation oximetry, transcutaneous carbon dioxide measurement thermography, skin and muscle near-infrared spectroscopy (NIRS), sublingual videomicroscopy, direct videomicroscopic observation of red cell flux in the nail fold capillaries, cerebral NIRS, retinal videomicroscopy, static retinal photography, and scleral videomicroscopy.[18-36] These techniques have all been used to measure blood flow in neonates and have demonstrated changes during the transitional period in the few days after birth.

Of all these sites, clearly the skin is the main site in neonates that is easily accessible and therefore has received most attention. However, it has been questioned as to how representative the skin is of the microcirculation in general, especially since the skin has some very specialist microvascular functions, principally thermoregulation. Yet, the skin is also a part of the wider microcirculation. Thus, whereas skin blood flow represents a variety of adaptive responses, including local thermal response, it also represents a general aspect of the microcirculation.[37] Many of the signals that govern microvascular response are systemic and thus affect all vascular beds to some degree. This may be particularly the case in the first few days of postnatal life in the preterm infant, where the ability for adequate locally adaptive responses in the dermal circulation is impaired.[38] Moreover, even in adults, significant and generalizable systemic microvascular changes have been documented in highly specialized peripheral sites, such as the nail folds.[39]

Whilst many techniques have been used in the past, some are too invasive or extremely difficult in the nonsedated neonate.[40] Others are indirect measures, such as temperature, color, oxygen saturation or digital reperfusion changes and are unreliable.[41] Other useful and emerging techniques such as NIRS are discussed in detail in Chapters 7 and 8. Despite the huge variety of potential techniques, the microvascular literature is dominated by the use of laser Doppler flowmetry. Therefore the main techniques that are discussed in this chapter are laser Doppler and videomicroscopy. We focus on the skin microvascular flow but some discussion of the circulation in the retina is also included, as the retina is a significant area of interest, particularly in the context of vascular programming.

Laser Doppler Imaging

There are currently two systems utilizing the laser Doppler technique. This chapter focuses on laser Doppler flowmetry (LDF); however, laser Doppler imaging (LDI) can also be used and may prove of increasing value in the neonatal field.[42] An LDI instrument maps the cutaneous blood flow of a larger area than the LDF, as it uses a scanning laser beam over the area of interest compared to LDF which measures a small volume (~1 mm^3) only. This leads to increased reproducibility for LDI over LDF.[43] LDI is also noncontact in nature, so can be used in a wide variety of clinical situations wherein skin contact is not possible or desirable.[44] However, LDI gives only a "snapshot" of the perfusion, which makes it harder to study the dynamics of dilator or constrictor responses. LDF, with its constant measure of perfusion, is more useful to study the dynamic changes occurring in the microcirculation (Fig. 11-1).[43] This may change with the recent introduction of laser speckle contrast instruments showing an excellent reproducibility to assess skin microvascular reactivity.[45] However, the ability to perform dynamic measures and the relative low cost has led to LDF being the most generally used technique.

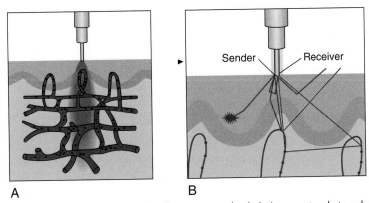

A   B

Figure 11-1 Principle of laser Doppler flowmetry method. **A,** Laser extends to subcapillary plexus. **B,** Principle of backscatter and Doppler shift is illustrated.[46]

B

Laser Doppler Flowmetry

Microvascular laser Doppler is the most established method of assessing the function of blood vessels of the peripheral microvasculature and skin tissues and has been used extensively in the newborn infant.[47,48] Laser Doppler flowmetry uses the Doppler shift of a low energy laser beam with a wavelength of 780 nm to quantify microvascular perfusion. The light is delivered to the tissue by a fiber-optic cable. In the tissue, the light is scattered by both stationary structures and moving blood cells. When scattered by the moving cells, the light frequency is shifted and the magnitude of the Doppler shift is proportional to the cell flux. The cell flux is defined as the product of the number and mean velocity of cells in the measuring volume of a few cubic millimeters. The output is picked up by fiber-optic receiving fibers in the same probe that delivered the original signal (see Fig. 11-1). After detection, the signal is processed and stored using proprietary software, which varies among the machines. Although directly proportional to tissue perfusion, laser Doppler measurements provide only a semiquantitative measure of blood flow expressed as arbitrary perfusion units (PU) of output voltage (1 PU = 10 mV) standardized by international agreement between manufacturers.[43,49,50] The difficulties with reproducibility seem to relate as much to the heterogeneous nature of the microvascular system as to the assessment method. When the recording site is standardized, the reproducibility of LDF is high, whereas when the recording site is varied, the technique shows poorer reproducibility.[51-53] Therefore the importance and clinical relevance of findings with laser Doppler rest with results being shown to be reproducible and across larger populations than in many other physiologic studies, and to be unaffected by other predictable modifiers such as changes in hematocrit.

The anatomy of the peripheral skin vascular bed is schematically drawn in Figure 11-2. Blood enters the skin through small arterioles, penetrating the subcutaneous tissue toward the skin surface. One artery often branches into several precapillary arterioles (30-80 µm), which pass into the venous plexuses that are organized parallel to the skin surface. Each arteriole can divide into eight to 10 capillary loops oriented perpendicular to the skin surface. In adults, one to three loops perfuse every skin papilla.[55] In neonates, however, this is much less organized and the arteriolar-venular anastomoses and the capillary loops are poorly developed with a less defined network. Formation of a more adult-type network occurs by approximately 4 months of age in the term newborn.[56] The preterm skin microcirculation may be even less well discriminated (Fig. 11-3).

Laser Doppler measurements from the skin surface thus measure flow, not only in the capillary loops, but also in most parts of the subpapillary plexus in children and adults. In the newborn, LDF measures the whole microcirculatory plexus and, therefore, should be less affected than in later age groups by thermoregulatory shunts and other adaptive capillary loop mechanisms.

Assessment of Skin Microcirculation Responses

LDF is a technique that has continued to develop over the past 20-30 years. Because of the limitations of LDF as a baseline measurement alone, active stimulations of the microvascular response to look at both endothelial and wider pathways have been studied. These stimuli include:

- Postocclusive hyperemia
- Thermal hyperemia
- Iontophoresis of vasoactive medication

Postocclusive Reactive Hyperemia

Postocclusive reactive hyperemia (PORH) is one of the methods used to assess microvascular reactivity with LDF. PORH is often used as a test of microvascular reactivity in conditions such as diabetes and has been linked to cardiovascular risk factors.[57-59] The test is performed by placing a sphygmomanometer cuff proximal to

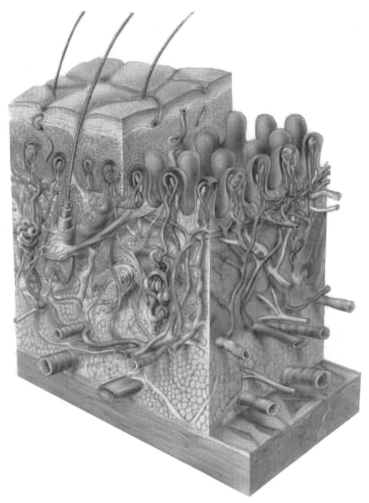

Figure 11-2 The microcirculation in adult skin. The vessel pattern is much less organized in the preterm neonate, with a 3-D network form, rather than these clearly defined capillary loops.[54] (See Expert Consult site for color image.)

an LDF probe placed on the neonate's limb. The cuff is then inflated to suprasystolic levels, holding for a designated length of time and then releasing the pressure as quickly as possible.[50] PORH presents with an increase in skin blood flow above baseline levels. This test is analogous to the tests assessing arterial flow-mediated vasodilation used to examine the adult macrovasculature and the phenomenon is thought to be mediated by the same endothelium-dependent pathways. There has been some debate about the length of the occlusion time required, balancing the need to obtain the best response with patient comfort and safety. While 3 minutes of occlusion time has been proposed as the best balance for adults, in the newborn only a 1-minute occlusion period is usually applied.[60]

The maximum increase in hyperemia-perfusion ($PORH_{max}$) is the most common derived variable from this test. Hyperemia-perfusion may be expressed as an absolute value, an increase above baseline, a percentage increase above baseline, or a percentage relative to baseline. In addition, the time to reach the maximum perfusion, the so-called time-to-peak (T_p) hyperemia, has been claimed to relate to the stiffness of the microvascular system.[50] While this latter is not currently widely used in the assessment of the neonate, it may be relevant to the long-term follow-up of premature infants and assessment of programming effects.[61]

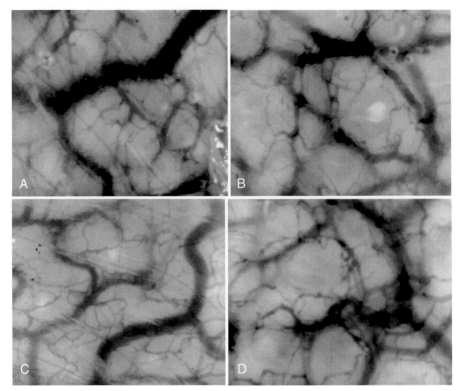

Figure 11-3 Stills taken from microvascular videos on infants showing developmental changes with increasing gestation. **A,** Male less than 28 weeks' gestation. **B,** Male at term. **C,** Female less than 28 weeks. **D,** Female at term. Note change from 3-D network to more planar structured plexus with maturity. All images acquired at 24 hours of postnatal age using Microscan (Amsterdam, The Netherlands) sidestream darkfield orthogonal polarized videomicroscope.

Local Thermal Hyperemia

Local thermal hyperemia is elicited by warming of the skin, which causes direct vasodilatation in the given area. Heating can be applied to the whole environment but in neonates it is usually applied to the area surrounding the LDF probe.[50] Several different thermostatically regulated probes are available and these LDF probes can be used both for ensuring a constant temperature at the site of the probe to reduce study variability as well as be used to elicit responses to thermal stimuli.[50,53] There are a number of different protocols used for this technique. In adults, applying a temperature change over a 20-minute period is the most common practice, but this is less suitable in the unstable preterm neonate and thus, for this patient population, shorter protocols have been evolved. These protocols often resemble the one described by Roustit and colleagues, with an initial rapid temperature increase to 40°C and then a sequential further increase to 44°C over a period of 5 minutes.[53] The maximum vasodilatation is then measured at the end of 1 minute at 44°C.

Two different mechanisms have been implicated in the response to thermal stimulation within the skin microvasculature. The initial response is mediated through the nociceptive nerve ending–dependent pathways and via neurogenic reflexes and locally released vasoactive substances such as calcitonin gene-related peptide and nitric oxide.[62] Interestingly, the involvement of this mechanism opens up the possibility of interaction of these assessments with assessment of pain in the newborn, an area of much current interest. On the other hand, the subsequent increase in microvascular blood flow over a longer period of time and/or at higher temperatures is likely to be mediated through the more classic endothelium-dependent nitric oxide pathways.[63]

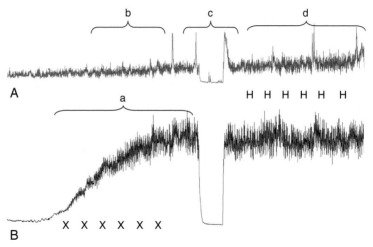

Figure 11-4   An example of LDF trace. Laser Doppler flowmetry trace acquired using Periflux 5000 system, Periont iontophoresis system, and Perisoft software (Perimed AB, Järfälla Sweden). Trace A is from a standard heated small angled probe; trace B is a simultaneous tracing from a larger heated iontophoresis probe. Section a demonstrates Ach iontophoresis response (X represents iontophoretic dose applied); section b, baseline trace; section c, occlusion and reperfusion; section d, thermal response (poor in this subject); (H represents surface temperature increments at skin surface; max 44°C).

Iontophoresis

Iontophoresis is the introduction of ions of soluble salts into the tissues of the body using a small direct electrical current. Clinically it is known most to pediatricians when used to drive in pilocarpine for sweat-testing in patients with suspected cystic fibrosis. However, it has been extensively investigated as a mode of drug delivery and it may be used to drive a whole variety of variously charged, soluble molecules into the skin; including a whole variety of vasoactive molecules and hormonal moderators of vascular control.[64,65] Acetylcholine (ACh) is the standard transdermal drug used in assessment of the microvasculature as a classic paradigm-test of selective endothelium-dependent vasodilators with relaxation dependent on non–nitric oxide, nonprostanoid endothelium-dependent hyperpolarization.[66,67]

Iontophoresis has been used with the LDI systems, where a patch of skin can be tested. However it is used more commonly with the LDF systems, where an iontophoresis laser Doppler probe may allow real-time monitoring of the physiological response, as illustrated in Figure 11-4.

Microvasculature of the Preterm Neonate Studied by LDF

Peripheral microvascular blood flow is subject to considerable changes during the first days of postnatal life, a period of marked circulatory vulnerability especially in preterm infants. Myogenic and neural control of skin blood flow must be rapidly established during this period to allow appropriate thermoregulation to take place.[68] There is an increasing body of recent work demonstrating the relationship between peripheral microvascular blood flow and measures of neonatal physiologic and cardiovascular stability in preterm infants during the immediate posttransitional period.

Previously published literature on baseline peripheral cutaneous blood flow was conflicting. Some authors found no influence of postmenstrual age on blood flow.[69] Other investigators reported an inverse relationship between baseline blood flow and increasing postmenstrual age, whereas a few reported a higher baseline flow with increasing postmenstrual age.[29,70-72] The apparent lack of consensus most likely reflected methodological differences, with different timing and methods used and patient groups included. However, using LDF and transcutaneous PO_2 methods in healthy term neonates during the first few days of life baseline skin blood flow had been shown to decrease.[73-75]

Interestingly, findings of recent studies suggest a different pattern of skin blood flow changes in the immediate postnatal period. Using heated probes, these studies take into account the thermal conditions and utilize standardized postfeeding timing for the assessment. For instance, in a large cohort of normal term infants, the authors' group has shown that changes in skin microvascular blood flow show a gender-specific dimorphic response during the first 24 hours after delivery with no further changes occurring after the first postnatal day.[76] Male infants demonstrate a significant increase in baseline blood flow from 6 to 24 hours after delivery, while female infants show no change in their peripheral baseline microvascular blood flow during this period. As a result of these different patterns, female infants have lower peripheral baseline microvascular blood flow at 24 hours of age compared to their male counterparts.[76]

Previous studies of neonatal microvascular adaptation have reported significant changes both with gestational and postnatal age. Gestational age has been described to have a variable influence on microvascular function with blood flow reported to decrease, increase, and remain unchanged with increasing gestational age.[77-79]

Although clinical observations support an important role for alterations in microvascular function in the pathologic events associated with septicemia and polycythemia, it is the process of cardiovascular adaptation following birth preterm that is perhaps the greatest interest.[80,81] Given the fact that most preterm infants that are going to die do so in the first 72 hours following delivery, it is the influence of the short-term adaptation in microvascular blood flow that is potentially of the most importance and clinical relevance.[82]

Indeed, there is evidence that the changes in early microvascular flow are of clinical significance. Despite evidence from the animal literature and observational data in human neonates, the relationships between peripheral microvascular blood flow and measures of neonatal physiologic and cardiovascular stability in the immediate postnatal period had not been characterized until recently.[83] The authors' group studied the relationship between LDF-derived basal peripheral microvascular blood flow, clinical illness severity, and measures of cardiovascular function in the preterm neonate.[84] The findings of this study showed for the first time that LDF measurements of microvascular blood flow in premature infants exhibited significant relationships with both clinical illness severity (Fig. 11-5A) and concomitant measures of cardiovascular function, in particular blood pressure (Fig. 11-5B).

These studies led to further explorations as to what the nature of these associations was and whether there could be further detail to strengthen the association. The questions specifically addressed have included whether these associations between peripheral skin blood flow and disease severity and certain hemodynamic parameters in the most immature infants are stronger than in those at lesser risk, and whether there is also a gender-specific difference in the microvascular findings as males are 1.6-2 times more likely to die during the first 48-72 hours than females.

Gestation Differences

Studies on a large cohort of premature infants revealed a significant inverse relationship between LDF-measured baseline microvascular blood flow at 24 and 72 hours of age and gestational age (Fig. 11-6).[85]

This relationship is further complicated by the demonstration of a close interaction of gestational age and gender of the infant (see later), although some parameters still appear to be related to gestational age alone. Interestingly, the effect of thermal stimulation was most marked in the more immature infants. This finding fits with previous work showing little response to thermal stimulation per se in the term newborn but is unlike the earlier studies, which demonstrated no difference in skin vasodilatation to local thermal stimulation between preterm and term infants.[75,86,87] Of note is that the previous studies only looked at infants born after 30 weeks'

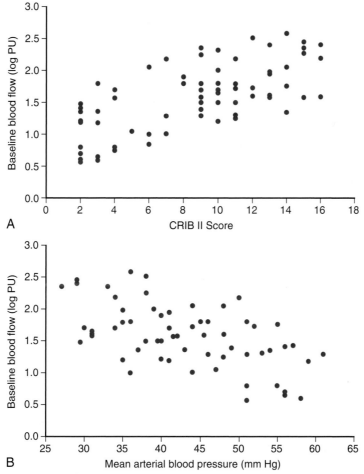

Figure 11-5   **A,** Relationship between baseline microvascular blood flow (log PU) at 24 hours of age and clinical illness severity determined by the CRIB-II score in infants of ≤ 32 weeks' gestation (n = 74); r^2 = 0.442; P < .001, multiple linear regression controlling for gestational age. **B,** Relationship between baseline microvascular blood flow (log PU) at 24 hours of age and mean arterial blood pressure (mm Hg); r^2 = −0.563, P < .001, multiple linear regression controlling for gestational age. See text for details. (From Stark MJ, Clifton VL, Wright IMR. Microvascular flow, clinical illness severity and cardiovascular function in the preterm infant. Arch Dis Child Fetal Neonatal Ed 2008;93(4):F271-F274, with permission.)

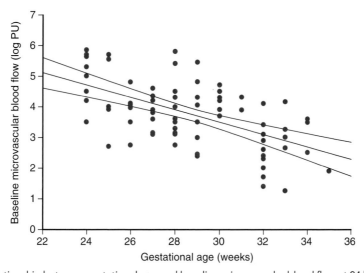

Figure 11-6   Relationship between gestational age and baseline microvascular blood flow at 24 hours of postnatal age for all infants of 24-36 weeks' gestational age (r = 0.624; P < .001, Spearman r). PU, laser Doppler perfusion units. See text for details. (From Stark MJ, Clifton VL, Wright IMR. Sex-specific differences in peripheral microvascular blood flow in preterm infants. Pediatr Res 2008;63:415-419, with permission.)

gestation or studied the subjects at the end of the first postnatal week of life.[86,87] More recent studies using different methods than LDF to investigate the changes in microvascular blood flow support the observations by Stark and colleagues as they show a thermal response in the preterm neonate as well.[85,88] Given the fact that we use data obtained largely before the widespread use of humidity to drive our incubator settings, it is possible that some of the vasodilatory effects of local thermal stimulation described more recently may be, at least in part, iatrogenic. However, no studies using thermal interventions have been performed to counter the demonstrated microvascular vasodilation.

Peripheral Microvascular Blood Flow and Neonatal Gender

Gender-related differences in respiratory and circulatory parameters have been observed following preterm birth with male gender being associated with higher morbidity and mortality.[89-92] As for morbidities, the need for cardiovascular support and the incidence of vasopressor-resistant hypotension have been demonstrated to be significantly higher in extremely preterm male infants during the first postnatal day.[90] Therefore abnormal regulation of peripheral microvascular blood flow resulting in vasodilation and decreased peripheral vascular resistance may contribute to the development of circulatory compromise following preterm birth (Chapters 1 and 12). Previous attempts to link clinical assessment of skin perfusion and early circulatory compromise had not excluded any gender-specific effect. Another study by the authors' group has investigated gender-specific differences in basal peripheral microvascular blood flow and the functional ability of the microvasculature to respond to vasoactive stimuli in preterm infants in the immediate newborn period and showed a significantly higher baseline flow in male than female infants, with the effect increasing with decreasing gestation.[93] The dimorphic response was lost by 72 hours. When the response to ACh delivered by iontophoresis at 24 hours of age was tested, the most immature infants (24-28 weeks' gestation), showed a significant ability to vasodilate above their already increased baseline flow. However, this effect was again limited to males. These gender-specific differences in microvascular function occur at a time of circulatory transition to the extrauterine environment and thus may influence the transitional circulation and contribute to the hypotension and low systemic blood flow most commonly recognized in the first postnatal day.[94] The underlying mechanisms resulting in this gender-specific dimorphic pattern of microvascular function have not been fully elucidated and are discussed further later.

Before moving on to consider the potential mechanisms involved in the regulation of peripheral blood flow during transition, we consider a specific disease state where similar dimorphic differences have been demonstrated in the microvasculature of both the infant and the mother. Recent studies using LDF of neonates born to mothers with mild-to-moderate late-gestation preeclampsia demonstrate significant differences compared to normal controls during the first 72 postnatal hours. Again the nature of this response is dimorphic; in term neonates born after preeclamptic pregnancy, female infants exhibit similar baseline microvascular blood flow at 6 hours of age to females of normotensive mothers followed by significantly greater microvascular blood flow at 24 and 72 hours. Conversely, male infants do not demonstrate a temporal change in blood flow in the presence of preeclampsia but were significantly more vasodilated than males of non-preeclamptic mothers at 6 hours of age.[76]

The transient nature of these findings supports differences in production or response to vasoactive mediators and/or neural control as opposed to structural differences being responsible. However, the underlying mechanisms have not been fully elucidated and warrant further investigation. Interestingly, these findings might lend support to the theory that the evolutionary reason for the persistence of preeclampsia is to sustain brain growth in the presence of restriction of placental blood supply and that the male and female fetus have different strategies to preserve growth and development.[95,96] This speculation might be further supported by available evidence that the male and female fetus have different effects on the maternal circulation. Indeed, studies using LDF in women have shown different microvascular responses depending on the sex of their fetus. The increased microvascular constriction, and lack of response to the vasodilator corticotropin releasing hormone seen in the mothers with a male fetus may support the view that, in the presence of placental compromise, there is an attempt by the male to improve the uteroplacental nutritional supply needed to support the maintained or, even increased, growth seen in late-gestation male fetuses of preeclamptic mothers.[97]

This series of studies shows developmental changes in peripheral microvascular blood flow and the relationship between microvascular blood flow and gestation, gender, clinical illness severity, and disease state. Thus, deviations in microcirculatory function might contribute to cardiovascular maladaptation in early neonatal life. Cardiovascular maladaptation and the resultant hypotension and low systemic and organ blood flow are common problems in the preterm infant, yet there is little clinical, outcome-based evidence showing improvement in short- or long-term morbidity and mortality in response to commonly used treatments (see also Chapters 1, 12, and 16). Therefore the importance of understanding the potential mechanisms of the response of the microvasculature to cardiovascular adaptation after preterm birth is of clinical relevance and warrants further investigation.[98]

Mechanisms of Preterm Microvascular Control

As with the microvasculature in any other situation, the basic control is reliant on a complex interplay of many different and often redundant mechanisms (for review, see reference 99). Broadly there are local controls acting either dependently or independently of the endothelium, and sympathetic, parasympathetic, and other nerve ending–related controls. There is no evidence that any of these mechanisms is absent in the preterm infant but the relative contribution and interplay among them is not well understood. A detailed discussion of these mechanisms and their interaction is beyond the scope of this chapter. Therefore, in the context of the observations described earlier, we focus on a group of vasodilators, the so-called gasotransmitters, as well as the most important vasoconstrictor mechanisms regulating microcirculation.

Vasodilators Regulating Microvascular Tone

The gasotransmitters represent small, freely permeable gas molecules produced in the vasculature throughout the body that have specific pathways of action to modulate, among others, microvascular control. The best characterized such molecule is nitric oxide (NO), produced from arginine by the action of nitric oxide synthase (NOS) in the endothelium. Via its second messenger, guanosine 3,5-cyclic monophosphate (cGMP), NO mediates vascular smooth muscle relaxation and thus plays an active role in the regulation of blood pressure in preterm and term infants.[100]

In preterm infants with respiratory distress syndrome (RDS), however, increased cGMP levels are present in the absence of upregulation of the NO pathway demonstrating the role of other cGMP-generating pathways in this high-risk population.[100,101] Indeed, carbon monoxide (CO)-mediated increases in cGMP have been demonstrated to also play a significant role in the regulation of blood pressure and cardiac function in both physiologic and pathologic conditions and have been proposed to contribute to low blood pressure in mechanically ventilated infants with RDS.[102,103]

Another currently accepted gasotransmitter is hydrogen sulfide (H_2S). Hydrogen sulfide, produced by two enzymes (cystathione gamma-lyase and cystathione beta-synthase) acts via a variety of cGMP independent smooth muscle pathways.[104,105] What little is known about this gasotransmitter in the context of the neonatal cardiovascular system is also discussed briefly.

B

Nitric Oxide

While NO has been shown to be of importance in sick preterm infants with RDS, a recent study by the authors' group suggests that NO is not as important in modulating peripheral blood flow during the first few postnatal days. According to the findings of this study, the urinary concentration of metabolites of NO does not suggest that NO becomes a significant contributor to the pattern of changes of microvascular blood flow described in sicker, more immature and male infants until after the first three postnatal days. This finding is similar to that of Krediet and colleagues, who examined NO production in preterm infants with and without RDS during the first postnatal week.[100] Taken together, these findings suggest that increased NO synthesis occurring after upregulation of the calcium-dependent, constitutive NOS may be an important regulator of baseline vascular tone after the first few postnatal days and that other mechanisms, such as the CO pathway, might be influencing peripheral vascular homeostasis in preterm neonates during the transitional period.

Carbon Monoxide

Approximately 85% of endogenous CO production can be ascribed to heme metabolism via the inducible heme-oxygenase (HO), also called heat-shock protein-32. Endogenous CO production is increased by oxidative stress and inflammation, known associations of poor outcome in the preterm neonate.[106,107] Carbon monoxide-induced vasorelaxation is endothelium independent, is not a consequence of tissue hypoxia, and is independent of any adrenergic effects. Carbon monoxide binds competitively to hemoglobin, in preference to oxygen, to form carboxyhemoglobin representing an in vivo "CO sink." Carboxyhemoglobin levels are elevated significantly during stress, sepsis, and shock in both adult and pediatric patients.[108,109] In preterm infants, CO-mediated upregulation of plasma cGMP levels has been proposed to result in increased vasodilation of the systemic vascular bed and increased CO levels are associated with hypotension and, via the augmented production of cGMP, have been implicated in the pathophysiologic processes of peri/intraventricular hemorrhage.[103,110] In addition, CO has been demonstrated to also decrease vascular tone by blocking the cytochrome P450-mediated production of the vasoconstrictor endothelin-1 (ET-1) and mediate vascular relaxation through the activation of potassium channels in a tissue-dependent manner.[111,112] These findings indicate that different signaling pathways mediate vasodilation induced by CO and that the relative contributions of these pathways depend on the vascular site. The effects of developmental factors on pathway expression remain largely unstudied.

In a recent study by the authors' group, arterial carboxyhemoglobin levels showed gestational age- and gender-specific differences during the first few postnatal days, as they were higher in boys and in the most immature infants.[113] In addition, a significant relationship between carboxyhemoglobin levels and microvascular perfusion was observed. These findings suggest that gender-specific differences in CO production in preterm infants in the immediate newborn period might contribute to the greater incidence of hemodynamic instability caused by dysregulated microvascular tone in male infants (Fig. 11-7). Finally, the authors also found that elevated carboxyhemoglobin levels at 72 hours of postnatal life were predictive of death during the first postnatal week (Fig. 11-8).

The underlying pathophysiologic processes that lead to ongoing elevated CO production in preterm neonates are yet to be fully elucidated. However, if CO-mediated increases in microvascular blood flow were indeed in the causal pathway for increased neonatal morbidity and mortality, a number of potential novel therapeutic approaches might become available.[114]

Hydrogen Sulfide

Hydrogen sulfide (H_2S) is the newest of the accepted gasotransmitters. Like NO, H_2S has suggested roles in many processes ranging from inflammatory response through to neural control. In this section, we focus only on its role in the control of the microvasculature and peripheral blood flow. Again, analogous to the production of NO, H_2S is largely produced from a freely available amino acid, cysteine, by enzyme

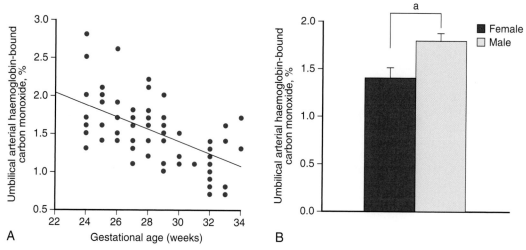

Figure 11-7 **A,** Correlation between umbilical arterial carboxyhemoglobin levels and gestational age for infants born between 24 and 34 weeks' gestation (r = 0.636; n = 66; *P* < .0001). **B,** Umbilical arterial carboxyhemoglobin levels in male and female infants. *P* < .032. See text for details. (From Stark MJ, Clifton VL, Wright IMR. Carbon monoxide is a significant mediator of cardiovascular status following preterm birth. Pediatrics 2009;124:277-284, with permission.)

systems that are demonstrably present in the endothelium of arteries and arterioles. As with NO, H_2S is only present for very short periods before it is converted to more stable and probably less active compounds and so is expected to exert most of its action locally. Hydrogen sulfide acts on vascular smooth muscle and causes vasodilatation via a number of specific pathways including the K_{ATP}–associated calcium channels.[105] Increased H_2S has been demonstrated in a number of disease states but there are almost no data in the human newborn.[115,116] Recent work has shown that H_2S also plays a role in the placental circulation suggesting that these pathways are active in gestational tissues.[117] We have recently demonstrated that the primary stable

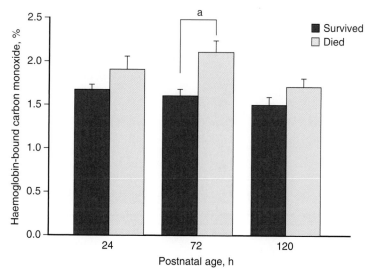

Figure 11-8 Arterial carboxyhemoglobin levels at 24, 72, and 120 hours of age in infants who survived and those who died in the first week of life after birth at gestational age of 24-34 weeks. *P* < .035. See text for details. (From Stark MJ, Clifton VL, Wright IMR. Carbon monoxide is a significant mediator of cardiovascular status following preterm birth. Pediatrics 2009;124:277-284, with permission.)

metabolite of total body H$_2$S production, urinary thiosulfate, is detectable in human newborns and is increased in neonates with lower gestation and higher microvascular flow (unpublished data). Clearly there are multiple redundant pathways modulating microvascular dilatation of which CO and H$_2$S are merely some. The different pathways that can control these effectors, their balance and their interaction remain a field of active research.

Vasoconstrictors Regulating Microvascular Tone

Homeostasis of vascular tone requires a finely regulated balance between vasodilatation and constriction. As discussed earlier, a number of vasodilators are increased with prematurity and in a gender-specific manner. The next question to be addressed is whether similar gestational and gender-specific differences exist in endogenously produced vasoconstrictors acting upon the microvasculature of the neonate.

The endogenous catecholamine, norepinephrine and the endothelially derived endothelin-1 (ET-1) are the most powerful vasoconstrictors known to be influenced by gestational age and their production and activity are altered in the pathophysiologic processes associated with prematurity.[118,119] Circulating epinephrine produced primarily by the adrenal medulla and norepinephrine, released mainly from networks of sympathetic nerves that enmesh blood vessels, especially arterioles, are the main sympathetic neurotransmitters regulating the cardiovascular system during transition and beyond.[118] Peripheral vascular resistance has previously been shown to correlate with the degree of sympatho-adrenal activation at birth.[120] Endothelin-1 is a potent vasoconstrictor also promoting the release of other downstream endothelium-dependent factors acting on the vascular smooth muscle.[121]

In recent studies both of these vasoconstrictors were found to have an altered pattern consistent with the balance of the endogenous vasodilators.[122] Normetanephrine (the primary urinary metabolite of norepinephrine) is increased in line with factors associated with good neonatal outcomes and with decreased baseline microvascular flow (Fig. 11-9). In this study, a complex interaction among endothelin, gender and time since administration of antenatal steroids was also demonstrated.[122] Many of the proposed mechanisms of the influence of gender upon outcomes of both microvascular control and of the risk of neonatal mortality involve the steroid pathways. Indeed, some recent data suggest that fetal steroid exposure and the

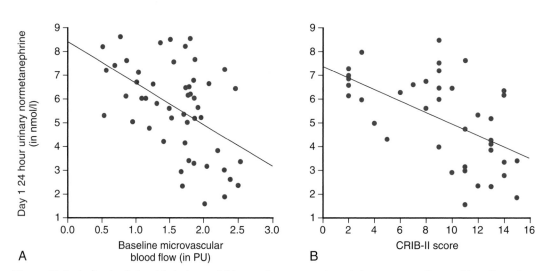

Figure 11-9   Indirect relationship between 24-hour urinary normetanephrine concentration and baseline microvascular tone **(A)** and CRIB-II score **(B)**. Normetanephrine is the primary urinary metabolite of norepinephrine. CRIB, clinical risk index for babies; PU, laser Doppler perfusion units. See text for details. (From Stark MJ, Hodyl NA, Wright IMR, Clifton V. The influence of sex and antenatal betamethasone exposure on vasoconstrictors and the preterm microvasculature. J Matern Fetal Neonatal Med 2011;24(10):1215-1220, with permission.)

related placental control by 11-beta-hydroxysteroid-dehydrogenase-2 may be significant factors.[123]

Most importantly, these systemic measures of both vasodilators and constrictors suggest a balance tipping in accordance with both known risk factors (gestation, gender, CRIB-II score) and with measured microvascular flow. This strongly supports that the microvascular flow in the skin is indeed reflective of overall microvascular tone. Some consideration, however, needs to be given to the nature of the increased flow and the interaction of the increased peripheral microvascular flow with central measures of cardiovascular function in the newborn (Chapter 1).

Videomicroscopy

Among the major forms of cardiovascular shock (Chapters 1 and 12), techniques assessing peripheral blood flow such as LDF may identify the presence of maldistributive of shock.[124] In maldistributive shock, high blood flow may be recorded in shunting vessels while there may actually be low blood flow in the nutritive components of the microvasculature. This clinical scenario is thus associated with high LDF blood flow and anaerobic metabolism and lactic acid accumulation. The potential for different growth patterns leading to different risks for maldistributive shock in the developing microvasculature is largely unstudied. Studies on lactic acid levels in premature babies have been inconclusive and our studies have also not shown any clear pattern of association of lactate with measured baseline microvascular flow.[125] Recent studies looking at blood flow distribution within the microvasculature have used sidestream darkfield orthogonal polarized light (SDOPL) videomicroscopy. Studies in babies with increased neonatal inflammatory markers, but without proven infection, have demonstrated increased flow with SDOPL videomicroscopy but blood flow distribution was not documented.[126] Our group has shown the structural maturation that could underlie different developmental risks for maldistribution (Fig. 11-3) but definitive studies are still underway. Another explanation for the apparent discrepancy between early low, centrally demonstrated, flow measures and high microvascular flow at 24 hours would be the temporal change with a period of low systemic perfusion followed by reperfusion.[127] Our recent human and animal data suggest, though, that this is not a significant effect.[128] Finally, another distributive scenario may contribute to this paradox. It is possible that a significant component to the increased microvascular flow may actually be on the venular side. This would lead to an apparent increase in flow by LDF assessment but with an accompanying significant increase in capacitance. Such an effect could decrease preload with associated decreased cardiac output.[129] Further videomicroscopic studies, in combination with direct cardiac output and blood pressure measurements (Chapters 1 and 6), may contribute to the clarification of this latter possibility.

Retinography and Cardiovascular Programming

In this chapter, we have focused so far on microvascular flow and its interaction with other hemodynamic measures and clinically relevant risk factors in the premature infant during the first few postnatal days. In most studies, microvascular differences between at risk groups and those at lesser risk are no longer evident by one week of age. However, there are concerns that the effects of the fetal and neonatal periods may have much longer lasting repercussions. The developmental origin of the health and disease model has demonstrated that early influences not only produce local and short-term effects but also long-term programming conditions.[130] Recent data suggest that some of the outcomes may be mediated by changes in the function of the microvasculature. The ARIC study demonstrated, using digital retinal photography (retinography), that microvascular changes were more common in a group of individuals who went on to develop metabolic disease, significantly before they developed changes in blood pressure or had metabolic changes.[131] Further studies have since shown microvascular changes at the age of 6-9 years, suggesting that these microvascular changes are markers, or even causal components, of the processes leading to the major health threats to our current society: obesity, hypertension, and diabetes.[132,133] Infants who have been born prematurely are at greater risk of developing hypertension and this is most marked in females.[134] It may be that those factors that protect girls from the adverse effects of microvascular dilatation in the first few days of postnatal life increase their later risks. Further cohort studies of infants using videomicroscopy and retinography may help to clarify this.

Future Applications in Neonatal Medicine

Apart from the potential to predict future metabolic and cardiovascular trajectory, what other future developments are likely to be seen in the area of microvascular physiology in the neonate? The establishment and clarification of novel mechanisms, such as the role and mechanism of action of newer gasotransmitters, have the potential for new treatments to influence these pathways. Further studies need to be undertaken to understand the specific microvascular effects of our current, less than ideal, treatment strategies and thus be able to factor the microvascular status and response into their use. Finally the development and understanding of easy, reliable measures of the status and function of the microvasculature, at both a clinical and research level, are likely to occur.

Conclusion

In this chapter we have discussed some of the tools and techniques necessary to understand more about the microvasculature in the newborn, specifically the preterm human infant. There is a significant pattern, in the first few days of postnatal life, of increased microvascular flow in premature infants with poorer outcome; specifically in those with male gender, earlier gestations and higher predictive clinical severity scores. We have demonstrated that this appears to be a systemic effect, associated with known vasomediators and have discussed the potential role of newer members of the vasomediator family, such as carbon monoxide and hydrogen sulfide. It is clear that much more work needs to be done, both to understand the microvascular function and effects, their hormonal modulators, their antecedents, and long-term consequences. Importantly, current and future studies should endeavor to include studying the physiology and pathophysiology of the microvasculature into research of the cardiovascular system of the newborn.

References

1. Guyton AC, Hall JE. The microcirculation and the lymphatic system: capillary fluid exchange, interstitial fluid, and lymph flow. In: Textbook of medical physiology. Philadelphia: WB Saunders/Elsevier; 2000:162-174.
2. Von der Weid PY, Rahman M, Imtiaz MS, et al. Spontaneous transient depolarizations in lymphatic vessels of the guinea pig mesentery: pharmacology and implication for spontaneous contractility. Am J Physiol Heart Circ Physiol. 2008;295(5):H1989-H2000.
3. Skapinker R, Rothberg AD. Postnatal regression of the tunica vasculosa lentis. J Perinatol. 1987;7(4):279-281.
4. McGregor ML, Bremer DL, Cole C, et al. HOPE-ROP Multicenter Group. High Oxygen Percentage in Retinopathy of Prematurity study. Retinopathy of prematurity outcome in infants with prethreshold retinopathy of prematurity and oxygen saturation >94% in room air: the high oxygen percentage in retinopathy of prematurity study. Pediatrics. 2002;110(3):540-544.
5. Rajappa M, Saxena P, Kaur J. Ocular angiogenesis: mechanisms and recent advances in therapy. Adv Clin Chem. 2010;50:103-121.
6. Wilkinson-Berka JL, Miller AG, Binger KJ. Prorenin and the (pro)renin receptor: recent advances and implications for retinal development and disease. Curr Opin Nephrol Hypertens. 2011;20(1):69-76.
7. Dyson RM, Palliser HK, Kelleher MA, et al. The guinea pig as an animal model for studying perinatal changes in microvascular function. Pediatr Res. 2012;71:20-24.
8. Newman JM, Dwyer RM, St-Pierre P, et al. Decreased microvascular vasomotion and myogenic response in rat skeletal muscle in association with acute insulin resistance. J Physiol. 2009;587(Pt 11):2579-2588.
9. Wauschkuhn CA, Witte K, Gorbey S, et al. Circadian periodicity of cerebral blood flow revealed by laser-Doppler flowmetry in awake rats: relation to blood pressure and activity. Am J Physiol Heart Circ Physiol. 2005;289(4):H1662-H1668.

10. Abu-Amara M, Yang SY, Quaglia A, et al. Effect of remote ischemic preconditioning on liver ischemia/reperfusion injury using a new mouse model. Liver Transpl. 2011;17(1):70-82.
11. Krouzecky A, Matejovic M, Radej J, et al. Perfusion pressure manipulation in porcine sepsis: effects on intestinal hemodynamics. Physiol Res. 2006;55(5):527-533.
12. Hammad FT, Davis G, Zhang XY, et al. Intra- and post-operative assessment of renal cortical perfusion by laser Doppler flowmetry in renal transplantation in the rat. Eur Surg Res. 2000;32(5): 284-288.
13. Taccone FS, Su F, Pierrakos C, et al. Cerebral microcirculation is impaired during sepsis: an experimental study. Crit Care. 2010;14(4):R140.
14. Treu CM, Lupi O, Bottino DA, et al. Sidestream dark field imaging. the evolution of real-time visualization of cutaneous microcirculation and its potential application in dermatology. Arch Dermatol Res. 2011;303(2):69-78.
15. Daudel F, Freise H, Westphal M, et al. Continuous thoracic epidural anesthesia improves gut mucosal microcirculation in rats with sepsis. Shock. 2007;28(5):610-614.
16. Hughes S, Brain S, Williams G, et al. Assessment of blood flow changes at multiple sites in rabbit skin using a 133Xenon clearance technique. J Pharmacol Toxicol Methods. 1994;32(1): 41-47.
17. Glenny RW, Bernard S, Brinkley M. Validation of fluorescent-labeled microspheres for measurement of regional organ perfusion. J Appl Physiol. 1993;74:2585-2597.
18. de Boode WP. Clinical monitoring of systemic hemodynamics in critically ill newborns. Early Hum Dev. 2010;86(3):137-141.
19. Brück K, Brück M, Lentis H. Temperature regulation in the newborn infant. Biol Neonate. 1961;3:65-119.
20. Oh W, Lind J. Body temperature of the newborn infant in relation to placenta infusion. Acta Paediatr Scand. 1967;172(suppl):137-145.
21. Strömberg B, Oberg PA, Sedin G. Transepidermal water loss in newborn infants. X. Effects of central cold-stimulation on evaporation rate and skin blood flow. Acta Paediatr Scand. 1983;72(5): 735-739.
22. Genzel-Boroviczény O, Christ F, Glas V. Blood transfusion increases functional capillary density in the skin of anemic preterm infants. Pediatr Res. 2004;56(5):751-755.
23. Wellhöner P, Rolle D, Lönnroth P, et al. Laser-Doppler flowmetry reveals rapid perfusion changes in adipose tissue of lean and obese females. Am J Physiol Endocrinol Metab. 2006;291(5): E1025-E1030.
24. Benaron DA, Parachikov IH, Friedland S, et al. Continuous, noninvasive, and localized microvascular tissue oximetry using visible light spectroscopy. Anesthesiology. 2004;100(6):1469-1475.
25. Vallée F, Mateo J, Dubreuil G, et al. Cutaneous ear lobe Pco_2 at 37°C to evaluate microperfusion in patients with septic shock. Chest. 2010;138(5):1062-1070.
26. Merla A, Di Romualdo S, Di Donato L, et al. Combined thermal and laser Doppler imaging in the assessment of cutaneous tissue perfusion. Conf Proc IEEE Eng Med Biol Soc. 2007;2007: 2630-2633.
27. De Felice C, Latini G, Vacca P, et al. The pulse oximeter perfusion index as a predictor for high illness severity in neonates. Eur J Pediatr. 2002;161:561-562.
28. Pellicer A, Bravo MC. Near-infrared spectroscopy. A methodology-focused review. Semin Fetal Neonatal Med. 2011;16(1):42-49.
29. Wu PYK, Wong WH, Guerra G. Peripheral blood flow in the neonate. Changes in total, skin, and muscle blood flow with gestational and postnatal age. Pediatr Res. 1980;14:1374-1378.
30. Top AP, Ince C, Schouwenberg PH, et al. Inhaled nitric oxide improves systemic microcirculation in infants with hypoxemic respiratory failure. Pediatr Crit Care Med. 2011 [Epub ahead of print].
31. Norman M, Herin P, Fagrell B, et al. Capillary blood cell velocity in full-term infants as determined in skin by videophotometric microscopy. Pediatr Res. 1988;23(6):585-588.
32. Bucher HU, Edwards AD, Lipp AE, et al. Comparison between near infrared spectroscopy and 133Xenon clearance for estimation of cerebral blood flow in critically ill preterm infants. Pediatr Res. 1993;33(1):56-60.
33. Baenziger O, Jaggi JL, Mueller AC, et al. Cerebral blood flow in preterm infants affected by sex, mechanical ventilation, and intrauterine growth. Pediatr Neurol. 1994;11(4):319-324.
34. Ahmad S, Wallace DK, Freedman SF, et al. Computer-assisted assessment of plus disease in retinopathy of prematurity using video indirect ophthalmoscopy images. Retina. 2008;28(10): 1458-1462.
35. Kandasamy Y, Smith R, Wright IM. Retinal microvasculature measurements in full-term newborn infants. Microvasc Res. 2011;82(3):381-384.
36. Ormerod LD, Fariza E, Webb RH. Dynamics of external ocular blood flow studied by scanning angiographic microscopy. Eye. 1995;9(Pt 5):605-614.
37. Johnson JM, Kellogg Jr DL. Local thermal control of the human cutaneous circulation. J Appl Physiol. 2010;109(4):1229-1238.
38. Fluhr JW, Darlenski R, Taieb A, et al. Functional skin adaptation in infancy—almost complete but not fully competent. Exp Dermatol. 2010;19(6):483-492.
39. Cutolo M, Sulli A, Smith V. Assessing microvascular changes in systemic sclerosis diagnosis and management. Nat Rev Rheumatol. 2010;6(10):578-587.
40. Kunzek S, Quinn MW, Shore AC. Does change in skin perfusion provide a good index to monitor the sympathetic response to a noxious stimulus in preterm newborns? Early Hum Dev. 1997;49(2):81-89.

11

41. Osborn DA, Evans N, Kluckow M. Clinical detection of low upper body blood flow in very premature infants using blood pressure, capillary refill time, and central-peripheral temperature difference. Arch Dis Child Fetal Neonatal Ed. 2004;89:F168-F173.

42. Millet C, Roustit M, Blaise S, et al. Comparison between laser speckle contrast imaging and laser Doppler imaging to assess skin blood flow in humans. Microvasc Res. 2011;82(2):147-151.

43. Rajan V, Varghese B, Van Leeuwen TG, et al. Review of methodological developments in laser Doppler flowmetry. Lasers Med Sci. 2009;24:269-283.

44. Turner J, Belch JJF, Khan F. Current concepts in assessment of microvascular endothelial function using laser Doppler imaging and iontophoresis. Trends Cardiovasc Med. 2008;184:109-116.

45. Roustit M, Millet C, Blaise S, et al. Excellent reproducibility of laser speckle contrast imaging to assess skin microvascular reactivity. Microvasc Res. 2010;80(3):505-511.

46. Perimed Instruments. Laser Doppler theory. http://www.perimed-instruments.com/support/theory/laser-doppler (accessed 31 Sept 2011).

47. Kubli S, Waeber B, Dalle-Ave A, et al. Reproducibility of laser doppler imaging of skin blood flow as a tool to assess endothelial function. J Cardiovasc Pharmacol. 2000;36:640-648.

48. Weindling M, Paize F. Peripheral haemodynamics in newborns: best practice guidelines. Early Hum Dev. 2010;86(3):159-165.

49. Smits GJ, Roman RJ, Lombard JH. Evaluation of laser-Doppler flowmetry as a measure of tissue blood flow. J Appl Physiol. 1986;61(2):666-672.

50. Cracowski JL, Minson CT, Salvat-Melis M, et al. Methodological issues in the assessment of skin microvascular endothelial function in humans. Trends Pharmacol Sci. 2006;27:503-508.

51. Agarwal SC, Allen J, Murray A, et al. Comparative reproducibility of dermal microvascular blood flow changes in response to acetylcholine iontophoresis, hyperthermia and reactive hyperaemia. Physiological Measurement. 2010;31:1-11.

52. Yvonne-Tee GB, Rasool AHG, Halim AS, et al. Reproducibility of different laser Doppler fluximetry parameters of postocclusive reactive hyperemia in human forearm skin. J Pharmacol Toxicol Methods. 2005;52;286-292.

53. Roustit M, Blaise S, Millet C, et al. Reproducibility and methodological issues of skin post-occlusive and thermal hyperemia assessed by single-point laser Doppler flowmetry. Microvasc Res. 2010;79;102-108.

54. Normal skin structure. http://www.rosaceainstitutetexas.com/skin_diagram.html. Texas Rosacea Institute. Accessed 8 September 2011.

55. Fagrell B. Peripheral vascular diseases. In: Shepard AP, Oberg PA, eds. Laser Doppler blood flowmetry. Norwell, MA: Kluwer Academic; 1990.

56. Perera P, Kurban AK, Ryan TJ. The development of the cutaneous microvascular system in the newborn. Br J Dermatol. 1970;82:86-91.

57. Yamamoto-Suganuma R, Aso Y. Relationship between post-occlusive forearm skin reactive hyperaemia and vascular disease in patients with type 2 diabetes—a novel index for detecting micro- and macrovascular dysfunction using laser Doppler flowmetry. Diabet Med. 2009;26(1):83-88.

58. Wilson SB, Jennings PE, Belch JJF. Detection of microvascular impairment in type I diabetics by laser Doppler flowmetry. Clin Physiol. 1992;12:195-208.

59. Strain WD, Chaturvedi N, Hughes A, et al. Associations between cardiac target organ damage and microvascular dysfunction. The role of blood pressure. J Hypertens. 2010;28;952-958.

60. Tee GBY, Rasool AHG, Halim AS, et al. Dependence of human forearm skin postocclusive reactive hyperemia on occlusion time. J Pharmacol Toxicol Methods. 2004;50:73-78.

61. Norman M. Preterm birth—an emerging risk factor for adult hypertension? Semin Perinatol. 2010;34:183-187.

62. Magerl W, Treede RD. Heat-evoked vasodilatation in human hairy skin; axon reflexes due to low-level activity of nociceptive afferents. J Physiol. 1996;497(Pt 3):837-848.

63. Minson CT, Berry LT, Joyner MJ. Nitric oxide and neurally mediated regulation of skin blood flow during local heating. J Appl Physiol. 2001;91(4):1619-1626.

64. Sekkat N, Kalia YN, Guy RH. Porcine ear skin as a model for the assessment of transdermal drug delivery to premature neonates. Pharm Res. 2004;21(8):1390-1397.

65. Clifton VL, Crompton R, Read MA, et al. Microvascular effects of corticotropin-releasing hormone in human skin vary in relation to estrogen concentration during the menstrual cycle. J Endocrinol. 2005;186(1):69-76.

66. Morris SJ, Shore AC. Skin blood flow responses to the iontophoresis of acetylcholine and sodium nitroprusside in man; possible mechanisms. J Physiol. 1996;496:531-542.

67. Buus NH, Simonsen H, Pilegaard HK, et al. NO, prostanoid and non-NO, non-prostanoid involvement in acetylcholine relaxation of isolated human small arteries. Br J Pharmacol. 2000;129:184-192.

68. Rutter N. The dermis. Semin Neonatol. 2000;5(4):297-302.

69. Beaufort-Krol GC, Suichies HE, Aarnoudse JG, et al. Postocclusive reactive hyperaemia of cutaneous blood flow in premature newborn infants. Acta Paediatr Scand Suppl. 1989;360:20-25.

70. Berg K, Celander O, Marild K. Circulatory adaptation in the thermoregulation of fullterm and premature newborn infants. Acta Paediatr Scand. 1971;60:278-284.

71. Riley ID. Hand and forearm blood flow in fullterm and premature infants. Clin Sci. 1954;13:317-320.

72. Celander O, Marild K. Reactive hyperemia in the foot and calf of the newborn infant. Acta Paediatr. 1962;51:544-552.

73. Ahlsten G, Ewald U, Tuvemo T. Impaired vascular reactivity in newborn infants of smoking mothers. Acta Paediatr Scand. 1987;76(2):248-253.

74. Strömberg B, Rieenfeld T, Sedin G. Laser Doppler measurement of skin blood flow in newborn infants. Int J Microcirc Clin Exp. 1984;3:326.

75. Suchies HE, Brouwer C, Aarnoudse JG, et al. Skin blood flow changes, measured by laser Doppler flowmetry, in the first week after birth. Early Hum Dev. 1990;23:1-8.

76. Stark MJ, Clifton VL, Wright IMR. Neonates born to mothers with preeclampsia exhibit sex-specific alterations in microvascular function. Pediatr Res. 2009;65:291-295.

77. Jahnukainen T, van Ravenswaaij-Arts C, Jalonen J, et al. Dynamics of vasomotor thermoregulation of the skin in term and preterm neonates. Early Hum Dev. 1993;33(2):133-143.

78. Celander O, Marild K. Regional circulation and capillary filtration in relation to capillary exchange in the foot and calf of the newborn infant. Acta Paediatr. 1962;51:385-400.

79. Martin H, Norman M. Skin microcirculation before and after local warming in infants delivered vaginally or by caesarean section. Acta Paediatr. 1997;86(3):261-267.

80. Poschl JM, Weiss T, Fallahi F, et al. Reactive hyperemia of skin microcirculation in septic neonates. Acta Paediatr. 1994;83:808-811.

81. Norman M, Fagrell B, Herin P. Skin microcirculation in neonatal polycythemia and effects of haemodilution. Interaction between haematocrit, vasomotor activity and perfusion. Acta Paediatr. 1993;82:672-677.

82. Kent AL, Wright IMR, Abdel-Latif ME. Mortality and adverse neurologic outcomes are greater in preterm male infants. Pediatrics. 2012;129(1):124-131.

83. Molnar J, Nijland MJ, Howe DC, et al. Evidence for microvascular dysfunction after prenatal dexamethasone at 0.7, 0.75, and 0.8 gestation in sheep. Am J Physiol Regul Integr Comp Physiol. 2002;283(3):R561-R567.

84. Stark MJ, Clifton VL, Wright IMR. Microvascular flow, clinical illness severity and cardiovascular function in the preterm infant. Arch Dis Child Fetal Neonatal Ed. 2008;93(4):F271-F274.

85. Stark MJ, Clifton VL, Wright IMR. Characterisation of microvascular function in newborn infants from 24-40 weeks gestation in the first week of life. Perinatal Society of Australia and New Zealand Annual Scientific Meeting. Perth, Western Australia: Blackwell: April 2006.

86. Beinder E, Trojan A, Bucher HU, et al. Control of skin blood flow in pre- and full-term infants. Biol Neonate. 1994;65:7-15.

87. Jahnukainen T, Lindqvist A, Jalonen J, et al. Reactivity of skin blood flow and heart rate to thermal stimulation in infants during the first postnatal days and after a two-month follow-up. Acta Paediatr. 1996;85:733-738.

88. Genzel-Boroviczény O, Seidl T, Rieger-Fackeldey E, et al. Impaired microvascular perfusion improves with increased incubator temperature in preterm infants. Pediatr Res. 2007; 61(2):239-242.

89. Khoury MJ, Marks JS, McCarthy BJ, et al. Risk factors affecting the sex differential in neonatal mortality; the role of respiratory distress syndrome. Am J Obstet Gynecol. 1985;151:777-782.

90. Elsmen E, Hansen Pupp I, Hellstrom-Westas L. Preterm male infants need more initial respiratory and circulatory support than females. Acta Paediatr. 2004;93:529-533.

91. Henderson-Smart DJ, Hutchinson JL, Donoghue DA, et al. Prenatal predictors of chronic lung disease in very preterm infants. Arch Dis Child Fetal Neonatal Ed. 2006;91(1):F40-F45.

92. Stevenson DK, Verter J, Fanaroff AA. Sex differences in outcomes of very low birthweight infants: the newborn male disadvantage. Arch Dis Child Fetal Neonatal Ed. 2000;83:F182-F185.

93. Stark MJ, Clifton VL, Wright IMR. Sex-specific differences in peripheral microvascular blood flow in preterm infants. Pediatr Res. 2008;63:415-419.

94. Osborn DA. Diagnosis and treatment of preterm transitional circulatory compromise. Early Hum Dev. 2005;81:413-422.

95. Chaline J. Increased cranial capacity in hominid evolution and preeclampsia. J Reprod Immunol. 2003;59:137-152.

96. Clifton VL. Sex and the human placenta: mediating differential strategies of fetal growth and survival. Placenta. 2010;31:S33-S39.

97. Stark MJ, Dierkx L, Clifton VL, et al. Alterations in the maternal peripheral microvascular response in pregnancies complicated by preeclampsia and the impact of fetal sex. J Soc Gynecol Investig. 2006;13(8):573-578.

98. Osborn DA, Paradisis M, Evans N. The effect of inotropes on morbidity and mortality in preterm infants with low systemic or organ blood flow. Cochrane Database Syst Rev. 2007;(1):CD005090.

99. Davis MJ, Hill MA, Kuo L. Local regulation of microvascular perfusion. Compr Physiol Supplement 9. In: Handbook of physiology: The cardiovascular system, microcirculation. Hoboken, NJ: Wiley-Blackwell, 2011;161-284.

100. Krediet TG, Valk L, Hempenius I, et al. Nitric oxide production and plasma cyclic guanosine monophosphate in premature infants with respiratory distress syndrome. Biol Neonate. 2002;82(3): 150-154.

101. Shaul PW. Ontogeny of nitric oxide in the pulmonary vasculature. Semin Perinatol. 1997;21(5): 381-392.

102. Chen YH, Yet SF, Perrella MA. Role of heme oxygenase-1 in the regulation of blood pressure and cardiac function. Exp Biol Med (Maywood). 2003;228(5):447-453.

103. van Bel F, Latour V, Vreman HJ: et al. Is carbon monoxide-mediated cyclic guanosine monophosphate production responsible for low blood pressure in neonatal respiratory distress syndrome? J Appl Physiol. 2005;98(3):1044-1049.

104. Wang R. Two's company, three's a crowd: can H2S be the third endogenous gaseous transmitter? FASEB J. 2002;16:1792-1798.
105. Szabó C. Hydrogen sulphide and its therapeutic potential. Nat Rev Drug Discov. 2007;6(11): 917-935.
106. Choi AM, Alam J. Heme oxygenase-1. Function, regulation, and implication of a novel stress-inducible protein in oxidant-induced lung injury. Am J Respir Cell Mol Biol. 1996;15(1):9-19.
107. Scott NM, Hodyl NA, Osei-Kumah A, et al. The presence of maternal asthma during pregnancy suppresses the placental proinflammatory response to an immune challenge in vitro. Placenta. 2011;32:454-461.
108. Moncure M, Braithwaite CEM, Samaha E. Carboxyhaemoglobin elevation in trauma victims. J Trauma. 1999;46(3):424-427.
109. Shi Y, Pan F, Li H, et al. Carbon monoxide concentration in paediatric sepsis syndrome. Arch Dis Child. 2003;88(10):889-890.
110. Van Bel F, Valk L, Uiterwaal CSPM, et al. Plasmaguanosine 3',5'-cyclic monophosphate and severity of peri/intraventricular haemorrhage in the preterm newborn. Acta Paedatr. 2002;91(4):434-439.
111. Coceani F, Kelsey L, Seidlitz E, et al. Carbon monoxide formation in the ductus arteriosus in the lamb: implications for the regulation of vascular tone. Br J Pharmacol. 1997;120(4):599-608.
112. Kaide JI, Zhang F, Wei Y, et al. Carbon monoxide of vascular origin attenuates the sensitivity of renal arterial vessels to vasoconstrictors. J Clin Invest. 2001;107(9):1163-1171.
113. Stark MJ, Clifton VL, Wright IMR. Carbon monoxide is a significant mediator of cardiovascular status following preterm birth. Pediatrics. 2009;124:277-284.
114. Dennery PA. Metalloporphyrins for the treatment of neonatal jaundice. Curr Opin Pediatr. 2005;17(2):167-169.
115. Jiang HL, Wu HC, Li ZL, et al. Changes of the new gaseous transmitter H2S in patients with coronary heart disease. Di Yi Jun Yi Da Xue Xue Bao. 2005;25:951-954.
116. Zhang J, Sio SW, Moochhala S, et al. Role of hydrogen sulfide in severe burn injury-induced inflammation in mice. Mol Med. 2010;16:417-424.
117. Herrera EA, Cindrova-Davies T, Niu Y, et al. Vasodilator effect of hydrogen sulphide in the perfused human placenta. Fetal Neonatal Physiological Society Proceedings. Brisbane, Queensland, Australia: University of Queensland; 2011:39.
118. Goldstein DS, Eisenhoffer G, Kopin IJ. Sources and significance of plasma levels of catechols and their metabolites in humans. Perspect Pharmacol. 2003;305:800-811.
119. Laforgia N, Difonzo I, Altomare M, et al. Cord blood endothelin-1 and perinatal asphyxia. Acta Paediatr. 2001;90:351-352.
120. Lagercrantz H, Edwards D, Henderson-Smart D, et al. Autonomic reflexes in preterm infants. Acta Pediatr Scand. 1990;79:721-728.
121. Molnar M, Hertelendy F. Signal transduction in rat myometrial cells; comparison of the actions of endothelin-1, oxytocin and prostaglandin F2a. Eur J Endocrinol. 1995;133:467-474.
122. Stark MJ, Hodyl NA, Wright IMR, et al. The influence of sex and antenatal betamethasone exposure on vasoconstrictors and the preterm microvasculature. J Matern Fetal Neonatal Med. 2011;24(10):1215-1220.
123. Stark MJ, Wright IMR, Clifton VL. Sex specific alterations in placental 11b-hydroxysteroid dehydrogenase 2 activity and early postnatal clinical course following antenatal betamethasone. Am J Physiol Regul Integr Comp Physiol. 2009;297:R510-R514.
124. den Uil CA, Klijn E, Lagrand WK, et al. The microcirculation in health and critical disease. Prog Cardiovasc Dis. 2008;51(2):161-170.
125. Hussain F, Gilshenan K, Gray PH. Does lactate level in the first 12 hours of life predict mortality in extremely premature infants? J Paediatr Child Health. 2009;45(5):263-267.
126. Weidlich K, Kroth J, Nussbaum C, et al. Changes in microcirculation as early markers for infection in preterm infants—an observational prospective study. Pediatr Res. 2009;66(4):461-465.
127. Kluckow M, Evans N. Superior vena cava flow in newborn infants; a novel marker of systemic blood flow. Arch Dis Child Fetal Neonatal Ed. 2000;82:F182-F187.
128. Wright IMR, Dyson RM, Latter J, et al. Microvascular blood flow changes from 6 to 24 hours in the preterm infant. J Paediatr Child Health. 2011;47(suppl 1):55.
129. Eiby YA, Lumbers ER, Headricks JP, et al. Coronary and aortic flow in response to changes in preload and afterload in the isolated preterm piglet heart. Fetal Neonatal Physiological Society Proceedings. Brisbane, Queensland, Australia: University of Queensland; 2011:54.
130. Nuyt AM. Mechanisms underlying developmental programming of elevated blood pressure and vascular dysfunction; evidence from human studies and experimental animal models. Clin Sci (Lond). 2008;114(1):1-17.
131. Sharrett AR, Hubbard LD, Cooper LS, et al. Retinal arteriolar diameters and elevated blood pressure; the Atherosclerosis Risk in Communities Study. Am J Epidemiol. 1999;150:263-270.
132. Li LJ, Cheung CY, Chia A, et al. The relationship of body fatness indices and retinal vascular caliber in children. Int J Pediatr Obstet. 2011;6(3-4):267-274.
133. de Jongh RT, Serné EH, IJzerman RG, et al. Microvascular function; a potential link between salt sensitivity, insulin resistance and hypertension. J Hypertens. 2007;25(9):1887-1893.
134. Kistner A, Jacobson L, Jacobson SH, et al. Low gestational age associated with abnormal retinal vascularization and increased blood pressure in adult women. Pediatr Res. 2002;51(6):675-680.

Clinical Presentations and Relevance of Neonatal Shock

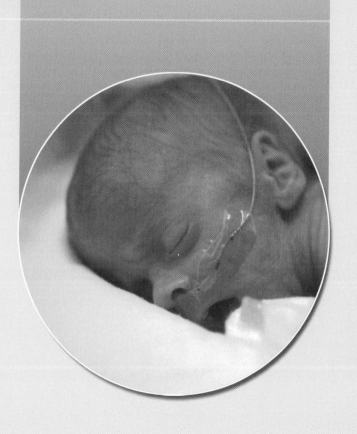

CHAPTER 12

Clinical Presentations of Neonatal Shock: The Very Low Birth Weight Neonate During the First Postnatal Day

Martin Kluckow, PhD, MBBS, FRACP,
Istvan Seri, MD, PhD, HonD

12

- Definition of Hypotension and Its Relationship to Low Systemic Perfusion
- The Transitional Circulation in the Very Low Birth Weight Infant
- Clinical Determinants of Blood Pressure in the Very Low Birth Weight Infant
- Assessment of Cardiovascular Compromise in the Shocked Very Low Birth Weight Infant
- Short- and Long-Term Effects of Cardiovascular Compromise/Shock in the Very Low Birth Weight Infant
- Treatment Options in the Management of Cardiovascular Compromise/Shock in the Very Low Birth Weight Infant
- Treatment of Very Low Birth Weight Neonates with Vasopressor-Resistant Shock
- Presentation and Management of Cardiovascular Compromise in the Very Low Birth Weight Infant on the First Postnatal Day
- Perinatal Depression with Secondary Myocardial Dysfunction and/or Abnormal Peripheral Vasoregulation
- Conclusion
- References

The birth of a very low birth weight (VLBW) infant creates a unique set of circumstances that can adversely affect the cardiovascular system resulting in cardiovascular compromise. The cardiovascular system of the fetus is adapted to an in utero environment that is constant and stable. The determinants of cardiac output, such as preload and afterload, are maintained in equilibrium without interference from the external factors that may affect a neonate born prematurely. Postnatal factors that can affect the cardiovascular function of the VLBW infant include perinatal asphyxia, positive pressure respiratory support, which may alter preload, and changes in afterload occurring with the rapid transition from the fetal circulation characterized by low systemic vascular resistance to the neonatal circulation with higher peripheral vascular resistance in the immediate transitional period. These changes of the transitional circulation, with predominantly systemic to pulmonary shunts at the atrial and ductal level through persisting fetal channels, can further reduce potential systemic blood flow (Fig. 12-1).

The situation is further complicated by the difficulty in assessing the adequacy of the cardiovascular system in the VLBW infant. The small size of the infant and the frequent presence of shunting at both ductal and atrial level preclude the use of many of the routine cardiovascular assessment techniques used in

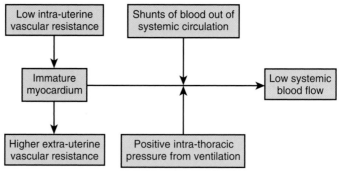

Figure 12-1 Suggested model of how the various external and internal influences on the cardiovascular system of the VLBW infant can result in low systemic blood flow.

children and adults to determine cardiac output. As a result, clinicians are forced to fall back on more easily measured parameters such as the blood pressure. However, blood pressure is but one measure of the cardiovascular system and changes in the blood pressure do not necessarily reflect changes in the cardiac output and subsequent changes in organ blood flow and tissue oxygen delivery (see Chapters 1 and 3).

Hypotension occurs in up to 30% of VLBW infants with between 16% and 52% of these infants receiving treatment with volume expansion and up to 39% receiving vasopressors.[1] More recent surveys of the management of extremely low birth weight (ELBW) infants have demonstrated treatment (fluid bolus or vasopressor administration) rates for hypotension up to 93% at 23 weeks' gestational age (GA) and up to 73% of infants at 27 weeks' GA.[2] Most treatment was commenced in the first 24 hours of postnatal life. Similarly, low systemic blood flow in the first 24 hours is seen in up to 35% of VLBW infants, but not all of these infants will have hypotension initially, though many will develop it.[3] Recent studies of the incidence of superior vena cava (SVC) flow show a reduced incidence (18-21% of ELBW infants) possibly reflecting changes in obstetrical management of the mother and delivery room, respiratory, and perhaps fluid management of the neonate.[4,5] There is a wide variation in the assessment and management of cardiovascular compromise both among institutions and individual clinicians.[1,2] As with many other areas in medicine where there is variation in practice with multiple treatment options, the lack of good evidence for both when to treat cardiovascular compromise and whether treatment benefits the long-term outcome of infants, underlies this uncertainty. This chapter explores the importance of the unique changes involved in the transitional circulation during the first postnatal day and how they impact upon the presentation, assessment and management of neonatal shock.

Definition of Hypotension and its Relationship to Low Systemic Perfusion

Hypotension can be defined as the blood pressure value where vital organ blood flow autoregulation is lost. If effective treatment is not initiated at this point, blood pressure may further decrease and reach a "functional threshold" when neuronal function is impaired, and then the "ischemic threshold" resulting in tissue ischemia with likely permanent organ damage (Chapter 1). Neither the blood pressure causing loss of autoregulation nor the critical blood pressure resulting in direct tissue damage has been clearly defined for the VLBW neonate in the immediate postnatal period.[6] The distinction between the three levels of hypotension is important because, although loss of autoregulation and cellular function *may* predispose to brain injury, reaching the ischemic threshold of hypotension by definition *is associated with direct tissue damage*. Finally, these thresholds may be affected by several factors including gestational and postmenstrual age, the duration of hypotension, and the presence of acidosis and/or infection.

Although the normal autoregulatory blood pressure range is not known, in clinical practice there are generally two definitions of early hypotension in wide-spread use:

- Mean blood pressure less than 30 mm Hg in any gestation infant in the first postnatal days. This definition is based on pathophysiologic associations between cerebral injury (white matter damage or intraventricular hemorrhage) and mean blood pressure less than 30 mm Hg and to a lesser degree on more recent data looking at maintenance of cerebral blood flow (CBF) measured by near-infrared spectroscopy (NIRS) over a range of blood pressures, suggesting a reduction in CBF when a particular mean blood pressure threshold is reached.[7-10] It is important to note that, although the 10th centile for infants of all gestational ages is at or above 30 mm Hg by the third postnatal day, in more immature infants the normal mean blood pressure is lower than 30 mm Hg during the first 3 days.[11] Therefore, it is too simplistic to use a single cutoff value for blood pressure across a range of gestation and postnatal ages.

- Mean blood pressure less than the gestational age in weeks during the first post-natal days, which roughly correlates with the 10th centile for age in tables of normative data.[7,12] This statistical definition has also been supported by professional body guidelines such as the Joint Working Group of the British Association of Perinatal Medicine.[13] Again this rule of thumb applies mainly in the first 24-48 hours of extra-uterine life—after this time there is a gradual increase in the mean blood pressure such that most premature infants have a mean blood pressure greater than 30 mm Hg and thus gestational age by postnatal day 3 (Chapter 3).[12]

The current definitions are not related to physiologic endpoints such as maintenance of organ blood flow or tissue oxygen delivery. However, most but not all studies using ^{133}Xe clearance or NIRS to assess changes in CBF found that the lower limit of the autoregulatory blood pressure range may be around 30 mm Hg even in the 1-day-old ELBW neonate.[10,14-16] Indeed, preterm neonates with a mean blood pressure at or above 30 mm Hg appear to have an intact static autoregulation of their CBF during the first postnatal day.[17] It is reasonable to assume that, although the gestational age–equivalent blood pressure value is below the CBF autoregulatory range, this value is still higher than the suspected ischemic blood pressure threshold for the VLBW patient population.[16]

A confounding finding to the straightforward-appearing blood pressure-CBF relationship has been provided by a series of studies using superior vena cava (SVC) flow measurements to indirectly assess brain perfusion in the VLBW neonate with a focus on the ELBW infant in the immediate postnatal period.[3,18] The findings of these studies suggest that, in the ELBW neonate, blood pressure in the normal range may not always guarantee normal vital organ (brain) blood flow. In the compensated phase of shock, by redistributing blood flow from nonvital organs (e.g., muscle, skin, kidneys, intestine), neuroendocrine compensatory mechanisms ensure that blood pressure and organ blood flow to vital organs (brain, heart, adrenals) are maintained within the normal range. With progression of the condition, shock enters its uncompensated phase and blood pressure and vital organ perfusion decrease. Since the immature myocardium of the ELBW neonate may not be able to compensate for the sudden increase in peripheral vascular resistance immediately following delivery, cardiac output may fall.[18,19] Yet, despite the decrease in cardiac output, many ELBW neonates maintain their blood pressure in the normal range by redistributing blood flow to the organs that are vital at that particular developmental stage (see Chapter 1). It is conceivable that the rapidly developing cerebral cortex and white matter of the ELBW neonate is not yet among the vital organs with appropriately developed autoregulatory capacity.[15,18,19] However, by the second postnatal day, normal blood pressure is highly likely to be associated with normal brain and systemic blood flow.[18,19] Thus the vasculature of the cerebral cortex and white matter of the ELBW neonate may mature rapidly and become a "high-priority" vascular bed soon after delivery.[19,20]

The Transitional Circulation in the Very Low Birth Weight Infant

The traditional understanding of the changes occurring in the transitional circulation of the preterm infant suggests that atrial and ductal shunts in the first postnatal hours are of little significance and are bi-directional or primarily right to left in direction as a result of the higher pulmonary vascular resistance expected in the newborn premature infant.[21] In contrast to this understanding, longitudinal studies using bedside noninvasive echocardiography show significant variability in the time taken for the preterm infant to transition from the in utero right ventricle–dominant, low resistance circulation to the bi-ventricular higher resistance postnatal circulation. Shortly after delivery, the severing of the umbilical vessels, the inflation of the lungs with air, and the associated changes in oxygenation lead to a sudden increase in the resistance in the systemic circulation and a lowering of resistance in the pulmonary circulation. Cardiac output now passes in a parallel fashion through the pulmonary and the systemic circulation except for the blood flow shunting through the closing fetal channels.

In normal full-term infants, the ductus arteriosus is functionally closed by the second postnatal day and the right ventricular pressure usually falls to adult levels by about 2-3 days after birth.[22,23] This constriction and functional closure of the ductus arteriosus is then followed by anatomical closure over the next two to three weeks. In contrast, in the VLBW infant there is frequently a failure of complete closure of both the foramen ovale and the ductus arteriosus in the expected time frame, probably due to immaturity of the mechanisms involved.[24,25] The persistence of the fetal channels leads to blood flowing preferentially from the aorta to pulmonary artery resulting in a relative loss of blood from the systemic circulation and pulmonary circulatory overload. Contrary to traditional understanding, this systemic to pulmonary shunting can occur as early as the first postnatal hours, with recirculation of 50% or more of the normal cardiac output back into the lungs.[26] The myocardium subsequently attempts to compensate by increasing the total cardiac output. There can be up to a 2-fold increase in the left ventricular (LV) output by one hour of age, resulting primarily from an increased stroke volume, rather than increased heart rate.[27] A significant proportion of this increased blood flow is likely to be passing through the ductus arteriosus.[28] There is a wide range of early ductal constriction, with some infants able to effectively close or minimize the size of the ductus arteriosus within a few hours of birth while others achieve an initial constriction, followed by an increase in size of the ductus and yet another group having a persistent large ductus arteriosus with no evidence of early constriction and subsequent limitation of shunt size.[29] In this early postnatal period both ductal and atrial shunts are frequently large in size and the direction of shunting is predominantly left to right, that is, systemic to pulmonary. This results in an increase in the pulmonary blood flow relative to the systemic blood flow and movement of blood flow away from the systemic circulation. Pulmonary blood flow can be more than twice the systemic blood flow as early as the first few postnatal hours which may be enough to cause clinical effects, such as reduced systemic blood pressure and blood flow, increases in ventilatory requirements, or even pulmonary hemorrhagic edema.[29]

In utero, the fetal communications of the foramen ovale and ductus arteriosus result in a lack of separation between the left and right ventricular outputs, making it difficult to quantitate their individual contributions. In addition to heart rate, the ventricular systolic function is determined by the physiologic principles of preload (distension of the ventricle by blood prior to contraction), contractility (the intrinsic ability of the myocardial fibers to contract), and afterload (the combined resistance of the blood, the ventricular walls and the vascular beds). The myocardium of the VLBW infant is less mature than that of a term infant with fewer mitochondria and less energy stores. This results in a limitation in the ability to respond to changes in the determinants of the cardiac output, in particular the afterload.[30] Consequently the myocardium of the VLBW infant, just like the fetal myocardium, is likely to be less able to respond to stresses that occur in the postnatal period such as increased peripheral vascular resistance with the resultant increase in afterload. There is a significant difference in the influence of determinants of cardiac output in the newborn premature infant with a dramatically increased afterload and changes in the preload caused by the inflation of the lungs. Furthermore, the effect of lung inflation on preload is different when lung inflation occurs by positive pressure ventilation rather than by the negative intrathoracic pressures generated by spontaneous breathing. The newborn ventricle is more sensitive to changes in the afterload, such that small changes can have large effects especially if the preload and contractility are not optimized.[30]

Failure of the normal transitional changes to occur in a timely manner can result in impairment of cardiac function leading to low cardiac output states and hypotension in the VLBW infant. As oxygen delivery is primarily related to both the oxygen content of the blood and to the volume of blood flow to the organ, delivery of oxygen to vital organs may be impaired where there is cardiovascular impairment.[31] Therefore, the timely identification and appropriate management of early low cardiac output states and hypotension are of vital importance in the overall care of the VLBW infant.

Physiologic Determinants of the Blood Pressure in the Very Low Birth Weight Infant (see also Chapter 1)

The product of cardiac output and peripheral vascular resistance determines arterial blood pressure. The main influences on the cardiac output are the preload or blood volume and myocardial contractility. The peripheral vascular resistance is determined by the vascular tone, which in the presence of an unconstricted ductus arteriosus may not only be the systemic peripheral vascular resistance, but is also contributed to by the pulmonary vascular resistance. Myocardial contractility is difficult to assess in the newborn as the accepted measures of contractility in the adult, such as the echocardiographic measure of fractional shortening, are adversely influenced by the asymmetry of the ventricles caused by the in utero right ventricular dominance. In this regard, use of load-independent measures of cardiac contractility, such as mean velocity of fractional shortening or LV wall stress indices, may provide more useful information (Chapter 5; Fig. 12-2).[32] Some studies have found a relationship between myocardial dysfunction and hypotension in the preterm infant while others have not, even though a similar measurement method was used. Similarly blood volume correlates poorly with blood pressure in hypotensive neonates.[33-36]

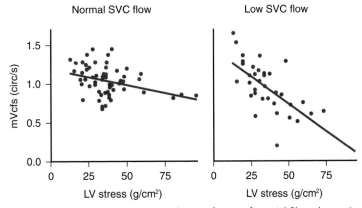

Figure 12-2 Relationship between mean velocity of circumferential fiber shortening (mVcfs) and LV wall stress at 3 hours in infants with low and normal SVC flows in the first 24 hours. Infants who developed low SVC flow had reduced LV contractility ($P = .02$). (Reproduced with permission from Osborn D, Evans N, Kluckow M. Diagnosis and treatment of low systemic blood flow in preterm infants. NeoReviews. 2004;5:e109-e121.)

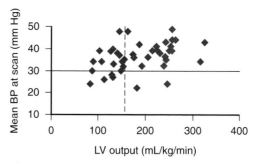

Figure 12-3 The weak relationship between mean systemic blood pressure and simultaneously measured left ventricular (LV) output. Some infants with a mean BP greater than 30 mm Hg have critically low cardiac output (<150 mL/kg/min) and conversely some infants with normal LV output have low mean blood pressure. (Reproduced with permission from Kluckow M, Evans N. Relationship between blood pressure and cardiac output in preterm infants requiring mechanical ventilation. J Pediatr. 1996;129:506-512.)

Due to the unique characteristics of the newborn cardiovascular system discussed earlier, systemic blood pressure is closely related to changes in the systemic vascular resistance. As systemic vascular resistance cannot be measured directly, the measurement of cardiac output or systemic blood flow becomes an essential element in understanding the dynamic changes occurring in the cardiovascular system of the VLBW infant.

In the absence of simple techniques to measure cardiac output and systemic vascular resistance (Chapter 6), clinicians have tended to rely on blood pressure as the sole assessment of circulatory compromise. However, in the VLBW neonate with a closed ductus arteriosus during the first 24-48 hours, there is only a weak relationship between mean blood pressure and cardiac output (Fig. 12-3).[34] Relying on measurements of blood pressure alone can lead the clinician to make assumptions about the underlying physiology of the cardiovascular system that may not be correct especially during the period of early transition with the fetal channels open. Indeed, many hypotensive preterm infants potentially have a normal or high left ventricular output.[34,37,38] One of the reasons for this apparent paradox relates to the presence of a hemodynamically significant ductus arteriosus, which causes an increase in left ventricular output while also causing a reduction in the overall systemic vascular resistance. Variations in the peripheral vascular resistance may cause a change in the underlying cardiac output that does not affect the blood pressure. This phenomenon makes it possible for two infants with the same blood pressure to have markedly different cardiac outputs. Thus the physiologic determinants of blood pressure may affect the blood pressure in multiple ways—acting via an effect on cardiac performance and thus cardiac output, altering the vascular resistance or sometimes altering both.

Clinical Determinants of Blood Pressure in the Very Low Birth Weight Infant

Gestational Age and Postnatal Age

Both gestational age and postnatal age are major determinants of the systemic blood pressure as can be seen by examining nomograms and tables of normal blood pressure data (see Chapter 3). Generally blood pressure is higher in more mature infants and progressively increases with advancing postnatal age. The reasons why blood pressure increases with postnatal age are unclear but are probably related to changes in the underlying vascular tone mediated by various humoral regulators and possibly up-regulation of receptors involved in myocardial responses. Simultaneously, there are temporal physical changes in the transitional circulation such as closure of the ductus arteriosus, which will affect both blood pressure and blood flow.

Use of Antenatal Glucocorticoid Therapy

There is evidence that sick VLBW infants have relative adrenocorticoid insufficiency and that this condition may be one of the underlying causes of cardiovascular dysfunction and the propensity to inflammation in these patients contributing to the pathogenesis of clinical conditions such as bronchopulmonary dysplasia.[39-41] Low cortisol levels have been documented in hypotensive infants requiring inotropic support.[42] The use of antenatal glucocorticoids to assist in fetal lung maturation may therefore have an additional effect of improving neonatal blood pressure. Likely mechanisms for this effect include the acceleration of adrenergic receptor expression and maturation of myocardial structure and function. The enhanced adrenergic receptor expression also increases the sensitivity of the myocardium and peripheral vasculature to endogenous catecholamines.[43] Randomized controlled trials of the use of antenatal glucocorticoids have shown variable effects on the neonatal blood pressure. In some, there was an increase in the mean blood pressure of VLBW infants in the treated group with a decreased need for inotropic support, while others have shown little difference between the mean blood pressures of infants whose mothers did or did not receive antenatal steroids.[44-47]

Blood Loss

Acute blood loss in the VLBW infant can result from prenatal events such as feto-maternal hemorrhage, antepartum hemorrhage or twin-twin transfusion syndrome, intrapartum events such as a tight nuchal cord resulting in an imbalance between blood flow to and from the fetus or postnatally from a large subgaleal hematoma or hemorrhage into an organ such as the liver or brain. Acute blood loss can result in significant hypotension but due to the immediate compensatory mechanisms of the cardiovascular system this effect may be delayed. Similarly, a drop in the infant's hemoglobin level can also be delayed following significant hemorrhage.

Positive Pressure Ventilation

Many VLBW infants are exposed to positive pressure respiratory support in the first postnatal days. Positive end-expiratory pressure (PEEP) or nasal continuous positive airway pressure (CPAP) is often utilized to reduce the atelectasis resulting from collapse of unstable alveoli when surfactant is lacking, particularly in more immature infants. Although surfactant deficiency is the main reason for provision of positive pressure support, there is also a contribution from sepsis and immaturity of the lungs without surfactant deficiency. The use of high ventilation pressures in the premature infant who has a relatively small chest can result in secondary interference with cardiac function. Function can be impaired by a reduction in the preload from reduced systemic or pulmonary venous return, or direct compression of cardiac chambers resulting in a reduced stroke volume or an increase in afterload. This latter scenario is particularly concerning for the right ventricle (RV) and may reduce cardiac output. As the right and left sides of the heart are connected in series, a reduction in the RV output will in turn result in a reduction in the LV cardiac output.

Studies in VLBW infants have shown a fall off in the systemic oxygen delivery if the PEEP was greater than 6 cm of water and a reduction in the cardiac output at a PEEP level of 9 cm water in mechanically ventilated infants.[48] A study of VLBW infants (mean gestational age 29 weeks) before and during treatment with mechanical ventilation for severe respiratory distress syndrome demonstrated a reduction in left ventricular dimensions and filling rate with a resultant decrease in the cardiac output by about 40% compared with control values. The addition of a packed cell blood transfusion prevented the decrease in ventricular size and reduction in cardiac output.[49] The blood pressure did not change significantly in the group where cardiac output dropped. In longitudinal clinical studies of blood pressure and blood flow, mean airway pressure has a consistently negative influence on both mean blood pressure and systemic blood flow.[18,34,50,51]

12

Patent Ductus Arteriosus (see also Chapter 13)

A patent ductus arteriosus (PDA) may not be recognized clinically in the first days after delivery as the flow through it is generally not turbulent and therefore no murmur is audible.[52] Despite this, the flow is almost always left to right or bidirectional with a predominantly left to right pattern.[26] A PDA is usually thought to be associated with a low diastolic BP but some data suggest that it can be associated with both low diastolic and systolic BP, making a PDA one of the possible causes of systemic hypotension.[53] As clinic detection of a PDA in the first postnatal days is difficult, an echocardiogram is required for early diagnosis.[52] The classic clinical signs of a murmur, bounding pulses and a hyperdynamic precordium, usually become evident only after the third postnatal day making clinical detection much more accurate at that time.[52]

Systemic Vascular Resistance

There is a reciprocal relationship between the systemic vascular resistance and cardiac output in the healthy term, preterm, and sick ventilated infant.[54] This relationship is particularly important when considering the use of vasopressor-inotropes such as dopamine in preterm infants where an increase in the peripheral vascular resistance can increase the blood pressure but have no impact on, or even decrease the cardiac output.[55] The peripheral resistance varies markedly in the preterm infant and can be affected by numerous factors, including environmental temperature, carbon dioxide level, the maturity of the sympathoadrenal system, patency of the ductus arteriosus, presence of vasoactive substances such as catecholamines, prostacyclin, and nitric oxide, and sepsis.[29,54,56] It is important to note that, in patients with a PDA, the left ventricle is exposed to the combined pulmonary and systemic vascular resistance. The potential variability of the peripheral resistance in VLBW infants means that significant changes in cardiac output or blood flow cannot be identified by measurement of the systemic blood pressure alone.

Assessment of Cardiovascular Compromise in the Shocked Very Low Birth Weight Infant

Because of the wide variation in blood pressure levels at varying gestations and postnatal ages, some authors have cautioned against the simplicity of just treating low BP alone but suggest that the clinician should look for some other evidence of hypoperfusion, such as decreased capillary return, oliguria, or metabolic acidosis.[57,58] The assessment of cardiovascular adequacy in the VLBW infant is more of a challenge than in infants and adults. Measures of cardiovascular function used in these groups, such as pulmonary wedge pressure, central venous pressure, and cardiac output measured via thermodilution, are impractical in the preterm infant due to their size and fragility and the frequent presence of cardiac shunting. Assessment usually consists of a mainly clinical appraisal of the perfusion via capillary refill time (CRT) and urine output and the documentation of the pulse rate and blood pressure. The acid-base balance and evidence of lactic acidosis are further adjuncts to this assessment but, unless serum lactate levels are serially monitored, monitoring changes in pH and base deficit may be misleading due to the increased bicarbonate losses through the immature kidneys. Indeed, the use of all of these parameters has limitations in the newborn and particularly in the VLBW infant.

Capillary Refill Time

Capillary refill time (CRT) is a widely utilized proxy of both cardiac output and peripheral resistance in neonates and normal values have been documented for this group of infants.[59] A number of confounding factors lead to the CRT being potentially inaccurate and these include the different techniques used (sites tested and pressing time), interobserver variability, ambient temperature, medications, and maturity of skin blood flow control mechanisms.[60] In addition, even in older children receiving intensive care, there is only a weak relationship between the CRT and other hemodynamic measures such as the stroke volume index.[61] A recent study investigating the relationship between a measure of systemic blood flow (superior vena cava (SVC) flow and CRT in VLBW infants showed that a CRT of ≥ 3 seconds had only 55% sensitivity and 81% specificity for predicting low systemic blood flow. However, a markedly increased CRT of 4 seconds or more was more closely correlated with low blood flow states.[62]

Urine Output

Following urine output is useful in the assessment of cardiovascular well-being in the adult; however, the immature renal tubule in VLBW infants is inefficient at concentrating the urine and therefore may be unable to appropriately reduce urine flow in the face of high serum osmolality.[63] As a result, even if the glomerular filtration rate is decreased markedly, there can be little or no change in urine output. In addition, accurate measurement of urine output is not easy in VLBW infants, generally requiring collection via a urinary catheter or via a collection bag, both techniques being invasive with significant potential complications.

Pulse Rate

A rising pulse rate is usually indicative of hypovolemia in the adult. The mechanism relies on a mature autonomic nervous system, with detection of reduced blood volume and then blood pressure via baroreceptors and subsequent increase in the heart rate in an attempt to sustain appropriate cardiac output. Neonates, especially preterm infants, have a faster baseline heart rate and immature myocardium and autonomic nervous system affecting the cardiovascular response to hypovolemia. There are many other influences on the heart rate in the immediate postnatal period so it cannot be relied upon as an accurate assessment of cardiovascular status.

Metabolic Acidosis/Lactic Acidosis

Tissue hypoxia, due to low arterial oxygen tension, inadequate blood flow, or a combination of these two factors, results in a switch to anaerobic metabolism at the cellular level. Reduced systemic blood flow may therefore result in an increase in the serum lactate. A combined lactate value of more than 4 mmol with prolonged capillary refill time more than 4 seconds predicts low SVC flow with 97% specificity.[64] Serum lactate levels have been correlated with illness severity and mortality in critically ill adults and in ventilated neonates with respiratory distress syndrome.[65-72] The normal lactate level in this group of infants is less than 2.5 mmoL/L and there is an association with mortality as the serum lactate level increases above this threshold.[70,71]

Blood Pressure (see also Chapter 3)

Invasive measurement of the arterial blood pressure using a fluid filled catheter and pressure transducer is usually performed either via an indwelling umbilical artery catheter in the descending aorta or a peripherally placed arterial catheter. There is a strong correlation between blood pressure obtained via a peripheral artery catheter and that obtained via the umbilical artery.[73] The agreement between direct and indirect (noninvasive) measures of blood pressure is generally also good.[74-78] However, the noninvasive technique is more problematic in the VLBW infant as it is more dependent on choice of the appropriate cuff size.[79] In the newborn, a cuff width-to-arm ratio between 0.45 and 0.55 increases the accuracy of indirect blood pressure measurements when compared with direct measures.[11] Accuracy of the invasive blood pressure measurement is dependent on proper use of the equipment, including accurate placement of the transducer at the level of the heart, proper calibration of the system, and avoidance of blockages, air bubbles, or blood clots in the catheter line.

Cardiac Output (see also Chapters 1, 5, 6, and 10)

Invasive hemodynamic measures such as pulmonary artery thermodilution and mixed venous oxygen saturation monitoring are commonly used in adult intensive care to allow accurate assessment of the cardiovascular system. The size of both term and preterm infants with the associated difficulty of placing intracardiac catheters has precluded the use of such measures, especially in the group of infants less than 30 weeks' gestation. Another issue specific to premature infants is the potential inaccuracy of the dye dilution and thermodilution method in the presence of intracardiac shunts through the ductus arteriosus and the foramen ovale. Noninvasive methods of measuring cardiac output such as echocardiography have become more popular, aided by improvements in picture resolution and reductions in ultrasound transducer size. Doppler ultrasound was first used to noninvasively measure the cardiac output in neonates in 1982 and subsequently has been validated against more invasive techniques in children, neonates, and VLBW infants.[80,81] The expected coefficient of variation using Doppler compares favorably to that of indicator-dilution and thermodilution (Chapters 5 and 6). Chapter 6 discusses other novel approaches such as impedance electrical cardiometry for the continuous beat-to-beat assessment of stroke volume and cardiac output in detail. Finally, another newer modality for measuring cardiac output is functional cardiac magnetic resonance imaging (MRI) which is envisaged to be predominantly a research tool at present (Chapter 10).[82]

Monitoring of Peripheral and Mucosal Blood Flow

Laser Doppler and visible light technology (T-Stat) are newer techniques currently being assessed for usefulness in directly assessing systemic vascular resistance in neonates.[83,84]

Pulse Oximeter Derived Perfusion Index

The perfusion index is derived from the plethysmographic signal of a pulse oximeter, using a ratio of the pulsatile component (arterial) and the nonpulsatile components of the light reaching the detector. The perfusion index is measured noninvasively, displayed continuously, and subsequently has potential as a marker of low systemic blood flow. Several studies have validated the perfusion index against other measures of systemic blood flow, including superior vena caval flow and found it to be reasonably predictive of low flow states.[85]

Systemic Blood Flow

Normal mean blood pressure does not guarantee normal LV output or CBF in preterm infants, even in the subgroup in whom the ductus arteriosus has closed (Fig. 12-3).[19,34,38] Further problems arise in assessing systemic blood flow in the preterm infant due to the persistence of elements of the fetal circulation as a result of failure or delay of the normal circulatory transition and closure of the fetal channels. Indeed, the assumption that the LV and RV outputs are identical is often incorrect in the VLBW infant. As discussed earlier, increased blood flowing through the PDA (ductal shunt) will be reflected in an increased LV output (up to 2-fold) and the blood flowing left to right through a patent foramen ovale (atrial shunt) will be reflected in an increased RV output (Fig. 12-4).[29]

Systemic blood flow falls dramatically in many extremely premature infants in the first hours of life and this reduction in flow is usually associated with an increase in peripheral vascular resistance. A substantial proportion of these infants will initially have a "normal" blood pressure (i.e., they are in "compensated shock"; see Chapter 1). Of the VLBW infants who initially develop low systemic blood flow, about 80% will subsequently develop systemic hypotension. Using hypotension to direct cardiovascular interventions, however, results in a considerable delay in infants with low systemic blood flow and some infants with low systemic blood flow not being recognized at all. Hypotension may also be associated with normal or even a high systemic blood flow as frequently occurs in the preterm infant with persisting hypotension after the first postnatal days or those with "hyperdynamic"

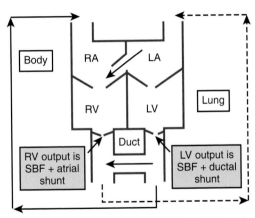

Figure 12-4 Diagram demonstrating the points where right and left ventricular output is measured using Doppler ultrasound. The RV output will consist of the combined systemic venous return and any left to right shunting across the foramen ovale. The LV output will consist of the total pulmonary venous return and the blood destined to cross the ductus arteriosus. (Reprinted with permission from Kluckow M, Evans N. Low systemic blood flow in the preterm infant. Semin Neonatol. 2001;6:75-84.)

sepsis. These infants generally have low systemic vascular resistance with peripheral vasodilation.

Short- and Long-Term Effects of Cardiovascular Compromise/Shock in the Very Low Birth Weight Infant

An important aim of intensive care management in VLBW infants is the maintenance of tissue oxygenation and avoidance of impaired cerebral perfusion (Chapters 2 and 16). CBF, which is important in determining cerebral oxygen delivery, is determined by the relationship between cerebral perfusion pressure, systemic blood flow, and the vascular resistance of the cerebral circulation. The process of cerebral autoregulation allows maintenance of a constant CBF in the face of variations in the blood pressure, systemic blood flow, and resistance (Chapters 1, 2, and 4). There is evidence that sick preterm infants may have lost the capability to autoregulate CBF, resulting in a pressure-passive cerebral circulation more vulnerable to fluctuations in blood pressure and in low CBF if there is systemic hypotension.[86] There is still controversy over the relationship between CBF and mean arterial blood pressure in preterm neonates. Tyszczuk found CBF was independent of mean blood pressure in infants between 24 and 34 weeks' gestation, suggesting preservation of autoregulation in some "hypotensive" infants.[16] In contrast, other groups have found significant relationships between mean arterial blood pressure and cerebral vascular oxygenation providing evidence of pressure passive cerebral circulation, in preterm infants who are hypotensive.[9,10] These authors have suggested an elbow or "cut point" at a mean blood pressure around 30 mm Hg when CBF begins to decline in very preterm infants.[10] In contrast to these observations, there is some evidence to support the concept that cardiac output and tissue oxygen extraction are the important regulatory factors in maintaining cerebral tissue oxygenation, as they appear to operate at a wide range of mean blood pressures. Indeed, the cerebral fraction of oxygen extraction is not related to blood pressure until very low levels (<20 mm Hg) of mean blood pressure have been reached, suggesting that sufficient oxygen to meet cerebral demand can be delivered, even in the presence of hypotension (Chapters 7 and 8).[19,31,87,88] This finding supports the concept that there is a difference between the "autoregulatory" and "ischemic" threshold of blood pressure with the latter being reached only when increasing fractional cerebral oxygen extraction cannot compensate for the decreased oxygen delivery anymore. In addition, the documented increase in the cardiac output (or systemic blood flow) in some VLBW infants with hypotension may be an additional compensatory mechanism preserving oxygen delivery to the brain.

Several studies have suggested that autoregulation is intact in many preterm babies but appears to be compromised in a subgroup who seem to be at particularly high risk of periventricular intraventricular hemorrhage (PIVH).[89,90] High coherence between mean arterial blood pressure and measures of CBF/oxygenation indicates impaired cerebral autoregulation and is associated with subgroup of preterm infants at high risk of adverse outcome (Chapters 1, 2, and 16).[91] It has been suggested that infants suffering severe PIVH are more likely to have blood pressure passive changes in CBF and oxygenation in the first postnatal days. [7-10,92]

Peri/Intraventricular Hemorrhage

A number of studies have described associations between low mean blood pressure and subsequent PIVH and neurological injury.[7,8,93-96] It was these observations of an association between systemic blood pressure and cerebral injury that led to current recommendations for treatment of blood pressure. Despite these statistical associations, a large population-based study has not found systemic hypotension to be an independent risk factor for PIVH in VLBW infants.[97] Furthermore, there is no evidence from appropriately designed, prospective, controlled clinical trials that treatment of hypotension decreases the incidence of PIVH and neurological injury.

Periventricular Leukomalacia

The potential relationship between low CBF and white matter injury due to the specific vulnerability of the periventricular white matter in the preterm infant has led to concerns that hypotension may be a precursor of white matter injury (Chapters 1, 2, and 16). Observational data again have shown a relationship between hypotension (often mean arterial blood pressure below 30 mm Hg) and adverse cranial ultrasound findings.[8] However, as with PIVH, larger population-based studies have failed to identify systemic hypotension as an independent risk factor for white matter injury.[98,99] It is conceivable that the pathogenesis of periventricular leukomalacia (PVL), just like that of PIVH, is multifactorial and, in addition to changes in cerebral perfusion pressure, factors such as specific or nonspecific inflammation and oxidant injury play a significant role in its development.

Long-Term Neurodevelopmental Outcome

Hypotension in VLBW infants has been correlated with longer-term adverse neurodevelopmental outcome.[95,96,100,101] There are no prospective studies evaluating the effect of untreated hypotension on any important long term outcomes; however there is a prospective study showing that hypotensive preterm infants had a significant increase in adverse neurodevelopmental outcome at term.[102] Several recent retrospective studies have raised the possibility that preterm infants treated for hypotension may have a worse outcome than untreated infants—it is unclear whether the effect is due to the treatment or other factors associated with hypotension.[58,96,103] Of note is that assessing all hypotensive patients as one group, regardless of their initial underlying physiology or response to treatment, is a significant further limitation of the retrospective studies. Interestingly, the findings of the only prospective randomized clinical trial addressing this issue revealed that hypotensive preterm VLBW neonates had a higher rate of severe PIVH compared with nonhypotensive controls.[103] However, the outcome of the hypotensive preterm neonates who responded to dopamine or epinephrine with an increase in blood pressure during the first postnatal day was the same as in the controls. Furthermore, there was no association between abnormal ultrasound findings and the use of vasopressors/inotropes. Finally, at 2- to 3-year follow-up, there was no difference in the rate of abnormal neurological outcome between survivors of the hypotensive and control groups. Although these findings provide some reassurance about the safety and potential benefits of vasopressors/inotropes for the treatment of early hypotension in VLBW neonates, the small sample size and the lack of an "untreated hypotensive group" limit the generalizability of the findings of this study.[103]

A study of systemic blood flow in VLBW infants demonstrated an independent relationship between low systemic blood flow (particularly the duration of the insult) and adverse neurodevelopmental outcome at 3 years of age.[104]

Treatment Options in the Management of Cardiovascular Compromise/Shock in the Very Low Birth Weight Infant

The appropriate management of shock in the VLBW infant will vary according to the underlying physiology. The clinician must take into account a number of possible factors including the infant's gestational age, postnatal age, measures of cardiovascular adequacy such as cardiac output or systemic blood flow if available, and associated pathologic conditions. An early echocardiogram can assist greatly in the diagnostic process by providing information about the presence, size, and direction of the ductus arteriosus shunt, presence of pulmonary hypertension, assessment of cardiac contractility, adequacy of venous filling, and measurement of cardiac output or systemic blood flow.

Before instituting specific treatment for hypotension potentially reversible causes such as a measurement error (transducer height in comparison to patient's right atrium, calibration of the transducer, air bubble, or blood clot in the measurement catheter), PDA hypovolemia from blood or fluid loss, pneumothorax, use of excessive mean airway pressure, sepsis, and adrenocortical insufficiency should be considered and managed appropriately. Therapeutic options that have a physiologic basis for efficacy and have been subjected to clinical trial include volume loading (with crystalloid or colloid), vasopressor/inotropes and inotropic agents, and hydrocortisone and other glucocorticoids. Table 12-1 suggests an approach to the use of these therapies according to the likely underlying mechanism of cardiovascular compromise and Table 12-2 summarizes the data regarding each individual intervention.

Closing the Ductus Arteriosus

A large and unconstricted ductus arteriosus has been associated with hypotension on the first postnatal day.[53] Early assessment of the ductus arteriosus in infants who are hypotensive for no obvious reason may demonstrate a large PDA that could be closed using a cyclooxygenase inhibitor such as indomethacin or ibuprofen. There are no trials of the use of cyclooxygenase inhibitors being used primarily to treat hypotension; however, there is some evidence that they assist in maintenance of normal systemic blood flow.[105] The trials of prophylactic indomethacin have shown a reduced incidence of PIVH—stabilization of the transitional circulation may be one mechanism for this effect. This effect, however, must be weighed against the potential of these agents to reduce CBF.[106] The hemodynamic effect of a large unconstricted PDA (>1.5 mm on color Doppler measurement) on the transitional circulation of the preterm infant can be significant and sometimes results in other complications such as the development of pulmonary hemorrhagic edema.[107,108] Use of a cyclooxygenase inhibitor to close a large unconstricted PDA associated with vasopressor/inotrope unresponsive hypotension should be considered during the first postnatal days (Chapter 13).[109] Alternatively, in infants with hypotension and a large PDA, dopamine at doses of 8-10 mcg/kg/min may increase systemic blood pressure and pulmonary vascular resistance resulting in a reduction of left to right shunt.[110]

Volume Expansion

Hypotension on the first postnatal day in the VLBW infant is rarely associated with absolute hypovolemia unless there has been significant perinatal blood loss. Hypovolemia should be suspected where there is pallor associated with tachycardia, especially in the setting of peripartum blood loss or a very tight nuchal cord. Infants with sepsis, particularly of later onset, can have significant absolute hypovolemia due to leakage of fluid into tissue spaces and may benefit from volume expansion.

Table 12-1   TREATMENT OPTIONS ACCORDING TO UNDERLYING MECHANISM OF
CARDIOVASCULAR COMPROMISE ON THE FIRST POSTNATAL DAY

Patient Group	Clinical Issues	Cardiovascular Parameters	Suggested Management
Extreme preterm infant during transitional period	Early low systemic blood flow	Normal or low BP Low blood flow/ cardiac output Large ductus arteriosus Higher systemic vascular resistance (unless born with chorioamnionitis) Poor myocardial contractility	Saline 10-20 mLs/kg Dobutamine 5-20 mcg/kg/ minute—adjust to blood flow Second-line: Add dopamine 5 mcg/kg/min titrate carefully to BP
VLBW infant with PDA	Low BP ± PDA signs	Low BP; Large PDA with left to right shunt	Indomethacin/ibuprofen first, then treatment of flow/pressure if required
VLBW infant with asphyxia	Myocardial damage Low systemic blood flow	Normal or low BP Poor myocardial contractility	Saline 10-20 mL/kg (care if myocardial function is affected) Dobutamine 5-20 mcg/ minute—adjust to blood flow Second-line: Add dopamine 5 mcg/kg/min titrate to BP (or low-dose epinephrine)
VLBW infant with suspected sepsis or chorioamnionitis—*High output*	High output cardiac failure secondary to sepsis	Normal or low BP High systemic blood flow Low systemic vascular resistance/capillary leak	Volume replacement—may require more than 20 mL/kg Dopamine 5 mcg/kg/min titrated to BP Second-line: Epinephrine 0.05 mcg/kg/min titrated to BP
VLBW infant with suspected sepsis or chorioamnionitis—*Low output*	Sepsis and poor myocardial function	Normal or low BP Normal or low systemic blood flow High systemic vascular resistance	Saline 10-20 mL/kg; dobutamine 15-20 mcg/ kg/min—adjust to blood flow Second-line: (low blood flow) epinephrine 0.05 mcg/kg/min Second-line: (hypotension) dopamine 5 mcg/kg/min titrate to BP (or epinephrine)
VLBW infant with acute fluid loss (intraventricular/ pulmonary hemorrhage)	Acute hypovolemia	Normal or low blood pressure Poor venous filling pressures	Volume replacement—may require more than 20 mLs/kg, including blood transfusion Dopamine 5 mcg/kg/min titrated to BP Second-line: Epinephrine 0.05 mcg/kg/min titrated to BP

Table 12-2 CARDIOVASCULAR INTERVENTIONS USED IN PRETERM INFANTS IN THE 1ST DAY

Intervention	Dose	Receptors/Effects	Indications	Considerations	Evidence
Volume (Normal saline or colloid)	10-20 mL/kg	Short term ↑ SBF	Hypovolemia suspected — perinatal blood loss, infant pale with ↑HR	No evidence of improved outcome. Excess fluid associated with increased mortality, PDA and CLD	Cohort[118] SR of RCTs[152]
Dobutamine	5-20 µg/kg/min	β: ↑ contractility, ↓ PVR/ SVR → ↑ SBF	1st line for low SBF Pulmonary hypertension Asphyxia	Corrects hypotension in 60%. Tachycardia if no volume expansion	SR of RCTs[118, 132]
Dopamine	2-10 mcg/kg/min	Dopamine: ↑ RBF and GFR. β: ↑ contractility, ↑ PVR/SVR α: ↑ SVR (± ↑ contractility) Net effect: ↑ BP, Ø or ↑ SBF (CBF)	Hypotension. Consider 2nd line for low SBF	In hypotensive infants may increase cerebral blood flow	SR of RCT[118, 132] RCT[120]
	>10µg/kg/min	α » β → ↑↑ SVR ↑↑ PVR Net effect: ↑↑ BP, Ø or ↓ SBF	Refractory hypotension Septic shock	May substantially reduce SBF	SR of RCT[118, 132]
Epinephrine	0.05-0.375 µg/kg/min	β > α: ↑ BP, ↑ SBF (CBF) ↑ SVR>PVR	Hypotension. Consider 2nd line for low SBF	In hypotensive infants may increase cerebral blood flow	RCT[120]
	>0.375 µg/kg/min	α > β: ↑↑ BP, ↑ SVR > PVR Net effect: ? ↓ SBF	Refractory hypotension Septic shock	May substantially reduce SBF	None in preterm
Hydrocortisone*	2-10 mg/kg/day in 2-4 divided doses	↑ SVR, ↑ BP, Ø or ↑ SBF∧	Refractory hypotension Adrenal insufficiency	Early steroids associated with intestinal perforation. High dose steroids ↑BSL	RCT[121] ∧ Prospective Observational[153]
Dexamethasone**	0.25 mg/kg single dose	↑ SVR, ↑ BP, unknown effect on SBF	Refractory hypotension Adrenal insufficiency	Early steroids associated with intestinal perforation. High dose steroids ↑BSL	RCT[154]
Milrinone	0.75µg/kg/min x 3 hours, then 0.2 µg/kg/min	Type III phosphodiesterase inhibitor: unknown effects on contractility; ↓SVR, ↓ PVR → ↑ SBF	Low SBF	May cause hypotension	RCT[5]

Modified from Osborn DA. Diagnosis and treatment of preterm transitional circulatory compromise. Early Hum Dev. 2005;81:413-422.
↑, increase; ↓, decrease; →, leads to; Ø, no change; BP, blood pressure; BSL, Blood sugar level; CBF, cerebral blood flow; CLD, chronic lung disease; GFR, glomerular filtration rate; HR, heart rate; PDA, patent ductus arteriosus; PVR, pulmonary vascular resistance; RBF, renal blood flow; RCT, randomized controlled trial; SBF, systemic blood flow; SR, systematic review; SVR, systemic vascular resistance.
*Recommended doses for low-dose hydrocortisone administration in VLBW neonates are 1 mg/kg/dose Q12 hours.
**Dexamethasone administration (even at low doses) to the VLBW neonates during the first postnatal week is NOT recommended.

12

Other clinical scenarios associated with absolute hypovolemia include infants with subgaleal hematomas or other intracavity hemorrhage. Studies of the relationship between the blood volume and blood pressure in premature infants show a poor correlation, suggesting that low blood volume is not synonymous with low blood pressure.[35,36,111] Similarly other groups have found that infants with hypotension and associated acidosis have reduced left ventricular output and impaired cardiac contractility.[33] The usefulness of volume expansion in this setting is questionable as it may lead to a worsening of cardiac function and cardiogenic failure. Routine use of volume expansion in preterm infants on the first day to improve outcome is not supported by the evidence.[112]

There appears to be little difference in the efficacy between crystalloid and colloid solutions in the treatment of systemic hypotension.[113,114] There have been concerns over the use of 5% albumin in older children and adults in intensive care settings and an association with increased morbidity.[115] Colloid solutions are more expensive than normal saline and are derived from donated blood with the associated risk of blood-borne infection. In the VLBW infant the increased capillary permeability may contribute to leakage of albumin into the extravascular compartment increasing tissue oncotic pressure and resulting in tissue fluid retention, impaired gas exchange in the lungs and potentially causing injury to the brain. Randomized trials have shown improvement in blood pressure in hypotensive infants given volume but no change in short or long term outcomes. In infants who have had an identified fluid loss such as a hemorrhage at the time of delivery or excessive transepidermal water loss with excessive weight loss from use of radiant heat, replacement with the type of fluid lost is appropriate. Volume expansion probably increases LV output, but it is less effective than inotropes at increasing the blood pressure. One trial showed dopamine to be more effective than plasma in improving the blood pressure in hypotensive preterm infants.[116] Observational studies have shown a short-term improvement in systemic blood flow after volume expansion.[62]

As the accurate diagnosis of absolute or relative hypovolemia is difficult in the neonate and hypovolemia results in reduced efficacy of vasopressor-inotropes, it is reasonable to initially treat hypotension with 10-20 mL/kg of normal saline solution over 30-60 minutes. Trials that have used a volume load before giving an inotrope (i.e., dobutamine) reported no reflex tachycardia in response to the inotrope, suggesting that volume load may lessen the reduction in preload that occurs with vasodilation potentially associated with the use of dobutamine. In an infant requiring positive pressure respiratory support, even if the infant is not hypovolemic, a volume load may increase the central venous pressure sufficiently to improve venous return to the heart. As there is an association between excess fluid administration in premature infants and adverse outcomes including increased incidence of PDA, necrotizing enterocolitis, chronic lung disease, and mortality, excessive and inappropriate administration of volume should be avoided.[117] If normalization of the blood pressure is not achieved with a single dose of volume replacement, then early initiation of a vasopressor-inotrope or an inotrope should be the next step considered.

Vasopressor-Inotropes, Inotropes, and Lusitropes

These agents have been used in neonates for many years in the treatment of hypotension. Vasopressor-inotropes, such as dopamine and epinephrine, increase both myocardial contractility and systemic vascular resistance (SVR), inotropes, such as dobutamine, increase myocardial contractility and exert a variable vasodilatory action on the periphery, and lusitropes, such as milrinone, work primarily as peripheral vasodilators with a variable degree of inotropy or no inotropic effect (Fig. 12-5). They were introduced without randomized and blinded trials and there is still no evidence that use of these treatments improves important neonatal outcomes such as death and disability. Studies of vasopressor-inotropes and inotropes have focused on the effect on blood pressure and only recently have the effects of these medications on cardiac output, the main determinant of oxygen delivery to tissues, been taken into account.[55,118] The mechanisms of action of these vasoactive agents are complex and affected by the developmental maturation of the cardiovascular and

+DOB's efficacy is independent of affinity for ARs ++DA also has serotoninergic actions	Adrenergic, Dopaminergic and Vasopressin Receptors					
	α₁/α₂ Vascular	β₁/β₂ Vascular	α₁ Cardiac	β₁/β₂ Cardiac	DA1/DA2 Vascular/Cardiac	V1a Vascular
Phenylephrine	++++	0	+	0	0	0
Norepinephrine	++++	0/+	++	++++	0	0
Epinephrine	++++	+++	++	++++	0	0
Dopamine++	++++	++	++	+++	++++	0
Dobutamine+	+/0	++	++	++++	0	0
Isuprenaline	0	+++	0	++++	0	0
Vasopressin	0	0	0	0	0	++++
PDE-III Inhibitors*	0	0	0	0	0	0
PDE-V Inhibitors**	0	0	0	0	0	0

Figure 12-5 Myocardial and vascular smooth muscle alpha- and beta-adrenergic, dopaminergic, serotoninergic, and vasopressor receptor-stimulatory effects of vasopressors, inotropes, and lusitropes. ARs, adrenergic receptors; DA, dopamine; DOB, dobutamine; PDE, phosphodieterase; V, vasopressin; *, milrinone, amrinone; **, sildenafil.

autonomic nervous systems. Consequently these agents can alter the relationship between the systemic blood pressure and systemic blood flow and, if only the blood pressure is monitored, a change in the blood flow may not be appreciated during treatment.

Dopamine

Dopamine is the most commonly used sympathomimetic amine for the treatment of hypotension in the VLBW infant. Dopamine is a precursor to both epinephrine and norepinephrine, but is also a naturally occurring catecholamine. The drug stimulates the cardiovascular alpha- and beta-adrenergic and dopaminergic receptors in a dose-dependent manner.[119] Manifestation of the hemodynamic actions of dopamine (and the other sympathomimetic amines) is affected by several factors. These include the level of expression of the adrenergic receptors and intracellular signaling systems, adrenal function, developmentally regulated maturity of the myocardium, and the dysregulated release of local vasodilators, such as endogenous nitric oxide and vasodilatory prostaglandins.[6] Fig. 12-6 illustrates the dose-dependent cardiovascular and renal actions of dopamine.

Potential cardiovascular and renal side effects of dopamine administration include tachycardia, hypertension and/or decreased systemic perfusion (at high doses) and increased urinary sodium, phosphorous, free water, and bicarbonate losses.[119] Dopamine also plays a role in the short-term physiologic regulation of sodium-potassium-ATPase activity and exerts certain endocrine and paracrine actions.[119] These effects include but are not limited to the temporary inhibition of prolactin, thyroid-stimulating hormone, growth hormone, and gonadotropin release from the pituitary and increased renin-angiotensin activity. Additionally, dopamine plays a role in the peripheral regulation of breathing and influences certain aspects of leukocyte function.[119] It is unclear whether these transient endocrine and paracrine dopaminergic actions have short- or long-term clinical significance in the preterm neonate.

Dopamine administered exogenously acts via dopaminergic and adrenergic receptors, with varying effects at different doses. At lower doses it acts via increasing

DOSE-DEPENDENT EFFECTS OF DOPAMINE IN NEONATES*

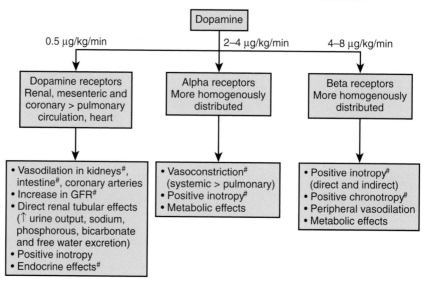

* Without adrenoreceptor downregulation
# Demonstrated effects in preterm neonates

Figure 12-6 In the preterm neonate, low doses of dopamine stimulate the dopaminergic receptors. At low-to-medium doses, effects of alpha-adrenergic receptor stimulation also appear. At medium-to-high doses (>8-10 mcg/kg/min), effects of both beta- and alpha-receptor stimulation dominate the hemodynamic response to the drug. However, this response is influenced by several factors (e.g., state of cardiovascular adrenergic receptor expression) regulated by the level of maturity and disease severity. See text for details. (Modified from Seri I. Management of hypotension and low systemic blood flow in the very low birth weight neonate during the first postnatal week. J Perinatol. 2006;26:S8-S13.)

myocardial contractility in a dose-dependent fashion, but at higher doses (>10 mcg/kg/min), peripheral vasoconstriction and increased afterload play an increasing role in its effect on blood pressure. It is this increase in the afterload that may also affect cardiac function, particularly in the very preterm infant in whom the immature ventricle may not be as capable of maintaining cardiac output with increasing peripheral vascular resistance. Accordingly, lower doses of dopamine or use of an inotrope may be prudent in the VLBW infant especially during the first postnatal days. Interestingly, though, low-to-medium doses of dopamine and epinephrine have recently been shown to be similarly effective at increasing both blood pressure and CBF in hypotensive VLBW neonates during the first postnatal day.[120] There is a significant degree of variability in response to dopamine dose between individual infants with gestational age and illness severity being important variables. Most infants have a cardiovascular response to dopamine in a dose range less than 20 mcg/kg/min with the majority of low birth weight infants responding to a dopamine dose of less than 10 mcg/kg/min.[55,121,122] Improvements in blood pressure and left ventricular function have been seen at doses as low as 2 mcg/kg/min.[56,123,124] In VLBW infants, dopamine should initially be commenced at a low to medium dose (2-5 mcg/kg/min) and increased according to the response of the blood pressure. Most clinicians are reluctant to increase the dose of dopamine to more than 20 mcg/kg/min due to concerns of excessive peripheral vasoconstriction, even though there is little evidence of harm if the treatment is for hypotension caused by vasodilation.[119,125] Addition of a second pharmacological agent is preferred. Tachyphylaxis to dopamine is common with low doses having a significant clinical effect initially, but with the need for increasing doses of dopamine or addition of another agent with time.[126]

CARDIOVASCULAR EFFECTS OF DOBUTAMINE IN NEONATES*

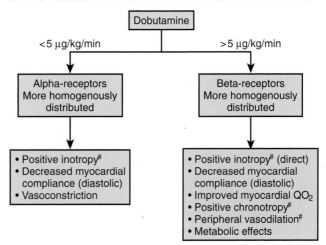

* Without adrenoreceptor downregulation
# Demonstrated effects in preterm neonates

Figure 12-7 In the preterm neonate, dobutamine increases cardiac output and exerts a variable degree of a peripheral vasodilatory effect. The cardiovascular response is influenced by several factors (e.g., state of cardiovascular adrenergic receptor expression) regulated by the level of maturity and disease severity. See text for details. (Modified from Seri I. Management of hypotension and low systemic blood flow in the very low birth weight neonate during the first postnatal week. J Perinatol. 2006;26:S8-S13.)

Dobutamine

Dobutamine is an inotropic synthetic sympathomimetic amine, which has complex cardiovascular actions, increasing myocardial contractility via stimulation of the myocardial adrenergic receptors.[127] In addition, it exerts a variable peripheral vasodilatory effect via the stimulation of the peripheral cardiovascular beta-adrenergic receptors.[128] In contrast to dopamine, dobutamine does not rely on the release of endogenous catecholamines for its positive inotropic action.[119] Although it also has some stimulatory effect on peripheral cardiovascular alpha-adrenergic receptors, its affinity to the peripheral cardiovascular beta-adrenergic receptors is higher. Due to these complex actions, the most frequently seen net cardiovascular effects of dobutamine are an increase in myocardial contractility and a variable degree of peripheral vasodilation.[128] These effects are present even in the preterm neonate and make dobutamine particularly suited to treatment of hypotension in neonates with associated myocardial dysfunction and low cardiac output.[55,129,130] Figure 12-7 illustrates the maturation-dependent cardiovascular actions of dobutamine. Cardiovascular response to dobutamine has been demonstrated via left ventricular performance at doses as low as 5 mcg/kg/min and increases in cardiac output and systemic blood flow at doses of 10-20 mcg/kg/minute.[55,118,131]

Cardiovascular side effects of dobutamine administration include tachycardia, undesirable decreases in blood pressure due to the drug's potential peripheral vasodilatory effects and, at higher doses, dobutamine may impair diastolic performance and thus compromise preload. This latter action is caused by a drug-induced decrease in the compliance of the myocardium as a result of a significant increase in the myocardial tone.

Dobutamine has been compared with dopamine in several randomized trials but, as with dopamine, has never been subjected to trial against placebo or no treatment in newborns. Systematic review of five randomized trials found that dopamine is better than dobutamine at increasing blood pressure in hypotensive preterm infants, but to date has not been better at improving clinical outcomes (including PIVH and PVL) in hypotensive preterm infants.[132] In contrast, in a randomized clinical trial using a crossover design in infants with low systemic blood flow in the first postnatal day, dobutamine administered at 10 and 20 mcg/kg/min was more effective at increasing blood flow than dopamine given at the same two doses.[118] Similarly, infants who received dobutamine as treatment for hypotension in another randomized trial were more likely to increase their cardiac output than infants who received dopamine, while dopamine was more effective at increasing blood pressure.[55] These findings can be explained by the differences in the effects on peripheral vascular resistance between the two drugs with dopamine significantly increasing SVR while dobutamine has little or even a decreasing effect on SVR. An understanding of the mechanisms of action of both of these drugs and their effect on the various vascular beds as well as that of the underlying pathogenesis of shock in the preterm infant is of utmost importance to guide the treatment of any cardiovascular compromise.

Epinephrine

Epinephrine is an endogenous catecholamine released from the adrenal gland medulla in response to stress. At low doses, it enhances myocardial contractility and causes some peripheral vasodilation via its beta-adrenergic effects. At higher doses, there is a significant alpha-adrenergic effect causing peripheral vasoconstriction and increased afterload. Administration of epinephrine results in increases in blood pressure and tissue perfusion by increasing cardiac output and systemic vascular resistance.[120] Figure 12-8 illustrates the dose-dependent cardiovascular actions of epinephrine.

Cardiovascular side effects of epinephrine include tachycardia, systemic hypertension and/or decreased systemic perfusion at medium to high doses as well as lactic acidosis due to the drug's potent metabolic actions.[120] As epinephrine is a more potent vasoconstrictor than dopamine, accidental purging of the infusion when changing the syringe or when priming the line may lead to significant and sudden increases in blood pressure and decreases in systemic perfusion. As these effects, especially in the VLBW neonate, may result in intracranial pathology, care must be taken when epinephrine is being administered. In addition, the drug-induced

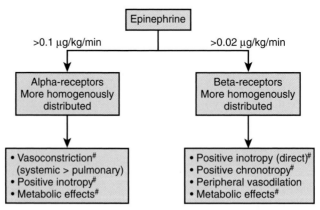

CARDIOVASCULAR EFFECTS OF EPINEPHRINE IN NEONATES*

* Without adrenoreceptor downregulation
# Demonstrated effects in preterm neonates

Figure 12-8   In the preterm neonate, at low to medium doses of epinephrine administration, effects of beta- and then alpha-adrenergic receptor stimulation become apparent. The cardiovascular response is influenced by several factors (e.g., state of cardiovascular adrenergic receptor expression, etc) regulated by the level of maturity and disease severity. See text for details. (Modified from Seri I. Management of hypotension and low systemic blood flow in the very low birth weight neonate during the first postnatal week. J Perinatol. 2006;26:S8-S13.)

increase in lactic acidosis may make it more difficult to assess the improvement in the hemodynamic status of the hypotensive preterm neonate receiving epinephrine and may prompt inappropriate volume administration, increases in epinephrine dose, or both.

There is only one published controlled trial of the use of epinephrine in neonates, but despite this epinephrine is often used in refractory hypotension in neonates.[133] In a single trial comparing low-moderate dose dopamine and low dose epinephrine in hypotensive very preterm infants in the first day, similar increases were reported in CBF and oxygenation as measured by near-infrared spectroscopy. Both vasopressor-inotropes were equally efficacious at increasing blood pressure. No other clinical benefits to either medication were reported.[120] No differences were found between groups at two-year neurodevelopmental follow-up.[103] As epinephrine at higher doses has a peripheral vasoconstrictive effect it may be of particular use in infants with pathologic peripheral vasodilation due to septic shock. The dose range used in neonates ranges from 0.05 to 2.6 mcg/kg/min or beyond.[133]

Milrinone

Milrinone is a phosphodiesterase-3 inhibitor and therefore it increases intracellular cyclic adenosine monophosphate (cAMP) concentrations. In the adult, it has both a positive inotropic effect (particularly improving myocardial diastolic function) and a peripheral vasodilatory effect. Although this combination of actions is potentially very efficacious in preterm infants in the first postnatal hours, where the immature myocardium is struggling against the increased afterload of the postnatal circulation, it is not known if milrinone acts as true inotrope in the neonate. Indeed, findings of studies in immature animal models show that class III phosphodiesterase inhibitors such as amrinone have minimal, no, or even negative inotropic effects.[134-136] It has been suggested that the developmentally regulated variation in the effect of phosphodiesterase inhibitors on myocardial contractility is a consequence of the developmental imbalance between class III and IV phosphodiesterases in the sarcoplasmic reticulum of the immature myocardium.[137] However, these negative inotropic effects exhibited in the neonatal puppies become positive within a few days after birth.[136] Indeed, milrinone has been shown to be effective in treatment of low cardiac output syndrome (LCOS) in infants post cardiac surgery by increasing cardiac output. LCOS in this patient population is associated with a rise in both systemic and pulmonary resistance.[138,139] The ability of the myocardium to adapt to an increased afterload is compromised by the effects of cardiac bypass, similarly to the myocardium of the preterm infant in transition, which may be compromised by the postnatal changes in afterload. In a multicenter randomized trial, there was a dose dependent reduction of incidence of LCOS when milrinone was used preventatively in infants after cardiac surgery.[140] A multicenter randomized controlled study of the use of milrinone in preterm infants using a modified dosing regime to prevent low blood flow demonstrated that the potential side effect of significant hypotension was not seen and all infants maintained adequate cardiac output when compared with historical controls.[5]

Vasopressin

There is limited evidence from uncontrolled clinical trials that VLBW infants with severe hypotension unresponsive to catecholamines may respond to vasopressin, particularly in the setting of sepsis. Doses used were 0.01-0.04 units/kg/hr. Potential side effects include splanchnic hypoperfusion, oliguria-anuria, and intraventricular hemorrhage.[141]

Treatment of Very Low Birth Weight Neonates with Vasopressor-Resistant Shock

More than 50% of hypotensive VLBW infants requiring dopamine at doses greater than 10 mcg/kg/min during the immediate postnatal period cannot be weaned off the drug for well over 3-4 days and many develop vasopressor-resistant hypotension.[6,39,142,143] These VLBW neonates with vasopressor dependence or with vasopressor-resistant hypotension often respond to relatively low doses of hydrocortisone with an improvement in blood pressure and urine output and frequently wean off vasopressor support within 24-72 hours.[6,39,142-145] The clinically relevant cellular mechanisms of vasopressor resistance, the characteristics of relative and absolute adrenal insufficiency, and the pharmacokinetics and side effects of corticosteroids (hydrocortisone and dexamethasone) in the preterm and term neonate are described in detail in Chapters 1 and 14.

Presentation and Management of Cardiovascular Compromise in the Very Low Birth Weight Infant on the First Postnatal Day

There are several different potential mechanisms that result in hypotension and/or decreased systemic blood flow on the first postnatal day. Each of these mechanisms needs to be considered individually when planning appropriate assessment and treatment:

- Delay in the adaptation of the immature myocardium to the sudden increase in systemic vascular resistance occurring at birth (transient myocardial dysfunction)
- Peripheral vasodilation and hyperdynamic myocardial function primarily in VLBW neonates born to mothers with chorioamnionitis
- Perinatal depression with secondary myocardial dysfunction and/or abnormal peripheral vasoregulation

    Some insight into the appropriate combination of therapies can be obtained by looking beyond just the measurement of blood pressure and beginning to assess other parameters that impact upon the cardiovascular adequacy. The underlying cause for cardiovascular compromise should be sought from the history, the physical examination, and by utilizing other available information such as that obtained from functional echocardiography.

Transient Myocardial Dysfunction

During the first postnatal day, VLBW neonates may present with shock because of the inability of the immature myocardium to pump against the increased peripheral vascular resistance occurring in the immediate period after delivery.[146] While attempting to maintain adequate perfusion pressure, the immature neonate's vasoconstrictive vasoregulatory response to decreased systemic perfusion may include cerebral vasoconstriction in addition to vasoconstriction in the vascular beds of the nonvital organs. The more immature the neonate, the higher the likelihood that systemic (and cerebral) hypoperfusion will occur during the first postnatal day.[3,18] Although a significant number of these patients will also be hypotensive, in others blood pressure may remain within the normal range. Thus, despite having "normal" blood pressure, some of these neonates may have a temporarily compromised CBF. Recognition of this presentation requires the ability to assess CBF at the bedside using functional echocardiography and/or NIR spectroscopy (Chapters 5 and 7).[3,9,16,19,118]

    Management of this presentation of circulatory compromise is difficult and findings in the literature are somewhat contradictory. In a series of studies using SVC blood flow as a surrogate measure of CBF in VLBW neonates during the first postnatal day, Evans et al. described the hemodynamics of systemic and cerebral hypoperfusion, the relationship between recovery from hypoperfusion and the development of PIVH, the weak relationship between SVC blood flow and systemic blood pressure, and the association between neurodevelopmental outcome at 3 years of age and low SVC blood flow during the first 24 postnatal hours.[3,18,34,104] In addition, this group performed a randomized blinded clinical trial with a crossover design to compare the effects of dopamine and dobutamine at 10 and 20 mcg/kg/min on SVC flow and blood pressure in VLBW neonates during the first postnatal day.[118] They found that dopamine improved systemic blood pressure more effectively in this group of infants, while dobutamine was better at increasing SVC flow at the two doses tested. Since pharmacodynamics rather than pharmacokinetics determine the cardiovascular response to these sympathomimetic amines, the limitation of this study was the lack of stepwise titration of the drugs in the search for the optimal hemodynamic response. Indeed, a recent study using continuous NIR spectroscopy monitoring to assess the relative changes in CBF demonstrated that, by stepwise titration of dopamine or epinephrine, both drugs are equally effective in the low-to-moderate dose range at improving blood pressure and CBF in VLBW neonates during the first postnatal day.[120] It is of note that, although the use of continuous NIRS monitoring to assess cerebral intravascular oxygenation and cerebral blood volume allows for data collection for a longer period of time (hours) and provides reliable information for the relative changes in these parameters, the absolute values are not known when one uses the continuous NIR spectroscopy measurements rather than intermittently checks for absolute CBF values with NIR spectroscopy.

Finally, findings using multiple (not continuous) measurements of CBF by NIR spectroscopy to assess the response of CBF and blood pressure to dopamine in ELBW neonates during the first two postnatal days suggest that these patients respond to moderate-to-high doses of dopamine with an increase in both the blood pressure and CBF.[10] However, although CBF returns to the presumed normal range as blood pressure normalizes, its autoregulation remains impaired. The authors also calculated the lower elbow of the autoregulatory curve in their patients and found that it is around 29 mm Hg. One of the limitations of the findings is that the bilinear regression analysis used in this study combines two small patient populations predefined by treatment criteria. The findings of this study also suggest that, once CBF autoregulation is lost in preterm neonates, it does not recover immediately after the normalization of the blood pressure with dopamine. Indeed, findings of an earlier study support this notion and indicate that, in sick preterm neonates, it may take up to 30-50 minutes or more for CBF autoregulation to recover after blood pressure has been normalized.[56] Another approach to the treatment of poor systemic perfusion in the 1-day-old VLBW neonate was investigated in a double blind randomized clinical trial using prophylactic milrinone within 6 hours of delivery in an attempt to prevent systemic hypoperfusion.[5] Prophylactic milrinone in a high-risk group of infants did not prevent low systemic blood flow in the first 24 hours. As there were minimal side effects (particularly hypotension) ascribed to milrinone, one might speculate that somewhat higher doses of milrinone would have been more effective in preventing low systemic blood flow.

In summary, treatment of the hypotensive 1-day old VLBW neonate remains complex even if systemic perfusion can be assessed by functional echocardiography. The use and stepwise titration of low-to-moderate dose dopamine or epinephrine to achieve mean blood pressure values somewhat higher than the gestational age of the patient is a preferred approach during the first postnatal day by most neonatologists especially if systemic perfusion can only be assessed by less reliable indirect signs of systemic hemodynamics such as urine output and CRT.[20,56,119,120] If there is evidence of myocardial dysfunction, dobutamine is the first-line medication and low-dose dopamine may be added if blood pressure decreases upon initiation of dobutamine administration. However, one must bear in mind that systemic vascular resistance should only be increased very carefully by dopamine as it may induce further decreases in the cardiac output secondary to the myocardial dysfunction. If assessment of systemic perfusion (SVC flow or ventricular output measures) is available, the systemic hemodynamic effects of the careful titration of a vasopressor-inotrope (dopamine or epinephrine) or an inotrope (dobutamine) can be followed.[3] Finally, it is important to note that it is not known whether the use of dopamine or dobutamine as the first-line vasoactive agent in the treatment of hypotension in the 1-day-old VLBW neonate has a more favorable impact on mortality and short- or long-term morbidity.

Vasodilation and Hyperdynamic Myocardial Function

Data indicate that VLBW neonates born after chorioamnionitis, especially if they also present with funisitis, develop hypotension and increased cardiac output within a few hours after delivery.[147] The presentation of hypotension with increased cardiac output suggests that systemic vascular resistance is lower in VLBW neonates born after chorioamnionitis. These alterations in the cardiovascular function correlate with cord blood interleukin-6 levels.[147] In addition, the presence of maternal fever or a neonatal immature-to-total (I/T) white blood cell ratio over 0.4 is associated with decreased left ventricular fractional shortening. In summary, these findings indicate that, in VLBW neonates born after chorioamnionitis, hypotension is primarily caused by vasodilation although a variable degree of myocardial dysfunction may also contribute to the hemodynamic disturbance especially in neonates with an increased I/T ratio.

Based on these findings, treatment of hypotension in the 1-day-old VLBW neonate born after chorioamnionitis should be tailored to address both components of the cardiovascular compromise (vasodilation and potential myocardial dysfunction). In these cases, dobutamine administration alone may lead to further decreases in systemic vascular resistance especially in patients with increased cardiac output and little or no myocardial compromise. Therefore, carefully titrated low-to-moderate doses of dopamine (or epinephrine) will likely be effective in these patients. However, dopamine or epinephrine at higher doses may increase systemic vascular resistance to levels where cardiac output may be compromised and, despite improving blood pressures, systemic blood flow may decrease. Thus, if functional echocardiography is not available, the indirect measures of tissue perfusion (urine output, CRT, base deficit, and/or serum lactate levels) should be carefully followed to monitor for the state of blood flow to the organs and vasopressor support needs to be adjusted accordingly.

Perinatal Depression with Secondary Myocardial Dysfunction and/or Abnormal Peripheral Vasoregulation

Perinatal asphyxia with secondary myocardial dysfunction occurs in both term and VLBW infants.[148] Administration of volume in this setting is common as the infant is often thought to be poorly perfused and hypotensive. There is however little evidence that this group of infants is hypovolemic unless there has been specific blood loss or a tight nuchal cord as discussed earlier.[149] The perfusion will usually improve with adequate resuscitation and respiratory support. Preterm infants with evidence of perinatal asphyxia and multiorgan dysfunction require careful management of fluid balance to prevent volume overload and subsequent cardiac failure—in this group inotropes such as dobutamine (and maybe milrinone) are probably of most use. Administration of excessive volume in the setting of asphyxia, with the added risk of an underlying myocardial injury being present, may result in fluid overload and cardiogenic heart failure.[150] In this situation, the judicious use of a vasopressor-inotrope such as dopamine or an inotrope such as dobutamine is preferable.[124,151] There is some suggestion that a hypoxic-ischemic insult may also impair proper peripheral vasoregulation resulting in an infant who is unable to adjust blood pressure in response to physiologic changes. However, direct evidence for this notion is lacking due to the difficulties in appropriately assessing peripheral vascular resistance.

Conclusion

The appropriate assessment and treatment of the VLBW infant with cardiovascular impairment or shock requires the clinician to obtain adequate information about the etiology and underlying physiologic determinants of the condition. The clinician should be aware of the physiologic changes that occur in areas such as myocardial

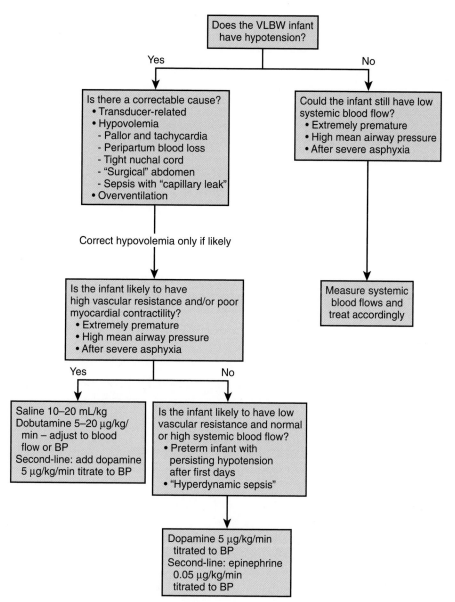

Figure 12-9 Treatment of cardiovascular compromise based on clinical findings. (Adapted from Subhedar NV. Treatment of hypotension in newborns. Semin Neonatol. 2003;8:413-423.)

function and vital organ blood supply allocation in the first postnatal days. An understanding of the actions of the therapeutic options available and the specific effects of these treatments on the circulation of the VLBW infant is also important (Table 12-2). Figure 12-9 shows an approach to the management of hypotension in the VLBW infant based on clinical information. The addition of a functional echocardiogram to the assessment process provides information about the size and shunt direction of the ductus arteriosus, the function of the myocardium and its filling as well as about the cardiac output and calculated peripheral vascular resistance. Figure 12-10 summarizes the approach to management of hypotension in the VLBW infant using the additional information provided by the functional echocardiogram.

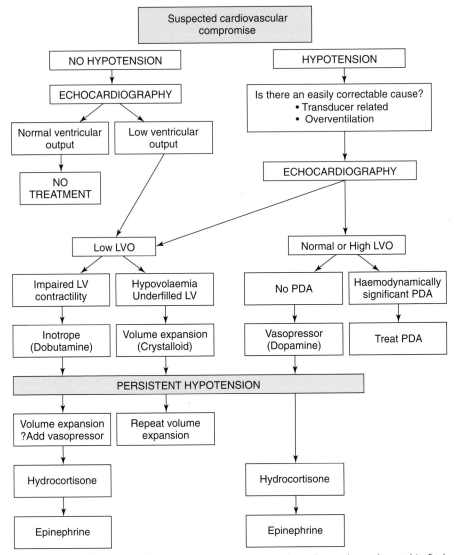

Figure 12-10 Treatment of cardiovascular compromise based on echocardiographic findings. (Adapted from Subhedar NV. Treatment of hypotension in newborns. Semin Neonatol. 2003;8:413-423.)

References

1. Al Aweel I, Pursley DM, Rubin LP, et al. Variations in prevalence of hypotension, hypertension, and vasopressor use in NICUs. J Perinatol. 2001;21:272-278.
2. Laughon M, Bose C, Allred E, et al. Factors associated with treatment for hypotension in extremely low gestational age newborns during the first postnatal week. Pediatrics. 2007;119:273-280.
3. Kluckow M, Evans N. Superior vena cava flow in preterm infants: a novel marker of systemic blood flow. Arch Dis Child Fetal Neonatal Ed. 2000;82:182-187.
4. Miletin J, Dempsey EM. Low superior vena cava flow on day 1 and adverse outcome in the very low birthweight infant. Arch Dis Child Fetal Neonatal Ed. 2008;93:F368-F371.
5. Paradisis M, Evans N, Kluckow M, et al. Randomized trial of milrinone versus placebo for prevention of low systemic blood flow in very preterm infants. J Pediatr. 2009;154:189-195.
6. Seri I. Circulatory support of the sick preterm infant. Seminars in Neonatology. 2001;6:85-95.
7. Watkins AM, West CR, Cooke RW. Blood pressure and cerebral haemorrhage and ischaemia in very low birthweight infants. Early Hum Dev. 1989;19:103-110.
8. Miall-Allen VM, de Vries LS, Whitelaw AG. Mean arterial blood pressure and neonatal cerebral lesions. Arch Dis Child. 1987;62:1068-1069.
9. Tsuji M, Saul JP, du Plessis A, et al. Cerebral intravascular oxygenation correlates with mean arterial pressure in critically ill premature infants. Pediatrics. 2000;106:625-632.

10. Munro MJ, Walker AM, Barfield CP. Hypotensive extremely low birth weight infants have reduced cerebral blood flow. Pediatrics. 2004;114:1591-1596.
11. Nuntnarumit P, Yang W, Bada-Ellzey HS. Blood pressure measurements in the newborn. Clin Perinatol. 1999;26:981-996.
12. Hegyi T, Carbone MT, Anwar M, et al. Blood pressure ranges in premature infants. I. The first hours of life. J Pediatr. 1994;124:627-633.
13. Development of audit measures and guidelines for good practice in the management of neonatal respiratory distress syndrome: report of a joint working group of the British Association of Perinatal Medicine and the research unit of the Royal College of Physicians. Arch Dis Child. 1992;67: 1221-1227.
14. Greisen G, Borch K. White matter injury in the preterm neonate: the role of perfusion. Developmental Neuroscience. 2001;23:209-212.
15. Greisen G. Autoregulation of cerebral blood flow in newborn babies. Early Hum Dev. 2005; 81:423-428.
16. Tyszczuk L, Meek J, Elwell C, et al. Cerebral blood flow is independent of mean arterial blood pressure in preterm infants undergoing intensive care. Pediatrics. 1998;102:337-341.
17. Seri I, Abbasi S, Wood DC, et al. Regional hemodynamic effects of dopamine in the sick preterm neonate. J Pediatr. 1998;133:728-734.
18. Kluckow M, Evans N. Low superior vena cava flow and intraventricular haemorrhage in preterm infants. Arch Dis Child Fetal Neonatal Ed. 2000;82:188-194.
19. Kissack CM, Garr R, Wardle SP, et al. Cerebral fractional oxygen extraction in very low birth weight infants is high when there is low left ventricular output and hypocarbia but is unaffected by hypotension. Pediatr Res. 2004;55:400-405.
20. Seri I. Hemodynamics during the first two postnatal days and neurodevelopment in preterm neonates. J Pediatr. 2004;145:573-575.
21. Friedman AH, Fahey JT. The transition from fetal to neonatal circulation: normal responses and implications for infants with heart disease. Semin Perinatol. 1993;17:106-121.
22. Mahoney LT, Coryell KG, Lauer RM. The newborn transitional circulation: a two-dimensional Doppler echocardiographic study. J Am Coll Cardiol. 1985;6:623-629.
23. Gentile R, Stevenson G, Dooley T, et al. Pulsed Doppler echocardiographic determination of time of ductal closure in normal newborn infants. J Pediatr. 1981;98:443-448.
24. Evans N, Iyer P. Longitudinal changes in the diameter of the ductus arteriosus in ventilated preterm infants: correlation with respiratory outcomes. Arch Dis Child Fetal Neonatal Ed. 1995;72: F156-F161.
25. Seidner SR, Chen YQ, Oprysko PR, et al. Combined prostaglandin and nitric oxide inhibition produces anatomic remodeling and closure of the ductus arteriosus in the premature newborn baboon. Pediatr Res. 2001;50:365-373.
26. Evans N, Iyer P. Assessment of ductus arteriosus shunt in preterm infants supported by mechanical ventilation: effects of interatrial shunting. J Pediatr. 1994;125:778-785.
27. Agata Y, Hiraishi S, Oguchi K, et al. Changes in left ventricular output from fetal to early neonatal life. J Pediatr. 1991;119:441-445.
28. Drayton MR, Skidmore R. Ductus arteriosus blood flow during first 48 hours of life. Arch Dis Child. 1987;62:1030-1034.
29. Kluckow M, Evans N. Low systemic blood flow in the preterm infant. Semin Neonatol. 2001; 6:75-84.
30. Teitel DF. Physiologic development of the cardiovascular system in the fetus. In: Polin RA, Fox WW, eds. Fetal and neonatal physiology. Philadelphia: WB Saunders; 1998:827-836.
31. Weindling AM, Kissack CM. Blood pressure and tissue oxygenation in the newborn baby at risk of brain damage. Biol Neonate. 2001;79:241-245.
32. Osborn D, Evans N, Kluckow M. Diagnosis and treatment of low systemic blood flow in preterm infants. NeoReviews. 2004;5:e109-e121.
33. Gill AB, Weindling. AM Echocardiographic assessment of cardiac function in shocked very low birthweight infants. Arch Dis Child. 1993;68:17-21.
34. Kluckow M, Evans N. Relationship between blood pressure and cardiac output in preterm infants requiring mechanical ventilation. J Pediatr. 1996;129:506-512.
35. Bauer K, Linderkamp O, Versmold HT. Systolic blood pressure and blood volume in preterm infants. Arch Dis Child. 1993;69:521-522.
36. Barr PA, Bailey PE, Sumners J, et al. Relation between arterial blood pressure and blood volume and effect of infused albumin in sick preterm infants. Pediatrics. 1977;60:282-289.
37. Lopez SL, Leighton JO, Walther FJ. Supranormal cardiac output in the dopamine- and dobutamine-dependent preterm infant. Pediatr Cardiol. 1997;18:292-296.
38. Pladys P, Wodey E, Beuchee A, et al. Left ventricle output and mean arterial blood pressure in preterm infants during the 1st day of life. Eur J Pediatr. 1999;158:817-824.
39. Ng PC, Lam CW, Fok TF, et al. Refractory hypotension in preterm infants with adrenocortical insufficiency. Arch Dis Child Fetal Neonatal Ed. 2001;84:F122-F124.
40. Watterberg KL. Adrenal insufficiency and cardiac dysfunction in the preterm infant. Pediatr Res. 2002;51:422-424.
41. Hanna CE, Jett PL, Laird MR, et al. Corticosteroid binding globulin, total serum cortisol, and stress in extremely low-birth-weight infants. Am J Perinatol. 1997;14:201-204.
42. Scott SM, Watterberg KL. Effect of gestational age, postnatal age, and illness on plasma cortisol concentrations in premature infants. Pediatr Res. 1995;37:112-116.

12

43. Sasidharan P. Role of corticosteroids in neonatal blood pressure homeostasis. Clin Perinatol. 1998;25:723-740.
44. Moise AA, Wearden ME, Kozinetz CA, et al. Antenatal steroids are associated with less need for blood pressure support in extremely premature infants. Pediatrics. 1995;95:845-850.
45. Demarini S, Dollberg S, Hoath SB, et al. Effects of antenatal corticosteroids on blood pressure in very low birth weight infants during the first 24 hours of life. J Perinatol. 1999;19:419-425.
46. LeFlore JL, Engle WD, Rosenfeld CR. Determinants of blood pressure in very low birth weight neonates: lack of effect of antenatal steroids. Early Hum Dev. 2000;59:37-50.
47. Leviton A, Kuban KC, Pagano M, et al. Antenatal corticosteroids appear to reduce the risk of post-natal germinal matrix hemorrhage in intubated low birth weight newborns. Pediatrics. 1993;91:1083-1088.
48. Trang TT, Tibballs J, Mercier JC, et al. Optimization of oxygen transport in mechanically ventilated newborns using oximetry and pulsed Doppler-derived cardiac output. Crit Care Med. 1988;16:1094-1097.
49. Maayan C, Eyal F, Mandelberg A, et al. Effect of mechanical ventilation and volume loading on left ventricular performance in premature infants with respiratory distress syndrome. Crit Care Med. 1986;14:858-860.
50. Skinner JR, Boys RJ, Hunter S, et al. Pulmonary and systemic arterial pressure in hyaline membrane disease. Arch Dis Child. 1992;67:366-373.
51. Evans N, Kluckow M. Early determinants of right and left ventricular output in ventilated preterm infants. Arch Dis Child Fetal Neonatal Ed. 1996;74:F88-F94.
52. Skelton R, Evans N, Smythe J. A blinded comparison of clinical and echocardiographic evaluation of the preterm infant for patent ductus arteriosus. J Paediatr Child Health. 1994;30:406-411.
53. Evans N, Moorcraft J. Effect of patency of the ductus arteriosus on blood pressure in very preterm infants. Arch Dis Child. 1992;67:1169-1173.
54. Fenton AC, Woods KL, Leanage R, et al. Cardiovascular effects of carbon dioxide in ventilated preterm infants. Acta Paediatr. 1992;81:498-503.
55. Roze JC, Tohier C, Maingueneau C, et al. Response to dobutamine and dopamine in the hypotensive very preterm infant. Arch Dis Child. 1993;69:59-63.
56. Seri I, Rudas G, Bors Z, et al. Effects of low-dose dopamine infusion on cardiovascular and renal functions, cerebral blood flow, and plasma catecholamine levels in sick preterm neonates. Pediatr Res. 1993;34:742-749.
57. Versmold HT, Kitterman JA, Phibbs RH, et al. Aortic blood pressure during the first 12 hours of life in infants with birth weight 610 to 4,220 grams. Pediatrics. 1981;67:607-613.
58. Dempsey EM, Al Hazzani F, Barrington KJ. Permissive hypotension in the extremely low birthweight infant with signs of good perfusion. Arch Dis Child Fetal Neonatal Ed. 2009;94:F241-F244.
59. Strozik KS, Pieper CH, Roller J. Capillary refilling time in newborn babies: normal values. Arch Dis Child Fetal Neonatal Ed. 1997;76:F193-F196.
60. Schriger DL, Baraff L. Defining normal capillary refill: variation with age, sex, and temperature. Annals of Emergency Medicine. 1988;17:932-935.
61. Tibby SM, Hatherill M, Murdoch IA. Capillary refill and core-peripheral temperature gap as indicators of haemodynamic status in paediatric intensive care patients. Arch Dis Child. 1999;80:163-166.
62. Osborn DA, Evans N, Kluckow M. Clinical detection of low upper body blood flow in very premature infants using blood pressure, capillary refill time, and central-peripheral temperature difference. Arch Dis Child Fetal Neonatal Ed. 2004;89:F168-F173.
63. Linshaw MA. Concentration of the urine. In: Polin RA, Fox WW, eds. Fetal and neonatal physiology. Philadelphia: WB Saunders; 1998:1634-1653.
64. Miletin J, Pichova K, Dempsey EM. Bedside detection of low systemic flow in the very low birth weight infant on day 1 of life. Eur J Pediatr. 2009;168:809-813.
65. Cady LDJ, Weil MH, Afifi AA, et al. Quantitation of severity of critical illness with special reference to blood lactate. Crit Care Med. 1973;1:75-80.
66. Peretz DI, Scott HM, Duff J, et al. The significance of lacticacidemia in the shock syndrome. Ann N Y Acad Sci. 1965;119:1133-1141.
67. Rashkin MC, Bosken C, Baughman RP. Oxygen delivery in critically ill patients. Relationship to blood lactate and survival. Chest. 1985;87:580-584.
68. Vincent JL, Dufaye P, Berre J, et al. Serial lactate determinations during circulatory shock. Crit Care Med. 1983;11:449-451.
69. Weil MH, Afifi AA. Experimental and clinical studies on lactate and pyruvate as indicators of the severity of acute circulatory failure (shock). Circulation. 1970;41:989-1001.
70. Beca JP, Scopes JW. Serial determinations of blood lactate in respiratory distress syndrome. Arch Dis Child. 1972;47:550-557.
71. Deshpande SA, Platt MP. Association between blood lactate and acid-base status and mortality in ventilated babies. Arch Dis Child Fetal Neonatal Ed. 1997;76:F15-F20.
72. Graven SN, Criscuolo D, Holcomb TM. Blood lactate in the respiratory distress syndrome: significance in prognosis. Am J Dis Child. 1965;110:614-617.
73. Butt WW, Whyte HW. Blood pressure monitoring in neonates: comparison of umbilical and peripheral artery measurements. J Pediatr. 1984;105:630-632.
74. Colan SD, Fujii A, Borow KM, et al. Noninvasive determination of systolic, diastolic and end-systolic blood pressure in neonates, infants and young children: comparison with central aortic pressure measurements. Am J Cardiol. 1983;52:867-870.

75. Emery EF, Greenough A. Non-invasive blood pressure monitoring in preterm infants receiving intensive care. Eur J Pediatr. 1992;151:136-139.
76. Kimble KJ, Darnall Jr RA, Yelderman M, et al. An automated oscillometric technique for estimating mean arterial pressure in critically ill newborns. Anesthesiology. 1981;54:423-425.
77. Lui K, Doyle PE, Buchanan N. Oscillometric and intra-arterial blood pressure measurements in the neonate: a comparison of methods. Australian Paediatric Journal. 1982;18:32-34.
78. Park MK, Menard SM. Accuracy of blood pressure measurement by the Dinamap monitor in infants and children. Pediatrics. 1987;79:907-914.
79. Dannevig I, Dale HC, Liestol K, et al. Blood pressure in the neonate: three non-invasive oscillometric pressure monitors compared with invasively measured blood pressure. Acta Paediatr. 2005;94:191-196.
80. Alverson DC, Eldridge M, Dillon T, et al. Noninvasive pulsed Doppler determination of cardiac output in neonates and children. J Pediatr. 1982;101:46-50.
81. Walther FJ, Siassi B, Ramadan NA, et al. Pulsed Doppler determinations of cardiac output in neonates: normal standards for clinical use. Pediatrics. 1985;76:829-833.
82. Groves AM. Cardiac magnetic resonance in the study of neonatal haemodynamics. Semin Fetal Neonatal Med. 2011;16:36-41.
83. Stark MJ, Clifton VL, Wright IM, et al. Microvascular flow, clinical illness severity and cardiovascular function in the preterm infant. Arch Dis Child Fetal Neonatal Ed. 2008;93:F271-F274.
84. Amir G, Ramamoorthy C, Riemer RK, et al. Visual light spectroscopy reflects flow-related changes in brain oxygenation during regional low-flow perfusion and deep hypothermic circulatory arrest. Journal of Thoracic & Cardiovascular Surgery. 2006;132:1307-1313.
85. Takahashi S, Kakiuchi S, Nanba Y, et al. The perfusion index derived from a pulse oximeter for predicting low superior vena cava flow in very low birth weight infants. J Perinatol. 2010;30: 265-269.
86. Lou HC, Lassen NA, Friis-Hansen B. Impaired autoregulation of cerebral blood flow in the distressed newborn infant. J Pediatr. 1979;94:118-121.
87. Victor S, Marson AG, Appleton RE, et al. Relationship between blood pressure, cerebral electrical activity, cerebral fractional oxygen extraction, and peripheral blood flow in very low birth weight newborn infants. Pediatr Res. 2006;59:314-319.
88. Wardle SP, Yoxall CW, Weindling AM. Peripheral oxygenation in hypotensive preterm babies. Pediatr Res. 1999;45:343-349.
89. Perlman JM, McMenamin JB, Volpe JJ. Fluctuating cerebral blood-flow velocity in respiratory-distress syndrome. Relation to the development of intraventricular hemorrhage. N Engl J Med. 1983;309:204-209.
90. Pryds O, Greisen G, Lou H, et al. Heterogeneity of cerebral vasoreactivity in preterm infants supported by mechanical ventilation. J Pediatr. 1989;115:638-645.
91. Wong FY, Leung TS, Austin T, et al. Impaired autoregulation in preterm infants identified by using spatially resolved spectroscopy. Pediatrics. 2008;121:e604-e611.
92. Pryds O, Greisen G, Lou H, et al. Heterogeneity of cerebral vasoreactivity in preterm infants supported by mechanical ventilation. J Pediatr. 1989;115:638-645.
93. Bada HS, Korones SB, Perry EH, et al. Mean arterial blood pressure changes in premature infants and those at risk for intraventricular hemorrhage. J Pediatr. 1990;117:607-614.
94. Cunningham S, Symon AG, Elton RA, et al. Intra-arterial blood pressure reference ranges, death and morbidity in very low birthweight infants during the first seven days of life. Early Hum Dev. 1999;56:151-165.
95. Grether JK, Nelson KB, Emery ES, et al. Prenatal and perinatal factors and cerebral palsy in very low birth weight infants. J Pediatr. 1996;128:407-411.
96. Fanaroff JM, Wilson-Costello DE, Newman NS, et al. Treated hypotension is associated with neonatal morbidity and hearing loss in extremely low birth weight infants. Pediatrics. 2006;117: 1131-1135.
97. Heuchan AM, Evans N, Henderson-Smart DJ, et al. Perinatal risk factors for major intraventricular haemorrhage in the Australian and New Zealand Neonatal Network, 1995-97. Arch Dis Child Fetal Neonatal Ed. 2002;86:F86-F90.
98. de Vries LS, Regev R, Dubowitz LM, et al. Perinatal risk factors for the development of extensive cystic leukomalacia. Am J Dis Child. 1988;142:732-735.
99. Perlman JM, Risser R, Broyles RS. Bilateral cystic periventricular leukomalacia in the premature infant: associated risk factors. Pediatrics. 1996;97:822-827.
100. Goldstein RF, Thompson Jr RJ, Oehler JM, et al. Influence of acidosis, hypoxemia, and hypotension on neurodevelopmental outcome in very low birth weight infants. Pediatrics. 1995;95:238-243.
101. Low JA, Froese AB, Galbraith RS, et al. The association between preterm newborn hypotension and hypoxemia and outcome during the first year. Acta Paediatr. 1993;82:433-437.
102. Martens SE, Rijken M, Stoelhorst GM, et al. Leiden Follow-Up Project on Prematurity. Is hypotension a major risk factor for neurological morbidity at term age in very preterm infants? Early Hum Dev. 2003;75:79-89.
103. Pellicer A, Bravo MC, Madero R, et al. Early systemic hypotension and vasopressor support in low birth weight infants: impact on neurodevelopment. Pediatrics. 2009;123:1369-1376.
104. Hunt RW, Evans N, Rieger I, et al. Low superior vena cava flow and neurodevelopment at 3 years in very preterm infants. J Pediatr. 2004;145:588-592.
105. Osborn DA, Evans N, Kluckow M. Effect of early targeted indomethacin on the ductus arteriosus and blood flow to the upper body and brain in the preterm infant. Arch Dis Child Fetal Neonatal Ed. 2003;88:F477-F482.

106. Patel J, Roberts I, Azzopardi D, et al. Randomized double-blind controlled trial comparing the effects of ibuprofen with indomethacin on cerebral hemodynamics in preterm infants with patent ductus arteriosus. Pediatr Res. 2000;47:36-42.

107. Kluckow M, Evans N. Early echocardiographic prediction of symptomatic patent ductus arteriosus in preterm infants undergoing mechanical ventilation. J Pediatr. 1995;127:774-779.

108. Kluckow M, Evans N. Ductal shunting, high pulmonary blood flow, and pulmonary hemorrhage. J Pediatr. 2000;137:68-72.

109. Sarkar S, Dechert R, Schumacher RE, et al. Is refractory hypotension in preterm infants a manifestation of early ductal shunting? J Perinatol. 2007;27:353-358.

110. Bouissou A, Rakza T, Klosowski S, et al. Hypotension in preterm infants with significant patent ductus arteriosus: effects of dopamine. J Pediatr. 2008;153:790-794.

111. Wright IM, Goodall SR. Blood pressure and blood volume in preterm infants. Arch Dis Child Fetal Neonatal Ed. 1994;70:F230-F231.

112. Randomised trial of prophylactic early fresh-frozen plasma or gelatin or glucose in preterm babies: outcome at 2 years. Northern Neonatal Nursing Initiative Trial Group. Lancet. 1996;348: 229-232.

113. Emery EF, Greenough A, Gamsu HR. Randomised controlled trial of colloid infusions in hypotensive preterm infants. Arch Dis Child. 1992;67:1185-1188.

114. So KW, Fok TF, Ng PC, et al. Randomised controlled trial of colloid or crystalloid in hypotensive preterm infants. Arch Dis Child Fetal Neonatal Ed. 1997;76:F43-F46.

115. Nadel S, De Munter C, Britto J, et al. Albumin: saint or sinner? Arch Dis Child. 1998;79:384-385.

116. Gill AB, Weindling AM. Randomised controlled trial of plasma protein fraction versus dopamine in hypotensive very low birthweight infants. Arch Dis Child. 1993;69:284-287.

117. Van Marter LJ, Leviton A, Allred EN, et al. Hydration during the first days of life and the risk of bronchopulmonary dysplasia in low birth weight infants. J Pediatr. 1990;116:942-949.

118. Osborn D, Evans N, Kluckow M. Randomized trial of dobutamine versus dopamine in preterm infants with low systemic blood flow. J Pediatr. 2002;140:183-191.

119. Seri I. Cardiovascular, renal and endocrine actions of dopamine in neonates and children. J Pediatr. 1995;126:333-344.

120. Pellicer A, Valverde E, Elorza MD, et al. Cardiovascular support for low birth weight infants and cerebral hemodynamics: a randomized, blinded, clinical trial. Pediatrics. 2005;115:1501-1512.

121. Bourchier D, Weston PJ. Randomised trial of dopamine compared with hydrocortisone for the treatment of hypotensive very low birthweight infants. Arch Dis Child Fetal Neonatal Ed. 1997;76: F174-F178.

122. Klarr JM, Faix RG, Pryce CJ, et al. Randomized, blind trial of dopamine versus dobutamine for treatment of hypotension in preterm infants with respiratory distress syndrome. J Pediatr. 1994;125:117-122.

123. Seri I, Tulassay T, Kiszel J, et al. Cardiovascular response to dopamine in hypotensive preterm neonates with severe hyaline membrane disease. Eur J Pediatr. 1984;142:3-9.

124. DiSessa TG, Leitner M, Ti CC, et al. The cardiovascular effects of dopamine in the severely asphyxiated neonate. J Pediatr. 1981;99:772-776.

125. Perez CA, Reimer JM, Schreiber MD, et al. Effect of high-dose dopamine on urine output in newborn infants. Crit Care Med. 1986;14:1045-1049.

126. Seri I, Evans J. Addition of epinepherine to dopamine increases blood pressure and urine output in critically ill extremely low birth weight infants with uncompensated shock. Pediatr Res. 1998;43:194A.

127. Ruffolo Jr RR. The pharmacology of dobutamine. American Journal of the Medical Sciences. 1987;294:244-248.

128. Noori S, Friedlich P, Seri I. Cardiovascular and renal effects of dobutamine in the neonate. NeoReviews. 2004;5:E22-E6.

129. Martinez AM, Padbury JF, Thio S. Dobutamine pharmacokinetics and cardiovascular responses in critically ill neonates. Pediatrics. 1992;89:47-51.

130. Robel-Tillig E, Knupfer M, Pulzer F, et al. Cardiovascular impact of dobutamine in neonates with myocardial dysfunction. Early Hum Dev. 2007;83:307-312.

131. Stopfkuchen H, Queisser-Luft A, Vogel K. Cardiovascular responses to dobutamine determined by systolic time intervals in preterm infants. Crit Care Med. 1990;18:722-724.

132. Subhedar NV, Shaw NJ. Dopamine versus dobutamine for hypotensive preterm infants. Cochrane Database of Systematic Reviews. 2003;CD001242.

133. Heckmann M, Trotter A, Pohlandt F, et al. Epinephrine treatment of hypotension in very low birthweight infants. Acta Paediatr. 2002;91:566-570.

134. Artman M, Kithas PA, Wike JS, et al. Inotropic responses change during postnatal maturation in rabbit. Am J Physiol. 1988;255(Part 2):H335-H342.

135. Klitzner TS, Shapir Y, Ravin R, et al. The biphasic effect of amrinone on tension development in newborn mammalian myocardium. Pediatr Res. 1990;27.

136. Binah O, Legato MJ. Developmental changes in the cardiac effects of amrinone in the dog. Circ Res. 1983;52:747-752.

137. Akita T, Joyner RW, Lu C, et al. Developmental changes in modulation of calcium currents of rabbit ventricular cells by phosphodiesterase inhibitors. Circulation. 1994;90:469-478.

138. Wernovsky G, Wypij D, Jonas RA, et al. Postoperative course and hemodynamic profile after the arterial switch operation in neonates and infants. A comparison of low-flow cardiopulmonary bypass and circulatory arrest. Circulation. 1995;92:2226-2235.

139. Chang AC, Atz AM, Wernovsky G, et al. Milrinone: systemic and pulmonary hemodynamic effects in neonates after cardiac surgery. Crit Care Med. 1995;23:1907-1914.
140. Hoffman TM, Wernovsky G, Atz AM, et al. Efficacy and safety of milrinone in preventing low cardiac output syndrome in infants and children after corrective surgery for congenital heart disease. Circulation. 2003;107:996-1002.
141. Bidegain M, Greenberg R, Simmons C, et al. Vasopressin for refractory hypotension in extremely low birth weight infants. J Pediatr. 2010;157:502-504.
142. Ng PC, Lee CH, Lam CW, et al. Transient adrenocortical insufficiency of prematurity and systemic hypotension in very low birthweight infants. Arch Dis Child Fetal Neonatal Ed. 2004;89: F119-F126.
143. Seri I, Noori S. Diagnosis and treatment of neonatal hypotension outside the transitional period. Early Hum Dev. 2005;81:405-411.
144. Helbock HJ, Insoft RM, Conte FA. Glucocorticoid-responsive hypotension in extremely low birth weight newborns. Pediatrics. 1993;92:715-717.
145. Seri I, Tan R, Evans J. Cardiovascular effects of hydrocortisone in preterm infants with pressor-resistant hypotension. Pediatrics. 2001;107:1070-1074.
146. Evans N, Seri I. Cardiovascular compromise in the newborn infant. In: Taeusch HW, Ballard RA, Gleason CA, eds. Avery's diseases of the newborn. Philadelphia: WB Saunders; 2004:398-409.
147. Yanowitz TD, Jordan JA, Gilmour CH, et al. Hemodynamic disturbances in premature infants born after chorioamnionitis: association with cord blood cytokine concentrations. Pediatr Res. 2002;51:310-316.
148. Cabal LA, Devaskar U, Siassi B, et al. Cardiogenic shock associated with perinatal asphyxia in preterm infants. J Pediatr. 1980;96(4):705-710.
149. Yao AC, Lind J. Blood volume in the asphyxiated term neonate. Biol Neonate. 1972;21:199-209.
150. Wyckoff MH, Perlman JM, Laptook AR. Use of volume expansion during delivery room resuscitation in near-term and term infants. Pediatrics. 2005;115:950-955.
151. Walther FJ, Siassi B, Ramadan NA, et al. Cardiac output in newborn infants with transient myocardial dysfunction. J Pediatr. 1985;107:781-785.
152. Osborn DA, Evans N. Early volume expansion for prevention of morbidity and mortality in very preterm infants. Cochrane Database of Systematic Reviews. 2004;CD002055.
153. Noori S, Friedlich P, Ebrahimi M, et al. Hemodynamic changes following low-dose hydrocortisone administration in vasopressor-treated preterm and term neonates. Pediatrics. 2006;118:
154. Gaissmaier RE, Pohlandt F. Single-dose dexamethasone treatment of hypotension in preterm infants. J Pediatr. 1999;34:701-705.

12

CHAPTER 13

The Very Low Birth Weight Neonate with Hemodynamically Significant Ductus Arteriosus During the First Postnatal Week

Ronald Clyman, MD, and Shahab Noori, MD, RDCS

During fetal life, increased pulmonary vascular resistance results in decreased pulmonary blood flow and diversion of the blood from the pulmonary to the systemic circulation through the wide-open ductus arteriosus (DA). As a consequence, the right ventricle contributes significantly to systemic blood flow—its output is about twice that of the left ventricle.[1] Ductal constriction or closure in utero results in increased pressure within the pulmonary vascular bed and increased hypertrophy and reactivity of the pulmonary vascular muscular layer.[2] This can lead to the development of pulmonary hypertension after birth or the development of fetal hydrops and fetal demise due to right ventricular failure.

The direction of flow in the patent ductus arteriosus depends on the relative resistances in the systemic and pulmonary circulation. The postnatal decrease in pulmonary resistance along with the increase in systemic vascular resistance results in changes of ductus flow from purely right-to-left in utero, to bidirectional during the transitional period, and to purely left-to-right thereafter. These changes occur over a short period of time; 52% of neonates less than 30 weeks' gestation have pure left-to-right ductal shunts, 43% predominantly left-to-right bidirectional shunts, and only 2% have pure right-to-left shunts by 5 hours of postnatal life.[3]

In term infants, closure of the patent ductus arteriosus (PDA) occurs within the first 48 hours after birth. Closure of the DA occurs in two phases: (1) "functional" narrowing of the lumen within the first hours after birth by smooth muscle constriction and (2) "anatomic remodeling," leading to occlusion of the residual lumen by extensive neointimal thickening and loss of muscle media smooth muscle over the next few days.

The rate and degree of initial "functional" closure is determined by the balance between factors that favor constriction (oxygen, endothelin, calcium channels, catecholamines, and Rho kinase) and those that oppose it (intraluminal pressure, prostaglandins [PGs], nitric oxide [NO], carbon monoxide, potassium channels, and cyclic adenosine monophosphate [cAMP] and cyclic guanosine monophosphate

[cGMP]). During the later part of gestation, the unique sensitivity of the fetal ductus arteriosus to the vasodilating effects of PGs, especially PGE_2, dominates ductus tone. Following delivery there are several events that promote ductus constriction:

1. An increase in arterial PO_2, which increases Ca^{++} induced constriction by (1) opening smooth muscle Ca^{++} channels, (2) increasing Rho kinase mediated Ca^{++} sensitization, and (3) inhibiting smooth muscle K^+ channels.
2. A decrease in ductus luminal blood pressure (due to the postnatal decrease in pulmonary vascular resistance.
3. A decrease in circulating PGE_2 (due to the loss of placental prostaglandin production and increase in its removal by the lungs).
4. A decrease in the number of PGE_2 receptors in the ductus wall.

The definitive "anatomic" closure of the ductus arteriosus requires remodeling of the tissue. This occurs following the initial functional constriction. In the full-term ductus, expansion of the neointima (by hyaluron, migrating smooth muscle cells, and proliferating endothelia) forms protrusions, or mounds, that permanently occlude the already constricted lumen.[4,5] The anatomic events that lead to permanent closure appear to be controlled by the degree of postnatal smooth muscle constriction. The stimulus for postnatal neointimal expansion appears to be tissue hypoxia.[6] In the full-term ductus the thickness of the ductus wall requires the presence of intramural vasa vasorum to provide oxygen to its outer half. During postnatal constriction, the intramural tissue pressure obliterates vasa vasorum flow in the muscle media. The ensuing profound ischemic hypoxia inhibits local PGE_2 and nitric oxide production, induces local production of hypoxia inducible factors like HIF-1α and vascular endothelial growth factor (which play critical roles in smooth muscle migration into the neointima), and produces smooth muscle apoptosis in the muscle media. In addition, monocytes/macrophages adhere to the ductus wall, and appear to be necessary for ductus remodeling.[7]

In contrast, preterm infants frequently fail to constrict their ductus or undergo anatomic remodeling after birth. The incidence of persistent PDA is inversely related to gestational age.[8] This is due to several mechanisms. The intrinsic tone of the extremely immature ductus (<70% of gestation) is decreased compared to the ductus at term.[9] This may be due to the presence of immature smooth muscle myosin isoforms, with a weaker contractile capacity, and to decreased Rho kinase expression and activity.[10-16] Calcium entry through L-type calcium channels also appears to be impaired in the immature ductus.[15-17] In addition, the potassium channels, which inhibit ductus contraction, change during gestation (switching from K_{Ca} channels [which are not regulated by oxygen tension] to K_V channels [which can be inhibited by increased oxygen concentrations]).[18-20] The reduced expression and function of the putative oxygen-sensing K_V channels in the immature ductus appear to contribute to ductus patency in several animal species.[16,18,20]

In most mammalian species, the major factor that prevents the preterm ductus from constricting after birth is its increased sensitivity to the vasodilating effects of PGE_2 and NO.[21] The increased sensitivity of the preterm ductus to PGE_2 is due to increased cyclic AMP signaling. There is both increased cyclic AMP production, due to enhanced PG receptor coupling with adenyl cyclase, and decreased cyclic AMP degradation by phosphodiesterase in the preterm ductus.[22,23] As a result, inhibitors of PG production (e.g., indomethacin, ibuprofen, and mefenamic acid) are usually effective agents in promoting ductus closure in the premature infant.

Premature infants also have elevated circulating concentrations of PGE_2 due to the decreased ability of the premature lung to clear circulating PGE_2.[24] In the preterm newborn, circulating concentrations of PGE_2 can reach the pharmacologic range during episodes of bacteremia and necrotizing enterocolitis, and are often associated with reopening of a previously constricted ductus arteriosus.[25]

The factors responsible for the changes that occur with advancing gestation are unknown. Prenatal administration of glucocorticoids significantly reduces the incidence of patent ductus arteriosus (PDA) in premature humans and animals.[26-31] Postnatal glucocorticoid administration also reduces the incidence of PDA.[32] However, postnatal glucocorticoid treatment also increases the incidence of several other neonatal morbidities.[32,33] The patient's genetic background also plays a significant role in determining persistent ductus patency. Several single nucleotide polymorphisms (SNPs) in candidate genes have been identified that are associated with PDA in preterm infants: ATR type 1, IFNγ, estrogen receptor-alpha PvuII, TFAP2B, PGI synthase, and TRAF1.[34-37] Recent studies suggest that an interaction between preterm birth and TFAP2B may be responsible for some of the PDAs that occur in preterm infants: TFAP2B is uniquely expressed in ductus smooth muscle, it regulates other genes that are important in ductus smooth muscle development, mutations in TFAP2B produce PDA in mice and humans, and TFAP2B polymorphisms are associated with preterm PDAs (especially those that are unresponsive to indomethacin).[37-39]

Nonsteroidal antiinflammatory drugs, like indomethacin, can effectively constrict and narrow the ductus lumen in 60-70% of preterm infants, but frequently fail to cause permanent anatomic closure.[25,40,41] Neointimal mounds are less well developed and often fail to occlude the lumen in preterm infants (especially those born before 28 weeks of gestation). The preterm ductus is a much thinner vessel than the full-term ductus. It has no need for vasa vasorum and is able to extract all the oxygen it requires just from its luminal blood flow (vasa vasorum first appear in the outer ductus wall after 28 weeks' gestation when the vessel wall thickness increases beyond 400 μm). As a result, unless the ductus lumen is completely obliterated, the preterm ductus is less likely to develop profound hypoxia as it constricts after birth. Without a strong hypoxic signal, neointimal expansion is markedly diminished, resulting in mounds that fail to occlude the residual lumen.[4,6,7,42]

Several neonatal morbidities have been associated with the presence of a persistent PDA (bronchopulmonary dysplasia [BPD], intraventricular hemorrhage [IVH], periventricular leukomalacia [PVL], and necrotizing enterocolitis [NEC]). Although these morbidities have been attributed to the hemodynamic consequences of the left-to-right PDA shunt, a cause-and-effect relationship has recently been questioned.[43]

This chapter discusses the effects of a PDA on the cardiovascular system, with special emphasis on how the premature heart copes with the increased preload and decreased peripheral vascular resistance that occurs in the presence of a PDA left-to-right shunt.

Signs and Symptoms of Patent Ductus Arteriosus

The degree of "PDA symptomatology" depends on the size and direction of the shunt, duration of ductal patency, extent of the "steal phenomenon," and adequacy of the compensatory mechanisms of the premature myocardium and other organs.

The direction of ductal shunt depends on the size of the DA and relative resistance in the pulmonary and systemic circulation.[3] In uncomplicated situations, the shunt pattern changes from bidirectional to left-to-right before complete closure of the DA. In the majority of preterm infants, the DA is open in the first few days of postnatal life. During this stage, the pulmonary and systemic hemodynamic effects of PDA appear to be well compensated. This explains why the specificity and sensitivity of the clinical diagnosis of PDA are low during the first few postnatal days.[44-46] With time, however, the classic signs and symptoms of PDA appear. These include the presence of a murmur, hyperactive left ventricular impulse, increased pulse pressure, and increased need for ventilatory support.[47] In most cases, the clinically silent PDA during the first few days goes undetected unless an echocardiogram is performed. Although color Doppler is very sensitive in diagnosing a PDA, the mere presence of ductal flow is a poor indicator of the hemodynamic disturbances that might be caused by the PDA. Although not well defined, a *hemodynamically significant PDA (hsPDA)* usually refers to a state in which the left-to-right shunt across the PDA has created a significant volume overload on the heart. An hsPDA is often associated with exhaustion of compensatory mechanisms, resulting in pulmonary edema and systemic hypoperfusion. Using echocardiographic measures, the left atrial to aortic root diameter ratio (LA:AO), the size of the DA, and/or estimation of the ductal flow have been used to define a hemodynamically significant PDA.[48-51] The LA:AO ratio estimates the significance of the PDA by assessing the degree of volume overload of the left side of the heart. Presuming normal mitral valve size and left ventricular function, the size of the left atrium is indicative of the left ventricular preload. However, this index does not necessarily reflect the degree of pulmonary overcirculation, since the presence of atrial level left-to-right flow (through a stretched patent foramen ovale [PFO] or atrial septal defect [ASD]) will reduce the left atrial diameter and the LA:AO ratio. In addition, a presumably normal LA:AO ratio does not say anything about the degree of steal phenomenon from the systemic circulation. In the presence of a nonrestricting PFO/ASD, a small left atrial diameter (lower preload) may, at least theoretically, interfere with the compensatory increase in LV output to offset the systemic steal phenomenon.[52]

Defining the size of the PDA by color Doppler is another more objective way to assess the hemodynamic significance of ductal patency. A PDA size ≥ 1.6 or ≥ 2 mm has been used as an indicator of a hemodynamically significant PDA. Kluckow and Evans showed that a ductal diameter of more than 1.6 mm at 5 hours of postnatal life predicts occurrence of hsPDA in preterm infants younger than 30 weeks' gestation.[51] However, flow velocity and ductus diameter are imperfect measures due to turbulence in ductus flow and other inaccuracies in their measurements.

More recently, diastolic flow velocity in the left pulmonary artery, transductal velocity ratio, ratio of left ventricular output to superior vena cava (SVC) flow, presence of holodiastolic retrograde flow in the descending aorta, and serum levels of B-type natriuretic peptide (BNP) have been used in an attempt to quantify the hemodynamic significance of the PDA.[53-58] Although BNP serum levels correlate well with echocardiographic markers of hsPDA, large variability in the proposed cutoff values and measurements have not made this test very useful for monitoring changes in left-to-right shunt.[58,59]

Cardiovascular Adaptation to Patent Ductus Arteriosus

Cardiac output is the result of the interactions among preload, afterload, myocardial contractility, and heart rate. Under normal conditions and in the absence of a PDA, the left cardiac output of a neonate is in the range of 150-300 mL/kg/min. Since blood flow to the lungs is increased in the presence of a PDA with a left-to-right shunt, venous return from the pulmonary circulation to the left atrium is also increased resulting in an increase in the preload of the left ventricle. Studies have consistently shown a higher left ventricle end-diastolic volume (preload) when the DA is open with a predominantly left-to-right shunting pattern. According to the Starling curve, the increase in myocardial muscle fiber stretch from higher preload augments stroke volume. Indeed, most studies have demonstrated a significantly increased left ventricular output in the presence of a PDA with predominantly left-to-right shunting.[60-69] In a lamb model, where ductus patency was mechanically regulated, stroke volume increased by 33%, 66%, and 97% as the ductus shunt increased by 31%, 50%, and 67% of the baseline left ventricular stroke volume, respectively. Preterm lambs with an open DA are able to increase their stroke volume when challenged with a fluid bolus, even though the degree of the increase is less than when the DA is closed.[63] In the presence of a PDA, the low-resistance pulmonary vascular bed is in parallel with the systemic vascular bed. This results in a reduction of left ventricle afterload, which, in combination with the increased preload, enhances the myocardium's ability to increase its stroke volume. However, in the clinical setting, the presence of a PFO significantly alters the effects of a PDA on left ventricular stroke volume by decompressing the left atrium. In the presence of a significant PFO flow, right ventricular output may even be higher than left ventricular output despite the presence of a significant left-to-right PDA shunt.[3]

There are significant differences in both the structure and function of the myocardium between preterm and term neonates and older children and adults. These differences put the immature myocardium at a disadvantage as far as contractility is concerned.[70] Furthermore, since perfusion to the myocardium takes place primarily during diastole, myocardial performance might be adversely affected if diastolic blood pressure is low in the presence of an hsPDA. Although some early studies suggested that myocardial ischemia may occur in the presence of an hsPDA, more recent studies indicate that myocardial perfusion and performance are well-maintained.[71]

Some authors have suggested that since the higher preload is associated with a greater stretch of myocardial fibers, myocardial contractility should actually increase in the presence of a PDA. They speculate that a lack of change in myocardial contractility, in the presence of a PDA, indicates deterioration of myocardial function. However, using a load-independent measure of myocardial contractility, Barlow and colleagues showed that hsPDA had no effect on contractility.[72] Similarly, contractility, assessed by a load-independent index, has been reported to remain unchanged after ligation of the DA.[73] On the other hand, a recent study found that cardiac troponin T, a marker of myocardial cell injury, is mildly elevated in preterm infants with a PDA during the first postnatal week.[74]

In the presence of a PDA, the increase in cardiac output is the result of an increase in stroke volume, since there is no change in heart rate. The increase in cardiac output may offset the systemic hemodynamic effects of the PDA, at least initially. However, in a number of very low birth weight (VLBW) infants, this compensatory mechanism may fail and systemic perfusion may become inadequate. When this occurs, signs and symptoms of tissue hypoperfusion may present in the form of poor peripheral perfusion and decreased urine output; ultimately, hypotension and lactic acidosis may develop.

Effects of Hemodynamically Significant Patent Ductus Arteriosus on Blood Pressure

Blood pressure is the product of the interaction between cardiac output and peripheral vascular resistance. In general, systolic blood pressure is primarily affected by changes in stroke volume while diastolic blood pressure is mainly reflective of changes in peripheral vascular resistance. Traditionally low diastolic blood pressure has been considered the hallmark of an hsPDA and many studies have supported this notion.[67,72] However, studies that specifically look at the relationship between blood pressure and PDA have shown similar decreases in both systolic and diastolic blood pressure (and therefore no change in the pulse pressure) at least during the first postnatal week (Fig. 13-1). Infants with an hsPDA and with birth weights

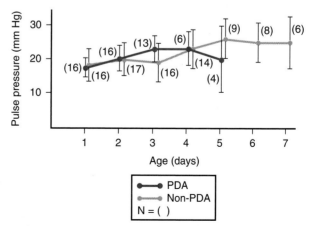

Figure 13-1 Similar pulse pressure in PDA and non-PDA preterm infants in first week of postnatal life. (From Ratner I, Perelmuter B, Toews W, et al. Association of low systolic and diastolic blood pressure with significant patent ductus arteriosus in the very low birth weight infant. Crit Care Med 1985;13:497-500.)

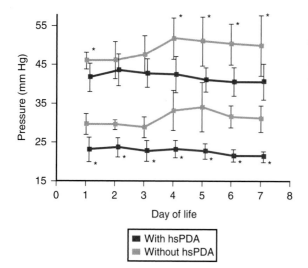

Figure 13-2 Changes in systolic and diastolic BP in infants <1000 g with and without an hsPDA during the first week of postnatal life. (From Evans N, Moorcraft J. Effect of patency of the ductus arteriosus on blood pressure in very preterm infants. Arch Dis Child 1992;67:1169-1173.)

between 1000-1500 g, have slight, but non-significant, decreases in systolic, diastolic and mean blood pressures.[75,76] In contrast, infants with birth weights <1000 g, with hsPDAs, have significantly lower systolic, diastolic and mean blood pressures and no change in the pulse pressures (Figs. 13-2 and 13-3).[76] Since stroke volume increases and vascular resistance decreases in the presence of an hsPDA, one might expect systolic blood pressure to be maintained despite the decrease in diastolic pressure. However, cardiac output, ductal shunt volume and peripheral resistance were not measured in these studies, making it difficult to determine the cause for the lack of a wide pulse pressure. In immature animals, a decrease in the diastolic and mean blood pressure occurs even when the shunt is small, whereas a significant decrease in systolic blood pressure has been documented only when the PDA shunt is moderate or large.[62]

Effects of Hemodynamically Significant Patent Ductus Arteriosus on Organ Perfusion

Despite the ability of the left ventricle to increase its output in the face of a left-to-right ductus shunt, organ blood flow distribution is significantly altered. Interestingly, redistribution of systemic blood flow occurs even with small shunts.[62] Blood

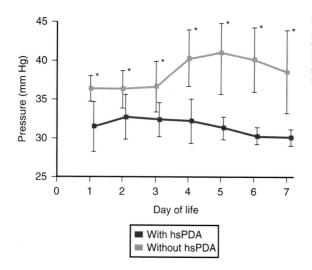

Figure 13-3 Changes in mean BP in infants <1000 g with and without an hsPDA during the first week of postnatal life. (From Evans N, Moorcraft J. Effect of patency of the ductus arteriosus on blood pressure in very preterm infants. Arch Dis Child 1992;67:1169-1173.)

	Ductus left-to-right shunt					
	Small (n = 18)		Moderate (n = 25)		Large (n = 20)	
	Closed	Open	Closed	Open	Closed	Open
Spleen (mL/min/100 g)	178 ± 133	110 ± 92*	216 ± 136	135 ± 100†	259 ± 155	106 ± 55‡
Gastrointestinal (mL/min/100 g)	74 ± 40	59 ± 34§	78 ± 41	54 ± 32‡	80 ± 39	34 ± 16‖
Adrenal (mL/min/100 g)	278 ± 142	218 ± 124§	322 ± 179	202 ± 109‖	300 ± 104	205 ± 208§
Carcass (mL/min/100 g)	9.5 ± 3.8	8.3 ± 2.8	9.2 ± 2.8	6.6 ± 1.8‖	7.7 ± 2.2	4.3 ± 1.5‖
Kidneys (mL/min/100 g)	160 ± 50	139 ± 64§	154 ± 73	113 ± 59‡	140 ± 48	88 ± 45‡
Liver (mL/min/100 g)	23 ± 13	18 ± 10*	28 ± 18	20 ± 12‡	30 ± 20	16 ± 12‖
Brain (mL/min/100 g)	40 ± 20	34 ± 15	37 ± 12	31 ± 10†	39 ± 8	28 ± 6‡
Heart (mL/min/100 g)	96 ± 47	114 ± 61	111 ± 47	123 ± 84	82 ± 36	83 ± 42
LV (mL/min/100 g)	102 ± 52	125 ± 73§	136 ± 61	152 ± 123	93 ± 41	97 ± 41
LV in/LV out	1.13 ± 0.49	1.03 ± 0.46§	1.22 ± 0.48	1.08 ± 0.32*	1.35 ± 0.48	1.09 ± 0.37†

Values represent mean ± SD.
Carcass = skin, skeletal muscle, bone; heart = total heart; LV = LV free wall; LV in/LV out = blood flow to inner third of LV divided by flow to outer two thirds.
*P <0.01, open vs closed.
†P <0.005
‡P <0.0005
§P <0.05
‖P <0.00005

Figure 13-4 Organ blood flow in preterm lamb with and without PDA. (From Clyman RI, Mauray F, Heymann MA, et al. Cardiovascular effects of a patent ductus arteriosus in preterm lambs with respiratory distress. J Pediatr 1987;111:579-587.)

flow to the skin, bone, and skeletal muscle is most likely to be affected first by the left-to-right ductal shunt. The most likely organs to be affected thereafter are the gastrointestinal tract and kidneys due to a combination of decreased perfusion pressure (ductal steal) and localized vasoconstriction. Mesenteric blood flow is decreased in both fasting and fed states in the presence of a PDA.[77] Significant decreases in blood flow to these organs may occur before there are signs of left ventricular compromise (Fig. 13-4).[66,67] In addition, treatment strategies used to facilitate closure of the PDA, such as indomethacin, may have an effect on organ blood flow independent of the hemodynamic changes associated with the presence of an hsPDA.

Although cerebral blood flow (CBF) has recently also been assessed by near infrared spectroscopy, blood flow velocity, measured by the Doppler technique, has been the primary mode used to assess organ blood flow in the human neonate. In animal models, organ blood flow has also been measured by the microsphere technique. Each of these techniques has significant limitations. Unfortunately, at the present time, we do not have the ability in the human neonate to continuously measure absolute blood flow to different organs.

Using the Doppler technique with ultrasonography, the amount of blood flowing through a vessel is a function of the vessel diameter (cross-sectional area) and mean blood flow velocity. Because of the small size of the neonatal vessels (e.g., anterior or middle cerebral artery), accurate measurement of vessel diameter is not possible. In addition, the Doppler technique assumes that the diameter of the vessel remains constant during the cardiac cycle, a notion that has been repeatedly challenged. Despite these limitations, Doppler velocity measurements and velocity-derived indices have been shown to have fairly good correlations with more invasive measures of organ blood flow.[78-80] The most commonly used Doppler indicators of organ blood flow are systolic, diastolic, and mean blood flow velocities, velocity time integral, pulsatility index (PI), and resistive index (RI). As the PI and RI are inversely related to flow, and directly related to vascular resistance, an increase in the PI or RI indicates a reduction in organ blood flow and/or an increase in the vascular resistance of the organ.

Cerebral Blood Flow

Although some studies suggest that CBF is maintained in the presence of an hsPDA, most studies have shown a decrease in flow and a disturbance in cerebral hemodynamics (Fig. 13-4).[61,62,67] Furthermore, indomethacin, the drug used for pharmacologic closure of the PDA, has a direct, albeit, transient vasoconstrictive effect on the cerebral circulation.[81,82]

Using the Doppler technique, Perlman and colleagues demonstrated a decrease in diastolic blood flow velocity in the anterior cerebral artery of preterm infants in the presence of hsPDA.[83] Similarly, Lemmers and colleagues reported that an hsPDA had a negative impact on cerebral oxygenation that resolved after treatment with indomethacin.[84] Investigators have also observed retrograde diastolic flow and increased PI in the anterior cerebral artery in the presence of a PDA.[85] In contrast, Shortland and colleagues found no difference in anterior CBF velocity between infants with or without a PDA[86]; however, they did report that there was a higher incidence of PVL in the subgroup of infants with retrograde blood flow in the anterior cerebral artery.[86] Correlations between an hsPDA (assessed by the LA:AO ratio) and both end-diastolic velocity and resistive index (RI) in the anterior cerebral artery have also been made in VLBW infants.[87] These data suggest that CBF progressively decreases as left-to-right shunts across the PDA become larger. In preterm lambs and humans, CBF is maintained at a constant level in the presence of a PDA, as long as left ventricular output is increased.[61,67] It appears that the increase in cardiac output, at least to a certain point, ensures adequate cerebral perfusion (albeit with an altered pattern) in patients with a PDA. Indeed, Baylen and colleagues reported a decrease in CBF when cardiac output was compromised in preterm lambs with a PDA.[68]

Furthermore, a significant PDA is an independent predictor of low superior vena cava (SVC) flow (a surrogate for low systemic blood flow and CBF) in preterm infants.[88] The effect of a PDA on SVC flow appears to be during the first 12 hours after birth (when the myocardium has not yet adjusted to the postnatal increase in afterload). This finding supports the notion that absence of a compensatory increase in cardiac output may be, at least in part, responsible for the low CBF associated with a PDA. However, the relationship between a PDA and SVC flow remains controversial as others have not found a similar adverse effect of a PDA on SVC flow.[89]

Superior Mesenteric and Celiac Artery Blood Flow

Intestinal hypoperfusion is a known risk factor for NEC. Studies evaluating blood flow to the abdominal organs in general and to the superior mesenteric artery (SMA) in particular have uniformly demonstrated a decrease in blood flow in the presence of an hsPDA. Diastolic flow reversal in the descending aorta has been reported as early as 4 hours after birth; flow reversal can be seen in 34% and 46% of the very preterm infants with a large PDA, at 12 and 24 hours after birth, respectively.[89] In addition, administration of indomethacin appears to directly reduce not only CBF but also intestinal blood flow.

Studies using preterm lambs, during the first 10 hours after delivery, demonstrate that even small ductal shunts (those less than 40% of the left ventricular cardiac output) cause significant reductions in blood flow to the abdominal organs (Fig. 13-5).[62] The decrease in organ blood flow occurs despite significant increases in cardiac output and is due to the combined effects of decreased perfusion pressure and localized vasoconstriction. Similar findings were also reported by other investigators.[68] In premature primates, mesenteric blood flow is decreased in both fasting and fed states in the presence of a PDA.[77] Despite the changes in blood flow, oxygen consumption, in the terminal ileum, appears to be unaffected by the presence of a PDA in preterm lambs.[66]

Similar findings have been reported in premature human infants. Martin and colleagues reported retrograde diastolic flow in the descending aorta of preterm infants with a large PDA; this resolved after closure of DA.[85] Similarly, Deeg and colleagues and Coombs and colleagues demonstrated a decrease in both the systolic and diastolic blood flow velocities in the superior mesenteric and celiac arteries in preterm infants with a PDA.[90,91] The diastolic blood flow abnormalities appeared to

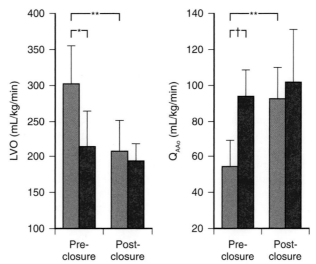

Figure 13-5 Left ventricular output (LVO) and blood flow volume of the abdominal aorta (QAAo) before and after closure of ductus arteriosus by mefenamic acid. Black bars represent the values for hsPDA group; open bars represent the values for group without hsPDA. Values are expressed as mean ± SD. *P < .002; **P < .001; †P < .0001. (From Shimada S, Kasai T, Konishi M, et al. Effects of patent ductus arteriosus on left ventricular output and organ blood flows in preterm infants with respiratory distress syndrome treated with surfactant. J Pediatr 1994;125:270-277.)

be greater in the superior mesenteric artery.[91] Using ultrasound, Shimada and colleagues assessed left cardiac output and abdominal aortic blood flow in VLBW infants before and after ductus closure and compared the findings to those obtained in patients without a PDA (Fig. 13-5).[67] Despite a significantly higher left ventricular cardiac output in the PDA group, blood flow in the abdominal aorta was significantly lower in the PDA group than in the control group. Abdominal aorta blood flow increased significantly after ductus closure. These changes in intestinal perfusion have led to concerns when feeding infants with a PDA. Although population-based studies have reported an association between a PDA and necrotizing enterocolitis (NEC), no randomized control trials (RCTs) have been designed to examine the effects of a *persistent* symptomatic PDA on NEC.[92-94] The PDA-related RCTs that have been performed to date only provide information about the effects of short-term exposure to a PDA since the PDAs in the control groups were treated and closed if they failed to close spontaneously within a few days of birth. These studies demonstrate that a limited exposure to a PDA does not increase the risk of NEC. Nor is there information about the advisability of continuing or stopping enteral feeding in the presence of a PDA. Currently there is great variability in feeding approaches among neonatologists when faced with an infant with a PDA.[95] There is evidence from one recent cohort-controlled trial about the effects of long-term exposure to a PDA. The investigators found that neither prolonged exposure to a PDA, nor the practice of feeding infants in the presence of a PDA, had an effect on the incidence of NEC.[96]

As mentioned earlier, indomethacin treatment of a PDA also affects mesenteric blood flow and compromises the premature intestine's ability to autoregulate its oxygen consumption.[66,91,97] On the other hand, ibuprofen, another non-selective cyclooxygenase inhibitor, mediates PDA closure without affecting mesenteric blood flow.[98] A recent metaanalysis comparing ibuprofen treatment of a PDA with indomethacin treatment suggests that ibuprofen may be associated with a lower incidence of NEC while being equally effective in producing PDA closure.[99]

Pulmonary Blood Flow

The decreased ability of the preterm infant to maintain active pulmonary vasoconstriction may be responsible, at least in part, for the pulmonary presentation of a "large" left-to-right PDA shunt in preterm infants relatively early after delivery.[100-102] Although dopamine has been reported to increase systemic vascular resistance more than pulmonary vascular resistance in preterm and term neonates (who lack intracardiac and extracardiac shunts associated with increased pulmonary blood flow), the drug appears to significantly increase pulmonary vascular resistance in preterm infants with a PDA and therefore may have variable effects on the direction and magnitude of ductal shunt and systemic blood pressure.[103-105] On the other hand, therapeutic maneuvers, like surfactant replacement, or prenatal conditions, such as intrauterine growth retardation, that lead to or are associated with an accelerated postnatal decrease in pulmonary vascular resistance can exacerbate the amount of left-to-right shunt and might result in pulmonary hemorrhage.[106-108] Randomized controlled trials have shown that early pharmacologic ductus closure decreases the incidence of significant pulmonary hemorrhage.[109-111] In addition to their ability to close the PDA, indomethacin and ibuprofen also increase the expression of alveolar epithelial sodium channels, which remove fluid from the lung's alveolar compartment. This effect may contribute to the decreased incidence of significant pulmonary hemorrhage in infants that are treated with prophylactic indomethacin immediately after birth.[109-111] Pharmacologic closure of the PDA with ibuprofen is also associated with improved lung development and alveolarization in premature baboons.[112]

In premature animals, a wide-open PDA increases the hydraulic pressures in the pulmonary vasculature; this, in turn, increases the rate of fluid transudation into the pulmonary interstitium.[113] Any increase in pulmonary microvascular perfusion pressure in premature infants with respiratory distress syndrome may also increase interstitial and alveolar lung fluid because of their low plasma oncotic pressures and increased capillary permeability. Leakage of plasma proteins into the developing lungs inhibits surfactant function and increases surface tension in the immature air sacs, which are already compromised by surfactant deficiency.[114] The increased FiO_2 and mean airway pressures required to overcome these early changes in compliance may contribute to the development of chronic lung disease.[115-117] Depending on the gestational age and the species examined, changes in pulmonary mechanics may occur as early as 1 day after birth or not before several days of exposure to the PDA left-to-right shunt.[112,118]

While it is true that preterm animals with a PDA have increased fluid and protein clearance into the lung interstitium, due to an increase in pulmonary microvascular filtration pressure, a simultaneous increase in lung lymph flow appears to eliminate the excess fluid and protein from the lung.[113] This compensatory increase in lung lymph acts as an "edema safety factor," inhibiting fluid accumulation in the lungs. As a result, there is no net increase in water or protein accumulation in the lung and there is no change in pulmonary mechanics.[117-121] This delicate balance between the PDA-induced fluid filtration and lymphatic reabsorption is consistent with the observation, made in human infants, that closure of the ductus arteriosus, within the first 24 hours after birth, has no effect on the course of the newborn's hyaline membrane disease. However, if lung lymphatic drainage is impaired, or alveolar epithelial permeability is altered, the likelihood of pulmonary and alveolar edema increases dramatically. After several days of mechanical ventilation, the residual functioning lymphatics are more easily overwhelmed by the same size ductus shunt that is well accommodated on the first day after delivery. As a result, it is not uncommon for infants with a persistent PDA to develop pulmonary edema and alterations in pulmonary mechanics at 7-10 days after birth. In these infants, improvement in lung compliance occurs following closure of the PDA.[117,122-126]

Not all of the changes associated with a PDA are necessarily detrimental to the immature infant with respiratory distress. The recirculation of oxygenated arterial blood through lungs that are not fully expanded can lead to improved levels of arterial PaO_2.[62,127] Conversely, decreases in systemic arterial O_2 content have been observed following PDA closure, despite the absence of any alterations in pulmonary mechanics.

Changes in Cardiac Function Following PDA Ligation

Infants who undergo surgical ligation of their PDA often develop a period of cardio-pulmonary deterioration usually becoming apparent 6-14 hours after the procedure, before their overall condition starts to improve. Approximately 25-30% of infants undergoing PDA ligation develop profound hypotension and receive vasopressors and/or inotropes and increased respiratory support.[128] Decreased gestational and postnatal age and increased ventilator support prior to surgery are the strongest predictors of the hemodynamic decompensation following ligation.[128-130]

The causes of this post-ligation deterioration are unknown. There are relatively few studies of the effects of PDA ligation on cardiac function. Most animal studies have been performed in the first 24 hours of birth, and, therefore, have limited applicability to clinical practice, where infants are exposed to a PDA for days or weeks before the surgery.[68,131] Although a recent study found beneficial effects of PDA ligation on left and right myocardial performance in 6-day-old preterm baboons, the study did not examine the changes in cardiac function in the 24 hours immediately following surgery.[132]

There is some evidence in preterm infants that the altered loading conditions (increased afterload and decreased preload) following PDA ligation may contribute to the clinical deterioration. Lindner and colleagues assessed cardiac function by measuring left ventricular output, stroke volume, and heart rate two days after PDA ligation and compared the findings to pre-ligation measurements.[65] They reported a significant decrease in left ventricular output and stroke volume without a significant change in heart rate. However, these findings are, at least in part, explained by the decrease in ventricular preload caused by the removal of ductal shunting leading to a decrease in the force of contraction and a reduction in left ventricular output. Thus, these changes would not necessarily indicate deterioration in cardiac function, since they represent a return to normal nonshunt conditions.

However, several other factors such as the prolonged exposure of the myocardium to volume overload prior to ligation or the sudden change in systemic vascular resistance following ligation, may impact cardiac performance after surgery in ways that cannot be explained by changes in preload alone. Most of the studies that have examined "ventricular performance" indices have examined them shortly after, that is, 1-2 hours after PDA ligation. No major impact of surgical ligation on left ventricular systolic performance has been noted at that time.[65,73,133] Kimball and colleagues observed an increase in systemic vascular resistance and a small decrease in left ventricular output but no change in myocardial contractility or afterload.[133] Similarly, Noori and colleagues found no change in contractility or afterload despite an increase in systemic vascular resistance and a decrease in left ventricular output shortly after ligation.[73] Although afterload is affected by changes in systemic vascular resistance, it is also affected by left ventricular diameter and wall thickness. Accordingly, Noori and colleagues speculated that, following PDA ligation the decrease in left ventricular diameter and the increase in wall thickness offset the effects of the increase in systemic vascular resistance on afterload. They also found no change in diastolic function, as assessed by indices derived from mitral inflow and tissue Doppler studies.[73]

While only some preterm infants develop significant myocardial dysfunction (Fig. 13-6), Noori and colleagues suggested that almost all demonstrate a transient, more subtle form of myocardial dysfunction, evidenced by deterioration in the myocardial performance index (MPI); a measure of both systolic and diastolic function).[73,134-136] This transient decrease appears to recover by 24 hours after the ligation.[73] These authors suggested that the decrease in stroke volume following ligation was due to both the acute volume unloading of the left ventricle and the transient deterioration in myocardial performance. They found that the degree of deterioration in global myocardial performance was directly related to the size of PDA prior to the ligation and suggested that the transient deterioration may be due to an abrupt decrease in myofibrillar length requiring "resetting" of the myocyte's Starling curve to adjust to the new loading condition. In summary, apart from a significant

13

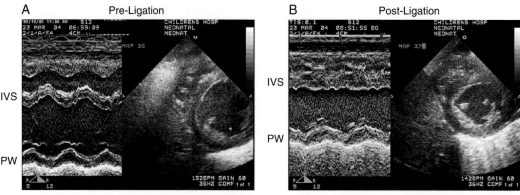

Figure 13-6   In some preterm infants after ligation there is a dramatic decrease in septal wall motion. **A,** Short axis view of the heart with M-mode tracing before ligation. The left ventricle (LV) is dilated and there is good motion of both the interventricular septum (IVS) and posterior wall (PW) of the ventricle. **B,** After ligation, the LV diameter is smaller but the IVS is essentially motionless. (From Noori S. Patent ductus arteriosus in the preterm infant: to treat or not to treat? J Perinatol 2010;30(Suppl):S31-S37.)

reduction in left ventricular stroke volume, no major change in systolic and diastolic function is apparent at 1-2 hours after the ligation.

These studies do not explain why some preterm infants develop profound hypotension 6-14 hours following PDA ligation. McNamara and colleagues recently reported their observations made at 1 and 8 hours after the operation with the latter time point being closer to the time of the actual clinical deterioration.[137] In contrast with the findings at 1 hour after ligation, these authors observed an increased incidence of diminished left ventricular performance defined as either a left ventricular output of less than 170 mL/kg/min or a fractional shortening of less than 25% 8 hours after ligation. Overall, 25% of their patients showed evidence of "decreased left ventricular performance." Based on these findings, they proposed that the observed alterations in myocardial function at 8 hours after the procedure might contribute to the post-ligation hypotension.

Although left ventricular output decreases after ligation, the change in "effective" left ventricular output (i.e., the portion of the left ventricular output supplying individual organs) is not known. At this time, it is unclear whether the post-ligation hypotension is the result of a decrease in "effective" left ventricular output due to myocardial dysfunction or a decrease in systemic vascular resistance following the initial increase in resistance that occurs when the ductus is ligated. Alterations in vasomotor tone due to anesthesia, down-regulation of cardiovascular adrenergic receptors, and/or relative adrenal insufficiency are all additional possible contributors to the post-ligation hemodynamic deterioration.[138,139]

Treatment

Surgical Ligation

Surgical ligation produces definitive ductus arteriosus closure; however, it is associated with its own set of morbidities: thoracotomy, pneumothorax, chylothorax, scoliosis, and infection.[140] The incidence of unilateral vocal cord paralysis (which increases the requirements for tube feedings, respiratory support and hospital stay) has been reported to be as high as 67% in infants with birth weights ≤ 1000 g, following PDA ligation.[141,142] As described earlier, approximately 25-30% of infants with birth weights ≤ 1000 g will require inotropic support for profound hypotension during the postoperative period.[128] In addition, neonatal transport to another facility may be required if surgical expertise is not readily available.

Early surgical ligation has recently been shown to be an independent risk factor for the development of bronchopulmonary dysplasia.[143,144] Early surgical ligation is associated with an increase in the expression of genes involved with pulmonary inflammation and decreases the expression of pulmonary epithelial sodium channels critical for alveolar water clearance.[145] These changes may contribute to the lack of improvement in pulmonary mechanics after PDA ligation. In addition, early surgical ligation impedes lung growth.[112,132,146] These findings raise the possibility that ductal ligation, while eliminating the detrimental effects of a PDA on lung development, may create its own set of problems that counteract many of the benefits derived from ductus closure.[143,144]

Indomethacin

Inhibition of prostaglandin synthesis with nonselective inhibitors of COX-1 and COX-2 (e.g., indomethacin and ibuprofen) appears to be an effective alternative to surgical ligation.[102] In most intensive care nurseries, indomethacin and ibuprofen have replaced surgery as the preferred therapy for closing a persistent PDA. However, both drugs have been associated with several potential adverse effects in the newborn.

Indomethacin produces significant reductions in renal, mesenteric, and CBF.[82,91,98,147-153] Indomethacin also reduces cerebral oxygenation.[153,154] Alterations in creatinine clearance and oliguria with variable responsiveness to dopamine or furosemide administration are common problems with indomethacin therapy.[155,156] Renal function returns towards normal after the initial doses of indomethacin or after drug discontinuation.[157] Some of indomethacin's actions on these organ systems are not due to the drug-induced inhibition of prostaglandin synthesis.[158-160]

Despite these complex organ-specific actions of indomethacin, none of the controlled, randomized trials examining the relationship between indomethacin and neonatal morbidity have found an increase in the incidence of necrotizing enterocolitis, gastrointestinal perforation, retinopathy of prematurity (ROP), chronic lung disease, or cerebral white matter injury following indomethacin treatment.[161] Although indomethacin, by itself, has not been shown to increase the incidence of gastrointestinal perforations, the combination of indomethacin *and* postnatal steroids, administered simultaneously, has been shown to increase the incidence of gastrointestinal perforations/necrotizing enterocolitis (Chapter 15).[33,162]

Indomethacin's cerebral vasoconstrictive effects are frequently cited as a concern for neonatologists.[152,163] However, a Cochrane systematic review found that indomethacin prophylaxis is more likely to decrease rather than increase the incidence of periventricular leukomalacia.[161] Furthermore, there is no evidence that prophylactic indomethacin has any adverse (or beneficial) effect on neurodevelopmental outcome at 18 months.[164] However, there is evidence that indomethacin administration might have longer-term benefits at 4.5 and 8 years of age.[165-167]

The postnatal age at which indomethacin is administered plays an important role in determining its effectiveness. Even when indomethacin concentrations have been maintained in the suggested therapeutic range, the drug's ability to produce ductal closure remains inversely proportional to the postnatal age at the time of treatment.[146,168-170] With advancing postnatal age, dilator prostaglandins play less of a role in maintaining ductus patency. As a result, indomethacin becomes less effective in producing PDA closure.[168] It appears that in some situations, prostaglandins may not be the dominant factors anymore for maintaining ductal patency.[171-173]

Recurrence of a symptomatic PDA can occur after initial successful treatment with indomethacin. The rate of reopening, which is greatest among the most immature infants, appears to be related to the timing and completeness of ductus closure after the initial treatment course.[40,117] Permanent anatomic closure requires tight constriction of the ductus lumen and the development of ductus wall hypoxia (see earlier). When the PDA is clinically closed after indomethacin treatment but there is still any evidence of luminal patency on the Doppler examination, the likelihood of the PDA becoming symptomatic later on is as high as 80% in preterm infants born at less than 28 weeks' gestation.[40] Unfortunately, there are limitations in the Doppler's ability to detect complete luminal closure. Even when there is no evidence of ductus patency on the Doppler/echocardiogram, a significant number of preterm infants will still have a tiny patent ductus lumen. The more immature the ductus (i.e., the thinner the ductus wall) the greater the likelihood that profound hypoxia and anatomic remodeling will not occur. Indeed, 23% of preterm neonates delivered before 26 weeks reopen despite echocardiographic evidence of closure, while only 9% of those delivered between 26 and 27 weeks will reopen if the ductus is closed by echocardiography. It has been speculated that early treatment produces a tighter degree of ductus constriction and as a result produces higher rates of ductus wall hypoxia and permanent closure.[40]

Ibuprofen

Ibuprofen is the other nonselective cyclooxygenase inhibitor that has been shown to close the ductus in animals and preterm infants.[174] It appears to be as effective as indomethacin in producing ductal closure in VLBW infants with a mean gestational age of 28 weeks.[99] In contrast to indomethacin, ibuprofen does not appear to affect mesenteric blood flow and has less of an effect on renal perfusion and function, and CBF.[98,153,158,160,175,176] Animal studies suggest that ibuprofen may have some cytoprotective effects in the intestinal tract.[177] Although individual studies have not found ibuprofen to be superior to indomethacin in the prevention of NEC, a recent metaanalysis suggests that ibuprofen may be associated with a lower incidence of NEC than indomethacin.[99] On the other hand, ibuprofen does not appear to have the same intracranial hemorrhage-sparing effect seen with indomethacin (see later). The optimal age-appropriate dosing schedule for ibuprofen is still under consideration.[178] Ibuprofen's effects on total and free serum bilirubin concentrations have raised some concerns about the safety of the higher dose regimens.[179,180]

Indomethacin and Intracranial Hemorrhage

Previous studies have shown that indomethacin, unlike ibuprofen, decreases the incidence of intracranial hemorrhage (ICH) in preterm infants and experimental animals. The effects of indomethacin on ICH do not appear to be due to its effects on ductus patency.[181,182] Indomethacin decreases CBF, decreases reactive post-asphyxial cerebral hyperemia, and accelerates maturation of the germinal matrix microvasculature.[183-185] Since most ICH occurs within the first 3 days after birth, one would expect to see beneficial effects only when indomethacin is given as a *prophylactic* strategy, that is, within the first 18 hours after birth. When prophylactic indomethacin is given to infants with preexisting normal cranial ultrasound findings, there is a significant reduction in both the incidence of all grades (I-IV) as well as the most severe grades (III, IV) of later ICH. The beneficial effects of prophylactic indomethacin are less dramatic when prophylactic indomethacin is administered to populations where the pretreatment ICH status is unknown.[117] Finally, as referred to earlier, although randomized controlled trials have not shown a beneficial effect of prophylactic indomethacin on neurodevelopmental outcome at 18 months, there is evidence for long-term benefits at 4.5 and 8 years.[164-167]

PDA and Neonatal Morbidity: To Treat or Not to Treat

Although a persistent PDA increases pulmonary hyperemia and pulmonary edema and decreases renal, mesenteric and cerebral perfusion, clear evidence is lacking for or against many of the approaches to PDA treatment.[43,186,187] A prolonged, persistent left-to-right shunt through a PDA shortens the life span of animals and humans.[188-192] In an neonatal intensive care unit where PDA ligation was not feasible, Brooks and colleagues reported a 4-fold increase in mortality in preterm infants with a persistent PDA.[190] Adjusting for perinatal factors, initial disease severity and pathologies associated with decreased survival, Noori and colleagues reported up to 8-fold rise in mortality among preterm infants with a persistent PDA.[192] On the other hand, preterm infants have a high rate of spontaneous PDA closure during the first 2 years. As a result, PDA early treatment runs the risk of exposing infants to drugs or procedures they might not need. Therefore, despite the association between persistent

PDA and decreased survival, there has been a growing debate about whether or not a persistent PDA needs to be treated during the neonatal period.[43]

Published randomized controlled trials (RCTs) provide only a limited amount of information to help guide current PDA treatment choices. Most RCTs were designed to assess the relationship between "timing" (initiation) of treatment and efficiency of PDA closure. Thus, these trials were not designed to address the question of whether or not to treat a symptomatic PDA during the neonatal period. As a result, the published RCTs are only useful for examining the effects of short-term (between 2 and 6 days) exposures to a PDA. RCTs that examined preterm infants whose PDA first became symptomatic when they were several days old, found that "early" PDA closure did not alter the incidence of serious neonatal morbidities, like BPD, NEC, or ROP, when compared with an approach that "delayed" PDA closure by 2-6 days.[193] On the other hand, using indomethacin as a "prophylactic" treatment (i.e., starting treatment within 12 hours of birth) appeared to have some benefits compared with waiting for "early" (usually 2-3 days after birth) PDA symptoms to appear before starting treatment. Individual RCTs (and their metaanalysis) demonstrate that indomethacin prophylaxis decreases the incidence of severe early pulmonary hemorrhage, severe grades of IVH, the risk of developing a symptomatic PDA, and the need for surgical PDA ligation.[109-111,161,164,194,195]

Although a "prophylactic" treatment approach has several short-term beneficial effects, it clearly results in over-treatment of infants who would normally close their ductus spontaneously.[196] Nemerofsky and colleagues observed that, in 67% of infants with birth weights greater than 1000 g, the ductus spontaneously closes by 7 days of postnatal life; in 94%, the ductus closes by the time of discharge.[197] On the other hand, the PDA closes by the time of discharge in only 30% of infants with a birth weight of 1000 g or less, and 60% will require treatment because of heart failure, acute renal impairment, or significant persistent or escalating respiratory support due to the PDA.[196,197] At this time, less than 30% of neonatologists in the United States use indomethacin prophylactically.[95]

Little information exists about the consequences of long-term exposure to a persistent, symptomatic, moderate-to-large PDA shunt. Only two small RCTs performed almost 30 years ago were designed to examine the effects of a *persistent* symptomatic PDA on neonatal pulmonary morbidity.[116,198] Both studies found that surgical closure of the PDA decreased the need for prolonged ventilatory support: significant pulmonary morbidity occurred in the group that was not allowed to have their PDA ligated when signs of congestive failure developed.[116,198] Whether these findings are still applicable in the setting of modern neonatal treatment (e.g., antenatal glucocorticoids, surfactant replacement therapy, "gentle" ventilation) has become a matter of controversy among neonatologists.[199] The role of a persistent PDA in the development of NEC is even more controversial (see earlier).

Although indomethacin and ibuprofen have been shown to be effective in producing ductal closure, the long-term benefits of ductal closure on the incidence and severity of BPD, NEC, or survival have yet to be established.[102,125,186,193,200,201] These uncertainties have resulted in several areas of controversy regarding PDA management: (1) whether or not to use indomethacin prophylaxis, (2) when to treat a moderate-to-large PDA, and (3) whether or not enteral feeding should be stopped in the presence of a PDA or during treatment of a PDA.[43,186,187,200,202] At this time, 95% of US neonatologists believe that a moderate-to-large PDA should be treated if it persists in infants born before 28 weeks who still require mechanical ventilation.[95] The number of neonatologists who treat a persistent PDA when it occurs in infants who do not require mechanical ventilation varies significantly by geographic region. Marked differences in the willingness of neonatologists to feed infants with a PDA account for much of the geographic variation in the rates of indomethacin use and PDA ligation. Seventy percent of US neonatologists believe that enteral feedings should be stopped in the presence of a PDA. In contrast, non-US neonatologists have exactly the opposite opinion: 70% believe that enteral feedings should continue in the presence of a PDA.[95]

The controversy about treatment really focuses on infants born before 28 weeks' gestation, or with birth weights of 1000 g or less, since only 30% will have a PDA that closes spontaneously and PDA-related symptoms will develop in 60% during their neonatal hospitalization.[196,197] Recently, a cohort-controlled study compared a "conservative" approach with a more "aggressive" approach for treatment of infants that failed to close their PDA after indomethacin treatment.[96] The "aggressive" approach used early surgical ligation (within 2 days) when the PDA failed to close after indomethacin treatment. The "conservative" approach continued feedings in the presence of a PDA and only ligated the PDA if cardiopulmonary compromise (persistent inotrope-dependent hypotension and/or persistent or escalating respiratory support) developed. There were no significant differences in the rates of BPD, sepsis, ROP, neurologic injury, or mortality between the two groups. The risk for NEC was significantly less in the conservatively treated infants, even though they received enteral feedings in the presence of a PDA. While the more conservative approach still resulted in eventual surgical ligation in the majority of infants born before 28 weeks' gestation in whom the PDA failed to close with indomethacin treatment, a significant number of infants did not receive surgery prior to hospital discharge, and the PDA ultimately closed spontaneously in several, despite initial treatment failure with indomethacin.[96] Further investigations are needed to determine which infants are most likely to benefit from surgical ligation and which infants might best be left untreated when pharmacologic approaches are no longer an option.

Conclusion

Patent ductus arteriosus is a common problem in preterm infants born at less than 30 weeks' gestational age. The shunt across the PDA is primarily left-to-right very soon after birth. If the DA remains open, it results in a progressive increase in pulmonary overcirculation and left-sided cardiac volume overload. Despite the immaturity of myocardium, the heart is capable of increasing cardiac output even in VLBW neonates. The compensatory increase in cardiac output is a result of an increased stroke volume without a significant change in heart rate. Because of the diversion of blood from the aorta to the pulmonary artery, the decrease in systolic, diastolic and mean blood pressure and the vasoconstriction that occurs in selected vascular beds, the increase in left ventricular output does not lead to an increase or even maintenance of *effective* left ventricular output. Both animal and human studies show compromised blood flow to several organs especially to the organs supplied by the aorta distal to the PDA.

References

1. Rudolph AM. Distribution and regulation of blood flow in the fetal and neonatal lamb. Circ Res. 1985;57:811-821.
2. Levin DL, Fixler DE, Morriss FC, et al. Morphologic analysis of the pulmonary vascular bed in infants exposed in utero to prostaglandin synthetase inhibitors. J Pediatr. 1978;92:478-483.
3. Evans N, Iyer P. Assessment of ductus arteriosus shunt in preterm infants supported by mechanical ventilation: effect of interatrial shunting. J Pediatr. 1994;125:778-785.
4. Clyman RI. Mechanisms regulating the ductus arteriosus. Biol Neonate. 2006;89:330-335.
5. Silver MM, Freedom RM, Silver MD, et al. The morphology of the human newborn ductus arteriosus: a reappraisal of its structure and closure with special reference to prostaglandin E1 therapy. Hum Pathol. 1981;12:1123-1136.
6. Kajino H, Goldbarg S, Roman C, et al. Vasa vasorum hypoperfusion is responsible for medial hypoxia and anatomic remodeling in the newborn lamb ductus arteriosus. Pediatr Res. 2002;51:228-235.
7. Waleh N, Seidner S, McCurnin D, et al. The role of monocyte-derived cells and inflammation in baboon ductus arteriosus remodeling. Pediatr Res. 2005;57:254-262.
8. Reller MD, Rice MJ, McDonald RW. Review of studies evaluating ductal patency in the premature infant. J Pediatr. 1993;122:S59-S62.
9. Kajino H, Chen YQ, Seidner SR, et al. Factors that increase the contractile tone of the Ductus Arteriosus also regulate its anatomic remodeling. Am J Physiol Regul Integr Comp Physiol. 2001;281:R291-R301.
10. Brown S, Liu X-T, Ramaekers F, et al. Differential maturation in ductus arteriosus and umbilical artery smooth muscle during ovine development. Pediatr Res. 2002;51:34A.

11. Sakurai H, Matsuoka R, Furutani Y, et al. Expression of four myosin heavy chain genes in developing blood vessels and other smooth muscle organs in rabbits. Eur J Cell Biol. 1996;69:166-172.
12. Colbert MC, Kirby ML, Robbins J. Endogenous retinoic acid signaling colocalizes with advanced expression of the adult smooth muscle myosin heavy chain isoform during development of the ductus arteriosus. Circ Res. 1996;78:790-798.
13. Reeve H, Tolarova S, Cornfield D, et al. Developmental changes in K+ channel expression may determine the O2 response of the ductus arteriosus. FASEB J. 1997;11:420A.
14. Kajimoto H, Hashimoto K, Bonnet SN, et al. Oxygen activates the Rho/Rho-kinase pathway and induces RhoB and ROCK-1 expression in human and rabbit ductus arteriosus by increasing mitochondria-derived reactive oxygen species. A newly recognized mechanism for sustaining ductal constriction. Circulation. 2007;115:1777-1788.
15. Clyman RI, Waleh NS, Kajino H, et al. Calcium-dependent and calcium-sensitizing pathways in the mature and immature ductus arteriosus. Am J Physiol Regul Integr Comp Physiol. 2007;293: R1650-R1656.
16. Cogolludo AL, Moral-Sanz J, Van der Sterren S, et al. Maturation of O2 sensing and signalling in the chicken ductus arteriosus. Am J Physiol Lung Cell Mol Physiol. 2009;297:L619-L630.
17. Thebaud B, Wu XC, Kajimoto H, et al. Developmental absence of the O2 sensitivity of L-type calcium channels in preterm ductus arteriosus smooth muscle cells impairs O2 constriction contributing to patent ductus arteriosus. Pediatr Res. 2008;63:176-181.
18. Waleh N, Reese J, Kajino H, et al. Oxygen-induced tension in the sheep ductus arteriosus: effects of gestation on potassium and calcium channel regulation. Pediatr Res. 2009;65:285-290.
19. Wu C, Hayama E, Imamura S, et al. Developmental changes in the expression of voltage-gated potassium channels in the ductus arteriosus of the fetal rat. Heart Vessels. 2007;22:34-40.
20. Thebaud B, Michelakis ED, Wu XC, et al. Oxygen-sensitive Kv channel gene transfer confers oxygen responsiveness to preterm rabbit and remodeled human ductus arteriosus: implications for infants with patent ductus arteriosus. Circulation. 2004;110:1372-1379.
21. Clyman RI, Waleh N, Black SM, et al. Regulation of ductus arteriosus patency by nitric oxide in fetal lambs. The role of gestation, oxygen tension and vasa vasorum. Pediatr Res. 1998;43:633-644.
22. Waleh N, Kajino H, Marrache AM, et al. Prostaglandin E2–mediated relaxation of the ductus arteriosus: effects of gestational age on g protein-coupled receptor expression, signaling, and vasomotor control. Circulation. 2004;110:2326-2332.
23. Liu H, Manganiello VC, Clyman RI. Expression, activity and function of cAMP and cGMP phosphodiesterases in the mature and immature ductus arteriosus. Pediatr Res. 2008;64:477-481.
24. Clyman RI, Mauray F, Heymann MA, et al. Effect of gestational age on pulmonary metabolism of prostaglandin E1 & E2. Prostaglandins. 1981;21:505-513.
25. Gonzalez A, Sosenko IR, Chandar J, et al. Influence of infection on patent ductus arteriosus and chronic lung disease in premature infants weighing 1000 grams or less. J Pediatr. 1996;128:470-478.
26. Collaborative Group on Antenatal Steroid Therapy. Prevention of respiratory distress syndrome: effect of antenatal dexamethasone administration. Publication No 85-2695. Washington, DC: National Institutes of Health; 1985:44.
27. Clyman RI, Ballard PL, Sniderman S, et al. Prenatal administration of betamethasone for prevention of patent ductus arteriosus. J Pediatr. 1981;98:123-126.
28. Clyman RI, Mauray F, Roman C, et al. Effects of antenatal glucocorticoid administration on the ductus arteriosus of preterm lambs. Am J Physiol. 1981;241:H415-H420.
29. Momma K, Mishihara S, Ota Y. Constriction of the fetal ductus arteriosus by glucocorticoid hormones. Pediatr Res. 1981;15:19-21.
30. Thibeault DW, Emmanouilides GC, Dodge ME. Pulmonary and circulatory function in preterm lambs treated with hydrocortisone in utero. Biol Neonate. 1978;34:238-247.
31. Waffarn F, Siassi B, Cabal L, et al. Effect of antenatal glucocorticoids on clinical closure of the ductus arteriosus. Am J Dis Child. 1983;137:336-338.
32. Group VONSS. Early postnatal dexamethasone therapy for the prevention of chronic lung disease. Pediatrics. 2001;108:741-748.
33. Watterberg KL, Gerdes JS, Cole CH, et al. Prophylaxis of early adrenal insufficiency to prevent bronchopulmonary dysplasia: a multicenter trial. Pediatrics. 2004;114:1649-1657.
34. Treszl A, Szabo M, Dunai G, et al. Angiotensin II type 1 receptor A1166C polymorphism and prophylactic indomethacin treatment induced ductus arteriosus closure in very low birth weight neonates. Pediatr Res. 2003;54:753-755.
35. Bokodi G, Derzbach L, Banyasz I, et al. Association of interferon gamma T+874A and interleukin 12 p40 promoter CTCTAA/GC polymorphism with the need for respiratory support and perinatal complications in low birthweight neonates. Arch Dis Child Fetal Neonatal Ed. 2007;92:F25-F29.
36. Derzbach L, Treszl A, Balogh A, et al. Gender dependent association between perinatal morbidity and estrogen receptor-alpha Pvull polymorphism. J Perinat Med. 2005;33:461-462.
37. Dagle JM, Lepp NT, Cooper ME, et al. Determination of genetic predisposition to patent ductus arteriosus in preterm infants. Pediatrics. 2009;123:1116-1123.
38. Ivey KN, Sutcliffe D, Richardson J, et al. Transcriptional regulation during development of the ductus arteriosus. Circ Res. 2008;103:388-395.
39. Zhao F, Weismann CG, Satoda M, et al. Novel TFAP2B mutations that cause Char syndrome provide a genotype-phenotype correlation. Am J Hum Genet. 2001;69:695-703.

40. Narayanan M, Cooper B, Weiss H, et al. Prophylactic indomethacin: Factors determining permanent ductus arteriosus closure. J Pediatr. 2000;136:330-337.
41. Weiss H, Cooper B, Brook M, et al. Factors determining reopening of the ductus arteriosus after successful clinical closure with indomethacin. J Pediatr. 1995;127:466-471.
42. Clyman RI, Seidner SR, Kajino H, et al. VEGF regulates remodeling during permanent anatomic closure of the ductus arteriosus. Am J Physiol. 2002;282:R199-206.
43. Laughon MM, Simmons MA, Bose CL. Patency of the ductus arteriosus in the premature infant: is it pathologic? Should it be treated? Curr Opin Pediatr. 2004;16:146-151.
44. Urquhart DS, Nicholl RM. How good is clinical examination at detecting a significant patent ductus arteriosus in the preterm neonate? Arch Dis Child. 2003;88:85-86.
45. Davis P, Turner-Gomes S, Cunningham K, et al. Precision and accuracy of clinical and radiological signs in premature infants at risk of patent ductus arteriosus. Arch Pediatr Adolesc Med. 1995;149:1136-1141.
46. Skelton R, Evans N, Smythe J. A blinded comparison of clinical and echocardiographic evaluation of the preterm infant for patent ductus arteriosus. J Paediatr Child Health. 1994;30:406-411.
47. Ellison RC, Peckham GJ, Lang P, et al. Evaluation of the preterm infant for patent ductus arteriosus. Pediatrics. 1983;71:364-372.
48. Johnson GL, Breart GL, Gewitz MH, et al. Echocardiographic characteristics of premature infants with patent ductus arteriosus. Pediatrics. 1983;72:864-871.
49. Iyer P, Evans N. Re-evaluation of the left atrial to aortic root ratio as a marker of patent ductus arteriosus. Arch Dis Child. 1994;70:F112-FF17.
50. Phillipos EZ, Robertson MA, Byrne PJ. Serial assessment of ductus arteriosus hemodynamics in hyaline membrane disease. Pediatrics. 1996;98:1149-1153.
51. Kluckow M, Evans N. Early echocardiographic prediction of symptomatic patent ductus arteriosus in preterm infants undergoing mechanical ventilation. J Pediatr. 1995;127:774-779.
52. Evans N. Diagnosis of patent ductus arteriosus in the preterm newborn. Arch Dis Child. 1993;68:58-61.
53. Suzumura H, Nitta A, Tanaka G, et al. Diastolic flow velocity of the left pulmonary artery of patent ductus arteriosus in preterm infants. Pediatr Int. 2001;43:146-151.
54. Davies MW, Betheras FR, Swaminathan M. A preliminary study of the application of the transductal velocity ratio for assessing persistent ductus arteriosus. Arch Dis Child Fetal Neonatal Ed. 2000;82:F195-F199.
55. El Hajjar M, Vaksmann G, Rakza T, et al. Severity of the ductal shunt: a comparison of different markers. Arch Dis Child Fetal Neonatal Ed. 2005;90:F419-F422.
56. Choi BM, Lee KH, Eun BL, et al. Utility of rapid B-type natriuretic peptide assay for diagnosis of symptomatic patent ductus arteriosus in preterm infants. Pediatrics. 2005;115:e255-e261.
57. Sanjeev S, Pettersen M, Lua J, et al. Role of plasma B-type natriuretic peptide in screening for hemodynamically significant patent ductus arteriosus in preterm neonates. J Perinatol. 2005;25:709-713.
58. Flynn PA, da Graca RL, Auld PA, et al. The use of a bedside assay for plasma B-type natriuretic peptide as a biomarker in the management of patent ductus arteriosus in premature neonates. J Pediatr. 2005;147:38-42.
59. Chen S, Tacy T, Clyman RI. How useful are B-type natriuretic peptide measurements for monitoring changes in patent ductus arteriosus shunt magnitude? J Perinatol. 2010;30:780-785.
60. Alverson DC, Eldridge MW, Johnson JD, et al. Effect of patent ductus arteriosus on left ventricular output in premature infants. J Pediatr. 1983;102:754-757.
61. Baylen BG, Ogata H, Oguchi K, et al. The contractility and performance of the preterm left ventricle before and after early patent ductus arteriosus occlusion in surfactant-treated lambs. Pediatr Res. 1985;19:1053-1058.
62. Clyman RI, Mauray F, Heymann MA, et al. Cardiovascular effects of a patent ductus arteriosus in preterm lambs with respiratory distress. J Pediatr. 1987;111:579-587.
63. Clyman RI, Roman C, Heymann MA, et al. How a patent ductus arteriosus effects the premature lamb's ability to handle additional volume loads. Pediatr Res. 1987;22:531-535.
64. Walther FJ, Kim DH, Ebrahimi M, et al. Pulsed Doppler measurement of left ventricular output as early predictor of symptomatic patent ductus arteriosus in very preterm infants. Biol Neonate. 1989;56:121-128.
65. Lindner W, Seidel M, Versmold HJ, et al. Stroke volume and left ventricular output in preterm infants with patent ductus arteriosus. Pediatr Res. 1990;27:278-281.
66. Meyers RL, Alpan G, Lin E, et al. Patent ductus arteriosus, indomethacin, and intestinal distension: effects on intestinal blood flow and oxygen consumption. Pediatr Res. 1991;29:569-574.
67. Shimada S, Kasai T, Konishi M, et al. Effects of patent ductus arteriosus on left ventricular output and organ blood flows in preterm infants with respiratory distress syndrome treated with surfactant. J Pediatr. 1994;125:270-277.
68. Baylen BG, Ogata H, Ikegami M, et al. Left ventricular performance and regional blood flows before and after ductus arteriosus occlusion in premature lambs treated with surfactant. Circulation. 1983;67:837-843.
69. Tamura M, Harada K, Takahashi Y, et al. Changes in left ventricular diastolic filling patterns before and after the closure of the ductus arteriosus in very-low-birth weight infants. Tohoku J Exp Med. 1997;182:337-346.
70. Noori S, Seri I. Pathophysiology of newborn hypotension outside the transitional period. Early Hum Dev. 2005;81:399-404.

71. Way GL, Pierce JR, Wolf RR, et al. ST depression suggesting subendocardial ischemia in neonates with respiratory distress syndrome and patent ductus arteriosus. J Pediatr. 1979;95:609-611.
72. Barlow AJ, Ward C, Webber SA, et al. Myocardial contractility in premature neonates with and without patent ductus arteriosus. Pediatr Cardiol. 2004;25:102-107.
73. Noori S, Friedlich P, Seri I, et al. Changes in myocardial function and hemodynamics after ligation of the ductus arteriosus in preterm infants. J Pediatr. 2007;150:597-602.
74. El-Khuffash AF, Molloy EJ. Influence of a patent ductus arteriosus on cardiac troponin T levels in preterm infants. J Pediatr. 2008;153:350-353.
75. Ratner I, Perelmuter B, Toews W, et al. Association of low systolic and diastolic blood pressure with significant patent ductus arteriosus in the very low birth weight infant. Crit Care Med. 1985;13:497-500.
76. Evans N, Moorcraft J. Effect of patency of the ductus arteriosus on blood pressure in very preterm infants. Arch Dis Child. 1992;67:1169-1173.
77. McCurnin D, Clyman RI. Effects of a patent ductus arteriosus on postprandial mesenteric perfusion in premature baboons. Pediatrics. 2008;122:e1262-e1267.
78. Raju TN. Cerebral Doppler studies in the fetus and newborn infant. J Pediatr. 1991;119:165-174.
79. Greisen G, Johansen K, Ellison PH, et al. Cerebral blood flow in the newborn infant: comparison of Doppler ultrasound and 133xenon clearance. J Pediatr. 1984;104:411-418.
80. Hansen NB, Stonestreet BS, Rosenkrantz TS, et al. Validity of Doppler measurements of anterior cerebral artery blood flow velocity: correlation with brain blood flow in piglets. Pediatrics. 1983;72:526-531.
81. Chemtob S, Beharry K, Rex J, et al. Prostanoids determine the range of cerebral blood flow autoregulation of newborn piglets. Stroke. 1990;21:777-784.
82. Laudignon N, Chemtob S, Bard H, et al. Effect of indomethacin on cerebral blood flow velocity of premature newborns. Biol Neonate. 1988;54:254-262.
83. Perlman JM, Hill A, Volpe JJ. The effect of patent ductus arteriosus on flow velocity in the anterior cerebral arteries: ductal steal in the premature newborn infant. J Pediatr. 1981;99:767-771.
84. Lemmers PM, Toet MC, van Bel F. Impact of patent ductus arteriosus and subsequent therapy with indomethacin on cerebral oxygenation in preterm infants. Pediatrics. 2008;121:142-147.
85. Martin CG, Snider AR, Katz SM, et al. Abnormal cerebral blood flow patterns in preterm infants with a large patent ductus arteriosus. J Pediatr. 1982;101:587-593.
86. Shortland DB, Gibson NA, Levene MI, et al. Patent ductus arteriosus and cerebral circulation in preterm infants. Dev Med Child Neurol. 1990;32:386-393.
87. Jim WT, Chiu NC, Chen MR, et al. Cerebral hemodynamic change and intraventricular hemorrhage in very low birth weight infants with patent ductus arteriosus. Ultrasound Med Biol. 2005;31:197-202.
88. Kluckow M, Evans N. Low superior vena cava flow and intraventricular haemorrhage in preterm infants. Arch Dis Child Fetal Neonatal Ed. 2000;82:F188-F194.
89. Groves AM, Kuschel CA, Knight DB, et al. Does retrograde diastolic flow in the descending aorta signify impaired systemic perfusion in preterm infants? Pediatr Res. 2008;63:89-94.
90. Deeg KH, Gerstner R, Brandl U, et al. [Doppler sonographic flow parameter of the anterior cerebral artery in patent ductus arteriosus of the newborn infant compared to a healthy control sample]. Klin Padiatr. 1986;198:463-470.
91. Coombs RC, Morgan MEI, Durin GM, et al. Gut blood flow velocities in the newborn: effects of patent ductus arteriosus and parenteral indomethacin. Arch Dis Child. 1990;65:1067-1071.
92. Cassady G, Crouse DT, Kirklin JW, et al. A randomized, controlled trial of very early prophylactic ligation of the ductus arteriosus in babies who weighed 1000 g or less at birth. N Engl J Med. 1989;320:1511-1516.
93. Dollberg S, Lusky A, Reichman B. Patent ductus arteriosus, indomethacin and necrotizing enterocolitis in very low birth weight infants: a population-based study. J Pediatr Gastroenterol Nutr. 2005;40:184-188.
94. Sankaran K, Puckett B, Lee DS, et al. Variations in incidence of necrotizing enterocolitis in Canadian neonatal intensive care units. J Pediatr Gastroenterol Nutr. 2004;39:366-372.
95. Jhaveri N, Soll RF, Clyman RI. Feeding practices and patent ductus arteriosus ligation preferences-are they related? Am J Perinatol. 2009;27:667-674.
96. Jhaveri N, Moon-Grady A, Clyman RI. Early surgical ligation versus a conservative approach for management of patent ductus arteriosus that fails to close after indomethacin treatment. J Pediatr. 2010;157:381-387.
97. Yanowitz TD, Yao AC, Werner JC, et al. Effects of prophylactic low-dose indomethacin on hemodynamics in very low birth weight infants. J Pediatr. 1998;132:28-34.
98. Pezzati M, Vangi V, Biagiotti R, et al. Effects of indomethacin and ibuprofen on mesenteric and renal blood flow in preterm infants with patent ductus arteriosus. J Pediatr. 1999;135:733-738.
99. Ohlsson A, Walia R, Shah S. Ibuprofen for the treatment of patent ductus arteriosus in preterm and/or low birth weight infants. Cochrane Database Syst Rev. 2010;CD003481.
100. Lewis AB, Heymann MA, Rudolph AM. Gestational changes in pulmonary vascular responses in fetal lambs in utero. Circ. Res. 1976;39:536-541.
101. Jacob J, Gluck G, DiSessa T, et al. The contribution of PDA in the neonate with severe RDS. J Pediatr. 1980;96:79-87.
102. Gersony WM, Peckham GJ, Ellison RC, et al. Effects of indomethacin in premature infants with patent ductus arteriosus: results of a national collaborative study. J Pediatr. 1983;102:895-906.

103. Seri I. Cardiovascular, renal and endocrine actions of dopamine in neonates and children. J Pediatr. 1995;126:333-344.
104. Liet JM, Boscher C, Gras-Leguen C, et al. Dopamine effects on pulmonary artery pressure in hypotensive preterm infants with patent ductus arteriosus. J Pediatr. 2002;140:373-375.
105. Bouissou A, Rakza T, Klosowski S, et al. Hypotension in preterm infants with significant patent ductus arteriosus: effects of dopamine. J Pediatr. 2008;153:790-794.
106. Raju TNK, Langenberg P. Pulmonary hemorrhage and exogenous surfactant therapy—a metaanalysis. J Pediatr. 1993;123:603-610.
107. Alpan G, Clyman RI. Cardiovascular effects of surfactant replacement with special reference to the patent ductus arteriosus. In: Robertson B, Taeusch HW, ed. Surfactant therapy for lung disease: lung biology in health and disease. New York: Marcel Dekker; 1995:531-545.
108. Rakza T, Magnenant E, Klosowski S, et al. Early hemodynamic consequences of patent ductus arteriosus in preterm infants with intrauterine growth restriction. J Pediatr. 2007;151:624-628.
109. Al Faleh K, Smyth J, Roberts R, et al. Prevention and 18-month outcome of serious pulmonary hemorrhage in extremely low birth weight infants: results of the trial of indomethacin prophylaxis in preterms. Pediatrics. 2008;121:e233-e238.
110. Domanico RS, Waldman JD, Lester LA, et al. Prophylactic indomethacin reduces the incidence of pulmonary hemorrhage and patent ductus arteriosus in surfactant treated infants < 1250 grams. Pediatr Res. 1994;35:331.
111. Clyman RI, Chorne N. PDA treatment: effects on pulmonary hemorrhage and pulmonary morbidity. J Pediatr. 2008;152:447-448.
112. McCurnin D, Seidner S, Chang LY, et al. Ibuprofen-induced patent ductus arteriosus closure: physiologic, histologic, and biochemical effects on the premature lung. Pediatrics. 2008;121: 945-956.
113. Alpan G, Scheerer R, Bland RD, et al. Patent ductus arteriosus increases lung fluid filtration in preterm lambs. Pediatr Res. 1991;30:616-621.
114. Ikegami M, Jacobs H, Jobe A. Surfactant function in respiratory distress syndrome. J Pediatr. 1983;102:443-447.
115. Brown E. Increased risk of bronchopulmonary dysplasia in infants with patent ductus arteriosus. J Pediatr. 1979;95:865-866.
116. Cotton RB, Stahlman MT, Berder HW, et al. Randomized trial of early closure of symptomatic patent ductus arteriosus in small preterm infants. J Pediatr. 1978;93:647-651.
117. Clyman RI. Commentary: Recommendations for the postnatal use of indomethacin. An analysis of four separate treatment strategies. J Pediatr. 1996;128:601-607.
118. Perez Fontan JJ, Clyman RI, Mauray F, et al. Respiratory effects of a patent ductus arteriosus in premature newborn lambs. J Appl Physiol. 1987;63:2315-2324.
119. Shimada S, Raju TNK, Bhat R, et al. Treatment of patent ductus arteriosus after exogenous surfactant in baboons with hyaline membrane disease. Pediatr Res. 1989;26:565-569.
120. Krauss AN, Fatica N, Lewis BS, et al. Pulmonary function in preterm infants following treatment with intravenous indomethacin. Am J Dis Child. 1989;143:78-81.
121. Alpan G, Mauray F, Clyman RI. Effect of patent ductus arteriosus on water accumulation and protein permeability in the premature lungs of mechanically ventilated premature lambs. Pediatr Res. 1989;26:570-575.
122. Gerhardt T, Bancalari E. Lung compliance in newborns with patent ductus arteriosus before and after surgical ligation. Biol Neonate. 1980;38:96-105.
123. Naulty CM, Horn S, Conry J, et al. Improved lung compliance after ligation of patent ductus arteriosus in hyaline membrane disease. J Pediatr. 1978;93:682-684.
124. Stefano JL, Abbasi S, Pearlman SA, et al. Closure of the ductus arteriosus with indomethacin in ventilated neonates with respiratory distress syndrome. Effects of pulmonary compliance and ventilation. Am Rev Respir Dis. 1991;143:236-239.
125. Yeh TF, Thalji A, Luken L, et al. Improved lung compliance following indomethacin therapy in premature infants with persistent ductus arteriosus. Chest. 1981;80:698-700.
126. Szymankiewicz M, Hodgman JE, Siassi B, et al. Mechanics of breathing after surgical ligation of patent ductus arteriosus in newborns with respiratory distress syndrome. Biol Neonate. 2004;85:32-36.
127. Dawes GS, Mott JC, Widdicombe JG. The patency of the ductus arteriosus in newborn lambs and its physiological consequences. J Physiol. 1955;128:361-383.
128. Moin F, Kennedy KA, Moya FR. Risk factors predicting vasopressor use after patent ductus arteriosus ligation. Am J Perinatol. 2003;20:313-320.
129. Harting MT, Blakely ML, Cox Jr CS, et al. Acute hemodynamic decompensation following patent ductus arteriosus ligation in premature infants. J Invest Surg. 2008;21:133-138.
130. Teixeira LS, Shivananda SP, Stephens D, et al. Postoperative cardiorespiratory instability following ligation of the preterm ductus arteriosus is related to early need for intervention. J Perinatol. 2008;28:803-810.
131. Taylor AF, Morrow WR, Lally KP, et al. Left ventricular dysfunction following ligation of the ductus arteriosus in the preterm baboon. J Surg Res. 1990;48:590-596.
132. McCurnin DC, Yoder BA, Coalson J, et al. Effect of ductus ligation on cardiopulmonary function in premature baboons. Am J Respir Crit Care Med. 2005;172:1569-1574.
133. Kimball TR, Ralston MA, Khoury P, et al. Effect of ligation of patent ductus arteriosus on left ventricular performance and its determinants in premature neonates. J Am Coll Cardiol. 1996;27: 193-197.

134. Noori S. Patent ductus arteriosus in the preterm infant: to treat or not to treat? J Perinatol. 2010;30(suppl):S31-S37.
135. Tei·C, Nishimura RA, Seward JB, et al. Noninvasive Doppler-derived myocardial performance index: correlation with simultaneous measurements of cardiac catheterization measurements. J Am Soc Echocardiogr. 1997;10:169-178.
136. Tei C, Ling LH, Hodge DO, et al. New index of combined systolic and diastolic myocardial performance: a simple and reproducible measure of cardiac function—a study in normals and dilated cardiomyopathy. J Cardiol. 1995;26:357-366.
137. McNamara PJ, Stewart L, Shivananda SP, et al. Patent ductus arteriosus ligation is associated with impaired left ventricular systolic performance in premature infants weighing less than 1000 g. J Thorac Cardiovasc Surg. 2010;140:150-157.
138. Ng PC, Lee CH, Lam CW, et al. Transient adrenocortical insufficiency of prematurity and systemic hypotension in very low birthweight infants. Arch Dis Child Fetal Neonatal Ed. 2004;89:F119-F126.
139. Seri I, Evans J. Controversies in the diagnosis and management of hypotension in the newborn infant. Curr Opin Pediatr. 2001;13:116-123.
140. Roclawski M, Sabiniewicz R, Potaz P, et al. Scoliosis in patients with aortic coarctation and patent ductus arteriosus: does standard posterolateral thoracotomy play a role in the development of the lateral curve of the spine? Pediatr Cardiol. 2009;30:941-945.
141. Smith ME, King JD, Elsherif A, et al. Should all newborns who undergo patent ductus arteriosus ligation be examined for vocal fold mobility? Laryngoscope. 2009;119:1606-1609.
142. Clement WA, El-Hakim H, Phillipos EZ, et al. Unilateral vocal cord paralysis following patent ductus arteriosus ligation in extremely low-birth-weight infants. Arch Otolaryngol Head Neck Surg. 2008;134:28-33.
143. Clyman R, Cassady G, Kirklin JK, et al. The role of patent ductus arteriosus ligation in bronchopulmonary dysplasia: reexamining a randomized controlled trial. J Pediatr. 2009;154:873-876.
144. Chorne N, Leonard C, Piecuch R, et al. Patent ductus arteriosus and its treatment as risk factors for neonatal and neurodevelopmental morbidity. Pediatrics. 2007;119:1165-1174.
145. Waleh N, McCurnin DC, Yoder BA, et al. Patent ductus arteriosus ligation alters pulmonary gene expression in preterm baboons. Pediatr Res. 2010 (Epub ahead of print).
146. Chang LY, McCurnin D, Yoder B, et al. Ductus arteriosus ligation and alveolar growth in preterm baboons with a patent ductus arteriosus. Pediatr Res. 2008;63:299-302.
147. Rennie JM, Doyle J, Cooke RWI. Early administration of indomethacin to preterm infants. Arch Dis Child. 1986;61:233-238.
148. Van Bel F, Van Zoeren D, Schipper J, et al. Effect of indomethacin on superior mesenteric artery blood flow velocity in preterm infants. J Pediatr. 1990;116:965-970.
149. Van Bel F, Van de Bor M, Stijnen T, et al. Cerebral blood flow velocity changes in preterm infants after a single dose of indomethacin: duration of its effect [see comments]. Pediatrics. 1989;84:802-807.
150. Austin NC, Pairaudeau PW, Hames TK, et al. Regional cerebral blood flow velocity changes after indomethacin infusion in preterm infants. Arch Dis Child. 1992;67:851-854.
151. Pryds O, Greisen G, Johansen KH. Indomethacin and cerebral blood flow in premature infants treated for patent ductus arteriosus. Eur J Pediatr. 1988;147:315-316.
152. Edwards AD, Wyatt JS, Richardson C, et al. Effects of indomethacin on cerebral haemodynamics in very preterm infants. Lancet. 1990;335:1491-1495.
153. Patel J, Roberts I, Azzopardi D, et al. Randomized double-blind controlled trial comparing the effects of ibuprofen with indomethacin on cerebral hemodynamics in preterm infants with patent ductus arteriosus [see comments]. Pediatr Res. 2000;47:36-42.
154. McCormick DC, Edwards AD, Brown GC, et al. Effect of indomethacin on cerebral oxidized cytochrome oxidase in preterm infants. Pediatr Res. 1993;33:603-608.
155. Brion LP, Campbell DE. Furosemide for symptomatic patent ductus arteriosus in indomethacin-treated infants (Cochrane Review). Cochrane Database Syst Rev. 2001;3:CD001148.
156. Barrington K, Brion LP. Dopamine versus no treatment to prevent renal dysfunction in indomethacin-treated preterm newborn infants. Cochrane Database Syst Rev. 2002;CD003213.
157. Seyberth HW, Rasher W, Hackenthal R, et al. Effect of prolonged indomethacin therapy on renal function and selected vasoactive hormones in very low birth weight infants with symptomatic patent ductus arteriosus. J Pediatr. 1983;103:979-984.
158. Malcolm DD, Segar JL, Robillard JE, et al. Indomethacin compromises hemodynamics during positive-pressure ventilation, independently of prostanoids. J Appl Physiol. 1993;74:1672-1678.
159. Chemtob S, Beharry K, Barna T, et al. Differences in the effects in the newborn piglet of various nonsteroidal antiinflammatory drugs on cerebral blood flow but not on cerebrovascular prostaglandins. Pediatr Res. 1991;30:106-111.
160. Speziale MV, Allen RG, Henderson CR, et al. Effects of ibuprofen and indomethacin on the regional circulation in newborn piglets. Biol Neonate. 1999;76:242-252.
161. Fowlie PW, Davis PG. Prophylactic intravenous indomethacin for preventing mortality and morbidity in preterm infants. Cochrane Database Syst Rev. 2010;CD000174.
162. Peltoniemi O, Kari MA, Heinonen K, et al. Pretreatment cortisol values may predict responses to hydrocortisone administration for the prevention of bronchopulmonary dysplasia in high-risk infants. J Pediatr. 2005;146:632-637.
163. Leffler CW, Busija DW, Fletcher AM, et al. Effects of indomethacin upon cerebral hemodynamics of newborn pigs. Pediatr Res. 1985;19:1160-1164.

164. Schmidt B, Davis P, Moddemann D, et al. Long-term effects of indomethacin prophylaxis in extremely-low-birth-weight infants. N Engl J Med. 2001;344:1966-1972.
165. Vohr BR, Allan WC, Westerveld M, et al. School-age outcomes of very low birth weight infants in the indomethacin intraventricular hemorrhage prevention trial. Pediatrics. 2003;111:e340-e346.
166. Ment LR, Vohr B, Allan W, et al. Outcome of children in the indomethacin intraventricular hemorrhage prevention trial. Pediatrics. 2000;105:485-491.
167. Ment LR, Vohr BR, Makuch RW, et al. Prevention of intraventricular hemorrhage by indomethacin in male preterm infants. J Pediatr. 2004;145:832-834.
168. Achanti B, Yeh TF, Pildes RS. Indomethacin therapy in infants with advanced postnatal age and patent ductus arteriosus. Clin Invest Med. 1986;9:250-253.
169. Brash AR, Hickey DE, Graham TP, et al. Pharmacokinetics of indomethacin in the neonate. N Engl J Med. 1981;305:67-72.
170. Thalji AA, Carr I, Yeh TF, et al. Pharmacokinetics of intravenously administered indomethacin in premature infants. J Pediatr. 1980;97:995-1000.
171. Cotton RB, Haywood JL, FitzGerald GA. Symptomatic patent ductus arteriosus following prophylactic indomethacin. A clinical and biochemical appraisal. Biol Neonate. 1991;60:273-282.
172. Chorne N, Jegatheesan P, Lin E, et al. Risk factors for persistent ductus arteriosus patency during indomethacin treatment. J Pediatr. 2007;151:629-634.
173. Waleh N, Hodnick R, Jhaveri N, et al. Patterns of gene expression in the ductus arteriosus are related to environmental and genetic risk factors for persistent ductus patency. Pediatr Res. 2010;68:292-297.
174. Coceani F, White E, Bodach E, et al. Age-dependent changes in the response of the lamb ductus arteriosus to oxygen and ibuprofen. Can J Physiol Pharmacol. 1979;57:825-831.
175. Mosca F, Bray M, Lattanzio M, et al. Comparative evaluation of the effects of indomethacin and ibuprofen on cerebral perfusion and oxygenation in preterm infants with patent ductus arteriosus. J Pediatr. 1997;131:549-554.
176. Chemtob S, Laudignon N, Beharry K, et al. Effects of prostaglandins and indomethacin on cerebral blood flow and cerebral oxygen consumption of conscious newborn piglets. Dev Pharmacol Ther. 1990;14:1-14.
177. Grosfeld JL, Kamman K, Gross K, et al. Comparative effects of indomethacin, prostaglandin E1, and ibuprofen on bowel ischemia. J Pediatr Surg. 1983;18:738-742.
178. Hirt D, Van Overmeire B, Treluyer JM, et al. An optimized ibuprofen dosing scheme for preterm neonates with patent ductus arteriosus, based on a population pharmacokinetic and pharmacodynamic study. Br J Clin Pharmacol. 2008;65:629-636.
179. Zecca E, Romagnoli C, De Carolis MP, et al. Does Ibuprofen increase neonatal hyperbilirubinemia? Pediatrics. 2009;124:480-484.
180. Ahlfors CE. Effect of ibuprofen on bilirubin-albumin binding. J Pediatr. 2004;144:386-388.
181. Ment LR, Duncan CC, Ehrenkranz RA, et al. Randomized low-dose indomethacin trial for prevention of intraventricular hemorrhage in very low birth weight neonates. J Pediatr. 1988;112:948-955.
182. Ment LR, Duncan CC, Ehrenkranz RA, et al. Randomized indomethacin trial for prevention of intraventricular hemorrhage in very low birth weight infants. J Pediatr. 1985;107:937-943.
183. Dahlgren N, Nilsson B, Sakabe T, et al. The effect of indomethacin on cerebral blood flow and oxygen consumption in the rat at normal and increased carbon dioxide tensions. Acta Physiol Scand. 1981;111:475-485.
184. Ment LR, Stewart WB, Scott DT, et al. Beagle puppy model of intraventricular hemorrhage: randomized indomethacin prevention trial. Neurology. 1983;33:179-184.
185. Ment LR, Stewart WB, Ardito TA, et al. Indomethacin promotes germinal matrix microvessel maturation in the newborn beagle pup. Stroke. 1992;23:1132-1137.
186. Clyman RI, Chorne N. Patent ductus arteriosus: evidence for and against treatment. J Pediatr. 2007;150:216-219.
187. Bose CL, Laughon M. Treatment to prevent patency of the ductus arteriosus: beneficial or harmful? J Pediatr. 2006;148:713-714.
188. Loftin CD, Trivedi DB, Tiano HF, et al. Failure of ductus arteriosus closure and remodeling in neonatal mice deficient in cyclooxygenase-1 and cyclooxygenase-2. Proc Natl Acad Sci U S A. 2001;98:1059-1064.
189. Campbell M. Natural history of persistent ductus arteriosus. Br Heart J. 1968;30:4-13.
190. Brooks JM, Travadi JN, Patole SK, et al. Is surgical ligation of patent ductus arteriosus necessary? The Western Australian experience of conservative management. Arch Dis Child Fetal Neonatal Ed. 2005;90:F235-F239.
191. Van Israel N, Dukes-McEwan J, French AT. Long-term follow-up of dogs with patent ductus arteriosus. J Small Anim Pract. 2003;44:480-490.
192. Noori S, McCoy M, Friedlich P, et al. Failure of ductus arteriosus closure is associated with increased mortality in preterm infants. Pediatrics. 2009;123:e138-e144.
193. Cooke L, Steer P, Woodgate P. Indomethacin for asymptomatic patent ductus arteriosus in preterm infants. Cochrane Database Syst Rev. 2003;CD003745.
194. Ment LR, Oh W, Ehrenkranz RA, et al. Low-dose indomethacin and prevention of intraventricular hemorrhage: a multicenter randomized trial. Pediatrics. 1994;93:543-550.
195. Bandstra ES, Montalvo BM, Goldberg RN, et al. Prophylactic indomethacin for prevention of intraventricular hemorrhage in premature infants. Pediatrics. 1988;82:533-542.

196. Koch J, Hensley G, Roy L, et al. Prevalence of spontaneous closure of the ductus arteriosus in neonates at a birth weight of 1000 grams or less. Pediatrics. 2006;117:1113-1121.
197. Nemerofsky SL, Parravicini E, Bateman D, et al. The ductus arteriosus rarely requires treatment in infants > 1000 grams. Am J Perinatol. 2008;25:661-666.
198. Kaapa P, Lanning P, Koivisto M. Early closure of patent ductus arteriosus with indomethacin in preterm infants with idiopathic respiratory distress syndrome. Acta Paediatr Scand. 1983;72:179-184.
199. Bose CL, Laughon MM. Patent ductus arteriosus: lack of evidence for common treatments. Arch Dis Child Fetal Neonatal Ed. 2007;92:F498-F502.
200. Knight DB. The treatment of patent ductus arteriosus in preterm infants. A review and overview of randomized trials. Semin Neonatol. 2001;6:63-73.
201. Yeh TF, Luken JA, Thalji A, et al. Intravenous indomethacin therapy in premature infants with persistent ductus arteriosus—a double blind controlled study. J Pediatr. 1981;98:137-145.
202. Amin SB, Handley C, Carter-Pokras O. Indomethacin use for the management of patent ductus arteriosus in preterms: a web-based survey of practice attitudes among neonatal fellowship program directors in the United States. Pediatr Cardiol. 2007;28:193-200.

13

CHAPTER 14

The Preterm Neonate with Cardiovascular and Adrenal Insufficiency

Erika F. Fernandez, MD, and Cynthia H. Cole, MD, MPH

Cardiovascular insufficiency as defined by hypotension and/or decreased systemic and organ blood flow has been associated with adrenal insufficiency in critically ill patients, including the newborn infant admitted to a newborn intensive care unit (NICU). The mechanisms that precipitate and fuel adrenal insufficiency and cardiovascular insufficiency in the newborn infant are complex and incompletely understood.

Adrenal insufficiency in critically ill patients is also known as "relative adrenal insufficiency," "functional adrenal insufficiency," or "critical illness related corticosteroid insufficiency," all of which are defined by inadequate corticosteroid activity for the degree of illness in a critically ill patient.[1-4] This inadequate activity may arise from corticosteroid tissue resistance or inadequate cortisol levels resulting from problems anywhere along the hypothalamus-pituitary-adrenal (HPA) axis. In this chapter, the term *adrenal insufficiency* (AI) is used to describe these ill patients in general and neonates in particular with inadequate corticosteroid activity and/or levels.

This chapter reviews AI and cardiovascular insufficiency, including proposed mechanisms for each and summarizes the available evidence that AI and cardiovascular insufficiency occur together in sick newborn patients. We also discuss the effects and proposed mechanisms by which corticosteroid therapy acts to resolve cardiovascular insufficiency.

Adrenal Insufficiency

In the mid-nineteenth century, Thomas Addison described manifestations of primary adrenal insufficiency as "general languor and debility, remarkable feebleness of the heart's action, irritability of the stomach ... occurring in connection with a diseased condition of the suprarenal capsules ..." (http://wehner.org/addison.htm). Now, more than 150 years after the original description of Addison's disease, these manifestations of AI extend to the recently described disorder of "relative" AI where there

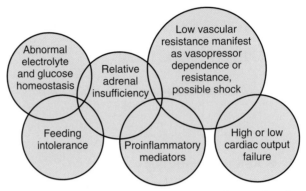

Figure 14-1   Characteristics of and relationship between relative adrenal insufficiency and vasopressor-resistant hypotension. Severe illness and cardiovascular instability are features of both RAI and VRH. RAI may or may not be associated with VRH and VRH may or may not be associated with RAI. RAI, relative adrenal insufficiency; VRH, vasopressor-resistant hypotension. See text for details.

is an inadequate corticosteroid activity to the level of illness. This disorder is not characterized by structural abnormality of the adrenal glands but by its transience as the majority of patients who recover return to normal HPA axis function and corticosteroid activity. The common terms used in ill patients with AI of "relative" or "functional" should not make one complacent about or underestimate the potentially life-threatening nature of this type of AI. Higher mortality rates occur in those whose adrenal response to stress is blunted as evidenced by trauma patients receiving etomidate during surgery.[5] Since the 1980s, AI has become increasingly recognized in sick premature and full-term neonates, infants, children, and adults.[6-27]

AI occurring in the presence of illness is often *characterized* by cardiovascular instability, inadequate random and/or stimulated cortisol levels for the degree of illness severity, and/or rapid clinical and hemodynamic improvement following corticosteroid therapy.[4,17,28-30] Cardiovascular instability, a key manifestation of AI, may present with decreased vascular resistance, vasopressor-dependent and vasopressor-resistant hypotension and, depending on myocardial function and the loading conditions of the heart, high or low cardiac output.[6-12,16,18,20,21,23,24,26,31-48] Other features, which are less likely to occur in critically ill patients whose electrolyte and fluid management is tightly controlled, include hyponatremia, hyperkalemia, hypoglycemia, metabolic acidosis, increased levels of proinflammatory markers, and feeding intolerance (Fig. 14-1).

The *spectrum of presentations and duration of AI* in neonates and other patient populations, and the determinants of the clinical presentation, are not known. For example, the presentation of hypotension with AI may be responsive, dependent, or resistant to vasopressor therapy.[6] Speculation about the duration of AI is based on treatment durations and cortisol levels. Hoen and colleagues and Annane and colleagues reported that AI and/or vasopressor dependency may be sustained for several days, even beyond one month, in adult septic or hemorrhagic-shock trauma patients.[6,49]

In *preterm infants,* Colasurdo and colleagues in an abstract reported about nine sick infants (gestational age 26 weeks) with clinical symptoms of AI, low cortisol levels (mean 251 ± 102 nmol/L) with reversal of signs within two days.[10] However, the duration of AI, based on cortisol data, varies in sick premature neonates. Ng and colleagues reported that inadequate cortisol response on postnatal day seven in sick, very low birthweight (VLBW) infants had resolved by day 14.[50] In contrast,

Guttentag and colleagues reported in an abstract that no increase in either cortisol or adrenocorticotrophic hormone (ACTH) occurred through 14 days in response to critical illness.[14] The duration of AI, based on the length of treatment, varies. Gaissmaier and Pohlandt reported that a single dose of dexamethasone was effective in reversing vasopressor-resistant hypotension in sick premature infants.[51] Yoder reported sustained improvement in cardiovascular status of premature baboons (gestational age equivalent to human at 26 weeks) with AI and vasopressor-resistant hypotension after 12-24 hours of hydrocortisone (two to four doses of 0.5-1.0 mg/kg every 6 hours) with no decrease in urinary free cortisol levels over the 2-week study.[52] Ng and colleagues reported 79% of preterm infants less than 32 weeks with refractory hypotension receiving hydrocortisone were off vasopressors by 72 hours of age compared with only 33% who were receiving placebo.[30] The duration of AI in extremely premature infants appears to be less than 1-2 weeks when it is defined by the short-term cardiovascular response to corticosteroid replacement therapy.

In *term ill infants*, an early study by Economou and colleagues found 4 of 15 infants were "low cortisol responders" relative to their illness and this state lasted through 5 days of age.[53] In a more recent study of critically ill newborn infants with refractory hypotension, Baker and colleagues used cortisol levels and the presence of hemodynamic stability to determine the duration of AI and thereby the duration of hydrocortisone replacement.[54] Term infants (n = 61) received 3.5 median days of hydrocortisone therapy, while the extremely preterm infants (n = 37) received the drug for a median of 15 days. In another study, 1-day-old term and late preterm ill infants with random low cortisol values (<15 μg/dL) received longer courses of treatment with hydrocortisone for hypotension compared to those with higher cortisol values (5 vs. 2.5 median days).[13] Evidence of AI has also been reported later in postnatal life (4-7 days of age) in ill newborn infants with respiratory distress or sepsis.[25] Infants with other diseases associated with hypotension include those born with congenital diaphragmatic hernia. Kamath and colleagues found a high incidence (67%) of low cortisol values (<15 μg/dL) in these infants, all of whom received hydrocortisone for a mean of 11 days.[55] Differences in presentation severity and duration of AI are likely to vary according to the level of immaturity, severity, etiology, and duration of the underlying disorders, and management and response to management.

Postulated mechanisms for AI include inadequate HPA axis response, limited adrenal reserve, adrenergic receptor insensitivity due to receptor down-regulation, proinflammatory cytokine-mediated suppression of the pituitary and adrenal glands, *glucocorticoid tissue resistance,* and limited adrenal perfusion (Fig. 14-2).[6,9,11,33,40,56-58] A limited capacity of the immature HPA axis, adrenal gland, and sympathoadrenal systems to respond to stress, coupled with increased illness severity, immaturity and/or slow transition to extra-uterine life, prolonged exposure to free radicals, and subsequent production of proinflammatory cytokines, set the stage for AI (and cardiovascular insufficiency) in acutely ill newborn infants.

The *overall incidence of AI in critically ill adult patients* is about 20% and is as high as 60% in patients with severe sepsis and septic shock.[59,60] In neonatal or pediatric critically ill patients, the incidence is less well understood because there is no consensus on diagnostic evaluation or diagnostic criteria.[17-19,36,44,49,61-69] Reported proportions of critically ill pediatric patients with "inadequate" cortisol response vary widely, from as low as 2% often up to 87%.[13,19,25,29,30,70,71] The proportions reported vary by patient characteristics, type of illness, choice of diagnostic test, dosage of stimulating agent, and diagnostic criteria for adequate or inadequate cortisol response.

The incidence of AI is influenced by *criteria for "adequate" and "inadequate" cortisol response or cortisol production.* In critically ill adults, proposed criteria for diagnosing AI are a change in total serum cortisol less than 9 μg/dL after cosyntropin ([1-24]ACTH; 250 μg) administration or a random total cortisol of less than 10 μg/dL (276 nmol/L).[60] A cortisol value of less than 10 μg/dL in ill adult patients has high predictive value (0.93) but low sensitivity (0.19) for AI.[59] The American College of

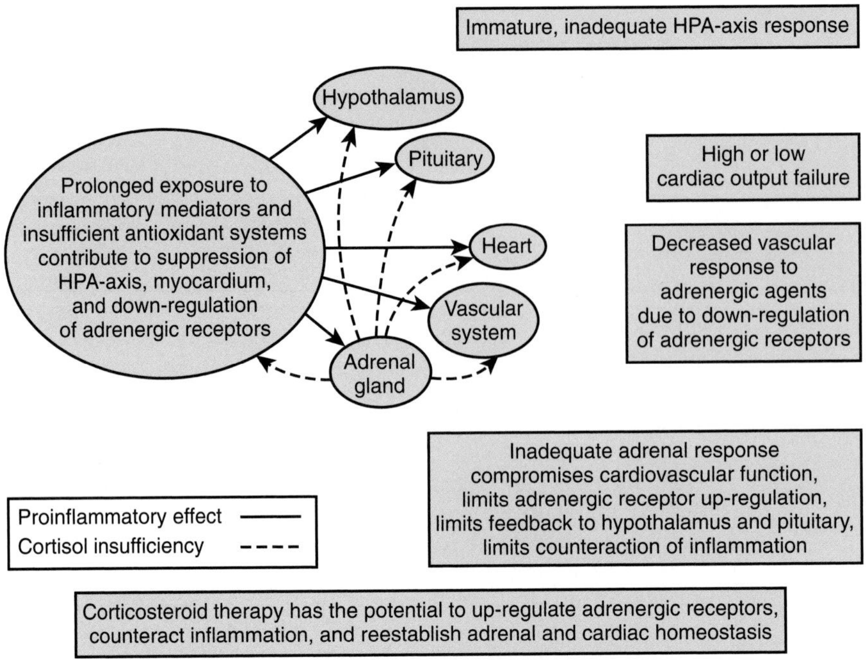

Figure 14-2 Effects of inflammation and immature antioxidant defense on the immature HPA axis and cardiovascular function. Corticosteroid treatment serves as hormone replacement therapy in RAI to counterbalance the cardiovascular and other organ system effects of inflammation in preterm neonates with immature HPA axis, cardiovascular function, and antioxidant defenses. RAI, relative adrenal insufficiency. See text for details.

Critical Care Medicine, in their most recent publication on clinical practice parameters for hemodynamic support of pediatric and neonatal septic shock, maintain "equipoise on the question of adjunctive steroid therapy and thus diagnosis of AI for pediatric and newborn septic shock (outside of classic AI) pending further trials."[64]

Devising diagnostic criteria for AI in infants is particularly challenging because there are the relatively little data available. The incidence of AI is greatly influenced by the choice of adrenal test. Neonatal investigators most often report isolated, random serum cortisol levels or stimulated serum cortisol levels at specific time points following corticotropin releasing hormone (CRH) or ACTH stimulation. Using random cortisol values at the time of stress, among VLBW infants, Korte and colleagues defined normal adrenal function as a random cortisol level of 15 μg/dL (414 nmol/L) and an inadequate serum cortisol as a serum cortisol level less than 5 μg/dL (<138 nmol/L).[18] In critically ill term and late preterm infants, Fernandez and colleagues showed that those with random cortisol values less than 15 μg/dL had higher blood pressure within 24 hours after hydrocortisone administration.[13] In addition, these infants demonstrated a decreased need for inotropes and lower heart rate after hydrocortisone compared to those with higher cortisol values. Debate remains on the use of random cortisol values as a diagnostic tool because total plasma cortisol can have marked hourly variability in both adults and neonates.[72,73] In addition, random cortisol values may not correlate with outcome, response to therapy, or severity of illness.[54,70,73]

To further test for AI, some investigators used CRH alone or CRH followed by ACTH.[16,50,74,75] Investigators more often selected ACTH as the stimulating agent with doses ranging from 0.1 to 62.5 μg/kg.[18,25,27,38,69,76-82] Adrenal stimulation with supraphysiologic ACTH doses can induce a compromised adrenal gland to produce an "adequate"-appearing cortisol level, and thus underestimate the diagnosis of AI.[18] However, ACTH doses of 0.1-0.2 μg/kg and 0.5-1.0 μg/kg are more likely to reveal "relative" AI than higher ACTH doses.[18,38,69,78,79] Even within the range of 0.1-1.0 μg/

kg, the proportion of sick premature infants with "inadequate" cortisol response (defined as <9 µg/dL) varies greatly. In a study of ventilated VLBW infants (gestational age <32 weeks and random serum cortisol levels <5 µg/dL (138 nmol/L), Korte and colleagues reported 64% and 37% of infants had inadequate cortisol response (<9 µg/dL) to cosyntropin at doses of 0.1 and 0.2 µg/dL, respectively.[18] In a trial of ventilated 3-week-old very preterm infants (gestational age 25 weeks), Watterberg and colleagues reported 21% and 2% of infants had inadequate cortisol response to 0.1 and 1.0 µg/kg ACTH, respectively.[69] In critically ill term infants, after giving 1 µg/kg of ACTH, Fernandez and colleagues found no infants with a cortisol value <18 µg/dL and all increment values were >9 µg/dL.[70] Additionally, there was no association between ACTH-stimulated cortisol values and severity of illness, need for vasopressor-inotropes, or days on mechanical ventilation. Soliman and colleagues, in a population of nonmechanically ventilated septic infants, found 0% with AI using an ACTH stimulation dose of 250 µg/1.73 m² and 13% with AI using 1 µg/1.73 m².[25] Those with lower stimulated cortisol values did have higher mortality.

Free cortisol and not the protein-bound cortisol is responsible for the physiologic effects at the cellular and receptor sites and may prove to be a better diagnostic tool for AI. However, the ability to measure free cortisol is not widely available as there are no available commercial tests. Yoder and colleagues chose to measure urinary free cortisol levels in 6-hourly blocked intervals in premature baboons (67% of term gestation, equivalent to ~28 weeks of human gestation) to define the ontogeny of cortisol release over the initial hours and days of postnatal life.[52] As noted by Yoder, urinary free cortisol levels are directly proportional to and highly correlated with plasma cortisol levels.[53] Moreover, urinary free cortisol avoids potential fluctuations seen in serum cortisol levels and the need for frequent blood sampling.[52]

The *lack of consensus on diagnostic evaluation and timing of evaluation* is further confounded by uncertainty about "adequate" and "inadequate" cortisol response or cortisol production across gestational and postnatal ages for different diagnostic evaluations.[18,69] More recent studies continue to complicate the utility of adrenal function tests. For instance, Miletin and colleagues found no correlation between superior vena cava flow and cortisol values or between cortisol and mean blood pressure values.[84] However, this finding might be explained by the lack of our ability to appropriately define the "normal range" for superior vena cava (SVC) blood flow since, similar to the "normal range" of blood pressure (Chapter 3), additional hemodynamic parameters affect the lower limit of the normal range of SVC flow in the individual patient (Chapters 1, 5, and 12). At present, the validity, reproducibility, and clinical importance of identifying inadequate cortisol response to illness or ACTH at different stimulating dosages (0.1, 0.2, 0.5, or 1.0 µg/kg ACTH) in terms of mortality, acute management, and longer outcomes is not clear in neonates. To further complicate the diagnosis, measurements of cortisol and ACTH stimulating tests may be influenced by the various procedures and the testing itself in acutely ill patients.[85] The validity and interpretation of adrenal function tests, especially in the midst of critical illness, is the subject of an ongoing debate among adult, pediatric, and neonatal critical care physicians.

Cardiovascular Insufficiency: Hypotension and Shock
(see also Chapter 1)

Vasopressor-dependent or vasopressor-resistant hypotension and shock are characterized by an acutely decreased vascular responsiveness to catecholamines. Decreased vascular responsiveness to adrenergic agents is due to down-regulation of adrenergic receptors.[86] Down-regulation of adrenergic receptors occurs within hours in clinical conditions of sustained sympathetic tone (including that caused by prolonged vasopressor therapy) and sustained exposure to inflammatory mediators, such as nitric oxide, tumor necrosis factor, and other inflammatory cytokines (interleukin [IL]-1,

IL-2, IL6, interferon gamma).[36,87-89] Thus multiple organ dysfunction may result, at least in part, from proinflammatory cytokine-mediated effects that decrease vascular reactivity and progress to vasopressor-resistant hypotension. Prolonged exposure to inflammatory mediators is one of the proposed mechanisms for both vasopressor-resistant hypotension (receptor down-regulation) and AI (suppression of adrenal and/or HPA axis). Severe illnesses in which decreased vascular responsiveness occurs include postnatal transition to extrauterine life, extreme prematurity, hypoxic-ischemic injury, respiratory disease, hemorrhage, sepsis, trauma, and major surgery.

Decreased vascular responsiveness to adrenergic stimulation is described in critically ill patients who did and did not meet study specific criteria for AI. Annane and colleagues observed worse vascular responsiveness in septic shock patients with AI compared to those without AI.[90] In contrast, Hoen and colleagues reported no difference in vascular responsiveness in adult hemorrhagic shock trauma patients with (n = 10) or without (n = 13) AI before hydrocortisone, and an increase in vascular reactivity after hydrocortisone appeared to be independent of adrenal reserve.[67] Indeed, several investigators documented improvement in vasopressor-dependent or vasopressor-resistant hypotension in patients with no evidence of AI by cortisol stimulation tests. It is clear that decreased vascular responsiveness due to down-regulation of adrenergic receptors is associated with vasopressor-resistant hypotension that responds to corticosteroid therapy. The scenario in which severe illness has components of decreased vascular responsiveness, due to inflammatory mediators, and concomitant cortisol insufficiency, corticosteroid therapy is critical to reestablish vascular responsiveness, counteract inflammation, and reestablish homeostasis.

The influence of specific precipitating events and mechanisms, and the temporal relationships that initiate vasopressor-resistant hypotension before AI, or vice versa, or both simultaneously are not known. It is clear though that insufficient cortisol activity in the presence of severe illness, or blocking the vascular effects of cortisol, results in profound hypotension.

Evidence of AI in Ill Preterm Infants

Colasurdo and Ward first described, in abstracts, ventilated, sick, extremely premature infants presenting with signs consistent with AI or "Addisonian crisis."[10,26] Ward's case series was prompted by prior observations of neonatal cases with unexplained cardiovascular collapse, abdominal distension, and renal failure prior to death. The specific manifestations reported in Colasurdo's and Ward's abstracts included hypotension, oliguria, hyponatremia, and cortisol values less than 15 μg/dL (414 nmol/L). All infants responded to hydrocortisone therapy. Subsequent investigations reported similar presentations of sick premature neonates with vasopressor-resistant hypotension, "low" serum cortisol levels, and rapid response to hydrocortisone or dexamethasone therapy. These case series and small studies provide most of the clinical and biochemical evidence that AI with vasopressor hypotension occurs in critically ill premature infants.* A recent randomized controlled trial (RCT) of hydrocortisone in hypotensive preterm infants found very low median cortisol values (<5 μg/dL) in enrolled infants.[30]

Contemporaneous with the studies in sick premature infants, investigators documented two intriguing observations regarding cortisol levels in well and sick premature infants. Many healthy premature infants, with no signs of AI, had random cortisol levels that were not detectable or below 5 μg/dL (138 nmol/L), a threshold considered to indicate AI.[14,16,18,23,27,30,77,80,91-94] Even more striking were observations that sick premature infants had serum cortisol levels similar to or lower than cortisol levels in well preterm or term infants.[16,18,26,27,30,50,74,77,92,93] The finding that sick premature infants did not have the expected increase in random cortisol levels commensurate with their illness acuity was additional evidence supportive of AI. Ng and

---

*References 7, 10, 12, 14, 16, 20, 21, 24-26, 37, 38, 41, 77, 91, 92.

colleagues reported normal pituitary response to hypothalamic cortisol–releasing hormone (hCRH) but absent adrenal response in sick premature infants with vasopressor-resistant hypotension and low serum cortisol values. These findings led Ng and colleagues to speculate that, in preterm neonates, the adrenal gland was responsible for AI.[20]

Additional evidence of AI in sick premature infants is supported by reported low random cortisol levels, elevated cortisol precursor in premature infants, with the highest precursor levels occurring in sick premature infants, and blunted response to ACTH stimulation.[14,18,76,77,92-95] Elevated cortisol precursors suggest that the adrenal gland responds to ACTH or other stimuli, but the adrenal enzyme system is not adequate to produce cortisol. As mentioned earlier, Guttentag and colleagues reported, in abstract, that sick extremely premature infants have inadequate random and stimulated cortisol levels through postnatal day 14, and that increasing precursor-to-cortisol ratios suggest the activity of other adrenal stimulants (e.g. IL-1, AII).[14] Watterberg and colleagues reported that compared to term infants, sick premature infants have higher cortisol precursor concentrations (17α-OH pregnenolone, 17α-OH progesterone, and 11-deoxycortisol) and low serum cortisol concentrations. Sick premature infants who developed chronic lung disease had elevated cortisol precursors compared with premature infants who recovered with no chronic lung disease.[94] In a small, prospective study of infants born at less than 30 weeks' gestation, Huysman and colleagues demonstrated that sick, ventilated infants, compared with less sick, nonventilated infants, had lower cortisol levels, elevated cortisol precursor 17-hydroxyprogesterone, and insufficient cortisol response to ACTH (0.5 µg/kg) stimulation.[38]

Insufficient adrenal function is also supported by studies of decreased adrenal response in sick premature infants. Korte and colleagues reported adrenal response to cosyntropin (ACTH) 0.1 vs. 0.2 µg/kg in 51 ventilated, premature infants of less than 32 weeks' gestation (birth weight <1.5 kg) who had baseline cortisol levels less than 5 µg/dL (138 nmol/L). Among these 51 infants, 64% and 37% had inadequate cortisol response (<9 µg/dL) to stimulation with either cosyntropin 0.1 or 0.2, respectively.[18] More recently, Watterberg and colleagues reported adrenal response to cosyntropin 0.1 vs. 1.0 µg/kg in premature infants (birth weight <1 kg and required ventilation) when tested at approximately 3 weeks of age.[69] Among 100 infants tested with cosyntropin at a dose of 0.1µg/kg, 21% had decreased cortisol response compared to 2% of 129 infants tested with cosyntropin at 1.0 µg/kg. A response curve based on cosyntropin 1.0 µg/kg indicated the 10th percentile response was 17 µg/dL (468 nmol/L). Cortisol response < 17 vs. ≥ 17 µg/dL was associated with more bronchopulmonary dysplasia and increased length of hospital stay.[69] Research by Watterberg and colleagues, Scott and colleagues, Huysman and colleagues, and others supports the notion that AI in sick, extremely premature infants is associated with increased pulmonary disease severity and subsequent chronic lung disease.[18,27,38,50,69,75,82,96-99]

Evidence of AI in Ill Late Preterm and Term Infants

There is growing evidence that a significant number of ill term and late preterm infants have AI.[13,25,40,53,55,80,100] In 1972, Gutai and colleagues were among the first authors to describe suboptimal cortisol responses to illness in a small number of stressed term newborn infants.[101] There was no difference in the median random cortisol value between 12 ill infants (5.2 µg/dL) and 28 normal newborns (4.1 µg/dL), and all infants responded to 5 units of ACTH appropriately. A subsequent study by Thomas and colleagues found 27% of ill term newborns studied had basal cortisol less than 2 µg/dL, and only 33% of those had an appropriate response to ACTH (>18 µg/dL).[80] In the first study to investigate cardiovascular responses to dexamethasone in full newborn infants with hypotension, Tanivit and colleagues found five of the seven infants had cortisol values less than 10 µg/dL.[71] All of these infants responded to glucocorticoid administration with prompt hemodynamic stabilization. In 2000, Pittinger described low cortisol values in sick infants with congenital diaphragmatic hernia and found 79% had random cortisol levels of less than 7 µg/dL.[100] Two of the four fatally ill patients had an inappropriately low cortisol response to cosyntropin. Soliman and colleagues found an overall increase in basal circulating cortisol concentration by 2- to 3-fold in newborns with sepsis and respiratory distress compared with healthy newborns.[25] Over 30% of these infants had cortisol values suggestive of AI (<15 µg/dL). Those with lower basal and peak cortisol responses to ACTH had higher mortality. In a larger, prospective, observational study of ill late preterm and term infants (n = 35) requiring mechanical ventilation, the median random cortisol level was 4.6 µg/dL, very low for the degree of illness and 74% had cortisol values <15 µg/dL.[70] These infants had relatively low ACTH values and appropriate cortisol responses to ACTH stimulation (1 µg/kg) suggesting secondary AI, a mechanism different for AI than what has been proposed in the ill VLBW infant.

The increased risk of serious short- and longer-term morbidity and mortality associated with AI in premature infants and the growing evidence in term newborns emphasize the need to recognize AI as a possible diagnosis. Studies in adults with AI implicate the hypothalamic-pituitary level is responsible for AI in some patients but that dysfunction at the adrenal level is the site primarily responsible for AI in most patients. Given the complex multisite mechanisms involved with AI, it is plausible that, in addition to the level of immaturity, inflammatory cytokines and/or other mediators may affect function at all levels of the HPA axis including problems at the level of the receptors. In summary, the level or levels of dysfunction within the HPA axis of newborn infants with AI is not completely understood and appears to depend on gestational age and type and severity of the underlying illness.

Cardiovascular Insufficiency and Adrenal Insufficiency in Ill Infants

Cardiovascular insufficiency is a recognized complication in sick infants and a key manifestation of AI. In addition to AI, other potential explanations for cardiovascular instability in sick infants include hypovolemia, severe anemia, myocardial dysfunction, abnormal regulation of vasomotor tone such as seen with sepsis, patent ductus arteriosus, hypoxic-ischemic injury, pulmonary hypertension, and anatomic abnormalities (Chapter 1). AI and the other etiologies of cardiovascular instability not infrequently occur simultaneously. Blood pressure has been found to positively correlate with cortisol production rate; that is, patients with low cortisol values are more likely to have low blood pressure.[34] In an RCT of hydrocortisone in hypotensive preterm newborn infants, their overall baseline median serum cortisol concentration was 3.3 and 4.1 µg/dL in the treated and placebo groups, respectively.[30] These values are thought to be low for the degree of illness even in preterm infants. In term infants, low median cortisol values have been reported to be in the range of 4.5-11.7 µg/dL in the face of refractory hypotension.[13,54,70] Attenuated cortisol response to adrenal stimulation and extremely high random cortisol levels may also represent a clinical presentation in which vasopressor-resistant hypotension is the predominant factor of the cardiovascular collapse. Infants with high random cortisol and low cortisol response to ACTH appear to have a greater risk for morbidity and mortality compared with infants with lower random cortisol levels.[81] Severely ill adults with high random cortisol (>34 mg/dL) and low cortisol response to ACTH stimulation (<9 µg/dL) are also noted to have extremely poor prognosis. Presentation of cardiovascular instability in sick infants may be recognized within a few hours to days following birth or later in the neonatal course.[7,12,13,20,25,41,45,70,94,102]

Cardiovascular compromise in the setting of AI may present as low systemic perfusion or hyperdynamic shock.[35] Characteristics of shock with low systemic perfusion include unchanged or decreased myocardial function and a compensatory increase in systemic vascular resistance to maintain perfusion pressure.

Relative or absolute hypovolemia may also be a contributing factor (Chapters 1 and 12). Hyperdynamic shock presents with high cardiac output and decreased systemic vascular resistance with advancing impairment of systemic and organ perfusion as the compensatory increase in cardiac output fails to maintain appropriate tissue oxygen delivery (Chapter 1). The specific presentation may depend upon myocardial immaturity and/or injury, prior fluid and electrolyte management, mineralocorticoid status, vasopressor therapy, and presence or absence of sepsis.[40] In preterm neonates, hypotension related to AI may occur with both presentations of shock.[103,104]

Alverson and Scott reported clinical, physiologic, and biochemical evidence linking cardiovascular insufficiency, increased morbidity (chronic lung disease), and increased mortality with low plasma cortisol levels in sick premature infants.[24,46,105] Alverson and colleagues reported, in an abstract, that 85 surfactant-treated, preterm infants (24 to 36 weeks' gestation) with left ventricular output (LVO) ≤ 180 mL//min/kg had greater mortality (6/14, 64%) during the first postnatal day compared with infants with an LVO of greater than 180 mL/min/kg (9/71, 13%) ($P = .001$).[3] Mortality was highest in infants less than 31 weeks' gestation who had lower LVO (9/10, 90%). Scott and colleagues measured serum cortisol values in 54 of the 85 infants reported by Alverson and colleagues. Infants with LVO ≤ 180 mL/min/kg had significantly lower cortisol values than infants with LVO greater than 180 mL/min/kg. In addition, infants with low LVO and low cortisol levels did not respond well to surfactant therapy. However, it should be kept in mind that LVO is influenced by left-to-right shunting at the level of the ductus arteriosus and, to a lesser extent, the foramen ovale during the first postnatal days and thus it does not appropriately represent systemic perfusion as long as these fetal channels are open.[103,104] In addition, the findings only reveal the presence of an association rather than causation. In separate reports, Scott and Watterberg described lower cortisol levels in preterm infants who required inotropic support and surfactant therapy than preterm infants not receiving vasopressor therapy.[23,99]

Among publications and abstracts on adrenal function and/or hydrocortisone's effect on vasopressor-resistant hypotension in sick infants or baboons, human reports and one baboon study have documented low cortisol values and vasopressor-resistant hypotension responsive to corticosteroid treatment.[10,12,20,24,26,30,37,51,52] Some studies report a similar presentation without cortisol data.[12,24,25,43,106] Vasopressor-resistant hypotension responded to corticosteroid therapy in all but two infants among reported neonates.[20] Responding infants weaned from vasopressor support often within 2-3 days. Other neonatal reports about the effect of hydrocortisone on blood pressure or other outcomes are not comparable to these studies due to different objectives and inclusion criteria that did not limit their study to infants with vasopressor-responsive hypotension and/or specific cortisol criteria. Efird and colleagues reported that prophylactic hydrocortisone therapy for 5 days (versus placebo) in extremely low birth weight infants reduced the use of vasopressors during the first two postnatal days.[107]

The study by Yoder and colleagues on very premature baboons provides the most direct evidence that AI, cardiovascular insufficiency, and prematurity are related.[52] In earlier studies, this group of investigators documented that the majority of extremely premature baboons, delivered at ~67% of baboon gestation (~26 weeks human gestation), required volume expansion and vasopressor therapy to treat hypotension, oliguria, and acid-base imbalance. Many of the premature baboons also required hydrocortisone to treat vasopressor-resistant hypotension.[108] Yoder and colleagues then demonstrated that decreased urinary free cortisol excretion in the first day of postnatal life correlated with decreased left ventricular function. Furthermore, hydrocortisone therapy (0.5-1.0 mg/kg/day for 1-2 days) corrected hypotension and left ventricular dysfunction, reduced vasopressor/inotrope use and mortality, and increased serum cortisol to levels comparable to cortisol levels seen in baboons with no evidence of AI or cardiovascular dysfunction through the end of the study at two weeks of extrauterine life.[52]

Mechanisms of Corticosteroids in the Treatment of Cardiovascular Insufficiency

The goal of corticosteroid therapy is to maintain homeostasis during stress, minimize organ dysfunction, and ensure appropriate tissue oxygen delivery. The HPA axis and the adrenergic and sympathetic nervous system are the primary mediators of stress response. Under normal conditions, all forms of stress increase ACTH and cortisol production.

The cardiovascular effects of corticosteroid maintain myocardial contractility, vascular tone, endothelial integrity, and vascular responsiveness to catecholamines and angiotensin II. Corticosteroids attenuate the proinflammatory cytokine response, reduce vascular permeability in the presence of acute inflammation, decrease the dysregulated production of nitric oxide (NO) and other vasodilators, and modulate free water distribution within the vascular compartment.[24,39,40,109-111]

Corticosteroids also modulate the immune response and counteract the inflammatory cascade. Acute exposure to inflammatory cytokines may increase affinity of glucocorticoid receptors. In addition, acute exposure to inflammatory cytokines (e.g., IL-1, IL-6, TNF-alpha) can activate the HPA axis, which decreases the inflammatory response, and may increase ligand affinity of glucocorticoid receptors. Cortisol feedback regulates the period for immunosuppressive and catabolic needs during stress. On the other hand, prolonged exposure to cytokines alters the response of the HPA axis. Low levels of ACTH have been documented in patients with severe sepsis. Chronic increase in IL-6 can suppress ACTH production and prolonged exposure to TNF-alpha may decrease adrenal function and CRH stimulation of ACTH production.

Corticosteroids exert their effects through genomic (slower) and non-genomic mechanisms.[40,110,111] Genomic actions of glucocorticoids reverse vasopressor-refractory hypotension by up-regulating cardiovascular α- and β-adrenergic receptors through synthesis and membrane-assembly of new receptor proteins, a process that occurs over hours. Other genomic effects include glucocorticoid mediation of the sympathetic nerve activity and maturational changes in Na^+, K^+-ATPase enzyme activity, myosin fibers, and other components of cardiac muscle.[40,112,113] However, the rapid response of the cardiovascular system to corticosteroids is thought to occur via non-genomic mechanisms through interaction with putative cell membrane-bound steroid receptors.[22] Via their genomic and non-genomic actions, corticosteroids rapidly sensitize the cardiovascular system to catecholamines. Corticosteroids exert their cardiovascular effects by increasing catecholamine levels through enhanced catecholamine synthesis and inhibition of catecholamine metabolism, by inhibition of prostacyclin and nitric oxide synthesis, by increasing intracellular calcium availability leading to enhanced myocardial and vascular smooth muscle cell contraction, and by improving capillary integrity (Chapters 1 and 12).

Corticosteroid Therapy for Cardiovascular Insufficiency

High-dose, short course, corticosteroid administration has shown no benefit and possible harm in critically ill adult patients with acute lung injury, acute respiratory distress syndrome (ARDS), and septic shock.[4,60] Instead, prolonged, low-dose corticosteroid therapy has shown beneficial effects on short-term mortality, ventilation-free days, length of intensive care unit stay, multiple organ dysfunction syndrome scores, lung injury scores, and shock reversal without increasing significant adverse events.[4,114,115]

Corticosteroids are recommended in adults with catecholamine refractory shock (norepinephrine or equivalent dose of inotrope > 0.05-0.1 µg/kg/min) or having ARDS for more than 48 hours.[60] In these adult patients, a course of stress-dose of hydrocortisone at a dose of 200-350 mg/day (about 3 mg/kg/day) is recommended for at least 7 days because rapid steroid tapers (2-6 days) have been associated with rebound inflammation, increased inflammatory mediators, and a need to reintroduce vasopressors and mechanical ventilation.[116,117]

Reversal of shock (withdrawal of vasopressors) in septic *adult patients* occurs earlier after receiving hydrocortisone vs. placebo (3.3 vs. 5.8 median days).[82] In a group of septic adults with higher severity of illness, the median time to vasopressor withdrawal with corticosteroids vs. placebo was 7 vs. 9 days, respectively.[6]

A 2007 Cochrane review on *corticosteroids for the treatment of hypotension in preterm infants* concluded that there was insufficient information to give any recommendations based on the two studies reviewed.[118] A more recent metaanalysis in preterm neonates with hypotension and vasopressor dependence, showed that hydrocortisone is effective in increasing blood pressure (seven studies, N = 144, r = 0.71, 95% CI = 0.18 to 0.92) and reducing vasopressor requirement (five studies, N = 93, r = 0.74, 95% CI = 0.0084-0.96).[119] The authors were not able to examine dosing strategy, adverse effects or any effect on medium- to long-term outcomes because of the limited data available. However, random effects meta-analysis found that the number of new studies needed to cancel out the effects of hydrocortisone on blood pressure increase and vasopressor requirement is 78 for blood pressure increase and 47 for reducing vasopressor requirement. Thus these selected cardiovascular effects of hydrocortisone in preterm infants with vasopressor resistance are robust with a large tolerance for future null results.

The *time to documented cardiovascular response to hydrocortisone* is often measured in hours in the ill newborn population. Helbock reported increase in blood pressure as early as 30 minutes and within 2 hours following hydrocortisone therapy (1 mg) in 25- to 26-week gestation infants with vasopressor-resistant hypotension.[37] Based on their case series, Helbock and Ng speculated that response time for reversal of vasopressor-resistant hypotension may be dose-related.[20,37] Gaissmaier and Pohlandt noted improvement in vasopressor-resistant hypotension in 4-8 hours following a single injection of dexamethasone.[51] Seri and colleagues and Noori and colleagues reported an increase in blood pressure within 2 hours following hydrocortisone and low-dose dexamethasone (0.1 mg/kg) administration, respectively.[24,43] Ng and colleagues showed a difference in the percentage of infants able to wean off vasopressors by 72 hours between those given hydrocortisone vs. placebo (79% vs. 33%, *P* = .001).[30] In 15 newborn infants, Noori and colleagues studied hemodynamics following hydrocortisone (2 mg/kg, followed by 1 mg/kg every 12 hours) and showed a significant increase in blood pressure at 6 hours, a parallel increase in systemic vascular resistance and a decrease in dopamine dosage without initial changes in stroke volume or left ventricular output.[103] The five term infants enrolled in this study showed no response in blood pressure to hydrocortisone but did have lower heart rate and received lower dopamine doses compared to baseline by 48 hours.

In seven *term ill newborn infants* given dexamethasone of 0.2 mg/kg/day, an increase in blood pressure was noted by 4 hours after initial dosing with a concomitant decrease in heart rate and vasopressor dosage.[71] Vasopressors were discontinued in all infants within 72 hours after initiating dexamethasone. In a larger study of ill late preterm and term neonates, there was a significant change in blood pressure over the first 24 hours after hydrocortisone and an overall decrease in vasopressor dose and heart rate within 12 hours.[13] However, there was no difference in blood pressure response between infants with high or low random cortisol values. In 12 term infants given hydrocortisone for low cardiac output syndrome after cardiac surgery, the blood pressure increased significantly 3 hours after hydrocortisone.[120] Baker found an increase in blood pressure starting at 2 hours and a decrease in the total inotrope dosage by 6 hours in a study of 117 critically ill term and preterm newborns.[54] Newborn infants appear to respond with improved hemodynamics to glucocorticoids within 2-6 hours of initiation of treatment.

Hydrocortisone dosing in infants. Pharmacokinetic data in newborn infants are sparse. In extremely low birth weight infants, in the first week of postnatal life, Watterberg and colleagues reported on six intubated infants who received 1.2-2.4 mg/kg/day of hydrocortisone. The mean serum half-life of hydrocortisone was 12.1 ± 5.8 hours (range 3.6-19).[120] In 1962, Reynolds and colleagues reported pharmacokinetics in five term infants after a bolus of 5 mg/kg hydrocortisone.[121]

Serum concentrations were evaluated with two different assay methods (Porter-Silber chromogen values and chromatography with isotope dilution), which showed similar results. Mean peak serum concentration (30-80 minutes after dose) was 557 µg/dL, and mean serum half-life was just under 4 hours (range 2.4-7.1 hours). This half-life is much longer than in adults, where elimination half-life has been reported to be 2 ± 0.3 hours.[122]

Doses as low as 1 mg/kg/day of hydrocortisone in preterm infants have been shown to increase blood pressure significantly.[81] Studies of vasopressor-dependent, critically ill newborn infants have used variable hydrocortisone dosing (2-3 mg/kg/day), and all have shown an increase in blood pressure, a decrease in volume and inotrope requirement, and a decrease in heart rate without confirmed increases in adverse events.[7,13,24,30,54,103,119]

Currently, there are insufficient data in neonates to recommend specific glucocorticoid interventions, particularly as related to criteria for treatment, type of glucocorticoid, dosage, and duration. This uncertainty is further fueled by the documented increases in spontaneous ileal perforations in premature neonates co-exposed to either hydrocortisone or dexamethasone and indomethacin as well as by the documented deleterious effects of early higher dose dexamethasone on neurodevelopment in preterm neonates.[81,123] There are encouraging recent studies on the long-term effects of hydrocortisone. A metaanalysis of three trials with a total of 411 children found that early low-dose hydrocortisone in preterm infants had no effect on the rate of cerebral palsy and survival without neurosensory or cognitive impairment.[97] In the largest of the three studies, there was a significantly lower incidence of cognitive deficits at 18-22 months in former preterm infants who received hydrocortisone early in life.[124] However, as none of the studies was designed to investigate long-term neurodevelopment as the primary outcome measure, the studies might have been underpowered and the findings need to be confirmed with appropriately designed CRTs.

Conclusion

Adequate HPA axis and adrenal function are vital to postnatal adaptation in extremely premature infants and critically ill late preterm and term newborn infants. Clinical, biochemical, and physiologic evidence indicates that AI and vasopressor-resistant hypotension are serious disorders in sick preterm and term infants, and that these conditions respond to corticosteroid therapy with improvements in the cardiovascular status. However, whether this improvement translates to improved mortality and/or morbidity is not known. Yet, recent findings provide important insight into AI and vasopressor-resistant hypotension and stimulate consideration of mechanisms for AI and vasopressor-resistant hypotension. Management of the critically ill hypotensive infant remains challenging and requires a better understanding of the pathophysiology of neonatal shock and improvements in our ability to evaluate cardiac output, organ blood flow, and tissue perfusion in real time at the bedside.

However, we still need to improve our understanding of the pathogenesis and epidemiology of AI and vasopressor-resistant hypotension especially in terms of determinants, mechanisms, and patterns, and their relationship with acute and long-term morbidity/mortality. Ultimately, we need to provide evidence that our interventions also improve clinically meaningful outcomes.

Another challenge is to improve diagnostic methods to assess adrenal function and vasopressor-resistant hypotension and criteria for treatment. We need to be able to determine which patient needs therapy and what evaluations provide reliable information early in the neonatal course? Are serum cortisol values the optimal measure of adrenal function? Can one improve diagnosis and prognosis by combining responses of different tests? Could serum or urine evaluations of adrenal function refine diagnosis? Will simultaneous measurements of inflammatory mediators improve our understanding and guide therapy? By improving our ability to establish accurate and timely diagnosis of AI, we will be able to target higher risk patients for investigational and clinical interventions and avoid unnecessary exposure of lower risk infants to glucocorticoid therapy. In addition, the more comprehensive issues to be addressed include identifying the factors influencing the choice of corticosteroid treatment and establishing the dosage, duration, and response to therapy of the individual patient.[125] We also need to find out whether corticosteroid regimens need to be adjusted according to disease severity or the response to treatment to maximize effectiveness and minimize harm. Only scientifically and ethically sound research and carefully designed studies will resolve these questions.

References

1. Cohen J, Venkatesh B. Relative adrenal insufficiency in the intensive care population; background and critical appraisal of the evidence. Anaesth Intensive Care. 2010;38:425-436.
2. Cooper MS, Stewart PM. Adrenal insufficiency in critical illness. J Intensive Care Med. 2007;22: 348-362.
3. Fernandez EF, Watterberg KL. Relative adrenal insufficiency in the preterm and term infant. J Perinatol. 2009;29(suppl 2):S44-S49.
4. Marik PE. Critical illness-related corticosteroid insufficiency. Chest. 2009;135:181-193.
5. de Jong FH, Mallios C, Jansen C, et al. Etomidate suppresses adrenocortical function by inhibition of 11 beta-hydroxylation. J Clin Endocrinol Metab. 1984;59:1143-1147.
6. Annane D, Sebille V, Charpentier C, et al. Effect of treatment with low doses of hydrocortisone and fludrocortisone on mortality in patients with septic shock. JAMA. 2002;288:862-871.
7. Bourchier D, Weston PJ. Randomised trial of dopamine compared with hydrocortisone for the treatment of hypotensive very low birthweight infants. Arch Dis Child Fetal Neonatal Ed. 1997;76:F174-F178.
8. Briegel J, Forst H, Kellermann W, et al. Haemodynamic improvement in refractory septic shock with cortisol replacement therapy. Intensive Care Med. 1992;18:318.
9. Caplan RH, Wickus GG, Reynertson RH, et al. Occult hypoadrenalism in critically ill patients. Arch Surg. 1994;129:456.
10. Colasurdo MA, HCa GJ, et al. Hydrocortisone replacement in extremely premature infants with cortisol insufficiency. Clin Res. 1989.
11. Cooper MS, Stewart PM. Corticosteroid insufficiency in acutely ill patients. N Engl J Med. 2003;348:727-734.
12. Fauser A, Pohlandt F, Bartmann P, et al. Rapid increase of blood pressure in extremely low birth weight infants after a single dose of dexamethasone. Eur J Pediatr. 1993;152:354-356.
13. Fernandez E, Schrader R, Watterberg K. Prevalence of low cortisol values in term and near-term infants with vasopressor-resistant hypotension. J Perinatol. 2005;25:114-118.
14. Guttentag SH, Rubin LP, Douglas R, et al. The glucocorticoid pathway in ill and well extremely low birthweight infants. Pediatric Res. 1991;77A.
15. Hanna CE, Jett PL, Laird MR, et al. Corticosteroid binding globulin, total serum cortisol, and stress in extremely low-birth-weight infants. Am J Perinatol. 1997;14:201-204.
16. Hanna CE, Keith LD, Colasurdo MA, et al. Hypothalamic pituitary adrenal function in the extremely low birth weight infant. J Clin Endocrinol Metab. 1993;76:384-387.
17. Ho JT, Al-Musalhi H, Chapman MJ, et al. Septic shock and sepsis: a comparison of total and free plasma cortisol levels. J Clin Endocrinol Metab. 2006;91:105-114.
18. Korte C, Styne D, Merritt TA, et al. Adrenocortical function in the very low birth weight infant: improved testing sensitivity and association with neonatal outcome. J Pediatr. 1996;128: 257-263.
19. Menon K, Ward RE, Lawson ML, et al. A prospective multicenter study of adrenal function in critically ill children. Am J Respir Crit Care Med. 2010;182:246-251.
20. Ng PC, Lam CW, Fok TF, et al. Refractory hypotension in preterm infants with adrenocortical insufficiency. Arch Dis Child Fetal Neonatal Ed. 2001;84:F122-F124.
21. Reynolds JW, Hanna CE. Glucocorticoid-responsive hypotension in extremely low birth weight newborns. Pediatrics. 1994;94:135-136.
22. Schneider AJ, Voerman HJ. Abrupt hemodynamic improvement in late septic shock with physiological doses of glucocorticoids. Intensive Care Med. 1991;17:436-437.
23. Scott SM, Watterberg KL. Effect of gestational age, postnatal age, and illness on plasma cortisol concentrations in premature infants. Pediatr Res. 1995;37:112-116.
24. Seri I, Tan R, Evans J. Cardiovascular effects of hydrocortisone in preterm infants with pressor-resistant hypotension. Pediatrics. 2001;107:1070-1074.
25. Soliman AT, Taman KH, Rizk MM, et al. Circulating adrenocorticotropic hormone (ACTH) and cortisol concentrations in normal, appropriate-for-gestational-age newborns versus those with sepsis and respiratory distress. Cortisol response to low-dose and standard-dose ACTH tests. Metabolism. 2004;53:209-214.
26. Ward RM R-DC. Addisonian crisis in extremely premature neonates. Clin Res. 1991.
27. Watterberg KL, Scott SM. Evidence of early adrenal insufficiency in babies who develop bronchopulmonary dysplasia. Pediatrics. 1995;95:120-125.
28. Annane D. Glucocorticoids in the treatment of severe sepsis and septic shock. Curr Opin Crit Care. 2005;11:449-453.

29. Langer M, Modi BP, Agus M. Adrenal insufficiency in the critically ill neonate and child. Curr Opin Pediatr. 2006;18:448-453.
30. Ng PC, Lee CH, Bnur FL, et al. A double-blind, randomized, controlled study of a "stress dose" of hydrocortisone for rescue treatment of refractory hypotension in preterm infants. Pediatrics. 2006;117:367-375.
31. Alverson D, Scott SM, Backstrom C, et al. Persistently low cardiac output during the first day of life predicts high mortality in preterm infants with respiratory distress syndrome. Pediatr Res. 1995;193A.
32. Annane D, Briegel J, Keh D, et al. Clinical equipoise remains for issues of adrenocorticotropic hormone administration, cortisol testing, and therapeutic use of hydrocortisone. Crit Care Med. 2003;31:2250-2251; author reply 2252-2253.
33. Annane D, Briegel J, Sprung CL. Corticosteroid insufficiency in acutely ill patients. N Engl J Med. 2003;348:2157-2159.
34. Arnold JD, Bonacruz G, Leslie GI, et al. Antenatal glucocorticoids modulate the amplitude of pulsatile cortisol secretion in premature neonates. Pediatr Res. 1998;44:876-881.
35. Briegel J, Forst H, Haller M, et al. Stress doses of hydrocortisone reverse hyperdynamic septic shock. a prospective, randomized, double-blind, single-center study. Crit Care Med. 1999;27:723-732.
36. Dimopoulou I, Tsagarakis S, Kouyialis AT, et al. Hypothalamic-pituitary-adrenal axis dysfunction in critically ill patients with traumatic brain injury. incidence, pathophysiology, and relationship to vasopressor dependence and peripheral interleukin-6 levels. Crit Care Med. 2004;32:404-408.
37. Helbock HJ, Insoft RM, Conte FA. Glucocorticoid-responsive hypotension in extremely low birth weight newborns. Pediatrics. 1993;92:715-717.
38. Huysman MW, Hokken-Koelega AC, De Ridder MA, et al. Adrenal function in sick very preterm infants. Pediatr Res. 2000;48:629-633.
39. Keh D, Boehnke T, Weber-Cartens S, et al. Immunologic and hemodynamic effects of "low-dose" hydrocortisone in septic shock. a double-blind, randomized, placebo-controlled, crossover study. Am J Respir Crit Care Med. 2003;167:512-520.
40. Lamberts SW, Bruining HA, de Jong FH. Corticosteroid therapy in severe illness. N Engl J Med. 1997;337:1285-1292.
41. Ng PC, Lee CH, Lam CW, et al. Transient adrenocortical insufficiency of prematurity and systemic hypotension in very low birthweight infants. Arch Dis Child Fetal Neonatal Ed. 2004;89:F119-F126.
42. Noori S, Seri I. Pathophysiology of newborn hypotension outside the transitional period. Early Hum Dev. 2005;81:399-404.
43. Noori S, Siassi B, Durand M, et al. Cardiovascular effects of low-dose dexamethasone in very low birth weight neonates with refractory hypotension. Biol Neonate. 2006;89:82-87.
44. Rivers EP, Gaspari M, Saad GA, et al. Adrenal insufficiency in high-risk surgical ICU patients. Chest. 2001;119:889-896.
45. Roze JC, Tohier C, Maingueneau C, et al. Response to dobutamine and dopamine in the hypotensive very preterm infant. Arch Dis Child. 1993;69:59-63.
46. Scott SM, Alverson DC, Backstrom C, et al. Positive effect of cortisol on cardiac output in the preterm infant. Pediatric Res. 1995;236A.
47. Seri I. Circulatory support of the sick preterm infant. Semin Neonatol. 2001;6:85-95.
48. Seri I, Tulassay T, Kiszel J, et al. Cardiovascular response to dopamine in hypotensive preterm neonates with severe hyaline membrane disease. Eur J Pediatr. 1984;142:3-9.
49. Hoen S, Asehnoune K, Brailly-Tabard S, et al. Cortisol response to corticotropin stimulation in trauma patients. influence of hemorrhagic shock. Anesthesiology. 2002;97:807-813.
50. Ng PC, Lam CW, Lee CH, et al. Reference ranges and factors affecting the human corticotropin-releasing hormone test in preterm, very low birth weight infants. J Clin Endocrinol Metab. 2002;87:4621-4628.
51. Gaissmaier RE, Pohlandt F. Single-dose dexamethasone treatment of hypotension in preterm infants. J Pediatr. 1999;134:701-705.
52. Yoder B, Martin H, McCurnin DC, et al. Impaired urinary cortisol excretion and early cardiopulmonary dysfunction in immature baboons. Pediatr Res. 2002;51:426-432.
53. Economou G, Andronikou S, Challa A, et al. Cortisol secretion in stressed babies during the neonatal period. Horm Res. 1993;40:217-221.
54. Baker CF, Barks JD, Engmann C, et al. Hydrocortisone administration for the treatment of refractory hypotension in critically ill newborns. J Perinatol. 2008;28:412-419.
55. Kamath BD, Fashaw L, Kinsella JP. Adrenal insufficiency in newborns with congenital diaphragmatic hernia. J Pediatr. 2010;156:495-497;e491.
56. Chrousos GP. The hypothalamic-pituitary-adrenal axis and immune-mediated inflammation. N Engl J Med. 1995;332:1351-1362.
57. Joosten KF, de Kleijn ED, Westerterp M, et al. Endocrine and metabolic responses in children with meningococcal sepsis: striking differences between survivors and nonsurvivors. J Clin Endocrinol Metab. 2000;85:3746-3753.
58. Meduri GU, Muthiah MP, Carratu P, et al. Nuclear factor-kappaB- and glucocorticoid receptor alpha- mediated mechanisms in the regulation of systemic and pulmonary inflammation during sepsis and acute respiratory distress syndrome. Evidence for inflammation-induced target tissue resistance to glucocorticoids. Neuroimmunomodulation. 2005;12:321-338.

59. Annane D, Maxime V, Ibrahim F, et al. Diagnosis of adrenal insufficiency in severe sepsis and septic shock. Am J Respir Crit Care Med. 2006;174:1319-1326.

60. Marik PE, Pastores SM, Annane D, et al. Recommendations for the diagnosis and management of corticosteroid insufficiency in critically ill adult patients: consensus statements from an international task force by the American College of Critical Care Medicine. Crit Care Med. 2008;36:1937-1949.

61. Angus M. One step forward: an advance in understanding of adrenal insufficiency in the pediatric critically ill. Crit Care Med. 2005;33:911-912.

62. Annane D. Time for a consensus definition of corticosteroid insufficiency in critically ill patients. Crit Care Med. 2003;31:1868-1869.

63. Arnold J, Leslie G, Bowen J, et al. Longitudinal study of plasma cortisol and 17-hydroxyprogesterone in very-low-birth-weight infants during the first 16 weeks of life. Biol Neonate. 1997;72: 148-155.

64. Brierley J, Carcillo JA, Choong K, et al. Clinical practice parameters for hemodynamic support of pediatric and neonatal septic shock: 2007 update from the American College of Critical Care Medicine. Crit Care Med. 2009;37:666-688.

65. Contreras LN, Arregger AL, Persi GG, et al. A new less-invasive and more informative low-dose ACTH test: salivary steroids in response to intramuscular corticotrophin. Clin Endocrinol (Oxf). 2004;61:675-682.

66. Dickstein G, Shechner C, Nicholson WE, et al. Adrenocorticotropin stimulation test: effects of basal cortisol level, time of day, and suggested new sensitive low dose test. J Clin Endocrinol Metab. 1991;72:773-778.

67. Hoen S, Mazoit JX, Asehnoune K, et al. Hydrocortisone increases the sensitivity to alpha1-adrenoceptor stimulation in humans following hemorrhagic shock. Crit Care Med. 2005;33: 2737-2743.

68. Marik PE, Zaloga GP. Adrenal insufficiency during septic shock. Crit Care Med. 2003;31: 141-145.

69. Watterberg KL, Shaffer ML, Garland JS, et al. Effect of dose on response to adrenocorticotropin in extremely low birth weight infants. J Clin Endocrinol Metab. 2005;90:6380-6385.

70. Fernandez EF, Montman R, Watterberg KL. ACTH and cortisol response to critical illness in term and late preterm newborns. J Perinatol. 2008;28:797-802.

71. Tantivit P, Subramanian N, Garg M, et al. Low serum cortisol in term newborns with refractory hypotension. J Perinatol. 1999;19:352-357.

72. Metzger DL, Wright NM, Veldhuis JD, et al. Characterization of pulsatile secretion and clearance of plasma cortisol in premature and term neonates using deconvolution analysis. J Clin Endocrinol Metab. 1993;77:458-463.

73. Venkatesh B, Mortimer RH, Couchman B, et al. Evaluation of random plasma cortisol and the low dose corticotropin test as indicators of adrenal secretory capacity in critically ill patients: a prospective study. Anaesth Intensive Care. 2005;33:201-209.

74. Bolt RJ, van Weissenbruch MM, Cranendonk A, et al. The corticotrophin-releasing hormone test in preterm infants. Clin Endocrinol (Oxf). 2002;56:207-213.

75. Ng PC, Wong GW, Lam CW, et al. The pituitary-adrenal responses to exogenous human corticotropin-releasing hormone in preterm, very low birth weight infants. J Clin Endocrinol Metab. 1997;82:797-799.

76. Bolt RJ, Van Weissenbruch MM, Popp-Snijders C, et al. Maturity of the adrenal cortex in very preterm infants is related to gestational age. Pediatr Res. 2002;52:405-410.

77. Hingre RV, Gross SJ, Hingre KS, et al. Adrenal steroidogenesis in very low birth weight preterm infants. J Clin Endocrinol Metab. 1994;78:266-270.

78. Karlsson R, Kallio J, Irjala K, et al. Adrenocorticotropin and corticotropin-releasing hormone tests in preterm infants. J Clin Endocrinol Metab. 2000;85:4592-4595.

79. Karlsson R, Kallio J, Toppari J, et al. Timing of peak serum cortisol values in preterm infants in low-dose and the standard ACTH tests. Pediatr Res. 1999;45:367-369.

80. Thomas S, Murphy JF, Dyas J, et al. Response to ACTH in the newborn. Arch Dis Child. 1986;61:57-60.

81. Watterberg KL, Gerdes JS, Cole CH, et al. Prophylaxis of early adrenal insufficiency to prevent bronchopulmonary dysplasia: a multicenter trial. Pediatrics. 2004;114:1649-1657.

82. Watterberg KL, Gerdes JS, Gifford KL, et al. Prophylaxis against early adrenal insufficiency to prevent chronic lung disease in premature infants. Pediatrics. 1999;104:1258-1263.

83. Trainer PJ, McHardy KC, Harvey RD, et al. Urinary free cortisol in the assessment of hydrocortisone replacement therapy. Horm Metab Res. 1993;25:117-120.

84. Miletin J, Pichova K, Doyle S, et al. Serum cortisol values, superior vena cava flow and illness severity scores in very low birth weight infants. J Perinatol. 2010;30:522-526.

85. Sweeney DA, Natanson C, Banks SM, et al. Defining normal adrenal function testing in the intensive care unit setting: a canine study. Crit Care Med. 2010;38:553-561.

86. Briegel J, Jochum M, Gippner-Steppert C, et al. Immunomodulation in septic shock: hydrocortisone differentially regulates cytokine responses. J Am Soc Nephrol. 2001;12(suppl 17):S70-S74.

87. Tsuneyoshi I, Kanmura Y, Yoshimura N. Lipoteichoic acid from Staphylococcus aureus depresses contractile function of human arteries in vitro due to the induction of nitric oxide synthase. Anesth Analg. 1996;82:948-953.

88. Tsuneyoshi I, Kanmura Y, Yoshimura N. Methylprednisolone inhibits endotoxin-induced depression of contractile function in human arteries in vitro. Br J Anaesth. 1996;76:251-257.

89. Tsuneyoshi I, Kanmura Y, Yoshimura N. Nitric oxide as a mediator of reduced arterial responsiveness in septic patients. Crit Care Med. 1996;24:1083-1086.

90. Annane D, Bellissant E, Sebille V, et al. Impaired pressor sensitivity to noradrenaline in septic shock patients with and without impaired adrenal function reserve. Br J Clin Pharmacol. 1998;46:589-597.

91. Heckmann M, Wudy SA, Haack D, et al. Reference range for serum cortisol in well preterm infants. Arch Dis Child Fetal Neonatal Ed. 1999;81:F171-F174.

92. Lee MM, Rajagopalan L, Berg GJ, et al. Serum adrenal steroid concentrations in premature infants. J Clin Endocrinol Metab. 1989;69:1133-1136.

93. al Saedi S, Dean H, Dent W, et al. Reference ranges for serum cortisol and 17-hydroxyprogesterone levels in preterm infants. J Pediatr. 1995;126:985-987.

94. Watterberg KL, Gerdes JS, Cook KL. Impaired glucocorticoid synthesis in premature infants developing chronic lung disease. Pediatr Res. 2001;50:190-195.

95. Linder N, Davidovitch N, Kogan A, et al. Longitudinal measurements of 17alpha-hydroxyprogesterone in premature infants during the first three months of life. Arch Dis Child Fetal Neonatal Ed. 1999;81:F175-F178.

96. Ng PC, Lee CH, Lam CW, et al. Early pituitary-adrenal response and respiratory outcomes in preterm infants. Arch Dis Child Fetal Neonatal Ed. 2004;89:F127-F130.

97. Peltoniemi O, Kari MA, Heinonen K, et al. Pretreatment cortisol values may predict responses to hydrocortisone administration for the prevention of bronchopulmonary dysplasia in high-risk infants. J Pediatr. 2005;146:632-637.

98. Scott SM, Cimino DF. Evidence for developmental hypopituitarism in ill preterm infants. J Perinatol. 2004;24:429-434.

99. Watterberg KL, Scott SM, Backstrom C, et al. Links between early adrenal function and respiratory outcome in preterm infants: airway inflammation and patent ductus arteriosus. Pediatrics. 2000;105:320-324.

100. Pittinger TP, Sawin RS. Adrenocortical insufficiency in infants with congenital diaphragmatic hernia: a pilot study. J Pediatr Surg. 2000;35:223-225; discussion 225-226.

101. Gutai J, George R, Koeff S, et al. Adrenal response to physical stress and the effect of adrenocorticotropic hormone in newborn infants. J Pediatr. 1972;81:719-725.

102. Pladys P, Wodey E, Beuchee A, et al. Left ventricle output and mean arterial blood pressure in preterm infants during the 1st day of life. Eur J Pediatr. 1999;158:817-824.

103. Noori S, Friedlich P, Wong P, et al. Hemodynamic changes after low-dosage hydrocortisone administration in vasopressor-treated preterm and term neonates. Pediatrics. 2006;118:1456-1466.

104. Seri I. Management of hypotension and low systemic blood flow in the very low birth weight neonate during the first postnatal week. J Perinatol. 2006;26(suppl 1):S8-13; discussion S22-13.

105. Palta M, Gabbert D, Weinstein MR, et al. Multivariate assessment of traditional risk factors for chronic lung disease in very low birth weight neonates. The Newborn Lung Project. J Pediatr. 1991;119:285-292.

106. Suominen PK, Dickerson HA, Moffett BS, et al. Hemodynamic effects of rescue protocol hydrocortisone in neonates with low cardiac output syndrome after cardiac surgery. Pediatr Crit Care Med. 2005;6:655-659.

107. Efird MM, Heerens AT, Gordon PV, et al. A randomized-controlled trial of prophylactic hydrocortisone supplementation for the prevention of hypotension in extremely low birth weight infants. J Perinatol. 2005;25:119-124.

108. Coalson JJ, Winter VT, Siler-Khodr T, et al. Neonatal chronic lung disease in extremely immature baboons. Am J Respir Crit Care Med. 1999;160:1333-1346.

109. Oppert M, Schindler R, Husung C, et al. Low-dose hydrocortisone improves shock reversal and reduces cytokine levels in early hyperdynamic septic shock. Crit Care Med. 2005;33:2457-2464.

110. Seri I, Evans JR. Why do steroids increase blood pressure in preterm infants? J Pediatr. 2000;136:420-421.

111. Shenker Y, Skatrud JB. Adrenal insufficiency in critically ill patients. Am J Respir Crit Care Med. 2001;163:1520-1523.

112. Segar JL, Lumbers ER, Nuyt AM, et al. Effect of antenatal glucocorticoids on sympathetic nerve activity at birth in preterm sheep. Am J Physiol. 1998;274:R160-167.

113. Wang ZM, Aizman R, Grahnquist L, et al. Glucocorticoids stimulate the maturation of H,K-ATPase in the infant rat stomach. Pediatr Res. 1996;40:658-663.

114. Annane D, Bellissant E, Bollaert PE, et al. Corticosteroids in the treatment of severe sepsis and septic shock in adults: a systematic review. JAMA. 2009;301:2362-2375.

115. Tang BM, Craig JC, Eslick GD, et al. Use of corticosteroids in acute lung injury and acute respiratory distress syndrome. a systematic review and meta-analysis. Crit Care Med. 2009;37:1594-1603.

116. Briegel J, Kellermann W, Forst H, et al. Low-dose hydrocortisone infusion attenuates the systemic inflammatory response syndrome. The Phospholipase A2 Study Group. Clin Investig. 1994;72:782-787.

117. Sprung CL, Annane D, Keh D, et al. Hydrocortisone therapy for patients with septic shock. N Engl J Med. 2008;358:111-124.

118. Subhedar NV, Duffy K, Ibrahim H. Corticosteroids for treating hypotension in preterm infants. Cochrane Database Syst Rev. 2007:CD003662.

119. Higgins S, Friedlich P, Seri I. Hydrocortisone for hypotension and vasopressor dependence in preterm neonates. A meta-analysis. J Perinatol. 2010;30:373-378.

120. Watterberg K, Cook K, Gifford K. Pharmacokinetics of hydrocortisone in extremely low birth weight infants in the first week of life. Pediatr Res. 1996;39:251A.
121. Reynolds JW, Colle E, Ulstrom RA. Adrenocortical steroid metabolism in newborn infants. V. Physiologic disposition of exogenous cortisol loads in the early neonatal period. J Clin Endocrinol Metab. 1962;22:245-254.
122. Czock D, Keller F, Rasche FM, et al. Pharmacokinetics and pharmacodynamics of systemically administered glucocorticoids. Clin Pharmacokinet. 2005;44:61-98.
123. Paquette L, Friedlich P, Ramanathan R, et al. Concurrent use of indomethacin and dexamethasone increases the risk of spontaneous intestinal perforation in very low birth weight neonates. J Perinatol. 2006;26:486-492.
124. Watterberg KL, Shaffer ML, Mishefske MJ, et al. Growth and neurodevelopmental outcomes after early low-dose hydrocortisone treatment in extremely low birth weight infants. Pediatrics. 2007;120:40-48.
125. Aucott SW. Hypotension in the newborn: who needs hydrocortisone? J Perinatol. 2005;25:77-78.

14

CHAPTER 15

Shock in the Surgical Neonate

Philippe S. Friedlich, MD, MS, Epi, MBA, Cathy Shin, MD, FACS, FAAP,
James Stein, MD, FACS, FAAP, Istvan Seri, MD, PhD, HonD

- Definition and Phases of Neonatal Shock
- Pathogenesis of Neonatal Shock
- Diagnosis of Circulatory Compromise and Shock
- Neonates with Surgical Condition and Shock
- References

A significant number of neonates are born with conditions that require surgery or develop such problems after birth. This chapter highlights the issues that are specific to cardiovascular compromise of patients requiring surgery in the neonatal period. The discussion focuses on review of the general pathophysiologic principles involved in the clinical management of shock in these patients and on the most frequently encountered surgical conditions that require urgent or emergent cardiovascular attention in the neonatal intensive care unit (NICU).

Definition and Phases of Neonatal Shock

The etiology, clinical presentations, phases, and pathophysiology of neonatal shock are discussed in Chapters 1 and 12 in detail. Here we briefly review the salient features of neonatal shock with special attention to their relevance to the neonate with surgical conditions.

Shock develops when O_2 delivery to the tissues is inadequate to satisfy cellular metabolic demand. Independent of the etiology, there are three phases of shock, with each phase being characterized by unique pathophysiologic changes of progressing severity. In the *compensated phase*, vital organ function is maintained by intrinsic neurohormonal compensatory mechanisms resulting in distribution of organ blood flow primarily to the heart, brain, and adrenal glands and away from the "nonvital" organs. Several hormones and local factors affecting myocardial function, organ blood flow distribution, capillary integrity, systemic and pulmonary vascular resistance, and cellular metabolism play a central role in the regulation of these specific hemodynamic changes. Stroke volume, central venous pressure, and urine output all decrease. However, blood pressure remains within normal limits because the increased myocardial contractility and heart rate maintain cardiac output close to the normal range. It is important to note that, since blood pressure is the function of blood flow and systemic vascular resistance, blood pressure alone, by definition, does not adequately reflect the status of organ blood flow and blood flow distribution. This notion is especially important in the nonacidotic extremely low birth weight preterm neonate with immature myocardium and compensated shock during the first postnatal day.[1-3] If the circulatory compromise advances, neonatal shock enters its *uncompensated phase* where failure of the neurohormonal compensatory mechanisms result in decreased myocardial contractility, stroke volume, and blood pressure with ensuing significant decreases in blood flow to all organs and the development of lactic acidosis. If treatment is delayed and/or the condition rapidly deteriorates as in cases with fulminant sepsis or asphyxia with multiorgan failure, neonatal shock enters its *irreversible phase,* wherein complete organ failure dominates the clinical picture and death occurs invariably.

Pathogenesis of Neonatal Shock

The clinical presentation, pathophysiology, and treatment of neonatal shock are significantly affected by the primary etiology of the condition. As discussed in Chapter 1 in detail, hypovolemia, myocardial dysfunction, or abnormal regulation of peripheral vascular tone are the primary etiological factors leading to shock in the neonate. In addition, in the critically ill neonate, more than one of these factors may be involved. For example, in a newborn with septic shock, the capillary leak-induced absolute hypovolemia, the relative hypovolemia associated with the abnormal regulation of vascular tone, and direct myocardial injury may all contribute to the development of the circulatory compromise.

Diagnosis of Circulatory Compromise and Shock

There is no universally accepted agreement on what the "gold standard" for the diagnosis of circulatory compromise in the neonate should be. Conventionally, blood pressure has been used as the gold standard. The major reason for this is that, in addition to heart rate, blood pressure is the only meaningful hemodynamic parameter that can be continuously monitored in absolute numbers (Chapter 3). The other hemodynamic parameters essential in the assessment of tissue perfusion such as cardiac output (systemic blood flow) and blood flow distribution to organs (e.g., cerebral, renal, intestinal, or pulmonary blood flow) can only be assessed in absolute numbers indirectly (i.e., using NIRS for continuous monitoring of tissue O_2 saturation [Chapters 7 and 8]) or as relative changes over time. In addition, the available monitoring techniques allowing for assessment of the hemodynamic parameters in the neonate (e.g., echocardiography [Chapter 5], near-infrared spectroscopy [Chapters 7 and 8], electrical impedance cardiometry [Chapters 6], magnetic resonance imaging [MRI; Chapters 9 and 10]) all have significant limitations and there are no data linking hemodynamic compromise and its treatment to changes in neonatal outcomes. Accordingly, the gestational- and postnatal age-dependent blood pressure range that "warrants intervention" is not known (see Chapter 3). Finally, even if we knew the normal blood pressure range, relying solely on blood pressure carries the inherent risk of overlooking the compensated phase of shock. The indirect and commonly used clinical signs of circulatory compromise, such as increased heart rate, slow skin capillary refill time, increased core peripheral temperature difference, low urine output, and acidosis, either have limitations in aiding the prompt diagnosis of circulatory compromise or, as in the very preterm neonate in the immediate postnatal period, are simply of limited clinical value (Chapters 1 and 12). Despite the limitations of these indirect measures of cardiovascular compromise, their combined use, and/or the changes in these measures occurring over time are predictive for outcome. For example, when blood pressure and capillary refill time are being assessed together or when there is evidence for worsening lactic acidosis, outcome becomes more predictable.[4,5]

Neonates with Surgical Condition and Shock

Respiratory Disorders

Congenital Diaphragmatic Hernia

Congenital diaphragmatic hernia (CDH) is a defect of the diaphragm thought to be due to an early failure of the pleuroperitoneal canal closure in early gestation resulting in a spectrum of pulmonary hypoplasia.[6] The incidence of CDH has been estimated between 1 in 3000 and 1 in 5000 live births.[7]

The defect allows the abdominal organs, such as the stomach and bowel, and occasionally the liver and spleen, to enter the thoracic cavity. These organs displace the heart and lung compromising pulmonary and, in severe cases, cardiac development in utero resulting in decreases in respiratory gas exchange, pulmonary blood flow and cardiac output and myocardial function after delivery. A major cause of hypoxemia associated with CDH is right-to-left shunting through the foramen ovale (FO) and/or patent ductus arteriosus (PDA) caused by the associated pulmonary hypertension. Persistent pulmonary hypertension in infants with CDH has many etiologies and significantly affects outcome of these neonates.

Prenatal factors affecting the severity of postnatal pulmonary hypertension in patients with CDH include the impact of the mediastinal shift and the malposition of the heart on fetal circulation and pulmonary and cardiac development.[8,9]

The neonatal heart is normally positioned on the left side of the thoracic cavity with the interventricular septum at a 45-degree angle to the midline sagittal plane. Indeed, Baumgart and colleagues have shown that cardiac malposition is common in neonates with CDH who require extracorporeal membrane oxygenation (ECMO) perioperatively.[9] The malposition of the heart is caused by the herniation of the abdominal viscera into the thorax resulting in a mediastinal shift, and pulmonary hypoplasia. Interestingly, the return of the heart to a more normal position after surgical repair of the diaphragm predicts a better outcome, whereas failure to return toward a normal axis after surgical repair has been associated with poor outcomes.[9]

In addition to causing malposition of the heart, CDH may affect the development of the heart itself. Indeed, an adequate left ventricular mass favors survival, whereas neonates with CDH and significant left ventricle hypoplasia are less likely to survive.[10] A redistribution of fetal cardiac output away from the left ventricle toward the right side may occur in infants with CDH based on the finding of a markedly increased pulmonary valve to aortic valve flow ratio compared with healthy fetuses.[11] The blood flow redistribution then seems to be associated with development of low left ventricular mass.[11]

Several additional mechanisms may contribute to the development of cardiovascular compromise in patients with severe CDH. For example, lung hypoplasia may diminish pulmonary blood flow returning to the left atrium during fetal life. By the mid to late third trimester, 22-24% of combined cardiac output normally circulates through the pulmonary vasculature in utero. However, fetal pulmonary blood flow may be reduced by as much as half when severe lung hypoplasia is present in patients with CDH.[12] There is also evidence that normal fetal pulmonary artery blood flow is necessary for normal pulmonary vascular and airway development and that diminished cardiac mass with severe CDH in utero may be used as an indicator of the severity of pulmonary hypoplasia.[13,14] Since a diminished left ventricle size in fetuses with CDH has been documented, it has been suggested that a decreased left ventricular mass is an intrinsic part of this anomaly.[14] As mentioned earlier, the extent of left ventricle hypoplasia may be a predictor of poor outcomes, as infants with the smallest left ventricular mass more frequently require preoperative ECMO support and often experience poor outcomes.[14] Furthermore, neonates with CDH often experience cardiac stun while receiving venoarterial (VA) ECMO support.[15] This phenomenon may be due to the inability of a relatively small left ventricle to adapt to the increased afterload effect of the aortic cannula.[15,16] Furthermore, the malposition of the cardiac angle within the thorax in the fetus may impede venous return to the right side of the heart from the umbilical circulation. Since umbilical flow returning from the placenta is normally directed by the ductus venosus across the foramen ovale into the left atrium, normal umbilical flow pattern contributes to left ventricular output and ventricle development.[17] As the shift in cardiac position in patients with CDH may redirect the venous return so that more blood stays in the right atrium, it could result in an imbalance between pulmonary and aortic blood flow.[10] Lastly, as a vicious cycle, the redistribution of cardiac output away from the left heart predisposes to the underdevelopment of the left ventricle, which in turn further

15

enhances redistribution of cardiac output away from the left heart resulting in poor outcome.[18]

In view of the complex pulmonary and cardiovascular problems facing the neonate with CDH, patients with prenatally diagnosed CDH should be delivered at centers with a multidisciplinary team available 24/7 and with the ability to deliver advanced modalities of respiratory and cardiovascular supportive therapies, including ECMO. After delivery, prenatally diagnosed infants or infants as soon as the diagnosis of CDH is suspected must not be ventilated by bag and mask and should be immediately intubated and ventilated using a low peak inspiratory pressure recommended not to exceed 24 cm H_2O to minimize the potential for the development of an air leak syndrome.[19] With a significant increase in the risk of air leak secondary to lung hypoplasia, the use of neuromuscular blockade and sedation has also been recommended to minimize both barotrauma and the possibility of bowel distension as well as to enhance decompression of the hollow abdominal organs displaced into the intrathoracic cavity.[20] Once the airway has been stabilized, appropriate arterial and central venous access established, and the patient has been transferred to the neonatal intensive care unit, right-to-left shunting is indirectly monitored by preductal and postductal pulse oximetry. In an attempt to decrease right-to-left shunting across the PDA and thus improve postductal oxygenation, cardiovascular support is usually also instituted with the judicious use of volume administration and, if appropriate, the continuous infusion of vasopressors/inotropes. Serial echocardiograms are essential in the assessment of the cardiac structure and function immediately following the stabilization of the patient and to gauge the response to treatments aimed at decreasing pulmonary vascular resistance and improving systemic blood flow. According to the general practice but without much supporting evidence, preductal arterial oxygen saturation is maintained around 90%. The utility of conventional versus high-frequency oscillatory ventilation has been extensively debated and remains unclear.[20,21] If hypoxemia resulting from pulmonary hypertension does not respond to the initial mechanical ventilatory methodologies, administration of inhaled nitric oxide (iNO), milrinone and, perhaps sildenafil are warranted.[22-24] Finally, if all else fails, the infant with CDH is managed using extracorporeal membrane oxygenation.[20]

The intraoperative and postoperative care of patients with congenital diaphragmatic hernia often includes the use of volume support in the form of colloids and/or crystalloids and vasoactive agents. There is very little and only anecdotal evidence of how much and what kind of volume and vasopressor/inotrope therapy to use.

More recently, the association between adrenal insufficiency, low cortisol levels, and neonates with CDH has been suggested.[25,26] Kamath and colleagues reported a 67% incidence of random cortisol level less than 15 μg/dL in 58 critically ill infants with CDH.[26] It may be therefore important for clinicians to screen CDH patients for adrenal insufficiency and evaluate the need for treatment when faced with vasopressor resistant hypotension.

Ideally, with the reduction of the defect and the return of abdominal contents into the peritoneum, improved venous return and thus cardiac preload will result in improvement of cardiac output and systemic and pulmonary blood flow. Some neonates with more severe pulmonary hypoplasia will experience a potentially fatal rebound pulmonary hypertensive crisis following ECMO and surgery with some responding to iNO while some of the nonresponders may respond to the addition of sildenafil to iNO.[24] Finally, it is uncertain if the recent improvement in survival rates of neonates with CDH translates into better long-term outcomes.[27]

Cystic Congenital Adenomatoid Malformation

The term *congenital cystic adenomatoid malformation* (CCAM) reflects the histopathologic features of the presentation.[28] It is believed that CCAM results from a cessation of bronchopulmonary maturation and concomitant overgrowth of mesenchymal elements at about the fifth and sixth weeks of gestation and produces the adenomatoid appearances of the anomaly.[29] There are two major classifications of CCAM. One classification divides the presentation into three types on the basis of histopathologic characteristics, while the other uses the size of the cysts within the mass to separate the macrocystic presentation (single or multiple cysts with a diameter > 5 mm) from the microcystic type with very small cysts and echodense homogeneous-appearing lungs.[29] As for the clinical presentation in the immediate postnatal period, many patients with CCAM are asymptomatic at birth.[29] However, since a small bronchial communication often exists within the CCAM, infections and overinflation of the cystic lesions frequently lead to respiratory pathology during infancy.

Antenatal ultrasound has increased the prenatal detection of CCAM and provides an opportunity to also identify fetuses that will remain asymptomatic after birth.[30,31] In general, the majority of CCAM lesions do not lead to significant abnormalities of lung or heart development in the fetus and regression and/or lack of growth of these lesions occurs frequently.[30,31]

A very small proportion of these malformations behave in a more aggressive fashion, forming a rapidly expanding space-occupying lesion. This may lead to the development of fetal hydrops due to the elevated central venous pressure caused by cardiac compression and altered hemodynamics.[32] In the hydropic fetus, Doppler study of the inferior vena cava often demonstrates a significantly greater degree of flow reversal with atrial contractions than occurs in normal fetuses.[32]

When faced with cardiopulmonary complications and when a large single cyst is involved, in utero drainage by thoracocentesis or placement of a thoracoamniotic shunt has had varying success for fetal salvage.[33] Similarly, in utero fetal surgery via maternal hysterotomy and fetal thoracotomy and lobectomy has been attempted but should be restricted to the most severe conditions and specialized fetal therapy centers.[33,34]

In the immediate postnatal period, patients with asymptomatic lesions can be safely followed with computed tomography scanning or MRI. The timing of the surgical management in asymptomatic cases is dictated by the potential development of recurrent infection.[35] In symptomatic lesions, respiratory distress is usually an acute postnatal event. Lobectomy remains the procedure of choice to prevent residual disease and recurrence in the remaining lobe.[35]

Vascular Tumors

Hepatic Vascular Tumors

The most common hepatic vascular anomalies in infancy are hepatic hemangioma and arteriovenous malformations (AVMs). These two disorders are biologically different yet exhibit similarities in their pathophysiology and clinical presentation, including fast flow hemodynamics. These lesions often manifest themselves in the neonatal period with hepatomegaly, congestive heart failure, and anemia.[36] Although liver hemangiomas often regress spontaneously, complications associated with liver hemangiomas still result in a mortality rate of up to 30%.[37] Unlike hemangiomas, AVMs are unlikely to regress spontaneously and have a higher, albeit not well-documented, mortality rate.[38]

Most cases of infantile hepatic hemangioma are benign vascular tumors and are the second most common liver tumors in infants after hepatoblastomas.[39] Infants with hepatic hemangioma especially with its capillary form (hemangioendothelioma) typically develop congenital hepatomegaly, congestive heart failure, and significant anemia.

The prenatal imaging techniques including ultrasound, color Doppler imaging, and ultrafast MRI provide critical information for early diagnosis and successful management of these conditions. Typical color Doppler flow pattern of hemangioma demonstrates enlarged vessels with high-flow velocity associated with corresponding abrupt changes in the vessel caliber and arteriovenous shunts.

Fetal hepatic hemangioma can result in nonimmune fetal hydrops and high-output cardiac failure due to the volume overload associated with the arteriovenous shunting. More than 55% of cases with in utero diagnosed hepatic hemangioma have been associated with fetal hydrops and mortality rate greater than 55%. In the absence of fetal hydrops, mortality rates are lower and estimated to be less than 30%.[39] The size, the enlargement, the side of the affected liver lobe, and the gestational age do not predict the likelihood of the development of hydrops.[39] The optimal prenatal and perinatal management strategies include the use of serial ultrasound and/or MRI monitoring of the fetus for signs of fetal hydrops. Postnatally, the diagnosis is confirmed or established by ultrasound, CT scan, and/or MRI with MRI being the preferred investigative modality as it can accurately define the extent and nature of the vascular lesion, alleviating the need of diagnostic arteriography.

Infantile hepatic hemangioendothelioma rarely presents with asymptomatic hepatomegaly. The classic manifestations are prominent massive hepatomegaly, out of proportion to the associated high-output cardiac failure resulting from the arteriovenous communications.[40] More than 50% of the cardiac output may be diverted to the hepatic hemangioendothelioma, resulting in severe cardiovascular compromise, and patients with severe congestive heart failure have a mortality rate approaching 70-90%.[41-43] The younger the age at presentation, the more severe are the cardiovascular symptoms.[44] Treatment of infantile hepatic hemangioendothelioma initially consists of supportive medical management and depends on the degree of shunting through intrahepatic arteriovenous fistulas along with the severity of the resultant congestive heart failure.[45,46] Progression of symptoms despite medical therapy is an indication for hepatic arteriography and embolization.[45,47] Neonates not responding to medical management have a poor prognosis for long-term survival.

Sacrococcygeal Teratoma

Sacrococcygeal teratoma is one of the most common tumors in newborns with an estimated incidence of 1 per 20,000 to 1 per 40,000 births.[48] Sacrococcygeal teratoma is defined as a neoplasm composed of tissue from either all three germ layers or multiple foreign tissues lacking organ specificity.[49] The American Academy of Pediatric Surgery Section classification uses a four-level staging classification based on the location, the ease of resection, and the malignant potential of these tumors.

Prenatal diagnosis of sacrococcygeal teratoma is usually established by ultrasonographic imaging or fetal MRI. Large, prenatally diagnosed sacrococcygeal teratomas usually are highly vascular and often lead to high output cardiac failure, resulting in hepatomegaly, placentomegaly, and nonimmune fetal hydrops.[50,51] As with liver AVMs, the development of fetal high-output failure in fetuses with sacrococcygeal teratoma is caused by the arteriovenous shunting within the tumor and/or occurs secondarily to hemorrhage within the tumor itself, leading to severe fetal anemia and poor outcomes.[52] When fetal hydrops develops in fetuses with sacrococcygeal teratoma, dilatation of the cardiac ventricular chambers and the inferior vena cava occurs due to the large venous return from the lower body.[53] Fetal intervention and resection have been attempted in fetuses whose courses were complicated with significant congestive heart failure and fetal hydrops.[52,54,55]

In the postnatal management of patients with sacrococcygeal teratoma, the clinical presentation of the hyperdynamic cardiovascular state should be anticipated and treated accordingly. Serial postnatal echocardiography is being used to assess cardiac function and response to management.

Finally, the long-term outcomes are variable for patients with sacrococcygeal teratoma. Prenatal diagnosis of sacrococcygeal teratoma prior to 30 weeks of gestation, especially with large tumors, tends to be associated with worse prognosis.[52,54] Recommendations for postnatal long-term monitoring include serial serum alpha-fetal protein levels and radiological examination every 3 months. Consideration for postsurgical chemotherapy regimen depends on the specific pathologic nature of the immature elements.[56]

Gastrointestinal Disorders

Several gastrointestinal neonatal surgical conditions may result in cardiovascular collapse or shock. Many of these disorders require prompt attention to initial fluid resuscitation as well as the coordination of care between the perinatal, obstetrical, and neonatal teams. With improvement in prenatal diagnosis, an increasing number of infants is diagnosed prenatally with correctible surgical malformations allowing for fetal intervention, planned delivery in a tertiary surgical center, and antenatal counseling using a multidisciplinary approach.

Gastroschisis and Omphalocele

Gastroschisis is a relatively frequently diagnosed fetal anomaly. The incidence of gastroschisis has been increasing worldwide and this condition primarily affects fetuses whose mothers are younger than 20 years of age.[57]

The effect of timing and mode of delivery on outcomes of neonates with gastroschisis is unclear. However, the present recommendations for delivery of these patients via the vaginal route in a tertiary care facility with close coordination of obstetrical, neonatal, and pediatric surgical care are supported by some evidence.[58]

The immediate postnatal management of the neonate with gastroschisis is directed toward preventing excessive fluid and sodium losses and hypothermia and trauma to the exteriorized intestines. In these patients, following stabilization and evaluation for anesthesia, the surgeons usually attempt primary closure if the abdominal cavity volume allows closure of the external fascia. Following abdominal closure of patients with smaller than anticipated abdominal cavity volume, the development of excessive abdominal wall tension can lead to compartment syndrome, including vena cava compression, compromised respiratory status, and on rare occasions, bowel ischemia. To avoid these complications, most surgeons estimate the intra-abdominal pressure with the use of a nasogastric or bladder catheter. If the estimated pressure is greater than 20 mm Hg, a silo is used to stage the closure of the abdominal wall. Because the tension associated with compartment syndrome after closure often leads to poor peripheral perfusion, metabolic acidosis, and decreased urine output, the immediate postsurgical management often includes significant fluid resuscitation. Following closure of large defects, the increased intraabdominal pressure often results in some degree of capillary leak, resulting in pulmonary and soft tissue edema. Recent recommendations favor performing the reduction over time to prevent potential complications of abdominal compartment syndrome and improve tolerance for early feeding and shorter hospital stay.[59,60] However, these recommendations are mainly experience- and not evidence-based.

Like for gastroschisis, the use of routine prenatal screening and fetal ultrasonography has led to significant proportions of omphalocele being detected by the early second trimester. However, unlike gastroschisis, omphalocele is a midline defect, so there is a relatively high incidence of associated anomalies and recognized genetic syndromes with omphalocele. Therefore prenatal diagnosis of fetuses with omphalocele includes a very careful evaluation for potential chromosomal anomalies as well as malformations of other organs.

To decrease the chance of omphalocele rupture, delivery by cesarean section is recommended. After delivery, trauma to the lesion must be avoided. In general, most small-to-medium size omphaloceles have good outcomes unless they are associated with severe cardiac, central nervous system, or other malformations. Giant omphaloceles present a challenge for medical and surgical management.

Necrotizing Enterocolitis

Necrotizing enterocolitis (NEC) is one of the most common gastrointestinal medical and/or surgical emergencies affecting preterm neonates. Due to the associated and often severe systemic inflammatory response syndrome, cardiovascular collapse, and respiratory failure, mortality rate of preterm infants with a birth weight less than 1500 g may be as high as 50%, and long-term gastrointestinal and nutritional complications often occur. The pathogenesis of NEC is multifactorial and likely includes significant decreases in gastrointestinal perfusion in general and mucosal perfusion in particular. Risk factors for NEC include but are not limited to prematurity, hypoxic ischemic insult, presence of a patent ductus arteriosus with "diastolic aortic steal," and time to full enteral feeding.

Medical management of infants with necrotizing enterocolitis includes decompression of the intestines, abstinence from enteral feedings, provision of broad-spectrum antibiotics and fluid resuscitation, and treatment of the respiratory and cardiovascular compromise.[61] Surgical care may include the placement of a temporary drain or formal laparotomy with intestinal resection as appropriate.[62] During laparotomy, the increased insensible and transmembranous fluid and electrolyte losses need to be addressed while in the preoperative and postoperative period the complex cardiovascular effects of the associated systemic inflammatory response syndrome require constant attention (see Chapters 1 and 12).

References

1. Kluckow M, Evans N. Relationship between blood pressure and cardiac output in preterm infants requiring mechanical ventilation. J Pediatr. 1996;129:506.
2. Kluckow M, Evans N. Superior vena cava flow in preterm infants: a novel marker of systemic blood flow. Arch Dis Child. 2000;82:F182.
3. Seri I, Evans J. Controversies in the diagnosis and management of hypotension in the newborn infant. Curr Opin Pediatr. 2001;13:116.
4. Osborn DA, Kluckow M, Evans N. Blood pressure, capillary refill, and central-peripheral temperature difference. Clinical detection of low upper body blood flow in very premature infants. Arch Dis Child Fetal Neonatal Ed. 2004;89(2):F168-F173.
5. Deshpande SA, Platt MP. Association between blood lactate and acid-base status and mortality in ventilated babies. Arch Dis Child Fetal Neonatal Ed. 1997;76:F15-F20.
6. Harrison MR, Adzick NS, Flake AW. Correction of congenital diaphragmatic hernia. VI. Hard lessons. J Pediatr Surg. 1993;28:1411-1418.
7. Puri P, Gorman F. Lethal nonpulmonary anomalies associated with congenital diaphragmatic hernia: Implications for early intrauterine surgery. J Pediatr Surg. 1984;19:29-32.
8. Ryan CA, Perreault T, Johnston-Hodgson A, et al. Extracorporeal membrane oxygenation and cardiac malformation. J Pediatr Surg. 1994;29:878.
9. Baumgart S, Paul JJ, Huhta JC. Cardiac malformation, redistribution of fetal cardiac output, and left heart hypoplasia reduce survival in neonates with congenital diaphragmatic hernia requiring extracorporeal membrane oxygenation. J Pediatr Surg. 1998;133:57-62.
10. Schwartz SM, Vermilion RP, Hirschl RB. Evaluation of left ventricular mass in children with left sided congenital diaphragmatic hernia. J Pediatr. 1994;125:447.
11. Rasanen J, Wood DC, Weiner S, et al. Role of the pulmonary circulation in the distribution of human fetal cardiac output during the second half of pregnancy. Circulation. 1996; 94:1068-1073.
12. Karamanoukian HL, Glick PL, Wilcox DT, et al. Pathophysiology of congenital diaphragmatic hernia. XI: anatomic and biochemical characterization of the heart in the fetal lamb CDH model. J Pediatr Surg. 1995;30:925-929.
13. Karamanoukian HL, O'Toole SJ, Rossman JR, et al. Can cardiac weight predict lung weight in patients with congenital diaphragmatic hernia? J Pediatr Surg. 1996;31:823-825.
14. Schwartz SM, Vermillion RP, Hirschl RB. Evaluation of left ventricular mass in children with left-sided diaphragmatic hernia. J Pediatr. 1994;125:447-451.
15. Martin GR, Short BL, Abbot C, et al. Cardiac stun in infants undergoing extracorporeal membrane oxygenation. J Thorac Cardiovasc Surg. 1991;101:607-611.
16. Martin GR, Short BL. Doppler echocardiographic evaluation of cardiac performance in infants on prolonged extracorporeal membrane oxygenation. Am JCardiol. 1988;62:929-934.
17. Kiserud T, Eik-Nes SH, Blaas HG, et al. Ultrasonographic velocimetry of the fetal ductus venosus. Lancet. 1991;338(8780):1412-1414.
18. Sharland GK, Lockhart SM, Heward AJ, et al. Prognosis in fetal diaphragmatic hernia. Am J Obstet Gynecol. 1991;166:9-13.
19. Finer NN, Tierney A, Etches PC, et al. Congenital diaphragmatic hernia: developing a protocolized approach. J Pediatr Surg. 1998;33:1331.
20. Ford JW. Neonatal ECMO: Current controversies and trends. Neonatal Netw. 2006;25:229-238.
21. Moya FR, Lally KP. Evidence-based management of infants with congenital diaphragmatic hernia. Semin Perinatol. 2005;29:112-117.
22. Kinsella JP, Abman SH. Inhaled nitric oxide therapy in children. Paediatr Respir Rev. 2005;6: 190-198.
23. Chen B, Lakshminrusimha S, Czech L, et al. Regulation of phosphodiesterase 3 in the pulmonary arteries during the perinatal period in sheep. Pediatr Res. 2009;66:682-687.
24. Noori S, Friedlich P, Seri I. Cardiovascular effects of sildenafil in neonates and infants with congenital diaphragmatic hernia. Neonatology. 2007;91:92-100.
25. Pittinger TP, Sawin RS. Adrenocortical insufficiency in infants with congenital diaphragmatic hernia: a pilot study. J Pediatr Surg. 2000;35(2):223-225.
26. Kamath BD, Fashaw L, Kinsella JP. Adrenal insufficiency in newborn with congenital diaphragmatic hernia. J Pediatr. 2010;156(3):495-497.
27. Chiu PP, Sauer C, Mihailovic A, et al. The price of success in the management of congenital diaphragmatic hernia: is improved survival accompanied by an increase in long-term morbidity? J Pediatr Surgery. 2006;41:888-892.

28. Chin KY, Tang MY. Congenital adenomatoid malformation of one lobe of a lung with general anasarca. Arch Pathol. 1949;48:221-229.
29. Bailey PV, Tracey Jr T, Connors RH, et al. Congenital bronchopulmonary malformations. Diagnostic and therapeutic considerations. J Thorac Cardiovasc Surg. 1990;99:597-603.
30. Van Leeuwen K, Teitelbaum DH, Hirschi RB, et al. Prenatal diagnosis of congenital cystic adenomatoid malformation and its potential postnatal presentation, surgical indications and natural history. J Pediatr Surg. 1999;34:794-798.
31. Marshall KW, Blane CE, Teitelbaum DH, et al. CCAM: impact of prenatal diagnosis and charging strategies in treatment of asymptomatic patient. AJR Am J Roentgenol. 2000;175:1551-1554
32. Mahle WT, Rychik J, Tian ZY, et al. Echocardiographic evaluation of the fetus with congenital cystic adenomatoid malformation. Ultrasound Obstet Gynecol. 2000;16:620-624.
33. Adzick NS, Harrison MR, Crombleholme TM, et al. Fetal lung lesions: management and outcome. Am J Obstet Gynecol. 1998;179:884-889.
34. Khosa JK, Leong SL, Borzi PA. Congenital cystic adenomatoid malformation of the lung: indications and timing of surgery. Pediatr Surg Int. 2004;20:505-508.
35. Keidar S, Ben-Sira L, Weinberg M, et al. The postnatal management of CCAM. Isr Med Assoc J. 2001;3:258-261.
36. Boon LM, Burrows PE, Paltiel HJ, et al. Hepatic vascular anomalies in infancy. A twenty-seven years experience. J Pediatr. 1996;129(3):346-354.
37. Cohen RC, Myers NA. Diagnosis and management of massive hepatic hemangiomas in childhood. J Pediatr Surg. 1986;21:6-9.
38. Mulliken JB, Young AE. Vascular birthmarks: hemangiomas and malformations. Philadelphia: WB Saunders; 1988.
39. Bartsch EMP, Paek BW, Yoshizawa J, et al. Giant fetal hepatic hemangioma. Fetal Diagn Ther. 2003;18:59-64.
40. Samuel M, Spitz L. Infantile hepatic hemangioendothelioma: the role of surgery. J Pediatr Surg. 1995;30(10):1425-1429.
41. Rocchini AP, Rosenthal A, Isenberg HJ, et al. Hepatic hemangioendothelioma: hemodynamic observation and treatment. Pediatrics. 1976;57:131-135.
42. Daller JA, Bueno J, Gutierrez J, et al. Hepatic hemangioendothelioma: clinical experience and management strategy. J Pediatr Surg. 1999;34:98-106.
43. Fishman SJ, Mulliken JB. Hemangiomas and vascular malformations of infancy and childhood. Pediatr Clin North Am. 1993;40:1177-1200.
44. Davenport M, Hansen L, Heaton ND, et al. Hemangioendothelioma of the liver in infants. J Pediatr Surg. 1995;30:44-48.
45. Holcomb GW, O'Neil JA, Mahboubi S, et al. Experience with hepatic hemangioendothelioma in infancy and childhood. J Pediatr Surg. 1988;23:661-666.
46. Fellows KE, Hoffer FA, Karkowitz RI, et al. Multiple collaterals to hepatic infantile hemangioendotheliomas and arteriovenous malformations: effects of embolization. Radiology. 1991;181:813-818.
47. Iyer CP, Stanley P, Mahour GH. Hepatic hemangiomas in infants and children: a review of 30 cases. Am Surg. 1996;62(5):356-360.
48. Isaacs HJ. Tumors of the fetus and newborns. Philadelphia: WB Saunders; 1997.
49. Mahour GH, Woolley MM, Trinedi SN. Sacrococcygeal teratoma: a 33 year experience. J Pediatr Surg. 1975;10:183-188.
50. Bond SJ, Harrison MR, Schmidt KG. Death due to high output cardiac failure in fetal coccygeal teratoma. J Pediatr Surg. 1990;25:1287-1291.
51. Grison ER, Gauderer MWL, Wolfson RN, et al. Antenatal diagnosis of sacrococcygeal teratoma: prognostic features. Pediatr Surg Int. 1998;3:173-175.
52. Flake AW. Sacrococcygeal teratoma. Semin Pediatr Surg. 1993;2:113-120.
53. Kapoor R, Saha MM. Antenatal sonographic diagnosis of fetal sacrococcygeal teratoma with hydrops. Aust Radiol. 1989;33:285-287.
54. Kuhlmann RS, Warsof SL, Levy DL, et al. Fetal sacrococcygeal teratoma. Fetal Ther. 1987;1: 95-100.
55. Adizick NS, Crombleholme TM, Morgan MA, et al. A rapidly growing fetal teratoma. Lancet. 1997;349:538.
56. Nair R, Pai SK, Saikia TK. Malignant germ cell tumors in childhood. J Surg Oncol. 1994;56: 186-190.
57. Wilson RD, Johnson MP. Congenital abdominal wall defects: an update. Fetal Diagn Ther. 2004;19(5):385-398.
58. Kitchanan S, Patole SK, Muller R, et al. Neonatal outcome of gastroschisis and exomphalos: a 10-year review. J Paediatr Child Health. 2000;6(5):428-430.
59. Bianchi A, Dickson AP. Elective delayed reduction and no anesthesia: 'minimal intervention management' for gastroschisis. J Pediatr Surg. 1998;33(9):1338-1340.
60. Kimble RM, Singh SJ, Bourke C, et al. Gastroschisis reduction under analgesia in the neonatal unit. J Pediatr Surg. 2001;36(11):1672-1674.
61. Thompson AM, Bizzarro MJ. Necrotizing enterocolitis in newborns: pathogenesis, prevention and management. Drugs. 2008;68:1227-1238.
62. Hunter CJ, Chokshi N, Ford HR. Evidence vs experience in the surgical management of necrotizing enterocolitis and focal intestinal perforation. J Perinatol. 2008;28(Suppl 1):S14-S7.

15

CHAPTER 16

Hemodynamics and Brain Injury in the Preterm Neonate

Adré J. du Plessis, MBChB, MPH

- **Magnitude of Problem**
- **Systemic and Cerebral Hemodynamic Vulnerability in Premature Infants**
- **The Premature Cardiovascular System**
- **Cerebral Hemodynamic Control in Premature Infants**
- **Evidence for an Association Between Systemic Hemodynamic Disturbances and Prematurity-Related Brain Injury: Current Status**
- **Resolving the Relationship Between Systemic Hemodynamics and Prematurity-Related Brain Injury: Obstacles to Progress**
- **Conclusion**
- **References**

The brain is more dependent upon a responsive circulatory supply of oxygen and energy substrate than any other organ in the body. For this reason, the maintenance of cerebral structural and functional integrity is often used as an indicator of appropriate systemic hemodynamic performance. This chapter reviews the evidence for the role of systemic hemodynamics in prematurity-related brain injury.

Despite more than 30 years of experience in treating "hypotension" in premature infants, there is very little direct evidence that hypotension causes brain injury in these infants, or that interventions to treat "hypotension" prevent such injury.[1,2] However, this chapter takes the stance that "a lack of evidence is not evidence of a lack" of a causative relationship and explores reasons for our ongoing ignorance in this important area. In doing so, we first discuss factors thought to predispose the immature brain to hemodynamic insult. This is followed by a discussion of ongoing challenges in defining and measuring cerebral hemodynamic insults and the onset of brain injury. Together, these factors conspire against establishing a temporal association between systemic hemodynamic changes and brain injury.

Magnitude of Problem

Prematurity-related brain injury is a problem of major and increasing public health concern.[3,4] Survivors of prematurity are at significant risk for long-term motor, cognitive, and behavioral dysfunction.[5-9] Both the incidence and severity of brain injury in premature infants are inversely related to gestational age.[10-18] Because advances in survival have been greatest among the sickest, smallest infants, that is, those at greatest risk for brain injury, it is perhaps not surprising that survivors of prematurity have become the fastest growing population of children who develop cerebral palsy.[5,19-24] Of major concern are the 25-50% of ex-preterm children who demonstrate potentially debilitating behavioral or learning problems by school age.[6-9]

Cerebrovascular insults leading to both hemorrhagic and hypoxic-ischemic injury have long been considered a leading cause of acute and long-term neurologic morbidity in this population.[25-30] Hypoxia-ischemia/reperfusion insults have been implicated in the causal pathway of both hemorrhagic and nonhemorrhagic forms of prematurity-related brain injury. Systemic hemodynamic impairment is commonly diagnosed and treated in the premature infant and is related inversely to gestational age at birth. This maturational association in premature infants between systemic hemodynamic disturbance and cerebrovascular injury has led to the notion that the relationship is causative. However, despite plausible extrapolations from human adult and supporting animal studies, establishing a causal link between systemic hemodynamic changes and brain injury in the human premature infant has been confounded by many difficult challenges.[31-34] This in turn continues to impede development of rational and effective interventions.

The principal forms of prematurity-related brain injury are germinal matrix-intraventricular hemorrhage (GM-IVH) and its complications, and injury to the parenchyma, particularly to the immature white matter (WM). At least in theory, a number of anatomic and physiologic features of the premature brain predispose it to cerebrovascular injury. The germinal matrices in the periventricular regions of the developing brain are supported by a profuse but transient vascular system of fragile thin-walled vessels with a deficient basal lamina, no muscularis layer, and a predisposition to hypoxia-ischemia/reperfusion injury increasing their vulnerability to rupture.[35-50] These germinal matrices are vulnerable to ischemic insults during hypoperfusion and to rupture during fluctuations in perfusion pressure, the so-called "water-hammer" effect.[35-37,42,51,52] Although the incidence has decreased in recent decades, GM-IVH continues to affect 15-20% of premature infants born at less than 1500 g, and almost half of those born at less than 750 g.[53-64] Both the acute and long-term complications of GM-IVH are more serious in the smallest, sickest infants.[57,65-74] The most serious complications of GM-IVH are periventricular hemorrhagic infarction, with an adverse long-term outcome rate exceeding 85%, and posthemorrhagic hydrocephalus, which has an adverse long-term outcome in up to 75% of cases.[65,66,75-80]

Incomplete arterial ingrowth into the developing brain parenchyma leaves undervascularized end zones in the premature cerebral WM that are susceptible to hypoxic-ischemic injury during periods of decreased perfusion pressure.[81-87] However, while parenchymal brain injury in the premature infant has a predilection for the developing WM, there is increasing recognition of injury and impaired development of gray matter structures.[88] Early autopsy studies described the classic WM lesion of prematurity as periventricular leukomalacia (PVL).[89,90] In its severe form, PVL consists of an area of infarction with necrotic cyst formation and a surrounding field of more selective injury to the immature oligodendrocytes with gliosis. The advent of cranial ultrasound (US) corroborated this predilection to WM injury in living premature infants with the typical cranial US features being a focal echogenic lesion often evolving into a cystic lesion, and atrophy/hypoplasia of the WM.[83,91] In recent years, the prevalence of cystic PVL has decreased significantly; however, recent MRI studies have described a high prevalence of diffuse noncystic WM injury to which cranial US is insensitive.[92-95] In some studies, this diffuse form of WM injury is detected by MRI in more than half of very premature infants.[92,94] Recent pathology and advanced MRI studies have expanded the spectrum of parenchymal lesions in survivors of prematurity by highlighting associations between WM injury and both injury and developmental disruption in both cortical and subcortical gray matter.[96]

Systemic and Cerebral Hemodynamic Vulnerability in Premature Infants

A prevailing paradigm for hemodynamically mediated brain injury in the premature infant centers on a confluence of insults emanating from an unstable immature cardiovascular system acting on a fragile cerebral vasculature with immature intrinsic cerebral autoregulation, and maturationally vulnerable cellular elements, particularly immature oligodendrocytes.[97,98]

The Premature Cardiovascular System

Many aspects of diagnosis and treatment of systemic hemodynamic disturbances in premature infants are based on principles originally established in adults and older children. However, important structural and functional differences exist between the mature cardiovascular system and that of the very premature infant, particularly during the early period of transition to extra-uterine life. First, in the premature infant the normal transition from the in utero "parallel circulation" to the postnatal circulation functioning "in series" is compromised by the delay of the normal postnatal closure of the fetal circulatory channels (the ductus arteriosus and foramen ovale) for days or even weeks. The persistence of ductal and foraminal patency, along with the decreasing pulmonary vascular resistance, results in pulmonary overcirculation and increased cardiovascular vulnerability in the postnatal period. Second, the premature myocardium and autonomic nervous system may be unprepared for the immediate postnatal challenges that confront them, compromising systemic blood flow. In certain pathophysiologic conditions, including extreme prematurity, the relationship between systemic blood pressure and blood flow becomes complex. After normal birth, the term infant experiences a brisk increase in cardiac output.[99] In the extremely premature infant, this early increase in cardiac output tends to be delayed[100-104]; in fact, 20-30% of these infants may experience periods of low superior vena cava (SVC) blood flow (a proposed surrogate of systemic blood flow) during the first 24 hours after birth, when the risk for brain injury is particularly high.[73,100-107] These low systemic blood flow states may be mediated by several mechanisms. First, maturation of the fetal sympathetic nervous system precedes that of the parasympathetic system, which remains underdeveloped in the premature infant.[108] This autonomic immaturity in the premature infant leaves the baroreflex and chemoreflex systems underdeveloped.[109,110] During periods of low systemic blood flow, the premature infant becomes particularly dependent on heart rate; however, with baseline sympathetic activity close to maximal, the ability to increase cardiac output by increasing heart rate alone is limited. Second, the immature myocardium has more mononuclear, that is, immature, myocytes with fewer contractile elements, mitochondria, and lower energy stores, resulting in impaired systolic and diastolic function. In addition, as its contractility is close to maximal under these circumstances, the immature myocardium has relatively limited ability to increase stroke volume. Positive pressure ventilation frequently used in extremely premature infants may further reduce cardiac output by increasing intrathoracic pressure, thus decreasing venous return. Third, the premature cardiovascular system is confronted at birth by a sudden and significant increase in systemic vascular resistance during the transition from the in utero parallel circulation with a low-resistance placental bed to the postnatal circulation in series with higher postnatal peripheral resistance.[100-104] Systemic vascular resistance also increases in the immediate postnatal period because of the increased release of catecholamines associated with labor and delivery. In addition, fluctuations in resistance may result from episodic sympathetic activation during oxyhemoglobin desaturation, suctioning, handling, hypocarbia, and hypercarbia, events that are common in neonatal critical care.

Oxygen delivery matching tissue oxygen demand is accomplished by adjustments of cardiac output and systemic vascular resistance (SVR) (independent variables), resulting in maintenance of normal perfusion pressure (blood pressure [BP]), the dependent variable (see Chapter 1). Therefore, to obtain accurate information about the circulation, at least two of these three variables need to be simultaneously monitored. As SVR can only be calculated and systemic blood flow cannot be accurately and continuously measured in the premature infant, we are left with continuous monitoring of BP, the dependent variable. The inability to appropriately monitor the cardiovascular status has resulted in a BP-based hemo-dynamic management in critically ill preterm infants. The resultant confusion in understanding and appropriately applying the principles of developmental cardio-vascular physiology to clinical care is largely responsible for the different and fre-quently opposing interpretations of the hemodynamic data.[1,2,100,101,111,112] Normal arterial BP may be defined broadly as the range of blood pressure required to maintain perfusion appropriate for the functional and structural integrity of the tissues (see Chapter 3). Blood pressure may be maintained by increasing peripheral resistance. In the extremely premature infant, the combination of increased periph-eral resistance and myocardial immaturity may translate into decreased systemic and organ blood flow. It is therefore not difficult to appreciate how the earlier definition of "normal BP" fails in this situation. Several approaches have been used in an attempt to define normal BP in premature infants (see Chapter 3 for details). Population-based studies have described statistical norms for BP in pre-mature infants without evidence of significant brain injury.[111-114] In these studies, BP increases with gestational age at birth as well as with postnatal age during the first week.[111,114-116] Others have tried to define the limits of normal BP by com-paring BP in premature infants with and without brain injury.[17,117-119] Despite these studies, the range of "normal BP" remains largely unknown for premature infants, and BP management continues to differ markedly between, and even within, centers. The lack of established normative data for BP notwithstanding, "hypoten-sion" remains commonly diagnosed and treated, especially in smaller and sicker premature infants.[111,120-122]

Cerebral Hemodynamic Control in Premature Infants

Several aspects of the immature hemodynamic physiology of the premature brain increase its vulnerability to cerebrovascular injury. First, unlike the mature brain where cerebral blood flow exceeds the ischemic threshold injury by 5-fold, the premature brain has significantly lower global and regional cerebral blood flow, especially in the WM.[123-134] This suggests a reduced margin of safety for cerebral perfusion, but has to be considered in the context of reduced oxygen metabolism in the premature brain.[135] In fact, a recent report suggests a relative cerebral hyper-oxygenation in stable premature infants.[136]

Under normal conditions, cerebral perfusion is maintained by a background perfusion pressure provided by the cardiovascular system, which is then "fine-tuned" within the cerebral vasculature by complex intrinsic autoregulatory mechanisms (see Chapter 2). These compensatory cerebral responses serve a transient, temporizing function. However, if cerebral insults are sustained, these responses eventually fail, leading to irreversible brain injury.[137] Cerebral pressure autoregulation maintains CBF relatively constant across a range of cerebral perfusion pressure called the autoregulatory plateau.[138-140] In addition to these upper and lower pressure bounds, cerebral pressure autoregulation also has a limited impulse-response time, on the order of 5-15 seconds.[141-146] Outside these pressure and temporal bounds, cerebral blood flow is pressure passive, with increased risk of cerebrovascular injury (see Chapter 2).

In animal models, cerebral pressure-flow autoregulation emerges during fetal life but is underdeveloped in the immature brain.[147-162] Specifically, with decreasing gestational age the autoregulatory plateau is narrower and lower, and normal resting BP is closer to the lower threshold of autoregulation.[148,152,156,163,164] Although cerebral pressure-flow autoregulation is well-characterized in children and adults, this is not the case for the newborn, least of all the sick premature infant.[132,139,140,165-174] Some studies in stable preterm infants have suggested a lower autoregulatory limit around 25-30 mm Hg[132,175,176]; however, in the sick premature infant the existence and limits of cerebral pressure autoregulation remain controversial.[168,169,173,177-181]

Evidence for an Association Between Systemic Hemodynamic Disturbances and Prematurity-Related Brain Injury: Current Status

Blood Pressure and Prematurity-Related Brain Injury

A variety of BP disturbances have been implicated in prematurity-related brain injury, including arterial hypotension or hypertension, cerebral venous hypertension, and/or fluctuating BP.[16-18,36,182-193] Early animal studies used a hypoperfusion-reperfusion model in newborn beagle puppies to induce GM-IVH. In these early studies, association between increased systemic BP and GM-IVH was found, especially following a period of hypotension.[32-34,155,194-201] Findings have not been consistent, with some studies implicating hypotension in the development of GM-IVH,[16,17,182-187] but other studies finding no such association.[112,118,119,169,202-204] Different mechanisms have been proposed for the role of "hypotension" in the pathogenesis of GM-IVH, apparently depending on the severity of hypotension and the integrity of cerebral pressure autoregulation. With intact pressure autoregulation, hypotension may trigger cerebral vasodilation, with the increased cerebral blood volume leading to the rupture of fragile vessels. Conversely, with disrupted cerebral pressure autoregulation, or with BPs below the autoregulatory plateau, there is greater variability in cerebral blood flow. In addition, during hypotension, hypoxic-ischemic injury to the vessel walls may further disrupt cerebral pressure autoregulation, and vessels may rupture with reperfusion. In addition to GM-IVH, systemic hypotension has also been implicated in the development of WM injury in immature animals, including fetal sheep, fetal rabbits, and premature nonhuman primates, as well as in premature infants.[16,17,31,117,119,129,167,205-216] However, other studies have shown no such relationship.[185,188,203,217] Unlike hypotension, sustained hypertension is not commonly diagnosed in premature humans; only occasional studies have implicated hypertension in the development of GM-IVH.[18,188] Fluctuating BP in premature infants, particularly during positive pressure ventilation, has been associated with GM-IVH in a number of reports, presumably through a "water-hammer" effect of fluctuations in perfusion of the fragile germinal matrix vessels.[16,18,172,183,192,193,218-220] However, the role of fluctuating cerebral perfusion in prematurity-related brain injury remains controversial, and several recent studies found no such association.[169,193] In summary, the role of systemic BP disturbances and impaired cerebral pressure-flow autoregulation in prematurity-related brain injury, particularly to the parenchyma, remains unresolved.

Recent studies using Doppler ultrasound and functional echocardiography have identified periods of low cardiac output and low "cerebral" perfusion in more than one third of premature infants during the early hours after birth, particularly in critically ill infants. These studies have made a number of important observations.[83] First, these low-flow states are not reliably detected by systemic BP measurements and do not respond to vasopressor-inotropes.[101-104,221] In addition, these low cardiac output states are associated with low SVC flow, suggesting decreased cerebral perfusion.[101,102,105,222-224] Up to 80% of these infants have their lowest SVC flow between 5 and 12 hours after birth. These periods of low SVC flow are associated with disturbed cerebral oxygenation by near-infrared spectroscopy.[225,226] Both the nadir and duration of low SVC flow are associated with severe GM-IVH and later adverse neurologic outcome.[101,102,224,226,227] In these infants, GM-IVH appears to develop *after* recovery of SVC flow, suggesting the hypoperfusion-reperfusion mechanism described in earlier animal models.[33,34,196]

In summary, the association between systemic BP disturbances, as currently measured and interpreted, and prematurity-related brain injury is controversial at best. A potential reason for this uncertainty might be a relative dissociation of systemic BP and blood flow during periods of critical illness in these infants.

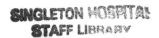

Resolving the Relationship Between Systemic Hemodynamics and Prematurity-Related Brain Injury: Obstacles to Progress

As discussed earlier, several fundamental and interrelated challenges continue to impede our understanding of the relationship between changes in systemic hemodynamics and brain injury in the premature infant. Some of these challenges are discussed next and can be summarized as lack of quantitative continuous measures of blood flow; lack of understanding of what constitutes significant "insult" dose and dosing; lack of hyperacute biomarkers for significant brain injury; distinguishing the role of other nonhemodynamic mechanisms of brain injury; and the variable response of the premature brain to insult and recovery. Although other factors no doubt obscure the field, resolution of these issues should provide considerable insight into the interaction between immature systemic and cerebral hemodynamics, and how this interaction might mediate injury to the immature brain.

Measurement of Relevant Hemodynamic and Metabolic Indices

Currently there are no established techniques for making continuous, quantitative measurements of systemic or cerebral blood flow in the fragile newborn infant although some advances have been made very recently (see Chapter 6). Arterial blood pressure, the only continuous systemic hemodynamic signal available in the premature infant, has several important limitations. First, unlike in the adult, there are no noninvasive techniques for acquiring continuous BP in the premature infant.[228] Continuous intra-arterial catheters are not without risk, particularly when used over prolonged periods. Second, the relationship between BP and systemic blood flow is not constant, particularly during periods of critical physiologic instability. For example, during the early hours after extremely premature birth, BP may be maintained through increased peripheral resistance, which may paradoxically decrease myocardial function and cardiac output. Arterial BP is often used as a surrogate for cerebral perfusion pressure because the effect of venous pressure is disregarded in many clinical situations. However, in premature infants requiring positive pressure ventilatory support with "low" arterial BP close to the lower threshold of cerebral pressure autoregulation, the effect of increased intrathoracic pressure may have a significant impact on cerebral perfusion. At present, techniques for monitoring cerebral perfusion pressure are not available.

Cardiac output is considered the gold standard measure of systemic blood flow. Although cardiac output measurements have provided valuable insights in premature infants, these measurements have important limitations in this population. First, measuring cardiac output requires some level of expertise, particularly in the small premature infant (see Chapters 5 and 6). Second, given the persistence of fetal shunts during the early period after premature birth, cardiac output measured in the proximal aortic or pulmonary arteries is limited as a measure of systemic tissue perfusion.

Similar challenges confront the measurement of continuous volemic cerebral blood flow (CBF) in critically ill humans, particularly in the premature infant. Cerebral artery Doppler measures continuous CBF velocity but not CBF, and its use over prolonged periods may raise significant safety concerns because of the risk of tissue warming.[127,145,180,192,229-233] In the absence of reliable techniques for *continuous* CBF measurement, a number of intermittent, so-called static approaches have been used over the past 3 decades to measure quantitative CBF in the premature infant.[101,102,105,179,222,223,234-238] These techniques have been largely based on the Fick principle, using tracers ranging from xenon-133 to oxyhemoglobin measured by near-infrared spectroscopy (NIRS) (see Chapters 4 and 7 for details).[179,234-238] These measures are based on the assumption of steady-state conditions during the measurement period (up to 15 minutes using the ^{133}Xenon clearance technique), an assumption that is particularly tenuous in the sick premature infant (Chapter 4). Another recently described approach used as a surrogate for CBF measurement is the intermittent measurement of SVC flow by Doppler ultrasound (Chapter 5). These studies have also shown that abnormally low SVC flow may be associated with acute and long-term neurologic morbidity.[101,102,105,222,223] However, this approach has several limitations (see Chapter 5). Finally, all of the so-called static measurements of CBF suffer from the inability to capture the dynamic nature of cerebral hemodynamics during the period of major physiologic change associated with transition from fetal to premature postnatal life.

The ability to measure the relationship between cerebral oxygen demand and supply would provide major insights into the mechanisms of brain injury in premature infants. This is particularly important because it has become increasingly clear that not only cerebral oxygen deficiency but also excessive cerebral oxygenation may be harmful to the immature brain. In fact, a recent study has suggested that in stable premature infants the premature brain might be "hyperoxygenated" at baseline compared with the mature brain.[136] In the absence of continuous CBF measures, quantitation of cerebral oxygen delivery is not possible. In order to circumvent this limitation, recent spatially resolved NIRS devices have been used to measure continuous cerebral tissue hemoglobin saturation as a surrogate measure of the adequacy of cerebral oxygen delivery (Chapters 7 and 8).[239] The rationale behind this approach is that normal autoregulatory mechanisms maintain appropriate cerebral oxygen delivery and cerebral oxygen extraction[137]; conversely, increasing cerebral oxygen extraction is interpreted as decreased oxygen delivery, presumably due to decreasing CBF. However, this approach too has several limitations, including the assumption that neurovascular coupling is intact in sick premature infants. Furthermore, cerebral oxygen extraction may actually decrease after significant brain insults. For these reasons, measures of cerebral tissue hemoglobin oxygenation may be misleading when considered in isolation.

Current bedside techniques are not only static in nature, but are also assumed to reflect global CBF. Currently there are no bedside techniques capable of measuring regional blood flow within the brain. This limitation may be particularly important in the premature infant. Not only is global CBF low in these infants with a reduced margin of safety, but blood flow is particularly low in the most vulnerable WM regions.[240] As such, measurement of global CBF may not detect dangerously low perfusion in these WM areas. Regional measurements of cerebral perfusion and metabolism are possible with techniques such as single photon emission computed tomography and positron emission tomography.[133,241,242] However, these techniques are not portable to the bedside and are confined to static, point measurements in time.

Characterizing "Significant" Systemic Hemodynamic Insults Is Difficult In Sick Premature Infants

Understanding the role of systemic hemodynamic factors in prematurity-related brain injury has been impeded by a fundamental lack of understanding of the "dose" of hemodynamic insult required to injure the premature brain. To a large degree we still think of cerebral "hypoxic-ischemic" insults in premature infants in terms of those insults capable of causing brain injury in more mature children and adults. However, hypoxic-ischemic insults capable of causing injury to the premature brain may be distinctly different from those injuring the mature brain. Data from adult animal and human studies are based on relatively well-defined insults such as cardiac arrest or vaso-occlusive stroke. In the adult, the symptoms for global and focal cerebral ischemia are relatively dramatic, allowing accurate timing of the onset and duration of insult and hence its relationship to ultimate injury. Conversely, in the extremely premature infant the risk period for hypoxic-ischemic brain insults may extend for weeks or months during the prolonged neonatal intensive care unit stay, and may include the initial pronounced transitional hemodynamic instability, as well as subsequent periods of decreased cerebral oxygen delivery, such as apnea and bradycardia, sustained diastolic hypotension associated with patent ductus arteriosus, recurrent infections with disturbed vascular resistance, hypotension and decreased systemic and organ blood flow, and sustained periods of positive pressure

16

ventilation with potential increases in venous drainage, among others. Presumably, injury thresholds exist for brief but severe, for mild but prolonged, and for repetitive hemodynamic insults, as well as for the cumulative impact of these insults. Even in the full-term infant, most forms of hypoxic-ischemic insult are relatively circumscribed, such as intrapartum asphyxia and postnatal cardiac arrest. After perinatal asphyxia in term infants, certain topographic patterns of injury have been described for different types of insult, such as severe transient and partial prolonged insults.[243-245] To date, no such relationships between insults and topography of cerebral injury have been described in the premature infant. The prolonged risk period for, and variety of, hemodynamic insults that might theoretically cause brain injury in the premature infant have made it difficult to design appropriate experimental models, or to monitor the human premature brain appropriately.

In addition to the unreliable association between systemic BP and CBF in newly born premature infants, most reported studies of the association between systemic BP and brain injury have used measures of systemic BP that are unsuited for exploring the complex hemodynamic changes during the fetal-neonatal circulatory transition. Measuring indices as crude as the lowest BP per day (in some cases multiple days) or BP averaged over prolonged periods is almost certainly inadequate to capture significant hemodynamic insults in this critically ill population.[112,203] Likewise, studies have used different definitions of "hypotension" (see Chapter 3) as well as different sampling times and durations.[16,17,112,118,119,183-187,202-204,246] The role of hemodynamic *fluctuations* in prematurity-related brain injury has been difficult to establish because fluctuating hemodynamics have been described in both normal and brain-injured term and premature newborns.[247-252]

Establishing a Temporal Relationship Between Systemic Hemodynamic Changes and Brain Insults

Establishing a biologically plausible temporal association between systemic hemodynamic disturbances and brain insult is an important step toward defining a causal relationship. This step is particularly challenging in the sick premature infant because the onset of brain injury is often unknown. Unlike older patients, premature infants rarely demonstrate acute signs at the onset of brain dysfunction, and therefore provide little or no clue to the timing of brain insult. Furthermore, neurodevelopmental deficits may only become evident months to years after the initial injury, sometimes as late as school age or beyond.[253-255] During this interval, multiple factors unrelated to the initial insult may significantly influence long-term outcome. The response to brain injury differs in important ways between mature and premature patients. Specifically, injury to the mature brain results in acute tissue destruction followed by atrophy and cicatricial changes. In the premature infant, brain injury precedes critical third-trimester events in brain development. The unfolding of these events after brain injury in individual infants may have implications for long-term outcome that are as or more important than the original cerebral injury. On the one hand, such normal third trimester developmental events may be derailed by acute injury resulting in acquired brain malformations (disruptions).[256] Conversely, the ameliorating effect of brain plasticity may play an important role in outcome. In addition, potentially injurious mechanisms other than hemodynamic insults may operate before (e.g., fetal inflammation), during (e.g., blood gas disturbances), and after (e.g., apnea and bradycardia) the immediate period of postnatal hemodynamic instability. Of particular importance is the role of infection and inflammation, now known to be associated with prematurity-related brain injury especially to the immature WM.[257-259] To date, no imaging markers have been identified that allow distinction between injury caused by such infection-inflammation and that caused by hemodynamic insults. Of course, these mechanisms may act in concert.

When challenged with the task of identifying the role of disturbed systemic hemodynamics in prematurity-related brain injury, it is critical that the potential impact of those modifying factors discussed earlier be identified and accounted for as well as possible. In order to minimize the impact of injury-related developmental disruption, reliable biomarkers of brain injury will be needed in the hyperacute period proximate to acute hemodynamic changes and before developmental disruption occurs. In trying to identify such biomarkers, it is useful to consider the sequence of brain responses on the road between insult and irreversible injury. At the onset of an emerging hemodynamic insult, the first response of the cerebral vasculature is to activate a compensatory response (e.g., hypotension elicits cerebral vasodilation).[137] If such compensatory mechanisms fail to maintain cerebral oxygen and substrate supply, loss of brain function follows (as detected by loss of electroencephalogram [EEG] activity), which might at first be an active compensatory "powering down" of neuronal activity to decrease demands.[260]

Finally, persistent or severe insults ultimately result in a loss of structural integrity and cell death.[111] Therefore, detecting a loss of compensatory responses, such as the development of cerebral pressure passivity, is a rational target for an early warning system of brain monitoring.

Identifying *acute structural injury* during periods of critical illness in these infants has been limited by the lack of sensitive portable neuroimaging, particularly for WM injury. For many years cranial US has been the principal imaging technique because infants were usually too ill to be transported to remote MRI scanners. Cranial US is sensitive to hemorrhage but remains insensitive to and delayed in its detection of diffuse WM injury, currently the leading cause of parenchymal brain injury. This has been confirmed not only at autopsy but also in several recent MRI studies that indicate that the majority of WM injury remains undetected by neonatal cranial ultrasound studies.[92,261,262] With the recent advent of MRI-compatible incubators safe transport of critically ill infants to MRI scanners is now feasible, and will hopefully advance detection of hyperacute brain injury.

Measures of *acute changes in brain function* have been difficult in the sick premature infant, in whom brain insults or even severe injury may remain clinically silent. Several studies have described the effect of hypotension on acute electrocortical function in premature infants, measured as changes in the amplitude, frequency, or continuity on the EEG.[113,128,263-265] Earlier studies in sick premature infants showed a decrease in EEG amplitude during hypotension.[263,266] More recently, Victor and colleagues found that in infants less than 30 weeks' gestation, EEG and cerebral oxygen extraction remained normal despite systemic BP levels as low as 23 mm Hg.[113] The use of EEG as a monitor of brain function has the advantage of being continuous, noninvasive, and relatively unobtrusive, especially utilizing the increasingly available limited-lead EEG techniques.[267] However, in extremely premature infants who are most at risk for brain injury, the background EEG has a relatively limited range of features and its reactivity to hemodynamic changes is in need of further exploration.

Intrinsic cerebrovascular systems aim to maintain brain oxygen/substrate delivery when systemic delivery fails.[137] These compensatory mechanisms are temporizing at best and, if systemic delivery does not recover, these mechanisms will collapse, elevating the risk for irreversible brain injury. For these reasons, a definition of systemic hypotension, using as a threshold the BP below which cerebral pressure-flow autoregulation begins to fail, appears logical.[111] Because the onset of cerebral pressure autoregulatory failure heralds an elevated risk for cerebrovascular injury at a point prior to irreversible injury, detection of cerebral pressure passivity might provide a sensitive cerebrovascular biomarker to relate to systemic BP changes. An association between failure of cerebral pressure-flow autoregulation and neonatal brain injury was first proposed three decades ago.[167,268] However, the presence and characteristics of pressure autoregulation in the sick premature infant remain controversial, in large part due to the ongoing lack of established techniques for detecting cerebral pressure passivity.[170,205,235,269] To date, most studies have used intermittent "static" measurements of CBF to study pressure autoregulation, with all their limitations for studying dynamic processes over time (discussed earlier). More recently, the NIRS hemoglobin difference (HbD) signal, which can be measured continuously, has been time-locked to measurements of systemic BP and applied to the study of cerebral pressure-flow autoregulation in immature animals and premature infants.[168,169,270-272] This approach identifies periods of pressure passivity using coherence function analysis to identify significant concordance between systemic BP and cerebral HbD changes. The magnitude of pressure passivity during these periods can then be measured using transfer gain analysis.[169] Using this approach, an association between cerebral pressure-passivity and brain injury has been described, as well as between the magnitude of pressure passivity and GM-IVH.[168,272] This approach has also highlighted the prevalence and dynamic nature of cerebral pressure flow autoregulation, with periods of pressure passivity interspersed with apparent autoregulation in most extremely premature infants.[169] Furthermore, these studies emphasized that cerebral pressure passivity could not reliably be predicted by the presence of blood pressure alone, suggesting that pressure autoregulation was affected by other influences as well.[169]

Limitations in using the onset of cerebral pressure passivity to define hypotension are several. In addition to the technical difficulties discussed earlier, this threshold may fluctuate despite constant BP, presumably due to other vasoactive factors such as hypoxemia, hypercarbia, inflammation, among others.[137,273-277] In addition, preceding insults (e.g., intrapartum) may temporarily abolish pressure autoregulation, making it unreliable as a criterion for "normative" definitions of hypotension. In summary, continuous monitoring for cerebral pressure passivity is clearly much needed. However, recent findings suggest that the notion of predictable gestational/postnatal age-related BP bounds between which cerebral perfusion is maintained constant is spurious (also see Chapter 3).[112]

Conclusion

It has long been accepted that a substantial component of the long-term neurodevelopmental burden in survivors of prematurity originates from neonatal brain injury resulting from systemic hemodynamic insults. However, despite compelling data from animal models, direct evidence of these mechanisms in premature humans remains limited. The role of hypotension in prematurity-related brain injury has been difficult to establish, as has the role for anti-hypotensive treatment in prevention of such injury. Consequently, there has been growing skepticism in some quarters about the rational basis for current practices, and the suggestion that less-aggressive intervention is warranted for hypotension in premature infants. This chapter has explored the fundamental challenges in both our understanding of systemic and cerebral hemodynamics, as well as the constraints of available technology for addressing these complex but critically important questions. Despite these many challenges, this chapter, along with other chapters in this book, also stresses the need for additional data before radical changes are made in our approach to hypotension in premature infants. The dictum "a lack of evidence for an association is not evidence for the lack of an association" has never been more valid.

References

1. Barrington KJ, Dempsey EM. Cardiovascular support in the preterm: treatments in search of indications. J Pediatr. 2006;148(3):289-291.
2. Dempsey EM, Barrington KJ. Treating hypotension in the preterm infant: when and with what: a critical and systematic review. J Perinatol. 2007;27(8):469-478.
3. Behrman R, Stith Butler A. Institute of Medicine Committee on Understanding Premature Birth and Assuring Healthy Outcomes Board on Health Sciences Outcomes: preterm birth: causes, consequences, and prevention. Washington, DC: The National Academies Press, 2007.
4. Martin JA, Kung HC, Mathews TJ, et al. Annual summary of vital statistics: 2006. Pediatrics. 2008;121(4):788-801.
5. Hagberg B, Hagberg G, Beckung E, et al. Changing panorama of cerebral palsy in Sweden. VIII. Prevalence and origin in the birth year period 1991-94. Acta Paediatr. 2001;90(3):271-277.
6. Schendel DE, Stockbauer JW, Hoffman HJ, et al. Relation between very low birth weight and developmental delay among preschool children without disabilities. Am J Epidemiol. 1997; 146(9):740-749.
7. Piecuch RE, Leonard CH, Cooper BA, et al. Outcome of extremely low birth weight infants (500 to 999 grams) over a 12-year period. Pediatrics. 1997;100(4):633-639.
8. Leonard CH, Piecuch RE. School age outcome in low birth weight preterm infants. Semin Perinatol. 1997;21(3):240-253.

9. O'Shea TM, Klinepeter KL, Goldstein DJ, et al. Survival and developmental disability in infants with birth weights of 501 to 800 grams, born between 1979 and 1994. Pediatrics. 1997; 100(6):982-986.

10. Fanaroff AA, Wright LL, Stevenson DK, et al. Very-low-birth-weight outcomes of the National Institute of Child Health and Human Development Neonatal Research Network, May 1991 through December 1992. Am J Obstet Gynecol. 1995;173:1423-1431.

11. Golden JA, Gilles FH, Rudelli R, et al. Frequency of neuropathological abnormalities in very low birth weight infants. J Neuropathol Exper Neurol. 1997;56:472-478.

12. Back SA, Gan X, Li Y, et al. Maturation-dependent vulnerability of oligodendrocytes to oxidative stress-induced death caused by glutathione depletion. J Neurosci. 1998;18(16):6241-6253.

13. Back SA, Luo NL, Borenstein NS, et al. Late oligodendrocyte progenitors coincide with the developmental window of vulnerability for human perinatal white matter injury. J Neurosci. 2001;21(4):1302-1312.

14. Back SA, Riddle A, McClure MM. Maturation-dependent vulnerability of perinatal white matter in premature birth. Stroke. 2007;38(2 Suppl):724-730.

15. Ment LR, Duncan CC, Ehrenkranz RA, et al. Intraventricular hemorrhage in the preterm neonate: timing and cerebral blood flow changes. J Pediatr. 1984;104(3):419-425.

16. Miall-Allen VM, de Vries LS, Whitelaw AG. Mean arterial blood pressure and neonatal cerebral lesions. Arch Dis Child. 1987;62(10):1068-1069.

17. Watkins AM, West CR, Cooke RW. Blood pressure and cerebral haemorrhage and ischaemia in very low birthweight infants. Early Hum Dev. 1989;19(2):103-110.

18. Gronlund JU, Korvenranta H, Kero P, et al. Elevated arterial blood pressure is associated with peri-intraventricular haemorrhage. Eur J Pediatr. 1994;153(11):836-841.

19. Hack M, Friedman H, Fanaroff AA. Outcomes of extremely low birth weight infants. Pediatrics. 1996;98(5):931-937.

20. Hack M, Fanaroff AA. Outcomes of children of extremely low birthweight and gestational age in the 1990's. Early Hum Dev. 1999;53(3):193-218.

21. McIntire DD, Bloom SL, Casey BM, Leveno KJ. Birth weight in relation to morbidity and mortality among newborn infants. N Engl J Med. 1999;340(16):1234-1238.

22. Darlow BA, Cust AE, Donoghue DA. Improved outcomes for very low birthweight infants: evidence from New Zealand national population based data. Arch Dis Child Fetal Neonatal Ed. 2003; 88(1):F23-F28.

23. Larroque B, Breart G, Kaminski M, et al. Survival of very preterm infants: Epipage, a population based cohort study. Arch Dis Child Fetal Neonatal Ed. 2004;89(2):F139-F144.

24. Anthony S, Ouden L, Brand R, et al. Changes in perinatal care and survival in very preterm and extremely preterm infants in The Netherlands between 1983 and 1995. Eur J Obstet Gynecol Reprod Biol. 2004;112(2):170-177.

25. Shalak L, Perlman JM. Hemorrhagic-ischemic cerebral injury in the preterm infant: current concepts. Clin Perinatol. 2002;29(4):745-763.

26. Khwaja O, Volpe JJ. Pathogenesis of cerebral white matter injury of prematurity. Arch Dis Child Fetal Neonatal Ed. 2008;93(2):F153-F161.

27. Volpe JJ. Brain injury in the premature infant—current concepts. Preven Med. 1994;23:638-645.

28. Volpe JJ. Brain injury in the premature infant: overview of clinical aspects, neuropathology, and pathogenesis. Semin Pediatr Neurol. 1998;5(3):135-151.

29. du Plessis AJ, Volpe JJ. Intracranial hemorrhage in the newborn infant. In: Burg FD, Ingelfinger JR, Wald ER, et al., eds. Gellis & Kagan's current pediatric therapy 16. Philadelphia: WB Saunders; 1999:304-308.

30. du Plessis AJ, Volpe JJ. Perinatal brain injury in the preterm and term newborn. Curr Opin Neurol. 2002;15(2):151-157.

31. Back SA, Riddle A, Hohimer AR. Role of instrumented fetal sheep preparations in defining the pathogenesis of human periventricular white-matter injury. J Child Neurol. 2006;21(7):582-589.

32. Ment LR, Stewart WB, Duncan CC, et al. Beagle puppy model of intraventricular hemorrhage. J Neurosurg. 1982;57(2):219-223.

33. Goddard J, Lewis RM, Alcala H, et al. Intraventricular hemorrhage—an animal model. Biol Neonate. 1980;37(1):39-52.

34. Goddard-Finegold J, Michael LH. Cerebral blood flow and experimental intraventricular hemorrhage. Pediatr Res. 1984;18(1):7-11.

35. Larroche JC. Intraventricular hemorrhage in the premature neonate. In: Korobkin R, Guilleminault C, eds. Advances in perinatal neurology. New York: SP Medical and Scientific Books; 1979:115.

36. Hambleton G, Wigglesworth JS. Origin of intraventricular haemorrhage in the preterm infant. Arch Dis Child. 1976;51(9):651-659.

37. Rorke LB. Pathology of perinatal brain injury. New York: Raven Press; 1982.

38. Nakamura Y, Okudera T, Fukuda S, et al. Germinal matrix hemorrhage of venous origin in preterm neonates. Hum Pathol. 1990;21(10):1059-1062.

39. Moody DM, Brown WR, Challa VR, et al. Alkaline phosphatase histochemical staining in the study of germinal matrix hemorrhage and brain vascular morphology in a very-low-birth-weight neonate. Pediatr Res. 1994;35:424-430.

40. Ghazi-Birry HS, Brown WR, Moody DM, et al. Human germinal matrix: venous origin of hemorrhage and vascular characteristics. Am J Neuroradiol. 1997;18(2):219-229.

41. Anstrom JA, Brown WR, Moody DM, et al. Subependymal veins in premature neonates: implications for hemorrhage. Pediatr Neurol. 2004;30(1):46-53.

42. Leech RW, Kohnen P. Subependymal and intraventricular hemorrhages in the newborn. Am J Pathol. 1974;77(3):465-475.

43. Pape KE, Wigglesworth JS. Haemorrhage, ischaemia and the perinatal brain. Philadelphia: JB Lippincott; 1979.

44. Kuban KC, Gilles FH. Human telencephalic angiogenesis. Ann Neurol. 1985;17(6):539-548.

45. Pinar MH, Edwards WH, Fratkin J, et al. A transmission electron microscopy study of human cerebral cortical and germinal matrix (GM) blood vessels in premature neonate (abstract). Pediatr Res. 1985;19(Part 2):394A.

46. Kamei A, Houdou S, Mito T, et al. Developmental change in type VI collagen in human cerebral vessels. Pediatr Neurol. 1992;8(3):183-186.

47. Oldendorf WH, Cornford ME, Brown WJ. The large apparent work capability of the blood-brain barrier: a study of the mitochondrial content of capillary endothelial cells in brain and other tissues of the rat. Ann Neurol. 1977;1(5):409-417.

48. Goldstein GW. Pathogenesis of brain edema and hemorrhage: role of the brain capillary. Pediatrics. 1979;64(3):357-360.

49. Takashima S, Tanaka K. Microangiography and vascular permeability of the subependymal matrix in the premature infant. Can J Neurol Sci. 1978;5(1):45-50.

50. Grunnet ML. Morphometry of blood vessels in the cortex and germinal plate of premature neonates. Pediatr Neurol. 1989;5(1):12-16.

51. Yakovlev PI, Rosales RK. Distribution of the terminal hemorrhages in the brain wall in stillborn premature and nonviable neonates. In: Angle CR, Bering Jr EA, eds. Physical trauma as an etiologic agent in mental retardation. Washington, DC: US Government Printing Office; 1970:67.

52. Gruenwald P. Subependymal cerebral hemorrhage in premature infants, and its relation to various injurious influences at birth. Am J Obstet Gynecol. 1951;61:1285-1292.

53. Ahmann PA, Lazzara A, Dykes FD, et al. Intraventricular hemorrhage in the high-risk preterm infant: incidence and outcome. Ann Neurol. 1980;7:118-124.

54. Holt PJ, Allan WF. The natural history of ventricular dilatation in neonatal intraventricular hemorrhage and its therapeutic implication. Ann Neurol. 1981;10:293.

55. Levene MI, Starte DR. A longitudinal study of post-haemorrhagic ventricular dilatation in the newborn. Arch Dis Child. 1981;56(12):905-910.

56. Lipscomb AP, Thorburn RJ, Reynolds EO, et al. Pneumothorax and cerebral haemorrhage in preterm infants. Lancet. 1981;1:414-416.

57. McMenamin JB, Shackelford GD, Volpe JJ. Outcome of neonatal intraventricular hemorrhage with periventricular echodense lesions. Ann Neurol. 1984;15:285-290.

58. Papile LA, Burstein J, Burstein R, et al. Incidence and evolution of subependymal and intraventricular hemorrhage: a study of infants with birth weights less than 1,500 gm. J Pediatr. 1978; 92:529-534.

59. Horbar JD, Badger GJ, Carpenter JH, et al. Trends in mortality and morbidity for very low birth weight infants, 1991-1999. Pediatrics. 2002;110(1 Pt 1):143-151.

60. Cust AE, Darlow BA, Donoghue DA. Outcomes for high risk New Zealand newborn infants in 1998-1999: a population based, national study. Arch Dis Child Fetal Neonatal Ed. 2003; 88(1):F15-F22.

61. Larroque B, Marret S, Ancel PY, et al. White matter damage and intraventricular hemorrhage in very preterm infants: the EPIPAGE study. J Pediatr. 2003;143(4):477-483.

62. Hamrick SE, Miller SP, Leonard C, et al. Trends in severe brain injury and neurodevelopmental outcome in premature newborn infants: the role of cystic periventricular leukomalacia. J Pediatr. 2004;145(5):593-599.

63. Davis DW. Cognitive outcomes in school-age children born prematurely. Neonatal Netw. 2003; 22(3):27-38.

64. Wilson-Costello D, Friedman H, Minich N, et al. Improved survival rates with increased neurodevelopmental disability for extremely low birth weight infants in the 1990s. Pediatrics. 2005;115(4): 997-1003.

65. du Plessis AJ. Posthemorrhagic hydrocephalus and brain injury in the preterm infant: dilemmas in diagnosis and management. Semin Pediatr Neurol. 1998;5(3):161-179.

66. Ventriculomegaly Trial Group. Randomised trial of early tapping in neonatal posthaemorrhagic ventricular dilatation: results at 30 months. Arch Dis Child Fetal Neonatal Ed. 1994;70(2): F129-F136.

67. Ment LR, Scott DT, Ehrenkranz RA, et al. Neurodevelopmental assessment of very low birth weight neonates: effect of germinal matrix and intraventricular hemorrhage. Pediatr Neurol. 1985; 1(3):164-168.

68. van de Bor M, Verloove-Vanhorick SP, Baerts W, et al. Outcome of periventricular-intraventricular hemorrhage at 2 years of age in 484 very preterm infants admitted to 6 neonatal intensive care units in The Netherlands. Neuropediatrics. 1988;19(4):183-185.

69. Lowe J, Papile L. Neurodevelopmental performance of very-low-birth-weight infants with mild periventricular, intraventricular hemorrhage. Outcome at 5 to 6 years of age. Am J Dis Child. 1990;144(11):1242-1245.

70. van de Bor M, Ensdokkum M, Schreuder AM, et al. Outcome of periventricular-intraventricular haemorrhage at five years of age. Dev Med Child Neurol. 1993;35(1):33-41.

71. Roth SC, Baudin J, McCormick DC, et al. Relation between ultrasound appearance of the brain of very preterm infants and neurodevelopmental impairment at eight years. Dev Med Child Neurol. 1993;35:755-768.

72. Levy ML, Masri LS, McComb JG. Outcome for preterm infants with germinal matrix hemorrhage and progressive hydrocephalus. Neurosurgery. 1997;41(5):1111-1117.

73. Perlman JM, Volpe JJ. Intraventricular hemorrhage in extremely small premature infants. Am J Dis Child. 1986;140(11):1122-1124.

74. Strand C, Laptook AR, Dowling S, et al. Neonatal intracranial hemorrhage. I. Changing pattern in inborn low-birth-weight infants. Early Hum Dev. 1990;23(2):117-128.

75. Bassan H, Benson CB, Limperopoulos C, et al. Ultrasonographic features and severity scoring of periventricular hemorrhagic infarction in relation to risk factors and outcome. Pediatrics. 2006;117(6):2111-2118.

76. Bassan H, Feldman HA, Limperopoulos C, et al. Periventricular hemorrhagic infarction: risk factors and neonatal outcome. Pediatr Neurol. 2006;35(2):85-92.

77. Bassan H, Limperopoulos C, Visconti K, et al. Neurodevelopmental outcome in survivors of periventricular hemorrhagic infarction. Pediatrics. 2007;120(4):785-792.

78. Guzzetta F, Shackelford G, Volpe S, et al. Periventricular intraparenchymal echodensities in the premature newborn: critical determinant of neurologic outcome. Pediatrics. 1986;78(6):995-1006.

79. de Vries LS, Roelants-van Rijn AM, Rademaker KJ, et al. Unilateral parenchymal haemorrhagic infarction in the preterm infant. Eur J Paediatr Neurol. 2001;5(4):139-149.

80. Volpe JJ. Intracranial hemorrhage: germinal matrix-intraventricular hemorrhage of the premature infant. In: Neurology of the newborn, 5th ed. Philadelphia: Saunders Elsevier; 2008:517-588.

81. De Reuck JL. Cerebral angioarchitecture and perinatal brain lesions in premature and full-term infants. Acta Neurol Scand. 1984;70(6):391-395.

82. Takashima S, Armstrong DL, Becker LE. Subcortical leukomalacia. Relationship to development of the cerebral sulcus and its vascular supply. Arch Neurol. 1978;35(7):470-472.

83. De Reuck J. The human periventricular arterial blood supply and the anatomy of cerebral infarctions. Eur Neurol. 1971;5(6):321-334.

84. De Reuck J. The cortico-subcortical arterial angio-architecture in the human brain. Acta Neurol Belg. 1972;72(5):323-329.

85. Rorke LB. Anatomical features of the developing brain implicated in pathogenesis of hypoxic-ischemic injury. Brain Pathol. 1992;2(3):211-221.

86. Takashima S, Tanaka K. Development of cerebrovascular architecture and its relationship to periventricular leukomalacia. Arch Neurol. 1978;35(1):11-16.

87. Nakamura Y, Okudera T, Hashimoto T. Vascular architecture in white matter of neonates: its relationship to periventricular leukomalacia. J Neuropathol Exp Neurol. 1994;53(6):582-589.

88. Volpe JJ. Encephalopathy of prematurity includes neuronal abnormalities. Pediatrics. 2005;116(1):221-225.

89. Banker B, Larroche J. Periventricular leukomalacia in infancy. Arch Neurol. 1962;7:386-410.

90. Armstrong D, Norman MG. Periventricular leucomalacia in neonates. Complications and sequelae. Arch Dis Child. 1974;49(5):367-375.

91. Nwaesei CG, Pape KE, Martin DJ, et al. Periventricular infarction diagnosed by ultrasound: a postmortem correlation. J Pediatr. 1984;105(1):106-110.

92. Maalouf EF, Duggan PJ, Counsell SJ, et al. Comparison of findings on cranial ultrasound and magnetic resonance imaging in preterm infants. Pediatrics. 2001;107(4):719-727.

93. Volpe JJ. Cerebral white matter injury of the premature infant-more common than you think. Pediatrics. 2003;112(1 Pt 1):176-180.

94. Dyet LE, Kennea N, Counsell SJ, et al. Natural history of brain lesions in extremely preterm infants studied with serial magnetic resonance imaging from birth and neurodevelopmental assessment. Pediatrics. 2006;118(2):536-548.

95. De Vries LS, Wigglesworth JS, Regev R, et al. Evolution of periventricular leukomalacia during the neonatal period and infancy: correlation of imaging and postmortem findings. Early Hum Dev. 1988;17(2-3):205-219.

96. Pierson CR, Folkerth RD, Billiards SS, et al. Gray matter injury associated with periventricular leukomalacia in the premature infant. Acta Neuropathol. 2007;114(6):619-631.

97. Oka A, Belliveau MJ, Rosenberg PA, et al. Vulnerability of oligodendroglia to glutamate: pharmacology, mechanisms, and prevention. J Neurosci. 1993;13(4):1441-1453.

98. Fern R, Moller T. Rapid ischemic cell death in immature oligodendrocytes: a fatal glutamate release feedback loop. J Neurosci. 2000;20(1):34-42.

99. Agata Y, Hiraishi S, Oguchi K, et al. Changes in left ventricular output from fetal to early neonatal life. J Pediatr. 1991;119(3):441-445.

100. Evans N, Osborn D, Kluckow M. Preterm circulatory support is more complex than just blood pressure. Pediatrics. 2005;115(4):1114-1115; author reply 1115-1116.

101. Kluckow M, Evans N. Low superior vena cava flow and intraventricular haemorrhage in preterm infants. Arch Dis Child Fetal Neonatal Ed. 2000;82(3):F188-F194.

102. Hunt RW, Evans N, Rieger I, et al. Low superior vena cava flow and neurodevelopment at 3 years in very preterm infants. J Pediatr. 2004;145(5):588-592.

103. Kluckow M, Evans N. Low systemic blood flow and hyperkalemia in preterm infants. J Pediatr. 2001;139(2):227-232.

104. Osborn D, Evans N, Kluckow M. Randomized trial of dobutamine versus dopamine in preterm infants with low systemic blood flow. J Pediatr. 2002;140(2):183-191.

105. Kluckow M, Evans N. Superior vena cava flow in newborn infants: a novel marker of systemic blood flow. Arch Dis Child Fetal Neonatal Ed. 2000;82(3):F182-F187.

106. Levene MI, Fawer CL, Lamont RF. Risk factors in the development of intraventricular haemorrhage in the preterm neonate. Arch Dis Child. 1982;57:410-417.

107. Paneth N, Pinto-Martin J, Gardiner J, et al. Incidence and timing of germinal matrix/intraventricular hemorrhage in low birth weight infants. Am J Epidemiol. 1993;137:1167-1176.

108. Chatow U, Davidson S, Reichman BL, et al. Development and maturation of the autonomic nervous system in premature and full-term infants using spectral analysis of heart rate fluctuations. Pediatr Res. 1995;37(3):294-302.

109. Drouin E, Gournay V, Calamel J, et al. Assessment of spontaneous baroreflex sensitivity in neonates. Arch Dis Child Fetal Neonatal Ed. 1997;76(2):F108-F112.

110. Andriessen P, Koolen AMP, Berendsen RCM, et al. Cardiovascular fluctuations and transfer function analysis in stable preterm infants. Pediatr Res. 2003;53(1):89-97.

111. McLean CW, Cayabyab R, Noori S, et al. Cerebral circulation and hypotension in the premature infant—diagnosis and treatment. In: Perlman JM, ed. Questions and controversies in neonatology—neurology. Philadelphia: Saunders/Elsevier; 2008:3-26.

112. Noori S, Stavroudis TA, Seri I. Systemic and cerebral hemodynamics during the transitional period after premature birth. Clin Perinatol. 2009;36:723-736.

113. Victor S, Marson AG, Appleton RE, et al. Relationship between blood pressure, cerebral electrical activity, cerebral fractional oxygen extraction, and peripheral blood flow in very low birth weight newborn infants. Pediatr Res. 2006;59(2):314-319.

114. Batton B, Batton D, Riggs T. Blood pressure during the first 7 days in premature infants born at postmenstrual age 23 to 25 weeks. Am J Perinatol. 2007;24(2):107-115.

115. Lee JM, Zipfel GJ, Choi DW. The changing landscape of ischaemic brain injury mechanisms. Nature. 1999;399(6738 Suppl):A7-14.

116. Northern Neonatal Nursing Initiative. Systolic blood pressure in babies of less than 32 weeks gestation in the first year of life. Arch Dis Child Fetal Neonatal Ed. 1999;80(1):F38-F42.

117. de Vries LS, Regev R, Dubowitz LM, et al. Perinatal risk factors for the development of extensive cystic leukomalacia. Am J Dis Child. 1988;142(7):732-735.

118. Limperopoulos C, Bassan H, Kalish LA, et al. Current definitions of hypotension do not predict abnormal cranial ultrasound findings in preterm infants. Pediatrics. 2007;120(5):966-977.

119. Weindling AM, Wilkinson AR, Cook J, et al. Perinatal events which precede periventricular haemorrhage and leukomalacia in the newborn. Br J Obstet Gynaecol. 1985;92(12):1218-1223.

120. Seri I, Abbasi S, Wood DC, et al. Regional hemodynamic effects of dopamine in the sick preterm neonate. J Pediatr. 1998;133(6):728-734.

121. Al-Aweel I, Pursley DM, Rubin LP, et al. Variations in prevalence of hypotension, hypertension, and vasopressor use in NICUs. J Perinatol. 2001;21(5):272-278.

122. Zubrow AB, Hulman S, Kushner H, et al. Determinants of blood pressure in infants admitted to neonatal intensive care units: a prospective multicenter study. Philadelphia Neonatal Blood Pressure Study Group. J Perinatol. 1995;15(6):470-479.

123. Powers WJ, Grubb Jr RL, Darriet D, et al. Cerebral blood flow and cerebral metabolic rate of oxygen requirements for cerebral function and viability in humans. J Cereb Blood Flow Metab. 1985;5(4):600-608.

124. Greisen G. Cerebral blood flow in preterm infants during the first week of life. Acta Paediatr Scand. 1986;75(1):43-51.

125. Greisen G. Cerebral blood flow in mechanically ventilated, preterm neonates. Dan Med Bull. 1990;37(2):124-131.

126. Greisen G. Thresholds for periventricular white matter vulnerability in hypoxia-ischemia. In: Lou H, Greisen G, Larsen J, eds. Brain lesions in the newborn. Copenhagen: Munksgaard; 1994:222-229.

127. Greisen G, Johansen K, Ellison PH, et al. Cerebral blood flow in the newborn infant: comparison of Doppler ultrasound and 133xenon clearance. J Pediatr. 1984;104(3):411-418.

128. Greisen G, Pryds O. Low CBF, discontinuous EEG activity, and periventricular brain injury in ill, preterm neonates. Brain Dev. 1989;11:164-168.

129. Pryds O, Christensen NJ, Friis HB. Increased cerebral blood flow and plasma epinephrine in hypoglycemic, preterm neonates. Pediatrics. 1990;85(2):172-176.

130. Pryds O, Greisen G, Friis-Hansen B. Compensatory increase of CBF in preterm infants during hypoglycaemia. Acta Paediatr Scand. 1988;77(5):632-637.

131. Pryds O, Greisen G, Johansen KH. Indomethacin and cerebral blood flow in premature infants treated for patent ductus arteriosus. Eur J Pediatr. 1988;147(3):315-316.

132. Pryds O, Andersen GE, Friis-Hansen B. Cerebral blood flow reactivity in spontaneously breathing, preterm infants shortly after birth. Acta Paediatr Scand. 1990;79(4):391-396.

133. Altman DI, Powers WJ, Perlman JM, et al. Cerebral blood flow requirement for brain viability in newborn infants is lower than in adults. Ann Neurol. 1988;24:218-226.

134. Borch K, Greisen G. Blood flow distribution in the normal human preterm brain. Pediatr Res. 1998;43(1):28-33.

135. Volpe JJ. Hypoxic-ischemic encephalopathy: biochemical and physiological aspects. In: Neurology of the newborn, 5th ed. Philadelphia: Saunders Elsevier; 2008:247-324.

136. Sorensen LC, Greisen G. The brains of very preterm newborns in clinically stable condition may be hyperoxygenated. Pediatrics. 2009;124(5):e958-e963.

137. du Plessis AJ. Cerebrovascular injury in premature infants: current understanding and challenges for future prevention. Clin Perinatol. 2008;35(4):609-641.

138. Busija DW. Cerebral autoregulation. In: Phillis JW, ed. The regulation of cerebral blood flow. Boca Raton, FL: Chemical Rubber Company; 1993:45-64.
139. Lassen NA. Cerebral blood flow and oxygen consumption in man. Physiol Rev. 1959;39(2):183-233.
140. Lassen N, Christensen M. Physiology of cerebral blood flow. Br J Anaesth. 1976;48:719-734.
141. Symon L, Held K, Dorsch NWC. A study of regional autoregulation in the cerebral circulation to increased perfusion pressure in normocapnea and hypercapnea. Stroke. 1973;4(2):139-147.
142. Kontos H, Wei E, Navari R, et al. Responses of cerebral arteries and arterioles to acute hypotension and hypertension. Am J Physiol. 1978;3(4):H371-H383.
143. Aaslid R, Lindegaard KF, Sorteberg W, et al. Cerebral autoregulation dynamics in humans. Stroke. 1989;20(1):45-52.
144. Florence G, Seylaz J. Rapid autoregulation of cerebral blood flow: a laser-Doppler flowmetry study. J Cereb Blood Flow Metab. 1992;12(4):674-680.
145. Panerai RB, Kelsall AW, Rennie JM, et al. Cerebral autoregulation dynamics in premature newborns. Stroke. 1995;26(1):74-80.
146. Zhang R, Zuckerman JH, Giller CA, et al. Transfer function analysis of dynamic cerebral autoregulation in humans. Am J Physiol. 1998;274:H233-H241.
147. Jones Jr MD, Sheldon RE, Peeters LL, et al. Regulation of cerebral blood flow in the ovine fetus. Am J Physiol. 1978;235(2):H162-H166.
148. Hernandez MJ, Brennan RW, Bowman GS. Autoregulation of cerebral blood flow in the newborn dog. Brain Res. 1980;184(1):199-202.
149. Camp D, Kotagal UR, Kleinman LI. Preservation of cerebral autoregulation in the unanesthetized hypoxemic newborn dog. Brain Res. 1982;241(2):207-213.
150. Tweed WA, Cote J, Wade JG, et al. Preservation of fetal brain blood flow relative to other organs during hypovolemic hypotension. Pediatr Res. 1982;16(2):137-140.
151. Tweed WA, Cote J, Pash M, et al. Arterial oxygenation determines autoregulation of cerebral blood flow in the fetal lamb. Pediatr Res. 1983;17(4):246-249.
152. Papile LA, Rudolph AM, Heymann MA. Autoregulation of cerebral blood flow in the preterm fetal lamb. Pediatr Res. 1985;19(2):159-161.
153. Tweed A, Cote J, Lou H, et al. Impairment of cerebral blood flow autoregulation in the newborn lamb by hypoxia. Pediatr Res. 1986;20:516-519.
154. Armstead WM, Leffler CW. Neurohumoral regulation of the cerebral circulation. Proc Soc Exp Biol Med. 1992;199(2):149-157.
155. Pasternak JF, Groothuis DR. Autoregulation of cerebral blood flow in the newborn beagle puppy. Biol Neonate. 1985;48(2):100-109.
156. Szymonowicz W, Walker AM, Yu VY, et al. Regional cerebral blood flow after hemorrhagic hypotension in the preterm, near-term, and newborn lamb. Pediatr Res. 1990;28(4):361-366.
157. Hohimer AR, Bissonnette JM. Effects of cephalic hypotension, hypertension, and barbiturates on fetal cerebral blood flow and metabolism. Am J Obstet Gynecol. 1989;161(5):1344-1351.
158. Young RS, Hernandez MJ, Yagel SK. Selective reduction of blood flow to white matter during hypotension in newborn dogs: a possible mechanism of periventricular leukomalacia. Ann Neurol. 1982;12(5):445-448.
159. Arnold BW, Martin CG, Alexander BJ, et al. Autoregulation of brain blood flow during hypotension and hypertension in infant lambs. Pediatr Res. 1991;29:110-115.
160. Monin P, Stonestreet BS, Oh W. Hyperventilation restores autoregulation of cerebral blood flow in postictal piglets. Pediatr Res. 1991;30(3):294-298.
161. Hascoet JM, Monin P, Vert P. Persistence of impaired autoregulation of cerebral blood flow in the postictal period in piglets. Epilepsia. 1988;29(6):743-747.
162. Del Toro J, Louis PT, Goddard-Finegold J. Cerebrovascular regulation and neonatal brain injury. Pediatr Neurol. 1991;7(1):3-12.
163. van Os S, Liem D, Hopman J, et al. Cerebral O2 supply thresholds for the preservation of electrocortical brain activity during hypotension in near-term-born lambs. Pediatr Res. 2005;57(3):358-362.
164. Van Os S, Klaessens J, Hopman J, et al. Cerebral oxygen supply during hypotension in near-term lambs: a near-infrared spectroscopy study. Brain Dev. 2006;28(2):115-121.
165. Heistad DD, Kontos HA. Cerebral circulation. In: Shepherd JT, Abboud FM, eds. Handbook of physiology. Bethesda, MD: American Physiological Society; 1983:137-182.
166. Gebremedhin D, Lange AR, Lowry TF, et al. Production of 20-HETE and its role in autoregulation of cerebral blood flow [see comments]. Circ Res. 2000;87(1):60-65.
167. Lou HC, Lassen NA, Friis-Hansen B. Impaired autoregulation of cerebral blood flow in the distressed newborn infant. J Pediatr. 1979;94(1):118-121.
168. Tsuji M, Saul JP, du Plessis A, et al. Cerebral intravascular oxygenation correlates with mean arterial pressure in critically ill premature infants. Pediatrics. 2000;106(4):625-632.
169. Soul JS, Hammer PE, Tsuji M, et al. Fluctuating pressure-passivity is common in the cerebral circulation of sick premature infants. Pediatr Res. 2007;61(4):467-473.
170. Pryds O. Control of cerebral circulation in the high-risk neonate. Ann Neurol. 1991;30:321-329.
171. Milligan DW. Failure of autoregulation and intraventricular haemorrhage in preterm infants. Lancet. 1980;1(8174):896-898.
172. Miall-Allen VM, de Vries LS, Dubowitz LM, et al. Blood pressure fluctuation and intraventricular hemorrhage in the preterm infant of less than 31 weeks' gestation. Pediatrics. 1989;83(5):657-661.

16

173. Ramaekers VT, Casaer P, Daniels H, et al. Upper limits of brain blood flow autoregulation in stable infants of various conceptional age. Early Hum Dev. 1990;24(3):249-258.

174. Verma PK, Panerai RB, Rennie JM, et al. Grading of cerebral autoregulation in preterm and term neonates. Pediatr Neurol. 2000;23(3):236-242.

175. van de Bor M, Walther FJ. Cerebral blood flow velocity regulation in preterm infants. Biol Neonate. 1991;59(6):329-335.

176. Munro MJ, Walker AM, Barfield CP. Hypotensive extremely low birth weight infants have reduced cerebral blood flow. Pediatrics. 2004;114(6):1591-1596.

177. Lou HC, Lassen NA, Friis-Hansen B. Low cerebral blood flow in the hypotensive distressed newborn. Acta Neurol Scand Suppl. 1977;64:428-429.

178. Lou HC, Skov H, Pedersen H. Low cerebral blood flow: a risk factor in the neonate. J Pediatr. 1979;95(4):606-609.

179. Younkin DP, Reivich M, Jaggi J, et al. Noninvasive method of estimating human newborn regional cerebral blood flow. J Cereb Blood Flow Metab. 1982;2(4):415-420.

180. Boylan GB, Young K, Panerai RB, et al. Dynamic cerebral autoregulation in sick newborn infants. Pediatr Res. 2000;48(1):12-17.

181. Anthony MY, Evans DH, Levene MI. Neonatal cerebral blood flow velocity responses to changes in posture. Arch Dis Child. 1993;69(3 Spec No):304-308.

182. Bada HS, Korones SB, Perry EH, et al. Frequent handling in the neonatal intensive care unit and intraventricular hemorrhage. J Pediatr. 1990;117(1):126-131.

183. Bada HS, Korones SB, Perry EH, et al. Mean arterial blood pressure changes in premature infants and those at risk for intraventricular hemorrhage. J Pediatr. 1990;117(4):607-614.

184. Low JA, Froese AB, Smith JT, et al. Hypotension and hypoxemia in the preterm newborn during the four days following delivery identify infants at risk of echosonographically demonstrable cerebral lesions. Clin Invest Med. 1992;15(1):60-65.

185. Perlman JM, Risser R, Broyles RS. Bilateral cystic periventricular leukomalacia in the premature infant: associated risk factors. Pediatrics. 1996;97(6 Pt 1):822-827.

186. Murphy DJ, Hope PL, Johnson A. Neonatal risk factors for cerebral palsy in very preterm babies: case-control study. BMJ. 1997;314(7078):404-408.

187. Fanaroff JM, Wilson-Costello DE, Newman NS, et al. Treated hypotension is associated with neonatal morbidity and hearing loss in extremely low birth weight infants. Pediatrics. 2006;117(4):1131-1135.

188. Trounce JQ, Shaw DE, Levene MI, et al. Clinical risk factors and periventricular leucomalacia. Arch Dis Child. 1988;63(1):17-22.

189. Cowan F, Thoresen M. The effects of intermittent positive pressure ventilation on cerebral arterial and venous blood velocities in the newborn infant. Acta Paediatr Scand. 1987;76(2):239-247.

190. Svenningsen L, Lindemann R, Eidal K. Measurements of fetal head compression pressure during bearing down and their relationship to the condition of the newborn. Acta Obstet Gynecol Scand. 1988;67(2):129-133.

191. Skinner JR, Milligan DWA, Hunter S, et al. Central venous pressure in the ventilated neonate. Arch Dis Child. 1992;67(SI):374-377.

192. Perlman JM, McMenamin JB, Volpe JJ. Fluctuating cerebral blood-flow velocity in respiratory-distress syndrome: relation to the development of intraventricular hemorrhage. N Engl J Med. 1983;309:204-209.

193. van Bel F, Van de Bor M, Stijnen T, et al. Aetiological role of cerebral blood-flow alterations in development and extension of peri-intraventricular haemorrhage. Dev Med Child Neurol. 1987;29(5):601-614.

194. Goddard J, Lewis RM, Armstrong DL, et al. Moderate, rapidly induced hypertension as a cause of intraventricular hemorrhage in the newborn beagle model. J Pediatr. 1980;96(6):1057-1060.

195. Pasternak JF, Groothuis DR, Fischer JM, et al. Regional cerebral blood flow in the beagle puppy model of neonatal intraventricular hemorrhage: studies during systemic hypertension. Neurology. 1983;33(5):559-566.

196. Goddard-Finegold J, Armstrong D, Zeller RS. Intraventricular hemorrhage following volume expansion after hypovolemic hypotension in the newborn beagle. J Pediatr. 1982;100(5):796-799.

197. Pasternak JF, Groothuis DR, Fischer JM, et al. Regional cerebral blood flow in the newborn beagle pup: the germinal matrix is a "low-flow" structure. Pediatr Res. 1982;16(6):499-503.

198. Pasternak JF, Groothuis DR. Regional variability of blood flow and glucose utilization within the subependymal germinal matrix. Brain Res. 1984;299(2):281-288.

199. Ment LR, Stewart WB, Petroff OA, et al. Thromboxane synthesis inhibitor in a beagle pup model of perinatal asphyxia. Stroke. 1989;20(6):809-814.

200. Goddard-Finegold J, Donley DK, Adham BI, et al. Phenobarbital and cerebral blood flow during hypertension in the newborn beagle. Pediatrics. 1990;86(4):501-508.

201. Reynolds ML, Evans CA, Reynolds EO, et al. Intracranial haemorrhage in the preterm sheep fetus. Early Hum Dev. 1979;3(2):163-186.

202. Meek JH, Tyszczuk L, Elwell CE, et al. Low cerebral blood flow is a risk factor for severe intraventricular haemorrhage. Arch Dis Child Fetal Neonatal Ed. 1999;81(1):F15-F18.

203. Dammann O, Allred EN, Kuban KC, et al. Systemic hypotension and white-matter damage in preterm infants. Dev Med Child Neurol. 2002;44(2):82-90.

204. D'Souza SW, Janakova H, Minors D, et al. Blood pressure, heart rate, and skin temperature in preterm infants: associations with periventricular haemorrhage. Arch Dis Child Fetal Neonatal Ed. 1995;72(3):F162-F167.

205. Lou H. The "lost autoregulation hypothesis" and brain lesions in the newborn: an update. Brain Dev. 1988;10:143-146.

206. Leffler CW, Busija DW, Beasley DG, et al. Postischemic cerebral microvascular responses to norepinephrine and hypotension in newborn pigs. Stroke. 1989;20(4):541-546.

207. Leffler CW, Busija DW, Mirro R, et al. Effects of ischemia on brain blood flow and oxygen consumption of newborn pigs. Am J Physiol. 1989;257(6 Pt 2):H1917-H1926.

208. Laptook A, Corbett R, Ruley J, et al. Blood flow and metabolism during and after repeated partial brain ischemia in neonatal piglets. Stroke. 1992;23:380-387.

209. Conger J, Weil J. Abnormal vascular function following ischemia-reperfusion injury. J Investig Med. 1995;43(5):431-432.

210. Blankenberg FG, Loh NN, Norbash AM, et al. Impaired cerebrovascular autoregulation after hypoxic-ischemic injury in extremely low-birth-weight neonates: detection with power and pulsed wave Doppler US. Radiology. 1997;205(2):563-568.

211. Matsuda T, Okuyama K, Cho K, et al. Induction of antenatal periventricular leukomalacia by hemorrhagic hypotension in the chronically instrumented fetal sheep. Am J Obstet Gynecol. 1999;181(3):725-730.

212. Reddy K, Mallard C, Guan J, et al. Maturational change in the cortical response to hypoperfusion injury in the fetal sheep. Pediatr Res. 1998;43(5):674-682.

213. Mallard C, Welin AK, Peebles D, et al. White matter injury following systemic endotoxemia or asphyxia in the fetal sheep. Neurochem Res. 2003;28(2):215-223.

214. Derrick M, Drobyshevsky A, Ji X, et al. A model of cerebral palsy from fetal hypoxia-ischemia. Stroke. 2007;38(2 Suppl):731-735.

215. Verney C, Rees S, Biran V, et al. Neuronal damage in the preterm baboon: impact of the mode of ventilatory support. J Neuropathol Exp Neurol. 2010;69(5):473-482.

216. Low JA, Froese AB, Galbraith RS, et al. The association between preterm newborn hypotension and hypoxemia and outcome during the first year. Acta Paediatr. 1993;82(5):433-437.

217. Bejar RF, Vaucher YE, Benirschke K, et al. Postnatal white matter necrosis in preterm infants. J Perinatol. 1992;12(1):3-8.

218. Fujimura M, Salisbury DM, Robinson RO, et al. Clinical events relating to intraventricular haemorrhage in the newborn. Arch Dis Child. 1979;54(6):409-414.

219. McDonald MM, Koops BL, Johnson ML, et al. Timing and antecedents of intracranial hemorrhage in the newborn. Pediatrics. 1984;74(1):32-36.

220. Perlman J, Thach B. Respiratory origin of fluctuations in arterial blood pressure in premature infants with respiratory distress syndrome. Pediatrics. 1988;81(3):399-403.

221. Kluckow M, Evans N. Relationship between blood pressure and cardiac output in preterm infants requiring mechanical ventilation. J Pediatr. 1996;129(4):506-512.

222. Kluckow M, Evans N. Low systemic blood flow in the preterm infant. Semin Neonatol. 2001;6(1):75-84.

223. Miletin J, Dempsey EM. Low superior vena cava flow on day 1 and adverse outcome in the very low birthweight infant. Arch Dis Child Fetal Neonatal Ed. 2008;93(5):F368-F371.

224. Evans N, Kluckow M, Simmons M, et al. Which to measure, systemic or organ blood flow? Middle cerebral artery and superior vena cava flow in very preterm infants. Arch Dis Child Fetal Neonatal Ed. 2002;87(3):F181-F184.

225. Moran M, Miletin J, Pichova K, et al. Cerebral tissue oxygenation index and superior vena cava blood flow in the very low birth weight infant. Acta Paediatr. 2009;98(1):43-46.

226. Kissack CM, Garr R, Wardle SP, et al. Cerebral fractional oxygen extraction in very low birth weight infants is high when there is low left ventricular output and hypocarbia but is unaffected by hypotension. Pediatr Res. 2004;55(3):400-405.

227. Osborn DA, Evans N, Kluckow M. Hemodynamic and antecedent risk factors of early and late periventricular/intraventricular hemorrhage in premature infants. Pediatrics. 2003;112(1 Pt 1):33-39.

228. Wesseling KH. Finapress, continuous noninvasive finger artery pressure based on the method of Penaz. In: Meyer-Sabellek W, Anlauf M, Gotzen R, eds. Blood pressure measurement. Darmstadt, Germany: Steinkopff Verlag; 1990:161-172.

229. Perlman JM, Volpe JJ. Cerebral blood flow velocity in relation to intraventricular hemorrhage in the premature newborn infant. J Pediatr. 1982;100(6):956-959.

230. Rennie JM, South M, Morley CJ. Cerebral blood flow velocity variability in infants receiving assisted ventilation. Arch Dis Child. 1987;62(12):1247-1251.

231. van Bel F, de Winter PJ, Wijnands HBG, et al. Cerebral and aortic blood flow velocity patterns in preterm infants receiving prophylactic surfactant treatment. Acta Paediat. 1992;81(6):504-510.

232. Hansen NB, Stonestreet BS, Rosenkrantz TS, et al. Validity of Doppler measurements of anterior cerebral artery blood flow velocity: correlation with brain blood flow in piglets. Pediatrics. 1983;72(4):526-531.

233. Thoresen M, Haaland K, Steen PA. Cerebral Doppler and misrepresentation of flow changes. Arch Dis Child. 1994;71(2):F103-F106.

234. Edwards A, Richardson C, Cope M, et al. Cotside measurement of cerebral blood flow in ill newborn infants by near infrared spectroscopy. Lancet. 1988;ii:770-771.

16

235. Tyszczuk L, Meek J, Elwell C, et al. Cerebral blood flow is independent of mean arterial blood pressure in preterm infants undergoing intensive care. Pediatrics. 1998;102:337-341.
236. Meek JH, Tyszczuk L, Elwell CE, et al. Cerebral blood flow increases over the first three days of life in extremely preterm neonates. Arch Dis Child Fetal Neonatal Ed. 1998;78(1):F33-F37.
237. Lassen NA. Control of cerebral circulation in health and disease. Circ Res. 1974;34(6):749-760.
238. Greisen G, Pryds O. Intravenous 133Xe clearance in preterm neonates with respiratory distress. Internal validation of CBF infinity as a measure of global cerebral blood flow. Scand J Clin Lab Invest. 1988;48(7):673-678.
239. Shimizu N, Gilder F, Bissonnette B, et al. Brain tissue oxygenation index measured by near infrared spatially resolved spectroscopy agreed with jugular bulb oxygen saturation in normal pediatric brain: a pilot study. Childs Nerv Syst. 2005;21(3):181-184.
240. Borch K, Lou HC, Greisen G. Cerebral white matter blood flow and arterial blood pressure in preterm infants. Acta Paediatr. 2010;99(10):1489-1492.
241. Park C, Spitzer A, Desai H, et al. Brain SPECT in neonates following extracorporeal membrane oxygenation: Evaluation of technique and preliminary results. J Nucl Med. 1992;33:1943-1948.
242. Powers W. Cerebral blood flow and metabolism in newborn infants: what can they teach us about stroke? Stroke. 1993;24(12):133-134.
243. Barkovich AJ, Westmark K, Partridge C, et al. Perinatal asphyxia: MR findings in the first 10 days. AJNR Am J Neuroradiol. 1995;16(3):427-438.
244. Pasternak JF. Hypoxic-ischemic brain damage in the term infant. Lessons from the laboratory. Pediatr Clin North Am. 1993;40(5):1061-1072.
245. Pasternak JF, Gorey MT. The syndrome of acute near-total intrauterine asphyxia in the term infant. Pediatr Neurol. 1998;18:391-398.
246. Goldstein RF, Thompson Jr RJ, Oehler JM, et al. Influence of acidosis, hypoxemia, and hypotension on neurodevelopmental outcome in very low birth weight infants. Pediatrics. 1995;95(2):238-243.
247. Urlesberger B, Trip K, Ruchti JJ, et al. Quantification of cyclical fluctuations in cerebral blood volume in healthy infants. Neuropediatrics. 1998;29(4):208-211.
248. Mullaart RA, Hopman JCW, Dehaan AFJ, et al. Cerebral blood flow fluctuation in low-risk preterm newborns. Early Hum Dev. 1992;30(1):41-48.
249. Dimitriou G, Greenough A, Kavvadia V, et al. Blood pressure rhythms during the perinatal period in very immature, extremely low birthweight neonates. Early Hum Dev. 1999;56(1):49-56.
250. von Siebenthal K, Beran J, Wolf M, et al. Cyclical fluctuations in blood pressure, heart rate and cerebral blood volume in preterm infants. Brain Dev. 1999;21(8):529-534.
251. Andriessen P, Schoffelen RL, Berendsen RC, et al. Noninvasive assessment of blood pressure variability in preterm infants. Pediatr Res. 2004;55(2):220-223.
252. Cunningham S, Deere S, McIntosh N. Cyclical variation of blood pressure and heart rate in neonates. Arch Dis Child. 1993;69(1 Spec No):64-67.
253. Bhutta AT, Cleves MA, Casey PH, et al. Cognitive and behavioral outcomes of school-aged children who were born preterm: a meta-analysis. JAMA. 2002;288(6):728-737.
254. Msall ME, Tremont MR. Measuring functional outcomes after prematurity: developmental impact of very low birth weight and extremely low birth weight status on childhood disability. Ment Retard Dev Disabil Res Rev. 2002;8(4):258-272.
255. Allin M, Matsumoto H, Santhouse AM, et al. Cognitive and motor function and the size of the cerebellum in adolescents born very pre-term. Brain. 2001;124(Pt 1):60-66.
256. Messerschmidt A, Brugger PC, Boltshauser E, et al. Disruption of cerebellar development: potential complication of extreme prematurity. AJNR Am J Neuroradiol. 2005;26(7):1659-1667.
257. Kadhim H, Tabarki B, Verellen G, et al. Inflammatory cytokines in the pathogenesis of periventricular leukomalacia. Neurology. 2001;56(10):1278-1284.
258. Volpe JJ. Neurobiology of periventricular leukomalacia in the premature infant. Pediatr Res. 2001;50(5):553-562.
259. Yoon BH, Romero R, Yang SH, et al. Interleukin-6 concentrations in umbilical cord plasma are elevated in neonates with white matter lesions associated with periventricular leukomalacia. Am J Obstet Gynecol. 1996;174(5):1433-1440.
260. Martin ED, Fernandez M, Perea G, et al. Adenosine released by astrocytes contributes to hypoxia-induced modulation of synaptic transmission. Glia. 2007;55(1):36-45.
261. Hope PL, Gould SJ, Howard S, et al. Precision of ultrasound diagnosis of pathologically verified lesions in the brains of very preterm newborn infants. Dev Med Child Neurol. 1988;30:457-471.
262. Paneth N, Rudelli R, Monte W, et al. White matter necrosis in very low birth weight infants: neuropathologic and ultrasonographic findings in infants surviving six days or longer. J Pediatr. 1990;116:975-984.
263. Greisen G, Pryds O, Rosen I, et al. Poor reversibility of EEG abnormality in hypotensive, preterm neonates. Acta Paediatr Scand. 1988;77(6):785-790.
264. Kurtis PS, Rosenkrantz TS, Zalneraitis EL. Cerebral blood flow and EEG changes in preterm infants with patent ductus arteriosus. Pediatr Neurol. 1995;12(2):114-119.
265. Victor S, Appleton RE, Beirne M, et al. The relationship between cardiac output, cerebral electrical activity, cerebral fractional oxygen extraction and peripheral blood flow in premature newborn infants. Pediatr Res. 2006;60(4):456-460.
266. Greisen G, Pryds O. Low CBF, discontinuous EEG activity, and periventricular brain injury in ill, preterm neonates. Brain Dev. 1989;11(3):164-168.

267. Hellstrom-Westas L, de Vries L, Rosen I. An atlas of amplitude-integrated EEG's in the newborn. New York: Parthenon Publishing; 2003.

268. Lou HC, Lassen NA, Friis-Hansen B. Is arterial hypertension crucial for the development of cerebral haemorrhage in premature infants? Lancet. 1979;1(8128):1215-1217.

269. Lou HC. Autoregulation of cerebral blood flow and brain lesions in newborn infants. Lancet. 1998;352(9138):1406.

270. Soul JS, du Plessis AJ, Walter GL, et al. Near-infrared spectroscopy monitoring detects changes in cerebral blood flow in an animal model of acute hydrocephalus (abstr). Ann Neurol. 1998;44(3):535.

271. Bassan H, Gauvreau K, Newburger JW, et al. Identification of pressure passive cerebral perfusion and its mediators after infant cardiac surgery. Pediatr Res. 2005;57(1):35-41.

272. O'Leary H, Gregas MC, Limperopoulos C, et al. Elevated cerebral pressure passivity is associated with prematurity-related intracranial hemorrhage. Pediatrics. 2009;124(1):302-309.

273. Kety SS, Schmidt CF. The effects of altered arterial tensions of carbon dioxide and oxygen on cerebral blood flow and cerebral oxygen consumption of normal young men. J Clin Invest. 1948; 27(4):484-492.

274. Wyatt JS, Edwards AD, Cope M, et al. Response of cerebral blood volume to changes in arterial carbon dioxide tension in preterm and term infants. Pediatr Res. 1991;29:553-557.

275. Yamashita N, Kamiya K, Nagai H. CO_2 reactivity and autoregulation in fetal brain. Child's Nerv Syst. 1991;7:327-331.

276. Dietz V, Wolf M, Keel M, et al. CO_2 reactivity of the cerebral hemoglobin concentration in healthy term newborns measured by near infrared spectrophotometry. Biol Neonate. 1999;75(2):85-90.

277. Leahy FA, Cates D, MacCallum M, et al. Effect of CO_2 and 100% O_2 on cerebral blood flow in preterm infants. J Appl Physiol. 1980;48(3):468-472.

16

SECTION D

Embryonic and Fetal Development

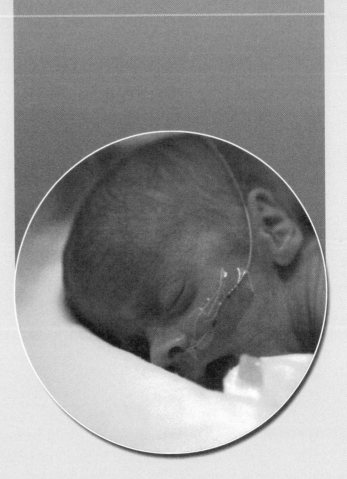

CHAPTER 17

The Genetics of Fetal and Neonatal Cardiovascular Disease

Wendy Chung, MD, PhD, Marko T. Boskovski, MD, Martina Brueckner, MD, Kwame Anyane-Yeboa, MD, and Punita Gupta, MD

GENETIC BASIS OF CONGENITAL HEART DISEASE
Wendy Chung, MD, PhD

- **Developments in Molecular Diagnostics for Congenital Heart Disease**
- **What Is Involved with Genetic Testing?**
- **What Is the Approach Used in Genetic Evaluation?**
- **How to Interpret Test Results**
- **References**

Congenital heart defects (CHD) occur in approximately 1% of live births and 10% of spontaneously aborted fetuses, making CHD the most common human congenital malformation. Heart defects occur together with other malformations in about 30% of cases.[1-4] The success of surgical repair of most lesions has resulted in approximately 1 million adult patients with CHD, many of whom are now of reproductive age.[5] In addition, with improved prenatal imaging techniques and experience, many cases of congenital heart disease are now diagnosed in the second trimester prenatally, offering important options to couples seeking guidance about long-term prognosis as they try to make informed decisions about prenatal and postnatal care.

Nonsyndromic CHD is usually classified as having complex or multifactorial inheritance, implying the interaction of multiple genetic and/or environmental factors as well as being genetically heterogeneous. Studies of risks for siblings and other relatives have demonstrated an increased risk compared to the background risk in the general population. Risk of CHD recurrence in a sibling ranges from 1% to 13%, depending upon the lesion and whether one considers only the same lesion or all CHD.[6] Twin studies have also shown a higher concordance in monozygotic twins (25%) than in dizygotic twins (5%).[7] These non-Mendelian risks have been considered to indicate multifactorial inheritance, but they are also consistent with variable expression, de novo genetic defects, and tissue mosaicism.

CHD occurs in all the complete trisomy syndromes seen in live births, in Turner syndrome (monosomy X), and in patients with partial aneuploidies (deletions or duplications) for almost every chromosome arm.[8] In these chromosomal syndromes there may be a predominant cardiac lesion (e.g., coarctation of the aorta in Turner syndrome, atrioventricular septal defects in Down syndrome, ventricular septal defect in trisomy 13, hypoplastic left heart in Jacobsen syndrome with 11q deletion) but there is great variability in the type of CHD that may occur. Clearly, there must be a large number of dosage-sensitive genes that affect heart development, since cytogenetically visible segmental aneuploidy (i.e., ~5 Mb of DNA) so often results in CHD. The population-based study of Ferencz and colleagues estimated that 13% of CHD cases were associated with karyotypic abnormalities.[9]

Table 17a-1   COMMON MICRODELETIONS ASSOCIATED WITH
CONGENITAL HEART DISEASE

Condition	Chromosome Region	Congenital Heart Disease
	1p36	ASVD, valvular anomalies, TOF, CoA, Ebstein anomaly
Williams-Beuren syndrome	7q11.23	Supravalvular AS, PPS
Jacobsen syndrome	11a23	VSD, AVSD, CoA, HLHS
DiGeorge syndrome	22q11.2	IAA type B, aortic arch anomalies, truncus arteriosus, TOF

AS, aortic stenosis; ASVD, atrial septal ventricular defects; AVSD, atrioventricular septal defect; CoA, coarctation of the aorta; HLHS, hypoplastic left heart syndrome; IAA, interrupted aortic arch; PPS, peripheral pulmonic stenosis; TOF, tetralogy of Fallot; VSD, ventricular septal defect.

The association between particular malformation syndromes and small visible deletions and/or translocations involving specific chromosomal bands led in the 1980s to the delineation of a group of "microdeletion" syndromes. The common deletions are 1-4 Mb in size, and are not visible with chromosome banding but are routinely detected by fluorescence in situ hybridization (FISH). A number of these microdeletion syndromes include specific types of CHD (e.g., conotruncal defects in deletion 22q11.2 (DiGeorge syndrome), supravalvular aortic stenosis and pulmonic stenosis in Williams syndrome (deletion 7q11.23), and right-sided heart defects in Alagille syndrome (deletion 20p11.2).[10] Molecular analysis of the deleted regions and studies of mouse models have identified specific genes associated with the heart defects in these syndromes: T-Box 1 (*TBX1*) in DiGeorge syndrome, *Elastin* (*ELN*) in Williams syndrome and *Jagged 1* (*JAG1*) in Alagille syndrome. In all these examples, the involvement of the gene has been proven by identifying heterozygous point mutations in patients with the characteristic type of CHD but no deletion. Identification of karyotypic aberrations has been instrumental in the discovery of genes such as *PROSIT240* as a cause of d-transposition of the great arteries (d-TGA) and *CHD7* as a major cause of CHARGE and suggest that this general strategy will be effective in identifying novel genes responsible for CHD.[11,12]

Recent molecular advances in DNA microarray copy number analysis have demonstrated that small copy number changes below the level of chromosome banding resolution may be causal in CHD.[12] As shown in Table 17a-1, the results suggest that (1) rates of de novo copy number changes (CNCs) are generally higher than expected in controls, and (2) cases with additional anomalies have higher rates of CNCs than those with isolated CHD.

In recent years, a number of genes have been implicated in the origins of CHD, by (1) analysis of microdeletions (Table 17a-1), (2) discovery of the genes mutated in syndromes segregating as Mendelian traits (Table 17a-2), and (3) analysis of development in model organisms, chiefly the mouse and zebrafish.[10,13-16] Table 17a-2 lists genes in which mutations have been associated with CHD in humans.

Heart development begins with the identification of a cardiac progenitor field, establishment of myocardial fate, and acquisition of chamber identity. Transcription factors, such as *NKX2.5*, *GATA4*, *GATA6*, and *TBX5*, guide the precursor cell population through the process of cardiac induction and the molecular cascade of fate commitment.[17-19] Furthermore, inductive (fibroblast growth factors [FGFs], bone morphogen proteins [BMPs], nodal family members) or repressive (retinoic acid [RA], canonical WNTs, NOTCH) signaling pathways modulate the function of these transcription factors and thereby alter the progression from early progenitor cell to the matured ventricular or atrial cardiomyocyte.[20] Disruption in this fine coordination of transcriptional networks and combinatorial molecular signaling leads to morphogenesis defects that result in CHD.

Table 17a-2 HUMAN GENE MUTATIONS ASSOCIATED WITH CONGENITAL HEART DISEASE

Gene	Associated Syndrome	Heart Defects
ACTC1		ASD, VSD
ACVR2B		Heterotaxy
ALK2		ASD, TGA, DORV, AVSD
ANKRD1		TAPVR
CFC1		Heterotaxy, TGA, TOF, TA, AVSD
CHD7	CHARGE	ASD, VSD, valve defects
CHDR7	Smith-Lemli-Opitz	ASD, VSD, AVSD
CITED2		VSD, ASD
CREBBP	Rubenstein-Taybi	ASD, VSD, HLHS
CRELD1		AVSD
ELN	Williams	PS, AS
EP300	Rubenstein-Taybi	
EVC1,2	Ellis-van Creveld	ASD
FOXH1		TOF
GATA4		AVSD, TOF, HRHS, PAPVR, PS
GATA6		TA, PS
GJA1		HLHS
HOXA1	Athabaskan brain stem dysgenesis	Conotruncal defects
JAG1	Alagille	PS, PA, TOF
KRAS	Noonan	AS, AVC
LEFTYA		Heterotaxy
MYH6		ASD
MYH7		ASD, Ebstein
NKX2.5	Holt-Oram	ASD, TOF, HLHS, CoA, IAA, heterotaxy, TGA, DORV, VSD, Ebstein, ASD
NKX2.6		TA
NODAL		Heterotaxy
NOTCH1		Biscuspid aortic valve, AS
NOTCH22	Alagille	
PTPN11	Noonan, LEOPARD	AS, AVC
RAF1	Noonan	AS, AVC
SEMA3E	CHARGE	ASD, VSD, valve defects
SOS1	Noonan	AS, AVC
TBX1	DiGeorge	Conotruncal spectrum
TBX20		ASD, VSD, MS, HLHS
TBX5	Holt-Oram	ASD, VSD, HLHS
TDGF1		TOF
TFAP2B		PDA
THRAP2		TGA
TLL1		ASD
ZFPM2		TOF
ZIC3		Heterotaxy, TGA, ASD, AVSD

AS, aortic stenosis; ASD, atrial septal defect; AVC, atrioventricular canal; ASVD, atrial septal ventricular defects; AVSD, atrioventricular septal defect; CoA, coarctation of the aorta; DORV, double outlet right ventricle; HLHS, hypoplastic left heart syndrome; HRHS, hypoplastic right heart syndrome; IAA, interrupted aortic arch; PAPVR, partial anomalous pulmonary venous return; PDA, patent ductus arteriosus; PPS, peripheral pulmonic stenosis; PS, pulmonic stenosis; TA, tricuspid atresia; TAPVR, total anomalous pulmonary venous return; TGA, transposition of the great arteries; TOF, tetralogy of Fallot; VSD, ventricular septal defect.

Table 17a-3 PUBLISHED STUDIES OF MICROARRAY ANALYSIS IN
CONGENITAL HEART DISEASE

Reference	No. Cases	Criteria	% De Novo
Thienpont[12]	60	CHD + other malformation or mental retardation	11.7%
Erdogan[22]	105	Isolated CHD	2.8%
Richards[25]	40	CHD, half with other malformations	7.5%
Lu[24]	108	CHD ± other malformations	20.4%
Greenway[23]	114	Isolated TOF	10%

Developments in Molecular Diagnostics for Congenital Heart Disease

The causes of congenital heart disease are diverse and incompletely understood, yet it is increasingly important to diagnose the cause to accurately predict prognosis, allowing families and providers to plan for the possibility of extracardiac manifestations and provide accurate information on recurrence risk. Evolving technologies that permit clinicians to request genetic testing in a nonselective manner have and will transform the conventional manner of clinical investigation of basis of congenital heart disease by permitting the parallel evaluation of multiple genetic etiologies.

Clinical genetic tests are especially complicated for disorders in which there may be several different genetic or nongenetic etiologies with the same clinical presentation. Genetic testing for these disorders is often not straightforward because the total number of genes that can be tested is often large. In these cases, detailed knowledge of the clinical features distinguishing each form is essential to making an informed decision about further investigation. For CHD, several rare Mendelian forms have been elucidated. However, for any particular CHD lesion, mutations in any one of several genes can lead to phenocopies that are clinically indistinguishable. In addition, for CHD, the mutations may be "private," meaning that any particular family is likely to have unique mutation(s), and the private mutation(s) could occur at different regions in the gene from family to family.

To date, clinical genetic tests for CHD have been largely limited to karyotyping, FISH, and more recently chromosome microarrays (Table 17a-3). Whole-genome screening using chromosome microarray surveys the entire genome for copy number variations and is equivalent to performing a genome-wide FISH study. Bacterial artificial chromosome (BAC) arrays were once the most common clinical assay in this category, but the focus has shifted to oligonucleotide microarrays, now available through a large number of clinical laboratories. The resolution of the genome-wide microarrays can be quite high and ranges from 40,000 to over 1,000,000 oligonucleotide probes to identify abnormalities of copy number of single genes or chromosomal regions (deletions, duplications) to generate a high-resolution molecular karyotype. For many clinicians, a chromosome microarray is now a front-line tool, even before a karyotype, because of the improved resolution of a chromosome microarray (routinely at least <1Mb) relative to a karyotype (>5 Mb).[21] However, only a karyotype is able to provide structural information about the chromosome (i.e., location of duplicated material) and identify balanced rearrangements such as balanced translocations. Laboratories are currently utilizing two types of oligonucleotide chromosome microarrays: (1) one that includes single nucleotide polymorphisms (SNPs) or (2) oligonucleotides designed only to quantify copy number. The advantage of the single nucleotide polymorphisms oligonucleotide microarray analysis (SOMA) is the ability to detect uniparental disomy because parentally distinguishable genotypes are generated in addition to microdeletions (either of which can be mechanisms causing Angelman syndrome). Oligonucleotide microarray analysis is now routinely covered by insurance companies and has approximately a 10-20% yield in children with CHD.[12,22-25] The yield increases as the number of noncardiac clinical features increases, including dysmorphic features, intrauterine growth restriction/failure to thrive, noncardiac birth defects, and a family history significant for other similarly affected children or a history of recurrent miscarriages in the parents (usually associated with one parent who is a balance translocation carrier).

With the recent advances of the chromosome microarray analysis, we are only now beginning to define many novel genetic syndromes associated with recurrent deletions and duplications. With increasing experience, these new syndromes will be better defined and additional details will be available regarding associated clinical features, range of severity of symptoms, and penetrance. In addition, it should be noted that we are also now only beginning to define the normal genomic architecture and benign polymorphic deletions and duplications that are present in the genome. Therefore, it is not uncommon to receive a test report from a chromosome microarray analysis that identifies a deletion or duplication variant of unknown clinical significance. In such cases, it has not been clearly established whether this copy number variant (CNV) is a normal benign polymorphism or a pathogenic disease-associated mutation. To distinguish between these two possibilities, it is recommended that the parents be tested for the CNV. If both parents are normal, the CNV is interpreted to be disease-associated because the CNV arises de novo. If one of the parents is affected, the CNV may be pathogenic if it is inherited from the affected parent. With time and additional population characterization, the number of test reports with variants of unknown clinical significance should decrease significantly.

The other major advance in oligonucleotide microarray analysis is in the detection of small deletions or duplications involving only portions of single genes associated with a given phenotype (i.e., an exon array). This type of test will increasingly replace the more cumbersome method of multiple ligation probe amplification (MLPA). These types of mutations are generally of the order of 500-100,000 base pairs and are routinely "invisible" to molecular methods that rely on polymerase chain reaction (PCR) amplification followed by sequence analysis. Increasingly, exon arrays are being designed to complement sequence-based tests for clinical conditions involving only a menu of single genes. The yields for these types of exon arrays are not always known because this technology has only recently become available.

Sequence-based testing of specific genes has become a burgeoning field in the last several years. In contrast to the methods described earlier, this approach targets much smaller changes in the DNA sequence, down to individual nucleotides. There are two distinct approaches to this testing, depending upon whether or not it is a specific known mutation (or several specific known mutations) for which the patient is at risk. In that case, analysis can be targeted to look for only those known mutation(s). Targeted mutation testing is widespread, but is limited in application to those conditions for which specific mutations account for the majority of patients with a clinical diagnosis. When the majority of patients are likely to have a "private" mutation as is the case for CHD, testing must examine the entire gene, nucleotide by nucleotide, and this represents a greater challenge.

The conventional technique for sequencing a gene involves PCR amplification of each exon and its splice junctions, followed by dideoxy sequencing. The sequence obtained is compared with the published reference sequence, and any nucleotide changes are then interpreted. In the context of laboratory diagnostics, the cost of a sequencing test is generally linearly related to the size of the gene. Performing comprehensive genetic testing for large genes or a large number of genes is less feasible, in that the cost of a test is much higher, and can become prohibitively high. This has created the need for new approaches in genetic testing that can increase capacity and reduce the cost of sequence based testing. A new generation of sequencing instruments has been introduced into the clinical genetic diagnostic arena. The so-called next-generation sequencing platforms are based on highly parallel data generation, and such instruments have the ability to produce up to 100 Gb per sequencing run. Next-generation instruments generate massive amounts of sequence data and greatly reduce the cost of sequencing per base when compared with capillary dideoxy sequencing. This capacity provides great potential to resequence and analyze large amounts of DNA for mutations and will facilitate the development of genetic test panels for common indications. There are no currently available test panels for CHD, but as the databases providing reference sequences on normal individuals increase, panels will likely become available for testing for many genes for CHD in parallel. There are even methods available to sequence the exome or the 1.6% of the genome encoding protein products as well as complete sequencing of the entire human genome. Although the cost of generating these sequence data are falling quite rapidly, the informatics required to analyze the vast amount of data and distinguish normal from disease-causing human genetic variation are not yet sufficiently advanced to use these methods for clinical diagnostics yet. However, with the next decade, this will likely be a clinical testing option.

What Is Involved with Genetic Testing?

Genetic testing in a symptomatic patient is described as "diagnostic." The number of genetic conditions associated with CHD is large. The impetus to identify a specific cause for a fetus/child's CHD disorder is more than academic. In general, diagnosis of a genetic cause clarifies prognosis and eliminates the need for further diagnostic evaluation. In many situations, treatment and monitoring will be altered by the molecular diagnosis. Families generally pursue genetic evaluation to clarify prognosis and calculate the risk of having additional similarly affected children in the family and determine methods to avoid recurrence within the family if the risk is high. The issue of risk of recurrence for the parents, siblings, and other family members as well as the patient him/herself is often of concern to the family. Usually, the immediate concern is the risk of recurrence to the parents. Many cases of CHD are the result of de novo mutations. If this is proven after testing the parents' blood, then the risk of recurrence to the parents is less than 1%, and any recurrence is due to undetectable gonadal mosaicism. In such families, prenatal testing with chorionic villus sampling or amniocentesis is appropriate to provide reassurance to the parents that they will not have another affected child while allowing them to conceive naturally and have other biological children. There is a significant risk for recurrence if (1) a parent is a balanced translocation carrier of a balanced chromosomal disorder, (2) a mother is a carrier for an X-linked condition, (3) both parents are carriers for an autosomal recessive condition, or (4) a parent who carries an autosomal dominant disorder. Parents have multiple options to plan future children including adoption, use of donor egg or donor sperm to remove the genetic contribution of the parent transmitting the mutation, prenatal testing (either chorionic villus sampling at 10-12 weeks of gestation or amniocentesis after 16 weeks of gestation), or preimplantation genetic diagnosis (PGD). Donor sperm is practically easier than donor egg. Donors of sperm or eggs should not be genetically related to the parents unless they are found not to carry the familial mutation. PGD can be performed for most families but requires development of an assay specific to the family in many cases. PGD requires in vitro fertilization and has only a 25% success rate/cycle in couples without fertility issues and may not be covered in part or wholly by insurance. PGD should be viewed as significantly risk reducing but is associated with rare errors in ~2% of cases. Thus, PGD usually avoids the necessity to terminate an affected pregnancy, but the process should be carefully considered by couples prior to initiation. PGD is available in the United States, but is not available in all countries. Attitudes toward these family planning options vary by culture in part based upon religious beliefs and acceptability of pregnancy termination. For other family members, their risk of recurrence should first be defined by genetic testing for the familial mutations. For those found to carry the familial mutation, similar reproductive options are available. Affected patients able and interested in having children should be carefully counseled about their options as well as risks to the mother if she has a history of CHD. Notably, although a genetic condition may have been de novo in the affected patient, there may be a significant risk of recurrence, as high as 50%, for their children.

What Is the Approach Used in Genetic Evaluation?

A genetic evaluation consists of review of the patient's history and medical records and documentation of at least a three-generation pedigree to identify patterns of inheritance. The evaluation includes a physical examination for growth, birth defects, and dysmorphic features, development of a differential diagnosis, counseling of the patient and the family of the options for genetic testing and the implications of these genetic test results. In certain circumstances, a thorough evaluation may include an echocardiogram in parents who are clinically asymptomatic to evaluate the presence of clinically silent structural heart disease to allow for accurate interpretation of genetic test results.

Genetic counseling should be nondirective and respect the beliefs and values of the patient and family. Patients and families should receive genetic counseling prior to genetic testing to understand what condition(s) are being tested, the medical implications for the patient and family, and any financial obligations to cover a portion or all of the cost of testing, which can amount to several thousand dollars. Children with appropriate mental capacity should provide assent for genetic testing.

An updated list of genetic tests available and laboratories performing testing is available at genetests.org and is an excellent resource for clinicians. Only Clinical Laboratory Improvement Amendment (CLIA) certified clinical laboratories should be used for clinical diagnosis of patients. In some cases it may be appropriate to perform tiered testing, that is, testing for the most likely locations of mutations and then proceeding to more extensive testing only when necessary. Such a strategy can result in significant savings in the cost of testing but result in longer turnaround times for testing in some cases.

How to Interpret Test Results

Results of genetic tests can be positive (i.e., pathogenic and disease associated), negative (i.e., failure to find a pathogenic mutation), or variant of unknown significance (i.e., ambiguous). All positive tests should be confirmed by the laboratory by methods such as sequencing the complementary strand of DNA for sequence-based tests or using an independent method of confirmation such as FISH or qPCR for chromosome microarrays. Negative test results only indicate that the method used did not identify a mutation but does not guarantee that (1) there is not a mutation that was not detectable by the method used by the laboratory or (2) there may not be a genetic cause due to a mutation in another gene that was not tested. For example, standard sequence-based genetic tests fail to identify large deletions in genes and when clinically suspected other methods such as multiple ligation primer amplification (MLPA), quantitative PCR, and/or exon oligonucleotide hybridization should be considered. Ambiguous test results are more likely to occur when clinical tests are first offered because there is less experience with the normal genetic variation in the gene or genome, especially across ethnic groups. In cases of variants of unknown significance, when the variants are shown to be de novo, they are assumed by the laboratory to be pathogenic. Thus testing of the parents is often the next step to clarify interpretation. For recessive conditions, it is helpful to know whether variants are in cis (on the same copy of the gene) or trans (each variant is on a different copy of the genes) which can also readily be determined by testing of the parents. In some cases it is necessary to track the variant through the family and demonstrate its consistent association with disease in affected family members. In such cases testing of the parents and more extended family members may be necessary. With experience in testing multiple affected patients as well as normal controls,

17

laboratories should be able to improve their interpretation of test results and decrease the number of variants of unknown significance.

References

1. Hoffman JI. Incidence of congenital heart disease. II. Prenatal incidence. Pediatr Cardiol. 1995;16:155-165.
2. Hoffman JI, Kaplan S. The incidence of congenital heart disease. J Am Coll Cardiol. 2002;39: 1890-1900.
3. Genetic and environmental risk factors of major cardiovascular malformations. *The Baltimore-Washington Infant Study 1981-1989.* Mt. Kisco, NY: Futura Publishing; 1997.
4. Ferencz C, Rubin JD, Loffredo C, et al. Epidemiology of congenital heart disease. The Baltimore-Washington Study 1981-1989. Mt. Kisco, NY: Futura Publishing; 1993.
5. Brickner ME, Hillis LD, Lange RA. Congenital heart disease in adults. First of two parts. N Engl J Med. 2000;342:256-263.
6. Marino B, Digilio MC. Congenital heart disease and genetic syndromes: specific correlation between cardiac phenotype and genotype. Cardiovasc Pathol. 2000;9:303-315.
7. Nora JJ, Gilliland JC, Sommerville RJ, et al. Congenital heart disease in twins. N Engl J Med. 1967;277:568-571.
8. van Karnebeek CD, Hennekam RC. Associations between chromosomal anomalies and congenital heart defects: a database search. Am J Med Genet. 1999;84:158-166.
9. Ferencz C, Neill CA, Boughman JA, et al. Congenital cardiovascular malformations associated with chromosome abnormalities: an epidemiologic study. J Pediatr. 1989;114:79-86.
10. Grossfeld PD. The genetics of congenital heart disease. J Nucl Cardiol. 2003;10:71-76.
11. Muncke N, Jung C, Rudiger H, et al. Missense mutations and gene interruption in PROSIT240, a novel TRAP240-like gene, in patients with congenital heart defect (transposition of the great arteries). Circulation. 2003;108:2843-2850.
12. Thienpont B, Mertens L, de Ravel T, et al. Submicroscopic chromosomal imbalances detected by array-CGH are a frequent cause of congenital heart defects in selected patients. Eur Heart J. 2007; 28:2778-2784.
13. Gelb BD. Genetic basis of syndromes associated with congenital heart disease. Curr Opin Cardiol. 2001;16:188-194.
14. Gelb BD. Genetic basis of congenital heart disease. Curr Opin Cardiol. 2004;19:110-115.
15. Gruber PJ, Epstein JA. Development gone awry: congenital heart disease. Circ Res. 2004;94: 273-283.
16. Srivastava D, Olson EN. A genetic blueprint for cardiac development. Nature. 2000;407: 221-226.
17. Bruneau BG. The developmental genetics of congenital heart disease. Nature. 2008;451:943-948.
18. Dunwoodie SL. Combinatorial signaling in the heart orchestrates cardiac induction, lineage specification and chamber formation. Semin Cell Dev Biol. 2007;18:54-66.
19. Solloway MJ, Harvey RP. Molecular pathways in myocardial development: a stem cell perspective. Cardiovasc Res. 2003;58:264-277.
20. Srivastava D. Making or breaking the heart: from lineage determination to morphogenesis. Cell. 2006;126:1037-1048.
21. Miller DT, Adam MP, Aradhya S, et al. Consensus statement: chromosomal microarray is a first-tier clinical diagnostic test for individuals with developmental disabilities or congenital anomalies. Am J Hum Genet. 2010;86:749-764.
22. Erdogan F, Larsen LA, Zhang L, et al. High frequency of submicroscopic genomic aberrations detected by tiling path array comparative genome hybridisation in patients with isolated congenital heart disease. J Med Genet. 2008;45:704-709.
23. Greenway SC, Pereira AC, Lin JC, et al. De novo copy number variants identify new genes and loci in isolated sporadic tetralogy of Fallot. Nat Genet. 2009;41:931-935.
24. Lu XY, Phung MT, Shaw CA, et al. Genomic imbalances in neonates with birth defects: high detection rates by using chromosomal microarray analysis. Pediatrics. 2008;122:1310-1318.
25. Richards AA, Santos LJ, Nichols HA, et al. Cryptic chromosomal abnormalities identified in children with congenital heart disease. Pediatr Res. 2008;64:358-363.

THE DEVELOPMENTAL BIOLOGY AND GENETICS UNDERLYING HUMAN HETEROTAXY

Marko T. Boskovski, Martina Brueckner

- Left-Right Asymmetric Heart Anatomy
- Theoretical Considerations in the Development of Chiral Asymmetry
- The Left-Right Organizer Is a Conserved Ciliated Signaling Center
- Structure and Function of Cilia

- **Asymmetric Gene Expression Downstream from the Left-Right Organizer**
- **Clinical Implications: Genetics of Heterotaxy**
- **References**

The heart is the most strikingly asymmetric organ in the vertebrate body, and normal cardiac function is dependent on the precise coordination of anteroposterior (AP), dorsoventral (DV), and left-right (LR) spatial information during development. This chapter discusses how global LR asymmetry is created and outlines the current understanding of interpretation of global LR positional cues by the developing heart. First, we focus on the mechanism by which the LR axis is initiated and how cilia are central to the determination of LR asymmetry. Then, we detail a pathway of asymmetric gene expression that propagates the earliest LR asymmetry observed at the node across the embryo to the developing heart. Finally, we address the link between genetic control of LR asymmetry development and the genetics of human heterotaxy syndrome.

Left-Right Asymmetric Heart Anatomy

The cardiac lineage is specified at gastrulation, when cells located at the middle to rostral primitive streak ingress and migrate anteriorly and spread laterally, to form the two outwardly symmetrical heart fields. These paired cardiac primordia meet and fuse at the midline from anterior to posterior to form the primitive heart tube. The primitive heart tube initially consists of three layers: an inner endothelium and an outer myoepicardial mantle separated by a complex layer of extracellular matrix called cardiac jelly. The first outward evidence of LR asymmetry in the whole embryo becomes apparent while the primitive heart tube is still forming, when a complex series of bending and rotational movements coordinate in looping morphogenesis (Fig. 17b-1).

Cardiac progenitors are identified as cardiac inflow, ventricles, and outflow during gastrulation as they migrate from the primitive streak through the lateral plate mesoderm. The left ventricle, AV canal, and atria arise from the first heart field, while the right ventricle and outflow develop primarily from the second heart field.[26] The first and second heart fields can be identified by a series of molecular markers, including Nkx2.5 in the first heart field and Isl-1 in the second heart field.[27] Information identifying morphological "right" and "left" ventricles starts as AP and medio-lateral information that is initially laid down in the organization of the first and second heart fields. Specification of ventricular fate is via a complex network of transcriptional regulation. To establish a morphologic left ventricle, the bHLH transcription factor Hand1 is controlled by Nkx2.5 in the first heart field. Hand1 expression becomes restricted to the left ventricle, and inactivation of Hand1 at the heart tube stage results in left ventricular hypoplasia.[28] The morphologic right ventricle arises from the Isl-1 expressing cells of the second heart field, and Isl-1 regulates several factors essential for formation of the right ventricle, including the bHLH transcription factor Hand2 and the forkhead box H1 gene Foxh1.[29] Notably, no LR asymmetry has been observed in expression of the genes controlling cardiac chamber formation. Heart looping then imposes geometric LR asymmetry on the initially symmetrical heart tube. Looping (shown in Fig. 17b-1) consists of movements and cell shape changes that are different between the greater curvature and lesser curvatures, located at the right and left lateral edge of the linear heart tube. While the outer curvature grows, the inner curvature remodels so the sum of the two events leads to proper alignment between the inflow, ventricles, and outflow. As looping progresses, the outflow becomes positioned ventrally and rightward of the dorsal and leftward inflow. The right and left ventricles achieve their normal relationships, and the AV cushions and conotruncus are aligned normally.

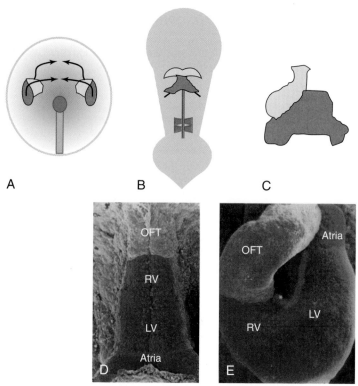

Figure 17b-1   Diagram outlining the organization of the heart tube through heart looping. **A-C,** Schematic representation of the heart fields and their contributions to the looping heart. The first heart field is shown in yellow, the second heart field in blue. **A,** Gastrulating embryo; the left and right heart fields are forming and migrating to the midline. **B,** Early somite embryo; the left and right heart fields have fused at the midline. The heart begins to beat. **C,** The straight heart tube rotates and bends to the right to form the normal D-loop. **D-E,**Scanning electron micrographs corresponding to **B** and **C.** Derivatives of the first heart field are in blue, the second heart field in yellow. The greater curvature is highlighted in red, the lesser curvature in green. (See Expert Consult site for color image.)

Theoretical Considerations in the Development of Chiral Asymmetry

The vertebrate body plan is outwardly symmetrical about the midline, the left side being a mirror image of the right. This outward symmetry belies elaborate internal LR asymmetries. For example, in all normal vertebrates, the heart tilts to the left, the liver is on the right, and the stomach and spleen are on the left. The LR axis is unique in that it is defined with respect to the AP and DV axes. Therefore the embryo must have mechanisms to both create asymmetry and to consistently align the asymmetry with the existing AP and DV axes. This predicts that failure to create asymmetry results in retained bilateral symmetry, manifesting as left or right atrial isomerism. In contrast, inability to align the asymmetry manifests as random asymmetry, such as the 50% incidence of situs inversus totalis observed in patients with primary ciliary dyskinesia. Wilhelmi originally proposed that the organism has an underlying mechanism that generates random asymmetry.[30] Brown and Wolpert hypothesized that this asymmetry is biased in a consistent direction by the presence of a handed asymmetric molecule or macromolecular structure, which they represented by the letter "F," which can align with the AP and DV axes.[31] Extensive work in model systems including zebrafish, *Xenopus,* and mouse indicates that the initial handed reference structure is the cilium, a highly chiral organelle that is found on almost all cells. Specifically, cilia positioned on the ventral surface of a small

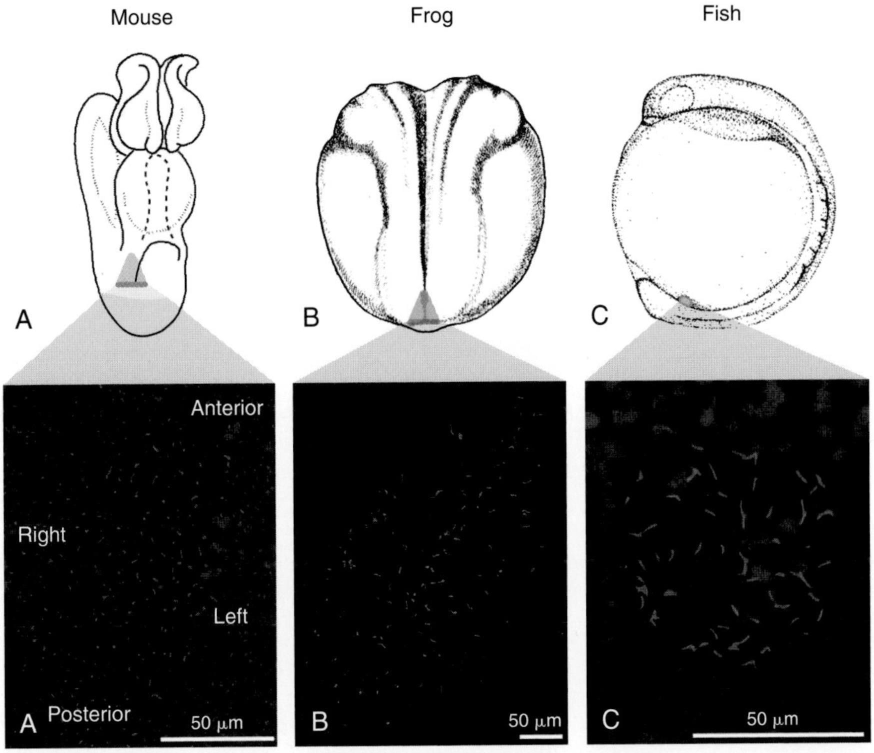

Figure 17b-2 Comparison of the LRO in different vertebrate species. **A-C,** Diagrams of developing mouse, frog, and fish embryos. The location of the LRO is outlined in red. **D-F,** Immunofluorescence pictures of the corresponding LRO. Monocilia are labeled with acetylated tubulin (red) and cell nuclei are labeled with Hoechst (blue). (See Expert Consult site for color image.)

population of left-right organizer (LRO) cells in the late gastrula embryo, prior to heart formation, orient the LR axis relative to the established AP and DV axes. The chirality of the cilium underlies the direction of flow of extracellular fluid across the LRO, and converts the local cellular asymmetry at the LRO to broader organismal LR asymmetry that is eventually communicated to the developing heart.

The LRO Is a Conserved Ciliated Signaling Center

LR axis development can be divided into three stages:
1. Asymmetric cilia-driven flow
2. Asymmetric gene expression
3. Asymmetric visceral morphogenesis

Despite the significantly different anatomy of various vertebrate species, central to the first stage of LR development is a conserved, homologous vertebrate structure called the Hensen's node in chick, node in mouse, posterior notochord (PNC) in rabbit, Kupffer's vesicle (KV) in fish, and gastrocoel roof plate (GRP) in frog, which we collectively refer to as the LRO (Fig. 17b-2).[32-36] The LRO forms during gastrulation and is composed of 50-250 monociliated cells. The synchronized beating of the cilia on these cells creates a leftward fluid flow (Fig. 17b-3) of the extracellular fluid, which is associated with an increase in intracellular calcium on the left of the LRO.[37-39] The calcium signal depends on sensory cilia displaying the polycystin-2 channel, indicating that cilia are required to both generate the earliest asymmetric signal (flow) and to transduce the extracellular flow signal to an intracellular calcium signal. This observation provided the first link between LR development and kidney development, and it is notable that mice lacking polycystin-2 develop right atrial isomerism and endocardial cushion defects.[40] Artificially applied flow can rescue the

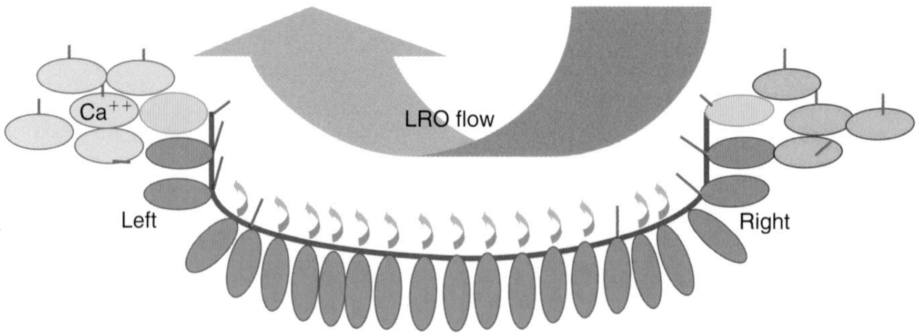

Figure 17b-3 Schematic of the mouse LRO. Motile cilia on pit cells (shown with thick red arrows on dark gray cells) generate leftward flow of extracellular fluid (shown as large red arrow). Sensory cilia on crown cells (shown as thin red arrows on light gray cells) transduce flow information into asymmetric signals, including increased intracellular calcium in the cells at the left. This leads to subsequent asymmetric gene expression.

phenotype of mice with paralyzed LRO cilia, and reversal of flow direction results in reversal of cardiac looping.[41] The second stage of LR development, asymmetric gene expression, then proceeds from the LRO.

There are several lines of evidence supporting that the LRO is a homologous structure that is conserved throughout vertebrate species. A ciliated LRO organizer has been identified in every major vertebrate model system (Fig. 17b-2), although it has been difficult to definitively identify the ciliated LRO in chick.[42] In each case, the cilia have been documented to be motile, and consequently, to produce leftward flow. Furthermore, it is always derived from the superficial mesoderm and has flanking expression of homologs of the gene *Nodal* (discussed later). Finally, mechanical destruction of LRO precursor cells in frog, or the LRO itself in zebrafish, yields laterality defects (i.e., situs inversus and heterotaxy) in the face of normal AP and DV development, indicating that the LRO is not only a conserved structure, but also one that is required for normal LR development.[35,43] The ciliated LRO has not actually been visualized in the human embryo; however, a combination of the remarkable conservation of a cilia-driven flow mechanism for initiating LR asymmetry in vertebrates, and the association between human ciliopathies (see later) and situs abnormalities, makes it highly likely that there is an LRO in the early human embryo also.

Structure and Function of Cilia

Essential for normal LRO function and subsequent normal LR development is the proper function of the LRO monocilia. Cilia, in general, are large, complex organelles that, depending on the tissue they are found in, protrude up to 20 µm beyond the cytoplasm.[44] They are composed of the ciliary axoneme surrounded by the ciliary membrane, which is contiguous with the plasma membrane. The axoneme comprises the microtubule skeleton consisting of nine microtubule (MT) doublets with attached intraflagellar transport (IFT) proteins. Since there is no protein synthesis in cilia, IFT proteins are required to selectively transport the structural and functional components of cilia from the cytoplasm into the axoneme, and to return products of ciliary signaling to the cytoplasm (Fig. 17b-4).

Cilia can be subdivided into epithelial cilia and primary cilia. Epithelial cilia, such as those found on the apical surface of epithelial cells of the trachea, choroid plexus, and oviduct, contain motor proteins, as well as a central pair of MTs linked by radial spokes to the outer nine doublets. The motor proteins—a combination of outer and inner arm dynein motors—along with their associated dynein regulatory proteins, hydrolyze ATP to generate ciliary movement. Typically there are many cilia per epithelial cell that arise from basal bodies beneath the cell membrane, which themselves originate from the template of the mother centriole. The concerted action

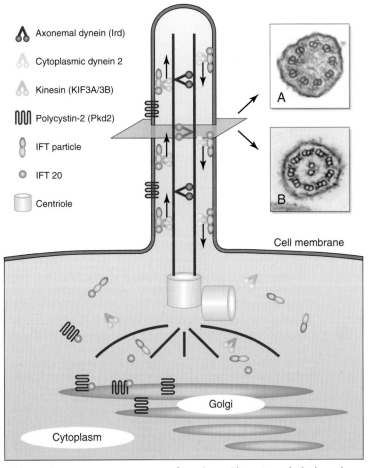

Figure 17b-4 Schematic representation of a cilium. The microtubule based structure is assembled at the basal body (epithelial cilia) or the mother centriole (monocilia). Proteins necessary for proper ciliary function go from the Golgi to the base of the cilium via IFT proteins where they are transported up the cilium in anterograde fashion by kinesin motor proteins, and down the cilium in retrograde fashion by the dynein motor proteins. **Inset A,** Electron micrograph (EM) of a monocilium lacking a central microtubule pair. **B,** EM of a motile epithelial cilium with a central microtubule pair.

of large numbers of closely spaced motile cilia transports surrounding fluid, such as tracheal secretions or cerebrospinal fluid.

In contrast to the highly specialized epithelial cilia, almost all cells (with the exception of a few myeloid and lymphoid lines) can carry primary cilia (also known as monocilia). As the name suggests, there is only one monocilium per cell, which arises directly from the mother centriole. Like the cilia found in ciliated epithelia, the axoneme of primary cilia is constructed on a scaffold consisting of nine MT doublets. Unlike the stereotypical arrangement of microtubules, motors and structural proteins found in epithelial cilia, the contents of monocilia are extremely varied. As such, monocilia can serve different functions depending on the proteins they are loaded with. For example, by displaying specialized receptors, these cilia are adapted to function as light photoreceptors in the retina, or as olfactory receptors in the nose. Primary cilia are also signaling centers at the interface between the cell and the extracellular environment. For example, they are essential for hedgehog signaling, and absent or defective cilia in mouse embryos result in a spectrum of defects including neural tube defects, polydactyly, and cardiac defects.[45,46]

In the LRO, there are two different types of primary cilia: motile and sensory (Fig. 17b-3). The motile primary cilia, which populate the center of the LRO, are equipped with dynein motor proteins, enabling them to create a leftward fluid flow and break LR symmetry. The nonmotile monocilia are more abundant at the lateral edge of the LRO in mouse and lack dynein motor proteins but contain polycystin-2, the product of the gene mutated in type 2 dominant polycystic kidney disease.[38] It is a cation channel that is required to sense the flow generated by the motile mono-cilia.[47] In the presence of leftward LRO flow, polycystin-2 induces an increase in calcium concentration on the left LRO border and therefore translates the LRO flow into an asymmetric calcium gradient.[38]

There is significant evidence to support the model outlined earlier that (1) flow generated by LRO monocilia is required for proper LR patterning and (2) sensory cilia detect this leftward flow. First, regarding the requirement for motile cilia at the LRO, altered function (i.e., mutations, knockdown, or knockout) of any of a number of ciliary genes including components of the dynein motor complex or genes necessary for ciliary biogenesis such as the IFTs results in LR patterning defects.[48-52] Initial evidence for a role of cilia in development of LR asymmetry came from study of patients with primary ciliary dyskinesia (PCD or Kartagener syndrome), which manifests as respiratory disease, male infertility, and a 50% incidence of situs inversus.[53] Respiratory compromise and male infertility in PCD are due to defective dynein function in the tracheal cilia and sperm axoneme, while randomization of situs solitus (SS) and situs inversus (SI) is secondary to improper LRO motile cilia function. Similarly, mice with a point mutation in the LR dynein (*lrd*) gene, which renders cilia immotile, also have randomization of SS and SI.[48] LRO flow in these mice is absent, but artificial application of leftward flow across the LRO can reestablish SS, while application of flow to the right can induce SI.[41] This indicates that LRO flow itself is the event that breaks LR symmetry. Second, regarding the requirement for sensory cilia at the LRO, mice that lack LRO flow due to immotile cilia have been shown to lack increased calcium levels on the left border of the LRO. This is also the case in mice with normal LRO flow that lack the *polycystin-2* gene, indicating that there are no asymmetric calcium levels in the absence of leftward LRO flow and that detection of LRO flow requires the presence of the polycystin-2 receptors in the surrounding sensory cilia.[38]

Asymmetric Gene Expression Downstream from the Left-Right Organizer

The result of asymmetric LRO flow is a downstream cascade of asymmetric gene expression that propagates the asymmetric signal throughout development and ultimately results in asymmetric organogenesis. This cascade is outlined by asymmetric expression of *Coco, Nodal, Lefty-1, Lefty-2,* and *PitX2,* all of which are observed prior to visible asymmetry of heart looping (Fig. 17b-5).

Nodal is a left-side determinant that is initially expressed symmetrically around the LRO.[52-57] It subsequently becomes asymmetrically expressed at both the LRO and the left lateral plate mesoderm (LPM), a structure lateral to the LRO. By default, in the absence of *Nodal* expression, both the left and right LPM specify right-sided organogenesis. In normal development peri-LRO *Nodal* expression induces its own expression at the left LPM through a positive feedback loop, thereby changing the default state of the left LPM from right- to left-sided organ development. With that in mind, complete absence of *Nodal* expression at both LPMs leads to the development of right atrial isomerism, while bilateral *Nodal* expression results in left atrial isomerism.

While leftward LRO flow is required for left LPM *Nodal* expression, *Nodal* itself does not directly respond to flow.[58] The transition from symmetric to asymmetric *Nodal* expression is mediated by *Coco*—a negative inhibitor of *Nodal*.[59-61] Before LRO flow is established, *Coco* and *Nodal* have overlapping, symmetric, peri-LRO patterns of expression. Unlike *Nodal, Coco* is directly inhibited by LRO flow. As a result, *Coco* is suppressed on the left, but still maintained on the right. Consequently, Coco releases its negative inhibition of the coexpressed *Nodal* protein, such that *Nodal* becomes asymmetrically expressed on the left, but not the right.[58]

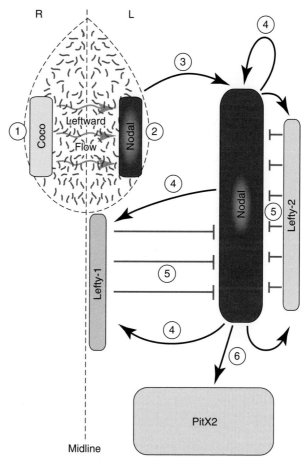

Figure 17b-5 Schematic representation of the asymmetric gene cascade. *1*, At the LRO, leftward flow inhibits *Coco* (shown in pink) expression on the left but not on the right. *2*, *Coco* inhibits *Nodal* (shown in dark gray) expression on the right but not the left. *3*, Left-sided *Nodal* expression at the LRO induces *Nodal* expression at the left LPM. *4*, *Nodal* induces its own expression, as well as the expression of *Lefty-1* and *Lefty-2* (shown in light red). *5*, *Lefty-1* and *Lefty-2* contain the expression of *Nodal* to the LPM. *6*, Left-sided *Nodal* expression induces left-sided *PitX2* expression (shown in light gray).

Lefty-1 and *Lefty-2* are also *Nodal* inhibitors that are responsible for keeping the *Nodal* positive feedback loop in control and its expression localized to the LPM.[62-64] They are induced by *Nodal* and are expressed at the midline (*Lefty-1*) and the left LPM (*Lefty-2*). In the absence of either gene, *Nodal* expression begins normally in the left LPM, but subsequently leaks to the other side.

The feedback inhibition of *Lefty-1* and *Lefty-2* not only limits the area of *Nodal* expression, but also the time. In the mouse, *Nodal* is present for only 6 hours. Once *Nodal* expression at the LPM ceases, it passes on the left-side determinant baton to another asymmetrically expressed gene *PitX2*.[65-67] *PitX2* is induced by *Nodal* at the LPM. However, it persists much longer, and once *Nodal* disappears its expression is maintained by *Nkx2*. As a left side determinant, similar to *Nodal*, complete absence of *PitX2* yields right atrial isomerism, while bilateral presence results in left atrial isomerism.

Clinical Implications: Genetics of Heterotaxy

Human heterotaxy is characterized by two salient features: a high degree of genetic heterogeneity combined with tremendous phenotypic variability.[68] In addition, the complexity of the associated heart disease results in a high degree of lethality prior to reproductive age, thus limiting the number of extended pedigrees.[69,70] Familial cases of heterotaxy (Htx) have shown tremendous phenotypic variability within many Htx pedigrees, with the coexistence of situs solitus, situs inversus, and isomerism syndromes within one family. This suggests the interaction of Htx genetic defects with modifiers and/or epigenetic factors. Although these features complicate attempts to delineate the genetic contributions to heterotaxy, the wealth of gene information gleaned from study of LR development in model organism systems provides a singular opportunity to dissect the underlying genetic etiology.

Currently, gene mutations have been associated with 10-20% of cases of Htx.[71,72] These can be divided into syndromes with a known genetic etiology that have Htx as an associated feature and isolated Htx cases with an identified single-gene mutation. Consistent with the prominent role cilia play in the development of LR asymmetry, syndromes associated with defects in cilia structure and function can manifest with Htx as part of the clinical spectrum (Table 17b-1).

Primary Ciliary Dyskinesia

The syndrome with the most prominent association with Htx is PCD (Kartagener syndrome). PCD consists of sinopulmonary disease, male infertility, and a 50% incidence of abnormal cardiac situs.[53] A minimum of 6.5% of patients with PCD have intracardiac disease consistent with Htx.[73] PCD is caused by mutations in genes affecting function of motile cilia in the airway, the sperm flagellum, and the motile cilia found on the LR organizer during development. At this time, defects in 12 distinct genes have been associated with PCD (Table 17b-1), and the repertoire is increasing as genomic analysis of affected patients becomes more sophisticated. Inheritance is predominantly recessive, although rare dominant and X-linked pedigrees have been identified.

Bardet-Biedl Syndrome

Bardet-Biedl syndrome (BBS) is a rare genetic disorder characterized by renal and hepatic cystic disease, retinitis pigmentosa, polydactyly, developmental delay, and obesity. The cardiac manifestation is rare situs inversus. Fourteen BBS genes have been identified to date, and they all focus on biogenesis and function of the centriole upon which the cilium is built.

Other syndromes that have been classified as "ciliopathies" include cardiac disease that is part of the Htx spectrum.[74] These include Meckel-Gruber syndrome, short-rib polydactyly syndrome and Ellis-van Creveld syndrome. Ellis-van Creveld syndrome is a skeletal dysplasia associated with a high incidence of common atrium and systemic and pulmonary venous anomalies that are frequently seen in the context of Htx. Mutations in two genes, *EVC* and *EVC2*, underlie approximately 70% of cases; *EVC* and *EVC2* interact at the cilium to affect hedgehog signaling.[75] Dextrocardia has been seen in the context of VACTERL-H syndrome, and one possible molecular etiology for VACTERL-H is a deletion encompassing the *Zic3* gene, which also causes X-linked nonsyndromic heterotaxy.[76]

Nonsyndromic Htx

A single large pedigree and several sporadic cases of Htx are caused by mutations in the gene encoding the zinc-finger transcription factor ZIC3, and sporadic cases of Htx have been attributed to mutations affecting the nodal cofactor CRIPTO, the growth factor LEFTY1, the Activin Receptor 2B, the TGF-β growth factor GDF1, the ciliary axonemal dynein LRD, and the ciliary signaling protein Inversin.[71,77-80] Overall, however, candidate gene analysis has defined a clear genetic cause for less than 10% of human Htx. Recently, copy number variations (CNVs) resulting in duplication or deletion of five additional Htx genes have been identified in individual patients with Htx.[81] Notably, three of the five genes identified by this approach can be linked to cilia function, further strengthening the support for ciliary dysfunction underlying a significant proportion of human Htx. Also, the overall burden of genic CNVs in Htx patients was almost twice that observed in controls, suggesting that subtle

Table 17b-1   SYNDROMIC HETEROTAXY

Syndrome	Cardiac Disease	Other Clinical Features	Gene(s) and References	Molecular/Cellular Ontology
Primary ciliary dyskinesia (PCD)	Situs inversus totalis (50%), heterotaxy (6.5%)	Chronic sinusitis, bronchiectasis, neonatal respiratory distress, male infertility Occasional: female infertility, retinopathy	DNAI1[82] DNAI2[83] DNAH5[49,84,85] DNAH11[86,87] RSPH9[88] RSPH4A[88] LRRC50[89,90] RPGR[91] TXNDC3[92] KTU[93] CCDC40[94] CCDC39[95]	Structure and function of motile cilia
Bardet-Biedl syndrome (BBS)	Rare situs inversus, up to 50% with minor cardiac abnormalities	Renal abnormalities, polydactyly, retinal dystrophy, hearing loss, obesity, developmental delay, hypogonadism	BBS1,2,4,5,7-10,12[96] Arl6(BBS3)[97] TRIM32 (BBS11)[98] BBS14[99]	Centriole/basal body structure and function
Meckel-Gruber syndrome	20% CHD including rare situs inversus	Encephalocele, polydactyly, polycystic kidneys, hepatic abnormalities	MKS1[100] TMEM216 (MKS2)[101] TMEM67 (MKS3)[102] RPGRIP1L CC2D2A[103]	Primary cilium and basal body
Nephronophthisis	Situs inversus, VSD	Cystic kidney disease, retinal degeneration	NPHP1[104] INVS (NPHP2)[105] NPHP3[106] NPHP4[107] NPHP5[108] CEP290 (NPHP6)[109] GLIS2 (NPHP7)[110] NEK8 (NPHP8)[111]	Cilium, centriole, cell cycle
VACTERL-H	VSD, dextrocardia (rare)	Vertebral anomalies, anal atresia, tracheoesophageal fistula, limb abnormalities, hydrocephalus, renal hypoplasia	Zic3[76]	Unknown
Ellis-van-Creveld syndrome	Atrio-ventricular canal, common atrium, LSVC[112]	Short ribs, polydactyly, ectodermal dysplasia, renal abnormalities	EVC1, EVC2[75,113,114]	Hedgehog signaling, cilium

increase or decrease in gene dosage for a wide range of genes may have the ability to perturb the development of LR asymmetry.

If one adds up all genes associated with human syndromic and nonsyndromic Htx, and also considers genes that have been implicated in LR development in model organisms, the total list of Htx candidate genes currently stands at more than 125 genes. This suggests that Htx is actually not a specific genetic diagnosis, but a manifestation of a broad range of developmental disorders that affect the development of LR asymmetry. The specific cardiac disease resulting from any individual gene defect is likely due to the summation of effects on LR development and for some Htx genes also direct effects on cardiac morphogenesis. The clinical manifestations observed in Htx patients are further complicated by prominent effects on the development and function of other organ systems; for example, many of the genes affecting LR development through their role in cilia also have critical effect(s) on kidney development and function. Thus eventually the clinical care of patients with Htx may be dictated by both the anatomy and physiology of the structural heart disease, and by the specific cardiac and extracardiac manifestations of the underlying genetic defect. Hopefully such individually tailored care will improve the long-term outcome for patients with this challenging form of congenital heart disease.

References

26. Evans SM, et al. Myocardial lineage development. Circ Res. 2010;107(12):1428-1444.
27. Moretti A, et al. Multipotent embryonic isl1+ progenitor cells lead to cardiac, smooth muscle, and endothelial cell diversification. Cell. 2006;127(6):1151-1165.
28. McFadden DG, et al. The Hand1 and Hand2 transcription factors regulate expansion of the embryonic cardiac ventricles in a gene dosage-dependent manner. Development. 2005;132(1):189-201.
29. Buckingham M, Meilhac S, Zaffran S. Building the mammalian heart from two sources of myocardial cells. Nat Rev Genet. 2005;6(11):826-835.
30. Wilhelmi H. Experimentelle Untersuchungen ueber situs inversus viscerum. Archive der Entwicklungsmechanik. 1921;48:517-532.
31. Brown NA, Wolpert L. The development of handedness in left/right asymmetry. Development. 1990;109(1):1-9.
32. Pagan-Westphal SM, Tabin CJ. The transfer of left-right positional information during chick embryogenesis. Cell. 1998;93(1):25-35.
33. Sulik K, et al. Morphogenesis of the murine node and notochordal plate. Dev Dyn. 1994;201(3):260-278.
34. Feistel K, Blum M. Three types of cilia including a novel 9+4 axoneme on the notochordal plate of the rabbit embryo. Dev Dyn. 2006;235(12):3348-3358.
35. Essner JJ, et al. Kupffer's vesicle is a ciliated organ of asymmetry in the zebrafish embryo that initiates left-right development of the brain, heart and gut. Development. 2005;132(6):1247-1260.
36. Schweickert A, et al. Cilia-driven leftward flow determines laterality in Xenopus. Curr Biol. 2007;17(1):60-66.
37. Nonaka S, et al. Randomization of left-right asymmetry due to loss of nodal cilia generating leftward flow of extraembryonic fluid in mice lacking KIF3B motor protein. Cell. 1998;95(6):829-837.
38. McGrath J, et al. Two populations of node monocilia initiate left-right asymmetry in the mouse. Cell. 2003;114(1):61-73.
39. Sarmah B, et al. Inositol polyphosphates regulate zebrafish left-right asymmetry. Dev Cell. 2005;9(1):133-145.
40. Pennekamp P, et al. The ion channel polycystin-2 is required for left-right axis determination in mice. Curr Biol. 2002;12(11):938-943.
41. Nonaka S, et al. Determination of left right patterning of the mouse embryo by artificial nodal flow. Nature. 2002;418(6893):96-99.
42. Essner JJ, et al. Left right development: conserved function for embryonic nodal cilia. Nature. 2002;418(6893):37-38.
43. Blum M, et al. Xenopus, an ideal model system to study vertebrate left-right asymmetry. Dev Dyn. 2009;238(6):1215-1225.
44. Silverman MA, Leroux MR. Intraflagellar transport and the generation of dynamic, structurally and functionally diverse cilia. Trends Cell Biol. 2009;19(7):306-316.
45. Caspary T, Larkins CE, Anderson KV. The graded response to Sonic Hedgehog depends on cilia architecture. Dev Cell. 2007;12(5):767-778.
46. Eggenschwiler JT, Anderson KV. Cilia and developmental signaling. Annu Rev Cell Dev Biol. 2007;23:345-373.
47. Nauli SM, et al. Polycystins 1 and 2 mediate mechanosensation in the primary cilium of kidney cells. Nat Genet. 2003;6:6.
48. Supp DM, et al. Targeted deletion of the ATP binding domain of left-right dynein confirms its role in specifying development of left-right asymmetries. Development. 1999;126(23):5495-5504.
49. Ibanez-Tallon I, Gorokhova S, Heintz N. Loss of function of axonemal dynein Mdnah5 causes primary ciliary dyskinesia and hydrocephalus. Hum Mol Genet. 2002;11(6):715-721.
50. Marszalek JR, et al. Situs inversus and embryonic ciliary morphogenesis defects in mouse mutants lacking the KIF3A subunit of kinesin-II. Proc Natl Acad Sci U S A. 1999;96(9):5043-5048.
51. Nonaka S, et al. Randomization of left-right asymmetry due to loss of nodal cilia generating leftward flow of extraembryonic fluid in mice lacking KIF3B motor protein [erratum Cell 1999;99(1):117]. Cell. 1998;95(6):829-837.
52. Huangfu D, et al. Hedgehog signalling in the mouse requires intraflagellar transport proteins. Nature. 2003;426(6962):83-87.
53. Afzelius BA. A human syndrome caused by immotile cilia. Science. 1976;193(4250):317-319.
54. Lowe LA, et al. Conserved left-right asymmetry of nodal expression and alterations in murine situs inversus [see comments]. Nature. 1996;381(6578):158-161.

55. Zhou X, et al. Nodal is a novel TGF-beta-like gene expressed in the mouse node during gastrulation. Nature. 1993;361(6412):543-547.
56. Long S, Ahmad N, Rebagliati M. The zebrafish nodal-related gene southpaw is required for visceral and diencephalic left-right asymmetry. Development. 2003;130(11):2303-2316.
57. Levin M, et al. A molecular pathway determining left-right asymmetry in chick embryogenesis. Cell. 1995;82(5):803-814.
58. Schweickert A, et al. The Nodal inhibitor Coco is a critical target of leftward flow in Xenopus. Curr Biol. 2010;20(8):738-743.
59. Marques S, et al. The activity of the Nodal antagonist Cerl-2 in the mouse node is required for correct L/R body axis. Gene Dev. 2004;18(19):2342-2347.
60. Hashimoto H, et al. The Cerberus/Dan-family protein Charon is a negative regulator of Nodal signaling during left-right patterning in zebrafish. Development. 2004;131(8):1741-1753.
61. Esteban CR, et al. The novel Cer-like protein Caronte mediates the establishment of embryonic left-right asymmetry. Nature. 1999;401(6750):243-251.
62. Meno C, et al. Mouse Lefty2 and zebrafish antivin are feedback inhibitors of nodal signaling during vertebrate gastrulation. Mol Cell. 1999;4(3):287-298.
63. Cheng AM, et al. The lefty-related factor Xatv acts as a feedback inhibitor of nodal signaling in mesoderm induction and L-R axis development in xenopus. Development. 2000;127(5): 1049-1061.
64. Bisgrove BW, Essner JJ, Yost HJ. Regulation of midline development by antagonism of lefty and nodal signaling. Development. 1999;126(14):3253-3262.
65. Yoshioka H, et al. Pitx2, a bicoid-type homeobox gene, is involved in a lefty-signaling pathway in determination of left-right asymmetry. Cell. 1998;94(3):299-305.
66. Ryan AK, et al. Pitx2 determines left-right asymmetry of internal organs in vertebrates. Nature. 1998;394(6693):545-551.
67. Campione M, et al. The homeobox gene Pitx2: mediator of asymmetric left-right signaling in vertebrate heart and gut looping. Development. 1999;126(6):1225-1234.
68. Taketazu M, et al. Spectrum of cardiovascular disease, accuracy of diagnosis, and outcome in fetal heterotaxy syndrome. Am J Cardiol. 2006;97(5):720-724.
69. Anagnostopoulos PV, et al. Improved current era outcomes in patients with heterotaxy syndromes. Eur J Cardiothorac Surg. 2009;35(5):871-878.
70. Cohen MS, et al. Controversies, genetics, diagnostic assessment, and outcomes relating to the heterotaxy syndrome. Cardiol Young. 2007;17(Suppl 2):29-43.
71. Belmont JW, et al. Molecular genetics of heterotaxy syndromes. Curr Opin Cardiol. 2004; 19(3):216-220.
72. Sutherland MJ, Ware SM. Disorders of left-right asymmetry: heterotaxy and situs inversus. Am J Med Genet C Semin Med Genet. 2009;151C(4):307-317.
73. Kennedy MP, et al. Congenital heart disease and other heterotaxic defects in a large cohort of patients with primary ciliary dyskinesia. Circulation. 2007;115(22):2814-2821.
74. Quinlan RJ, Tobin JL, Beales PL. Modeling ciliopathies: primary cilia in development and disease. Curr Top Dev Biol. 2008;84:249-310.
75. Ruiz-Perez VL, Goodship JA. Ellis-van Creveld syndrome and Weyers acrodental dysostosis are caused by cilia-mediated diminished response to hedgehog ligands. Am J Med Genet C Semin Med Genet. 2009;151C(4):341-351.
76. Chung B, et al. From VACTERL-H to heterotaxy: variable expressivity of ZIC3-related disorders. Am J Med Genet A. 2011;155(5):1123-1128.
77. Bisgrove BW, Morelli SH, Yost HJ. Genetics of human laterality disorders: insights from vertebrate model systems. Annu Rev Genomics Hum Genet. 2003;4:1-32.
78. Gebbia M, et al. X-linked situs abnormalities result from mutations in ZIC3 [see comments]. Nat Genet. 1997;17(3):305-308.
79. Karkera JD, et al. Loss-of-function mutations in growth differentiation factor-1 (GDF1) are associated with congenital heart defects in humans. Am J Hum Genet. 2007;81(5):987-994.
80. van Bon BW, et al. Transposition of the great vessels in a patient with a 2.9 Mb interstitial deletion of 9q31.1 encompassing the inversin gene: clinical report and review. Am J Med Genet A. 2008;146A(9):1225-1229.
81. Fakhro KA, et al. Rare copy number variants in congenital heart disease patients identify genes in left-right patterning. Proc Natl Acad Sci U S A. 2011;108(7):2915-2920.
82. Guichard C, et al. Axonemal dynein intermediate-chain gene (DNAI1) mutations result in situs inversus and primary ciliary dyskinesia (Kartagener syndrome). Am J Hum Genet. 2001;68(4): 1030-1035.
83. Loges NT, et al. DNAI2 mutations cause primary ciliary dyskinesia with defects in the outer dynein arm. Am J Hum Genet. 2008;83(5):547-558.
84. Hornef N, et al. DNAH5 mutations are a common cause of primary ciliary dyskinesia with outer dynein arm defects. Am J Respir Crit Care Med. 2006;174(2):120-126.
85. Olbrich H, et al. Mutations in DNAH5 cause primary ciliary dyskinesia and randomization of left-right asymmetry. Nat Genet. 2002;30(2):143-144.
86. Bartoloni L, et al. Mutations in the DNAH11 (axonemal heavy chain dynein type 11) gene cause one form of situs inversus totalis and most likely primary ciliary dyskinesia. Proc Natl Acad Sci U S A. 2002;99(16):10282-10286.
87. Schwabe GC, et al. Primary ciliary dyskinesia associated with normal axoneme ultrastructure is caused by DNAH11 mutations. Hum Mutat. 2008;29(2):289-298.

17

88. Castleman VH, et al. Mutations in radial spoke head protein genes RSPH9 and RSPH4A cause primary ciliary dyskinesia with central-microtubular-pair abnormalities. Am J Hum Genet. 2009; 84(2):197-209.

89. Duquesnoy P, et al. Loss-of-function mutations in the human ortholog of Chlamydomonas reinhardtii ODA7 disrupt dynein arm assembly and cause primary ciliary dyskinesia. Am J Hum Genet. 2009;85(6):890-896.

90. Escudier E, et al. Ciliary defects and genetics of primary ciliary dyskinesia. Paediatr Respir Rev. 2009;10(2):51-54.

91. Moore A, et al. RPGR is mutated in patients with a complex X linked phenotype combining primary ciliary dyskinesia and retinitis pigmentosa. J Med Genet. 2006;43(4):326-333.

92. Duriez B, et al. A common variant in combination with a nonsense mutation in a member of the thioredoxin family causes primary ciliary dyskinesia. Proc Natl Acad Sci U S A. 2007;104(9): 3336-3341.

93. Omran H, et al. Ktu/PF13 is required for cytoplasmic pre-assembly of axonemal dyneins. Nature. 2008;456(7222):611-616.

94. Becker-Heck A, et al. The coiled-coil domain containing protein CCDC40 is essential for motile cilia function and left-right axis formation. Nat Genet. 2011;43(1):79-84.

95. Merveille AC, et al. CCDC39 is required for assembly of inner dynein arms and the dynein regulatory complex and for normal ciliary motility in humans and dogs. Nat Genet. 2011;43(1):72-78.

96. Janssen S, et al. Mutation analysis in Bardet-Biedl syndrome by DNA pooling and massively parallel resequencing in 105 individuals. Hum Genet. 2011;129(1):79-90.

97. Wiens CJ, et al. Bardet-Biedl syndrome-associated small GTPase ARL6 (BBS3) functions at or near the ciliary gate and modulates Wnt signaling. J Biol Chem. 2010;285(21):16218-16230.

98. Chiang AP, et al. Homozygosity mapping with SNP arrays identifies TRIM32, an E3 ubiquitin ligase, as a Bardet-Biedl syndrome gene (BBS11). Proc Natl Acad Sci U S A. 2006;103(16):6287-6292.

99. Kim SK, et al. Planar cell polarity acts through septins to control collective cell movement and ciliogenesis. Science. 2010;329(5997):1337-1340.

100. Kyttala M, et al. MKS1, encoding a component of the flagellar apparatus basal body proteome, is mutated in Meckel syndrome. Nat Genet. 2006;38(2):155-157.

101. Valente EM, et al. Mutations in TMEM216 perturb ciliogenesis and cause Joubert, Meckel and related syndromes. Nat Genet. 2010;42(7):619-625.

102. Smith UM, et al. The transmembrane protein meckelin (MKS3) is mutated in Meckel-Gruber syndrome and the wpk rat. Nat Genet. 2006;38(2):191-196.

103. Mougou-Zerelli S, et al. CC2D2A mutations in Meckel and Joubert syndromes indicate a genotype-phenotype correlation. Hum Mutat. 2009;30(11):1574-1582.

104. Hildebrandt F, et al. A novel gene encoding an SH3 domain protein is mutated in nephronophthisis type 1. Nat Genet. 1997;17(2):149-153.

105. Otto EA, et al. Mutations in INVS encoding inversin cause nephronophthisis type 2, linking renal cystic disease to the function of primary cilia and left-right axis determination. Nat Genet. 2003;34(4):413-420.

106. Olbrich H, et al. Mutations in a novel gene, NPHP3, cause adolescent nephronophthisis, tapeto-retinal degeneration and hepatic fibrosis. Nat Genet. 2003;34(4):455-459.

107. Mollet G, et al. The gene mutated in juvenile nephronophthisis type 4 encodes a novel protein that interacts with nephrocystin. Nat Genet. 2002;32(2):300-305.

108. Otto EA, et al. Nephrocystin-5, a ciliary IQ domain protein, is mutated in Senior-Loken syndrome and interacts with RPGR and calmodulin. Nat Genet. 2005;37(3):282-288.

109. Valente EM, et al. Mutations in CEP290, which encodes a centrosomal protein, cause pleiotropic forms of Joubert syndrome. Nat Genet. 2006;38(6):623-625.

110. Attanasio M, et al. Loss of GLIS2 causes nephronophthisis in humans and mice by increased apoptosis and fibrosis. Nat Genet. 2007;39(8):1018-1024.

111. Otto EA, et al. NEK8 mutations affect ciliary and centrosomal localization and may cause nephronophthisis. J Am Soc Nephrol. 2008;19(3):587-592.

112. Hills CB, et al. Ellis-van Creveld syndrome and congenital heart defects: presentation of an additional 32 cases. Pediatr Cardiol. 2011;32(7):977-982.

113. Ruiz-Perez VL, et al. Mutations in a new gene in Ellis-van Creveld syndrome and Weyers acrodental dysostosis. Nat Genet. 2000;24(3):283-286.

114. Ruiz-Perez VL, et al. Mutations in two nonhomologous genes in a head-to-head configuration cause Ellis-van Creveld syndrome. Am J Hum Genet. 2003;72(3):728-732.

GENETICS OF CONGENITAL HEART DISEASE

Kwame Anyane-Yeboa, MD, Punita Gupta, MD

- **Nonsyndromic Congenital Heart Disease**
- **Syndromic Congenital Heart Disease**
- **References**

Cardiac malformations present at birth are an important component of pediatric cardiovascular disease and constitute a major percentage of clinically significant birth defects, with an estimated prevalence of 4-50 per 1000 live births. The true prevalence, however, may be much higher. Advances in medical and surgical care of children with congenital heart disease (CHD) have resulted in more than 85% of affected individuals surviving into adulthood and reaching a reproductive age.[115] Information regarding the genetic basis of CHD is rapidly accumulating. It is imperative for many disciplines within the medical community, including adult cardiologists, surgeons, internists, and obstetricians, to acquire knowledge in this arena in order to select the adults with CHD for genetic counseling, genetic screening, and career planning and reproductive options.

Congenital heart defects can be related to an abnormality of an infant's chromosomes (5-6%), single gene defects (3-5%), or environmental factors (2%). The contributions of teratogens such as alcohol, anticonvulsants medications, lithium, and maternal medical conditions such as poorly managed phenylketonuria, rubella, systemic lupus erythematosus (SLE) and diabetes mellitus to CHD is well established, but the number of teratogens that can potentially cause CHD is unknown. In 85-90% of cases, there is no identifiable cause for the heart defect, and most CHDs were viewed to occur as isolated cases. On the basis of studies of recurrence and transmission risks, a hypothesis of multifactorial etiology was proposed. The factors are usually both genetic and environmental, where a combination of genes from both parents, in addition to unknown environmental factors, produces the trait or condition. However, the risk increases when either parent has CHD, when another first degree relative or sibling has CHD, or when there is consanguinity in the family. When there is unequal sex incidence, the risk is greater among relatives of the more rarely affected sex. This phenotype could be explained by the polygenic model in which recurrence in siblings and offspring of the affected individuals is generally 3-5%. Not all forms of isolated CHD have recurrence risks that fit the polygenic model. In many studies the transmission rate for the lesion is 1.9-3.5% higher if the affected parent is the mother rather than the father. This discrepancy strongly suggests genetic heterogeneity as a possible explanation.

In the past decade, molecular genetic studies have exploited these observations of families with multiple affected individuals and have provided insights into the genetic basis of several forms of CHD. Most of the known causes of CHD are sporadic genetic changes, either focal mutations, deletion, or addition of segments of DNA. Large chromosomal abnormalities such as trisomies 21, 13, and 18 cause about 5-8% of cases of CHD,[116] with trisomy 21 being the most common genetic cause. Small chromosomal abnormalities also frequently lead to CHD, and examples include microdeletion of the long arm of chromosome 22 (22q11, DiGeorge syndrome), the long arm of chromosome 1 (1q21), the short arm of chromosome 8 (8p23), and many other, less recurrent regions of the genome, as shown by high-resolution genome-wide screening (array comparative genomic hybridization). While chromosome analysis and fluorescence in situ hybridization (FISH), can diagnose aneuploidies and subtle structural abnormalities, in certain disorders, changes occur at the level of a single gene and must be detected by alternative techniques. Mutation analysis identifies changes in the coding sequence of the gene, including small deletions, insertions, or substitutions of nucleotides that alter the encoded amino acid and consequently protein structure. Most methods employ polymerase chain reaction (PCR)-based assays. More expensive exon-by-exon sequencing of genomic DNA has recently emerged. Additionally, newer, more cost-effective direct sequence analysis methods have become available.

The genes regulating the complex developmental sequence of the heart have only been partly elucidated. Some genes are associated with specific defects. For example, mutations of a heart muscle protein, α-myosin heavy chain (MYH6) are associated with atrial septal defects (ASDs). Several proteins that interact with MYH6 such as GATA4, TBX5, and NKX2-5 are also associated with cardiac defects.[117,118] It is now the standard of care to perform high-resolution array comparative genomic hybridization in patients with CHD and additional features suggestive of a chromosomal aberration as it can lead to an etiological diagnosis.[119] However, the interpretation of the imbalances detected must be done with caution, given the presence in the human genome of a high level of copy number variations. The challenge of the future is to define the pathogenesis of disease-causing mutations, which in turn will provide opportunities to develop diagnostic and therapeutic strategies as alternatives to those now used.

Recent studies on isolated CHD using array genomic comparative hybridization (aCGH) show a high incidence of deletions and duplications in the genome that do not correspond to common genomic variants. Edorgan and colleagues, in a study of 105 patients with CHD, identified such changes in 18 (17%).[120]

Many of those regions are likely to harbor genes that are important in the causation of CHD. Many similar studies in progress will in the future help elucidate the underlying molecular mechanisms for various congenital heart lesions.

Nonsyndromic Congenital Heart Disease

Atrial Septal Defect

ASD is the third most common congenital heart malformation and occurs as an isolated defect or as a feature of more complex syndromes. It accounts for 10% of all isolated congenital heart malformations. A complex multifactorial inheritance model involving alterations in multiple genes and interactions with environment factors has been suggested to account for the lower penetrance and variable expressivity of familial ASDs. Autosomal dominant transmission has also been observed in some families, with affected relatives having secundum ASD or other congenital heart lesions. Coexisting heart block has been observed in some of the affected relatives.

Mutations of a heart muscle protein, α-myosin heavy chain (MYH6) are associated with ASDs. Several proteins that interact with MYH6 are also associated with cardiac defects. The transcription factor GATA4 forms a complex with the TBX5, which interacts with MYH6.[121] Another factor, the homeobox (developmental) gene, NKX2-5 also interacts with MYH6.[122] Mutations in these genes have been associated with human ASDs, notably the secundum ASDs (ASDII) (Table 17c-1).

Matsson and colleagues analyzed the ACTC1 gene in two large Swedish families segregating autosomal dominant secundum ASD and identified heterozygosity for a mutation in the 20 available affected individuals.[123] The authors studied 408 additional individuals referred for sporadic CHD and identified a 17-bp deletion in the ACTC1 gene in a 10-year-old girl with secundum ASD. The mutation was also identified in her clinically unaffected 43-year-old father, who was found to have an abnormal echocardiogram with a posteriorly deviated interventricular septum, believed to be associated with a spontaneously closed perimembranous ventricular septal defect (VSD), causing aortic valve regurgitation. Neither mutation was found in 580 control samples.

Ebstein Anomaly

Ebstein anomaly is rare and accounts for only 0.5% of all congenital heart malformations, with an incidence of 0.12 per 1000 live births. The cause of Ebstein anomaly is heterogeneous with most cases thought to be a multifactorial trait. An association between Ebstein anomaly with left ventricular noncompaction (LVNC) and mutations in MYH7 encoding β-myosin heavy chain has been reported. Dr. Alex V. Postma from Amsterdam along with additional members of his research team performed a multicenter study of cohorts from The Netherlands, Germany, and the United Kingdom.[124] They studied 141 Ebstein anomaly patients who were not related to each other for mutations in MYH7. In eight of the study participants, the researchers identified mutations in this gene. Six of these patients also suffered from the myocardial disease LVNC in addition to Ebstein anomaly. Ebstein anomaly has also been associated with in utero exposure to lithium.

Table 17c-1   SUMMARY OF DEFECTS AFFECTING THE CARDIOVASCULAR SYSTEM AND LIST OF INVOLVED GENES

Congenital Heart Disease	Phenotype	Involved Genes	Associated Diseases
Cyanotic heart disease	Transposition of the great arteries Tetralogy of Fallot Tricuspid atresia Pulmonary atresia Ebstein anomaly of the tricuspid valve Double outlet right ventricle Persistent truncus arteriosus Anomalous pulmonary venous connection	NKX2-5, THRAP2 NKX2-5, NOTCH1, TBX1, JAG1, NOTCH2 NKX2-5 PTPN11, JAG1, NOTCH2 NKX2-5 NKX2-5, THRAP2 TBX1	DiGeorge syndrome, Alagille syndrome Alagille syndrome DiGeorge syndrome
Left-sided obstruction defects	Hypoplastic left heart syndrome Mitral stenosis Aortic stenosis Aortic coarctation Interrupted aortic arch	NOTCH1 NOTCH1, PTPN11 NOTCH1, PTPN11 TBX1	DiGeorge syndrome
Septation defects	Atrial septation defects Ventricular septal defects Atrioventricular septal defects	NKX2-5, GATA4, TBX20, MYH6, TBX5 NKX2-5, GATA4, TBX20, MYH6, TBX5 PTPN11, KRAS, SOS1, RAF1, CRELD1	Holt-Oram syndrome Holt-Oram syndrome Noonan syndrome
Other congenital heart defects	Bicuspid aortic valve Patent ductus arteriosus	NOTCH1 TFAP2B	Char syndrome

Source: Modified from reference 165.

Patent Ductus Arteriosus

Isolated patent ductus arteriosus (PDA) is found in approximately 1 in 2000 full-term infants, constituting about 10% of all CHD, and is considerably more common in premature infants. PDAs in full-term infants presumably are multifactorial in origin. Environmental factors have been implicated, with in utero rubella infection being the most notable example. In those families where a single gene is suspected, however, the inheritance pattern has been interpreted as showing autosomal dominant and, in some cases autosomal recessive inheritance. Mutations in the TFAP2B gene and NOTCH1 genes have been identified in preterm infants with PDA (Table 17c-1).[125] There has also been a report of PDA and pulmonary valve stenosis in a patient with 18p deletion syndrome.[126] Char syndrome is an autosomal dominant disorder characterized by PDA, facial dysmorphism, and hand anomalies. A team of doctors and researchers from Mount Sinai School of Medicine, New York, and the University of Minnesota performed a genome scan with of 46 members of two unrelated families in which the disease was fully penetrant but the phenotype differed. Significant linkage was achieved with several polymorphic DNA markers mapping to chromosome 6p12-p21, which includes the TFAP2B gene.[127,128]

Coarctation of the Aorta

Aortic valve disease can be caused by mutation in the NOTCH1 gene, which maps to chromosome 9q (Table 17c-1).[129] Isolated coarctation of the aorta can be attributed to multifactorial inheritance, but a few families have been reported in which the transmission is autosomal dominant.[130] In such families, the recurrence risk is 50%. McBride and colleagues undertook a formal inheritance analysis of left ventricular outflow tract obstruction (LVOTO) in 124 families ascertained by an index case with aortic valve stenosis, coarctation of the aorta, or hypoplastic left heart.[131]

LVOTO malformations were noted in 30 relatives, along with significant congenital heart defects in two others, yielding a total of 32 (7.7%) of 413 relatives. Relative risk for first-degree relatives in this group was 36.9, with a heritability of 0.71 to 0.90. McBride and colleagues concluded that their data supported a complex but most likely oligogenic pattern of inheritance.[131]

Valvular Pulmonary Stenosis

Most types of valvular pulmonary stenosis fall into the multifactorial category, but a few families have been described with autosomal dominant transmission. In one family, a mother and her three children were affected. Two of the three affected children had other congenital heart lesions as well. A single causative gene has not been identified yet.[132]

Total Anomalous Pulmonary Venous Connections

Total anomalous pulmonary venous connection (TAPVC) accounts for 1.5% of all cardiovascular anomalies and has an incidence of 6.8/100,000 live births. The anomaly occurs as a feature of several syndromes, including cat eye syndrome, asplenia syndrome, and Holt-Oram syndrome. Isolated TAPVR is considered to be due to multifactorial causes. In 1960, the disorder was described in a father and daughter and referred to as the "scimitar syndrome," because of the radiographic appearance created by the anomalous vein draining the right lower lung and connecting the inferior vena cava.[133]

A large Utah-Idaho family was described in 1994, in which nonsyndromic TAPVC occurred as an autosomal dominant trait with incomplete penetrance and variable expression. There were 14 affected family members. The gene for TAPVC in this family has been mapped to 4p13-q12.[134] Other Utah families have not mapped to this chromosome locus, suggesting genetic heterogeneity in TAPVC. In an affected adult, recurrence in offspring is 50%, but reduced penetrance makes actual recurrence less than 50%.

Tetralogy of Fallot

Tetralogy of Fallot (TOF) is the most common cyanotic heart defect, occurring in approximately 400 per million live births and the most common cause of blue baby syndrome. It occurs slightly more often in males than in females. Its cause is thought to be due to environmental or genetic factors or a combination. TOF can be caused by mutations in the human homolog of rat Jagged-1 (JAG1) or in the NKX2-5 gene encoding the cardiac-specific homeobox.[135,136] Mutations in the ZFPM2, GDF1, GATA4, and TBX1 genes have been identified in sporadic cases of TOF (Table 17c-1).[137] Lambrechts and colleagues (2005) found that a haplotype of single nucleotide polymorphisms in the VEGF gene increased the risk for TOF.[138] VEGF was said to be the first modifier gene identified for TOF. Greenway and colleagues (2009) performed a genomewide survey of 114 subjects with TOF and their unaffected parents and identified 11 de novo copy number variants that were absent or extremely rare (less than 0.1%) in 2265 controls. They identified copy number variants at chromosome 1q21.1 in 1% of nonsyndromic sporadic TOF cases as well as at 3p25.1, 7p21.3 (gain), and 22q11.2 (loss). They concluded that their findings predicted at least 10% of sporadic nonsyndromic TOF cases result from de novo copy number variants.[137]

Tetralogy of Fallot is also a well-recognized feature of the 22q11 microdeletion syndrome and trisomy 21. Johnson and colleagues conducted a cytogenetic evaluation of 159 cases of tetralogy of Fallot.[139] A deletion (22q11) was identified in 14% who underwent FISH testing. Rauch and colleagues found that 22q11.2 deletion was the most common genetic anomaly among 230 patients with TOF, found in 7.4% of patients.[140] The second most common anomaly was trisomy 21, found in 5.2% of patients, which was often associated with atrioventricular septal defect. Other chromosomal aberrations or submicroscopic copy number changes were found in 3% of patients.

Digilio and colleagues (1997) calculated empiric risk figures for recurrence of isolated tetralogy of Fallot in families after exclusion of del(22q11).[141] Their results showed that the frequency of congenital heart defect was 3% in siblings, 0.5% in parents, 0.3% in grandparents, 0.2% in uncles or aunts, and 0.6% in first cousins and concluded that genes different from those located on 22q11 must be involved in causing familial aggregation of nonsyndromic tetralogy of Fallot in these cases.[134]

Transposition of Great Arteries

Transposition of the great arteries (TGA) can be both isolated or part of a syndrome. Deletions in the NKX2-5 and THRAP2 genes have been reported.[142] TGA can also be seen in chromosomal abnormalities such as trisomy 18 and 21. Rarely, it may be part of the 22q11 deletion syndrome. As CFC1 mutations have been identified in subjects with heterotaxy syndrome, all of whom had congenital cardiac malformations, including malposition of the great arteries. Goldmuntz and colleagues hypothesized that a subset of patients with similar types of CHD—namely, transposition of the great arteries and double-outlet right ventricle, in the absence of laterality defects—would also have CFC1 mutations.[143] They analyzed the CFC1 gene in patients with these cardiac disorders and identified two disease-related mutations in 86 patients.

Syndromic Congenital Heart Disease

Holt-Oram Syndrome

Holt-Oram syndrome is the most common of the "heart-hand syndromes," in which a CHD is associated with an upper limb deficiency. It is characterized by skeletal defects of the upper limb involving radial ray structures and may include hypoplasia or absence of the radius, absent thumb or triphalangeal fingerlike thumb, as well as anomalies of the scaphoid bone, humerus, and clavicle. The most common heart lesions are secundum ASD, VSD, and PDA. ASD alone or in combination with other heart lesions occurs in about 60% of patients. In addition, 17% have more complicated heart malformations such as tetralogy of Fallot or AV canal defect, and 6% have severe defects, including TAPVC, double outlet right ventricle, and hypoplastic left heart syndrome. Individuals with Holt-Oram syndrome with or without a congenital heart malformation are at risk for cardiac conduction disease. While individuals may present at birth with sinus bradycardia and first-degree atrioventricular (AV) block, AV block can progress unpredictably to a higher grade including complete heart block with and without atrial fibrillation.[144] Holt-Oram syndrome is not associated with dysmorphic facial features, extensive visceral malformations, lower limb anomalies, or cognitive deficiencies.

Mutations in the TBX5 gene on chromosome 12q24.1 account for more than 70% of individuals who meet the diagnostic criteria of Holt-Oram syndrome.[145] It is characterized by autosomal dominant inheritance with over 90% penetrance, with a prevalence of 1 per 100,000 live births. Recurrence in offspring is 50%. TBX5 is a T-box transcription factor that plays a critical role in organogenesis. To date, 34 different TBX5 mutations have been described in patients with Holt-Oram syndrome that are expected to produce truncated TBX5 proteins or no TBX5 at all. Based on these findings, TBX5 haploinsufficiency has been proposed as a mechanism underlying pathogenesis of Holt-Oram syndrome. It is interesting to note that increased TBX5 dosage, such as a chromosome 12q2 duplication, also results in Holt-Oram syndrome, suggesting that TBX5 dosage is critical to the development of the heart and limbs.[146] Additionally, genotype-phenotype correlations have been noted as missense mutations at the 5' end of the T-box have been reported to be associated with more serious cardiac defects, while missense mutations at the 3' end of the T-box are associated with more pronounced limb defects.[147] However, application of these population-based associations should be done cautiously, especially in individuals in whom mutations may not predict specific phenotypes.

Rarely, clinically typical Holt-Oram syndrome may be caused by mutations in the SALL4 gene, mutations that are usually associated with Duane-radial ray syndrome (DRRS, Okihiro syndrome) and acro-renal-ocular syndrome (AROS).[147]

17

Noonan Syndrome

Noonan syndrome is characterized by short stature, typical facial features, and congenital heart defects.

The main facial features are hypertelorism with down-slanting palpebral fissures, ptosis, low-set posteriorly rotated ears with a thickened helix, high arched palate, micrognathia, and a short neck with excess nuchal skin and a low posterior hairline. Additional features include neonatal feeding difficulties and failure to thrive, present in 63% of patients. Short stature is present in 60% of individuals with Noonan syndrome and webbed neck in 80% of recognized cases.[148]

Cryptorchidism at birth is present in about 77% of male patients. Chest deformities, which include superior pectus carinatum and inferior pectus excavatum, are present in 70-95% of cases with increased inter-nipple distance in 80%. Microcephaly is present in most individuals with Noonan syndrome, but macrocephaly may also be present. Mild motor delay attributable to muscular hypotonia is present in childhood and mild intellectual deficit is present in 15-35% of patients with Noonan syndrome. Lymphatic vessel dysplasia leading to lymphedema or lymphangiectasia can be seen in 20%. Up to 55% of cases have a mild-to-moderate bleeding tendency and there is no correlation between the results of coagulation tests and a history of easy bruising.

The most common congenital heart defect is pulmonary valve stenosis with dysplastic leaflets seen in 50-62% of cases. Hypertrophic obstructive cardiomyopathy with asymmetrical septum hypertrophy is present in 20% of patients. ASDs occur in 6-10% of cases, VSDs occur in 5% of cases, and persistent ductus arteriosus occurs in 3% of cases. Other congenital heart defects more often seen in Noonan syndrome are atrioventricular canal defect associated with subaortic obstruction and structural anomalies of the mitral valve.[149]

Noonan syndrome is inherited as an autosomal dominant trait and the incidence is estimated to between 1:1000 and 1:2500 live births. Many affected individuals have de novo mutations; however, an affected parent is recognized in 30-75% of families. Four genes are known to be associated with Noonan syndrome: PTPN11, KRAS, SOS1, and RAF1.[150-153] In approximately 50% of the patients with definite Noonan syndrome, a missense mutation is found in the PTPN11 gene on chromosome 12, which encodes for an enzyme, tyrosine protein phosphatase nonreceptor type II (SHP-2), an extracellular protein. This enzyme is required in several pathways that control diverse developmental processes including cardiac semilunar valvulogenesis, blood cell progenitor commitment, and differentiation, as well as modulating cellular proliferation, differentiation, migration, and apoptosis. The mutation results in a gain of function of SHP-2, which stimulates epidermal growth factor-mediated RAS/ERK/MAPK activation, increasing cell proliferation. These mutations are found in 59% of the familial cases and in 37% of the sporadic cases. The only reported deletion in PTPN11 was a three-nucleotide deletion (p.Gly60del) in a female infant with severe features of Noonan syndrome, including hydrops fetalis and juvenile myelomonocytic leukemia.[154] Less than 5% of patients were found to have mutations in the KRAS gene, 10-13% were found to have mutations in the SOS1 gene, and 3-17% in the RAF1 gene.

The Noonan syndrome phenotype in females overlaps greatly with that of Turner syndrome; therefore, chromosome studies must be ordered in all patients with suspected Noonan syndrome. PTPN11 and RAF1 mutations also cause LEOPARD syndrome, which resembles Noonan syndrome but has lentigines and deafness.[150] Mutations in KRAS are occasionally also seen in cardiofaciocutaneous syndrome, features of which overlap greatly with those of Noonan syndrome, but have a higher incidence of mental deficiency, structural central nervous system anomalies, skin pathology, and gastrointestinal problems. Because of the existing genetic heterogeneity and continued high percentage of mutation negative individuals, the discovery of additional genes in the future is likely.

Alagille Syndrome

Alagille syndrome is a multisystem disorder, the main features of which are intrahepatic cholestasis, CHD, skeletal and ocular anomalies. The clinical features are highly variable, even within families. In about 90% of patients, there is a history of prolonged neonatal jaundice resulting from paucity of intrahepatic and occasionally extrahepatic bile ducts. Cardiac lesions occur in about 85% of patients and are predominantly peripheral pulmonary stenosis but might include pulmonary valve stenosis, seen in 67% of individuals. The most common complex cardiac defect is tetralogy of Fallot, seen in 7-16% of individuals. Others include partial anomalous venous drainage, VSD, ASD, aortic stenosis, and coarctation of the aorta.[155] About 90% of Alagille patients have ocular anomalies which include anterior segment dysgenesis, particularly posterior embryotoxon, as well as pigmentary retinopathy. Bilateral optic disc drusen is found in 80% and unilateral drusen in 95%. The visual prognosis is good, although mild decreases in visual acuity may occur. Skeletal manifestations include hemivertebrae or butterfly vertebrae in about 30-90% of patients and short stature occurs in 50%. Typical facial features include a prominent forehead, deep-set eyes with moderate hypertelorism, pointed chin, and saddle or straight nose with a bulbous tip. These features give the face the appearance of an inverted triangle. Other features include renal abnormalities, pancreatic insufficiency, growth failure, intellectual disability, delayed puberty, and neurovascular accidents. The liver abnormalities resolve with age, but occasional individuals can have more severe hepatic problems requiring transplantation. Mortality is approximately 10%, with vascular accidents, cardiac disease, and liver disease accounting for most of the deaths.[136]

Alagille syndrome is an autosomal dominant trait with incomplete penetrance. The two genes associated with Alagille are JAG1 and NOTCH2. Sequence analysis of JAG1 detects mutations in more than 89% of individuals who meet clinical diagnostic criteria.[156] Microdeletion of 20p12, including the entire JAG1 gene, is seen in approximately 7% of affected individuals. Mutations in NOTCH2 are observed in less than 1% of individuals with Alagille syndrome.[157]

Approximately 30%-50% of individuals have an inherited mutation and about 50-70% have a de novo mutation. The parents of a child with a de novo mutation have a low but increased risk for recurrence because of the possibility of germline mosaicism. Prenatal testing for pregnancies at increased risk is possible if the JAG1 or NOTCH2 disease-causing mutation in an affected family member is known. Prenatal testing cannot predict the occurrence or severity of clinical manifestations.

VATER Association

VATER is a useful acronym for the nonrandom association of vertebral defects, anal atresia, tracheoesophageal fistula with esophageal atresia, and radial or renal dysplasia. The VATER association has been expanded to VACTREL which includes cardiac malformations and limb anomalies. Nearly all cases have been sporadic.[158]

Using a birth defects surveillance registry, Khoury and colleagues investigated the interrelation of the 6 components of the VACTERL association.[159] Of the 400 cases included in the registry, 50 cases were considered to have the VACTERL association. VSD was the most common cardiovascular defect (30%) and renal agenesis was the most common renal anomaly (30%); the most common limb defects were reduction deformities (34%) and polydactyly (20%).

VATER association shares phenotypic features with Fanconi anemia such as gastrointestinal atresias, skeletal, renal and cardiac abnormalities. They can be differentiated by chromosome breakage and diepoxybutane (DEB)-induced chromosome studies which have identified many of the genes associated with Fanconi anemia.

Other conditions that overlap with the VATER phenotype include Holt-Oram syndrome, Townes-Brocks syndrome, and the Mullerian duct aplasia, renal aplasia, cervicothoracic somite dysplasia (MURCS) association.[160]

Garcia-Barcelo and colleagues identified a heterozygous de novo 21-bp deletion in a polyalanine tract in the HOXD13 gene in a 17-year-old girl with many features of the VACTERL association.[161] Although the authors could not rule out a second mutation elsewhere in the genome as causative for the disorder, the findings suggested that the sonic hedgehog pathway may also be involved in the development of gut and genitourinary structures in addition to limb development. A few cases of parent-to-child transmission have been recorded with the VATER association. Thus although the recurrence risk for offspring is less than 1%, it is prudent to use ultrasound to monitor at-risk pregnancies.

CHARGE Association

CHARGE is an acronym that stands for *c*oloboma, *h*eart defects, choanal *a*tresia, *r*etarded growth and development, *g*enital abnormalities, and *e*ar anomalies. CHARGE syndrome is characterized by unilateral or bilateral coloboma of the iris, retina-choroid, and/or disc with or without microphthalmos (80-90% of individuals); unilateral or bilateral choanal atresia or stenosis (50-60%); cranial nerve dysfunction resulting in hyposmia or anosmia, unilateral or bilateral facial palsy (40%), impaired hearing and/or swallowing problems (70-90%); abnormal outer ears, ossicular malformations, Mondini defect of the cochlea, and absent or hypoplastic semicircular canals (>90%); cryptorchidism in males and hypogonadotrophic hypogonadism in both males and females; developmental delay; cardiovascular malformations (75-85%); growth deficiency (70-80%); orofacial clefts (15-20%); and tracheoesophageal fistula (15-20%).[162,163] Feeding difficulties are a major cause of morbidity in all age groups.

CHD7, encoding the chromodomain helicase DNA binding protein, is the only gene currently known to be associated with CHARGE syndrome.[164] Sequence analysis of the CHD7 coding region detects mutations in approximately 60-70% of individuals with CHARGE syndrome. It is inherited in an autosomal dominant manner although most cases are de novo in occurrence. If neither parent is affected, the empiric risk to siblings of a proband is approximately 1-2%, most likely attributable to germline mosaicism. Prenatal diagnosis for pregnancies at increased risk is possible if the disease-causing CHD7 mutation has been identified in an affected family member.[165]

Kabuki Syndrome

Kabuki syndrome is a congenital mental retardation syndrome with additional features, including postnatal dwarfism, dysmorphic facies characterized by long palpebral fissures with eversion of the lateral third of the lower eyelids, a broad and depressed nasal tip, large prominent earlobes, a cleft or high-arched palate, scoliosis, short fifth finger, persistence of fingerpads, dermatoglyphic abnormalities including increased digital ulnar loop and hypothenar loop patterns, radiographic abnormalities of the vertebrae, hands, and hip joints, and recurrent otitis media in infancy.[166] Congenital heart defects, including single ventricle with a common atrium, VSD, ASD, TOF, PDA, coarctation of aorta, aneurysm of aorta, transposition of great vessels, and right bundle branch block have been observed.[167]

Ng and colleagues identified 33 distinct MLL2 mutations (mapped to chromosome 12q12-q14) in 35 of 53 families (66%) with Kabuki syndrome.[168] In each of 12 cases for which DNA from both parents was available, the MLL2 variant was found to have occurred de novo. MLL2 mutations were also identified in each of two families in which Kabuki syndrome was transmitted from parent to child. None of the additional MLL2 mutations were found in 190 control chromosomes from individuals of matched geographic ancestry.

Down Syndrome

Down syndrome is one of the most frequent congenital birth defects, with an estimated incidence of 1/733 births, and the most common genetic cause of mental retardation. Approximately 95% of patients with Down syndrome have complete trisomy 21 in which there is an extra copy of chromosome 21. In rare cases, partial trisomy of chromosome 21 is present due to a chromosomal translocation or mosaicism.

It is unclear whether particular gene loci on chromosome 21 are sufficient to cause Down syndrome and its associated features. In 2009, Korbel and colleagues[169] assembled a high-resolution genetic map of Down syndrome phenotypes based on an analysis of 30 subjects carrying rare segmental trisomies of various regions of chromosome 21. They identified discrete regions of 1.8-16.3 Mb likely to be involved in the development of eight Down syndrome phenotypes, including acute mega-karyocytic leukemia, transient myeloproliferative disorder, Hirschsprung disease, duodenal stenosis, imperforate anus, severe mental retardation, Down syndrome-Alzheimer disease, and Down syndrome–specific CHD. This phenotypic map located Down syndrome–specific heart disease to a less than 2-Mb interval. Furthermore, this study provided evidence against the specific hypotheses of the presence of a single Down syndrome consensus region and the sufficiency of *DSCR1* and *DYRK1A*, or *APP*, in causing several severe Down syndrome phenotypes.

In 2008, Lyle 2009, Lyle and associates[170] reported the identification and mapping of 30 pathogenic chromosomal aberrations of chromosome 21 consisting of 19 partial trisomies and 11 partial monosomies for different segments of chromosome 21. Twenty-six of the 30 partial aneuploidies map within a 10-Mb region. They identified susceptibility regions for 25 phenotypes for Down syndrome and 27 regions for monosomy 21. Their data also argued against a single Down syndrome critical region.

Frequent features of Down syndrome include microbrachycephaly, sparse hair, midfacial hypoplasia with small nose, upslanted eyes with epicanthal folds and Brushfield spots in the irides, protruding tongue, single transverse palmar creases, fifth finger clinodactyly, brachydactyly, a gap between first and second toes, atlanto-axial instability, a hypoplastic pelvis, and joint laxity. Neurodevelopmental challenges include hypotonia, developmental delay, visual impairment, hearing loss, and moderate mental retardation. The mean intelligence quotient is usually in the 30-70 range, but there are occasional exceptions. The pathologic, metabolic, and neurochemical changes of Alzheimer disease are present in the brains of almost all individuals with Down syndrome, accounting for a progressive loss of cognitive function.

Approximately half of Down syndrome individuals are found to have a CHD, 60% of whom have some type of an AV canal defect and 30-40% a canal-type VSD.[171]

Additional CHDs may include an ASD, patent ductus arteriosus, tetralogy of Fallot, or double outlet right ventricle. Down syndrome individuals are 10-20 times more likely to develop acute leukemia than normal individuals. Hematologic abnormalities, autoimmunity, immunologic dysfunction, and thyroid disease are common.

Pregnancy is rare in women with Down syndrome, with 31 pregnancies reported in 27 women; these frequently are the result of sexual abuse.[172] About one third of the offspring have Down syndrome, one third are cytogenetically and phenotypically normal, and for reasons that are not clear, one third of the offspring have normal chromosomes but abnormal phenotype. Males with Down syndrome have normal spermatogenesis but usually do not reproduce owing to their low IQ. One case of a cytogenetically normal male infant that was fathered by a man with Down syndrome was reported by Sheridan and colleagues.[173]

Turner Syndrome

Turner syndrome is defined by a partially or completely absent X chromosome. Fifty percent of females with Turner syndrome have a 45,X karyotype. Less frequently there exist karyotype variations which include an isochromosome X, short arm or long arm deletion, ring chromosome and mosaicism, and a combination of cell lines such as 45,X and 46,XX. The heterogeneity of karyotypes results in a spectrum of phenotypes. Many reports indicate that mosaicism tends to moderate outcome and studies show that physical features such as cardiovascular symptoms and gonadal dysfunction tend to vary in frequency across the different karyotypes. In the Danish study in 1994, Gotzsche and associates reported a higher incidence of cardiovascular malformations among 45,X females—38% vs. 11% for mosaics.[174] One of the missing genes on the X chromosome is the short stature homeobox (*SHOX*) gene located on the pseudoautosomal region of the X-chromosome. *SHOX* has been identified as a candidate gene for short stature as well as for skeletal abnormalities associated with Turner syndrome, including high-arched palate, abnormal auricular development, cubitus valgus, genu valgum, and short metacarpals.[175] Other missing genes regulate ovarian development, which influences sexual characteristics.

The most common physical abnormalities affecting girls with Turner syndrome include short stature (more than 50% of cases), webbed neck (60% of cases), broad chest with wide-spaced nipples, hypertension, elevated hepatic enzymes, middle ear infection, perception hearing loss (50% of cases), micrognathia, cubitus valgus, poor thriving during the first postnatal year, estrogen deficiency, primary amenorrhea, and infertility as a result of streak gonads. Females with Turner syndrome also have significantly higher risks for certain diseases compared with the general population including hypothyroidism, diabetes, heart disease, osteoporosis, congenital malformations (heart, urinary system, face, neck, ears), neurovascular disease, cirrhosis of the liver, and colon and rectal cancers.

Cardiac abnormalities are considered the most serious medical problems associated with Turner syndrome. The most common CHDs are bicuspid aortic valve (approximately 15%) with/without aortic stenosis, mitral valve anomalies (<5%), coarctation of the aorta (approximately 10%), and rarely, hypoplastic left heart syndrome. Additional CHDs include partial anomalous pulmonary venous connection (13%) and ASD or VSD (5% each). Magnetic resonance imaging has identified additional vascular anomalies, notably elongation of the transverse arch (almost 50%), which may be accompanied by pseudocoarctation. Aortic root dilatation, aneurysm, dissection, and rupture in Turner syndrome are well established. Most cases of dissection in Turner syndrome have been associated with an underlying risk factor, such as bicuspid aortic valve and/or coarctation (69%) or hypertension (54%) with or without a CHD.[176] Compared to the Danish Registry estimate of aortic dissection (78/100,000) a prospective study by Matura and colleagues showed a much higher frequency of aortic dissection (618/100,000 Turner syndrome years).[177]

Spontaneous pregnancy is rare among women with Turner syndrome, but with the availability of assisted reproductive techniques such as donor egg and in vitro fertilization, pregnancy is increasingly pursued. There is no risk for Turner syndrome in offspring that result from using this method.

DiGeorge Syndrome

The 22q11.2 deletion syndrome encompasses the phenotypes previously called DiGeorge syndrome, velocardiofacial syndrome (Shprintzen syndrome), conotruncal anomaly face syndrome (CTAF), many cases of the autosomal dominant Opitz G/BBB syndrome, and Cayler cardiofacial syndrome (asymmetric crying facies). These syndromes have been incorporated into a group under the acronym CATCH 22 (conotruncal cardiac defect, abnormal face, thymic hypoplasia, cleft palate, hypocalcemia, microdeletion 22q11). The 22q11.2 deletion syndrome is the most commonly diagnosed chromosome deletion syndrome with an estimated prevalence between 1 in 4000 and 1 in 7000 live births and is calculated to be present in between 1.5% and 5% of children with a CHD.[178]

The phenotypic features are broad.[179] Characteristic facial features include narrow palpebral fissures, "hooded" eyelids, broad nasal root, bulbous nasal tip, overfolded external ears, and small mouth and chin. Individuals with the 22q11.2 deletion syndrome have a range of findings, including CHD (74% of individuals), particularly conotruncal malformations (tetralogy of Fallot, interrupted aortic arch, VSD, and truncus arteriosus); palatal abnormalities (69%), particularly velopharyngeal incompetence (VPI), submucosal cleft palate, and cleft palate; characteristic facial features (present in the majority of Caucasian individuals); and learning difficulties (70-90%). Seventy-seven percent of individuals have an immune deficiency regardless of their clinical presentation. Additional findings include hypocalcemia (50%), significant feeding problems (30%), renal anomalies (37%), hearing loss (both conductive and sensorineural), laryngotracheoesophageal anomalies, growth hormone deficiency, autoimmune disorders, seizures (without hypocalcemia), and skeletal abnormalities. Schizophrenia, major depression, and bipolar disease have been reported in 25-30% of adults with chromosome 22q11 deletion. Studies also suggest that 2-9% of patients with schizophrenia have chromosome 22q11 deletions. Routine psychiatric evaluations should be considered for all patients with chromosome 22q11 deletion.[180]

Deletion of genes in the DiGeorge chromosomal region (DGCR) is the only genetic defect known to be associated with deletion 22q11.2.[181] The 22q11.2 deletion syndrome is diagnosed in individuals with a submicroscopic deletion of chromosome 22 detected by FISH. Fewer than 5% of individuals with clinical symptoms of the 22q11.2 deletion syndrome have normal routine cytogenetic studies and negative FISH testing. A small percentage (<1%) of individuals with clinical findings of the 22q11.2 deletion syndrome have chromosomal rearrangements involving 22q11.2, such as a translocation between chromosome 22 and another chromosome, hence cytogenetic analysis is recommended at the time of FISH studies. Mutations in TBX1 have been found in individuals with DiGeorge syndrome who do not have a deletion.[182,183] It is still uncertain what other genes must be deleted since mutations in TBX1 do not account for the central nervous system manifestations of deletion 22q11.2 syndrome. Furthermore, some individuals with features of 22q11.2 deletion syndrome, including typical conotruncal cardiac anomalies, have not had either an identifiable deletion by FISH analysis or a TBX1 mutation.

The 22q11.2 deletion syndrome is a contiguous deletion syndrome inherited in an autosomal dominant manner. About 93% of probands have a de novo deletion of 22q11.2. Seven percent have inherited the deletion from a parent. Recommendations for the evaluation of parents of a proband include FISH testing because mildly affected adults, as well as normal adults with somatic mosaicism, have been identified.[180]

Williams Syndrome

The classic Williams syndrome phenotype comprises elastin arteriopathy, characteristic face, connective tissue abnormalities, growth and psychomotor retardation, behavioral abnormalities especially overfriendliness, and occasionally hypercalcemia in infancy. Facial features consist of broad brow, periorbital fullness, a stellate/lacy iris pattern, strabismus, short nose, full nasal tip, malar hypoplasia, long philtrum, full lips, wide mouth, malocclusion, small jaw, and prominent earlobes. Young children have epicanthal folds, full cheeks, and small, widely spaced teeth, while adults typically have a long face and neck, accentuated by sloping shoulders. Many adults are capable of holding simple supervised jobs, but independent living is usually restricted more by mental and adaptive limitations than by physical limitations. Overfriendliness, empathy, generalized anxiety, and attention deficit disorder are commonly observed.[184]

The growth pattern is characterized by prenatal growth deficiency, failure to thrive in infancy, and poor weight gain and linear growth in the first 4 years. The mean adult height is below the third centile. Endocrine abnormalities include idiopathic hypercalcemia (15%), hypercalciuria (30%), hypothyroidism (10%), and early (but not precocious) puberty (50%). An increased frequency of subclinical hypothyroidism, abnormal oral glucose tolerance tests, and diabetes mellitus is observed in adults with Williams syndrome. Renal malformations are found in about 18% of individuals and include renal agenesis or hypoplasia, duplicated kidney, and renal artery stenosis.

Cardiovascular disease is a common feature characterized by elastin arteriopathy, peripheral pulmonary stenosis, supravalvular aortic stenosis, and hypertension. Valvar aortic stenosis, bicuspid aortic valve, and mitral valve prolapse are also common. Other complications include connective tissue abnormalities, which result in hoarse voice, inguinal/umbilical hernia, bowel/bladder diverticula, rectal prolapse, joint limitation or laxity, and soft, lax skin.[185]

Contiguous gene deletions in the Williams-Beuren syndrome critical region (WBSCR) are known to be associated with Williams syndrome. A microdeletion of chromosome 7q11 encompassing the elastin (ELN) gene can be demonstrated in over 99% of individuals with the clinical diagnosis of Williams syndrome.[186] This is confirmed by chromosome studies and FISH using a probe specific for this region, or by targeted mutation analysis using real-time PCR or genomic microarray analysis. Despite at least 21 genes having been identified in the critical 1.5-Mb region in

17

humans, their individual contribution to the multisystem phenotype of Williams syndrome is unclear. So far, only the gene coding for elastin (*ELN*) has been proven to be causally involved. Intragenic deletions and translocations disrupting the elastin gene have been documented in dominant supravalvular aortic stenosis which lacks the cognitive, behavior, and phenotypic abnormalities of Williams syndrome. Except for a few cases that are caused by balanced chromosome translocations, all micro-deletion cases are sporadic. Transmission of the deletion from parents to their off-spring is limited by their intellectual capacity, although if it did occur it would be inherited in an autosomal dominant manner.[187]

Heterotaxy

Heterotaxy, also called *situs ambiguus, asplenia syndrome, Ivemark syndrome,* and *polysplenia syndrome,* is a complex congenital disorder characterized by the disruption of the normal left-right (LR) asymmetry of the thoracoabdominal organs, including the heart, lungs, liver, spleen, and stomach, thought to arise from disturbances in early developmental processes dependent on the establishment of the embryonic LR axis. Patients with segmental discordances in the asymmetric thoracoabdominal organs typically have complex cardiac and vascular abnormalities that are thought to involve partial or complete reversal of cardiac looping, LR patterning of the atria, or the failure of asymmetric remodeling of symmetric embryonic structures. Examples of congenital cardiovascular malformations that are highly suggestive of defects in embryonic LR patterning include dextrocardia, mesocardia, levo-transposition of great arteries, and atrial isomerisms. Other commonly associated cardiac defects, including pulmonic stenosis, pulmonary atresia, anomalous pulmonary venous return, interrupted inferior vena cava, persistent left superior vena cava, dextro-transposition of the great arteries (d-TGA), double-outlet right ventricle, VSD, ASD, single ventricle, hypoplastic left heart, and coarctation of the aorta, apparently can arise by more than one mechanism although they are often observed as part of the complex defects in heterotaxy.[188,189]

Mutations or chromosomal imbalances affecting ZIC3, CFC1, ACVR2B, LEFTY2, NKX2.5, CRELD1, NODAL, CRIPTO, and GDF1 have been associated with either heterotaxy or related cardiovascular malformations in humans.[190] In addition, a de novo reciprocal translocation t (6,18) (q21;q21) in a subject with heterotaxy was found to disrupt the SESN1 (PA26) locus. Currently, clinical genetic testing is available for Visceral Heterotaxy-1, X-linked, which tests for mutations in the ZIC3 gene, Visceral Heterotaxy-2, Autosomal, which tests for mutations in CFC1, and Visceral Heterotaxy-5, Autosomal, which tests for mutations in NODAL. Mutations in the remaining genes can be tested for on a research basis.

For most current information about genetic testing go to www.genetests.org.

References

115. Hoffman JI. Incidence of congenital heart disease. II. Prenatal incidence. Pediatr Cardiol. 1995;16: 155-165.
116. van Karnebeek CD, Hennekam RC. Associations between chromosomal anomalies and congenital heart defects: a database search. Am J Med Genet. 1999;84:158-166.
117. Goetz SC, Brown DD, Conlon FL. TBX5 is required for embryonic cardiac cell cycle progression. Development. 2006;133:2575-2584.
118. Marino B, Digilio MC. Congenital heart disease and genetic syndromes: specific correlation between cardiac phenotype and genotype. Cardiovasc Pathol. 2000;9:303-315.
119. Miller DT, Adam MP, Aradhya S, et al. Consensus statement: chromosomal microarray is a first-tier clinical diagnostic test for individuals with developmental disabilities or congenital anomalies. Am J Hum Genet. 2010;86:749-764.
120. Erdogan F, Larsen LA, Zhang L, et al. High frequency of submicroscopic genomic aberrations detected by tiling path array comparative genome hybridisation in patients with isolated congenital heart disease. J Med Genet. 2008;45(11):704-709.
121. Hirayama-Yamada K, Kamisago M, Akimoto K, et al. Phenotypes with GATA4 or NKX2.5 mutations in familial atrial septal defect. Am J Med Genet A. 2005;135A:47-52.
122. Posch MG, Perrot A, Berger F, et al. Molecular genetics of congenital atrial septal defects. Clin Res Cardiol. 2010;99:137-147.
123. Matsson H, Eason J, Bookwalter CS, et al. Alpha-cardiac actin mutations produce atrial septal defects. Hum Mol Genet. 2008;17:256-265.

17

124. Postma AV. Mutations in the sarcomere gene MYH7 in Ebstein's anomaly. Circ Cardiovasc Genet. 2011;4:43-50.
125. Dagle JM, Lepp NT, Cooper ME, et al. Determination of genetic predisposition to patent ductus arteriosus in preterm infants. Pediatrics. 2009;123:1116-1123.
126. Xie CH, Yang JB, Gong FQ, et al. Patent ductus arteriosus and pulmonary valve stenosis in a patient with 18p deletion syndrome. Yonsei Med J. 2008;49:500-502.
127. Satoda M, Zhao F, Diaz GA, et al. Mutations in TFAP2B cause Char syndrome, a familial form of patent ductus arteriosus. Nat Genet. 2000;25:42-46.
128. Sletten LJ, Pierpont ME. Familial occurrence of patent ductus arteriosus. Am J Med Genet. 1995;57:27-30.
129. Garg V, Muth AN, Ransom JF, et al. Mutations in NOTCH1 cause aortic valve disease. Nature. 2005;437:270-274.
130. Beekman RH, Robinow M. Coarctation of the aorta inherited as an autosomal dominant trait. Am J Cardiol. 1985;56:818-819.
131. McBride KL, Zender GA, Fitzgerald-Butt SM, et al. Linkage analysis of left ventricular outflow tract malformations (aortic valve stenosis, coarctation of the aorta, and hypoplastic left heart syndrome). Eur J Hum Genet. 2009;17(6):811-819.
132. Lamy M, de Grouchy J, Schweisguth O. Genetic and non-genetic factors in the etiology of congenital heart disease: a study of 1188 cases. Am J Hum Genet. 1957;9:17-41.
133. Neill CA, Ferencz C, Sabiston DC, et al. The familial occurrence of hypoplastic right lung with systemic arterial supply and venous drainage "scimitar syndrome." Bull Johns Hopkins Hosp. 1960;107:1-21.
134. Bleyl S, Nelson L, Ward K. A gene for familial total anomalous pulmonary venous return maps to chromosome 4p13-q12. Am J Hum Genet. 1995;56:408-415.
135. Goldmuntz E, Geiger E, Benson DW. NKX2.5 mutations in patients with tetralogy of Fallot. Circulation. 2001;104:2565-2568.
136. Kamath B, Bason L. Consequences of JAG1 mutations. J Med Genet. 2003;40(12):891-895.
137. Greenway SC, Pereira AC, Lin JC, et al. De novo copy number variants identify new genes and loci in isolated, sporadic tetralogy of Fallot. Nat Genet. 2009;41(8):931-935.
138. Lambrechts D, Devriendt K, Driscoll DA, et al. Low expression VEGF haplotype increases the risk for tetralogy of Fallot: a family based association study. J Med Genet. 2005;42:519-522.
139. Johnson MC, Hing A, Wood MK, et al. Chromosome abnormalities in congenital heart disease. Am J Med Genet. 1997;70:292-298.
140. Rauch R, Hofbeck M, Zweier C, et al. Comprehensive genotype-phenotype analysis in 230 patients with tetralogy of Fallot. J Med Genet. 2010;47:321-331.
141. Digilio MC, Marino B, Giannotti A, et al. Recurrence risk figures for isolated tetralogy of Fallot after screening for 22q11 microdeletion. J Med Genet. 1997;34:188-190.
142. Muncke N, Jung C, Rudiger H, et al. Missense mutations and gene interruption in PROSIT240, a novel TRAP240-like gene, in patients with congenital heart defect (transposition of the great arteries). Circulation. 2003;108:2843-2850.
143. Goldmuntz E, Bamford R, Karkera JD, et al. CFC1 mutations in patients with transposition of the great arteries and double-outlet right ventricle. Am J Hum Genet. 2002;70:776-780.
144. Sletten LJ, Pierpont ME. Variation in severity of cardiac disease in Holt-Oram syndrome. Am J Med Genet. 1996;65:128-132.
145. Heinritz W, Moschik A, Kujat A, et al. Identification of new mutations in the TBX5 gene in patients with Holt-Oram syndrome. Heart. 2005;91(3):383-384.
146. Basson CT, Huang T, Lin RC, et al. Different TBX5 interactions in heart and limb defined by Holt-Oram syndrome mutations. Proc Natl Acad Sci U S A. 1999;96:2919-2924.
147. Brassington AM, Sung SS, Toydemir RM, et al. Expressivity of Holt-Oram syndrome is not predicted by TBX5 genotype. Am J Hum Genet. 2003;73:74-85.
148. van der Burgt I. Noonan syndrome. Orphanet J Rare Dis. 2007;2:4.
149. Noonan JA. Noonan syndrome and related disorders. Prog Pediatr Cardiol. 2005;20:177-185.
150. Pandit B, Sarkozy A, Pennacchio LA, et al. Gain-of-function RAF1 mutations cause Noonan and LEOPARD syndromes with hypertrophic cardiomyopathy. Nat Genet. 2007;39:1007-1012.
151. Roberts AE, Araki T, Swanson KD. Germline gain-of-function mutations in SOS1 cause Noonan syndrome. Nat Genet. 2007;39:70-74.
152. Schubbert S, Zenker M, Rowe SL, et al. Germline KRAS mutations cause Noonan syndrome. Nat Genet. 2006;38:331-336.
153. Tartaglia M, Kalidas K, Shaw A, et al. PTPN11 mutations in Noonan syndrome: molecular spectrum, genotype-phenotype correlation, and phenotypic heterogeneity. Am J Hum Genet. 2002;70:1555-1563.
154. Yoshida R, Miyata M, Nagai T, et al. A 3-bp deletion mutation of PTPN11 in an infant with severe Noonan syndrome including hydrops fetalis and juvenile myelomonocytic leukemia. Am J Med Genet A. 2004;128A:63-66.
155. Emerick KM, Rand EB, Goldmuntz E, et al. Features of Alagille syndrome in 92 patients: frequency and relation to prognosis. Hepatology. 1999;29:822-829.
156. Krantz ID, Colliton RP, Genin A, et al. Spectrum and frequency of jagged1 (JAG1) mutations in Alagille syndrome patients and their families. Am J Hum Genet. 1998;62:1361-1369.
157. McDaniell R, Warthen D, Sanchez-Lara PA, et al. NOTCH2 mutations cause Alagille syndrome, a heterogeneous disorder of the notch signaling pathway. Am J Hum Genet. 2006;79(1):169-173.

158. Shaw-Smith C. Oesophageal atresia, tracheo-oesophageal fistula, and the VACTERL association: review of genetics and epidemiology. J Med Genet. 2006;43(7):545-554.
159. Khoury MJ, Cordero JF, Greenberg F, et al. A population study of the VACTERL association: evidence for its etiologic heterogeneity. Pediatrics. 1983;71:815-820.
160. Lopez AG, Fryns JP, Devriendt K. MURCS association with duplicated thumb. Clin Genet. 2002; 61:308-309.
161. Garcia-Barcelo MM, Wong KK, Lui VC, et al. Identification of a HOXD13 mutation in a VACTERL patient. Am J Med Genet A. 2008;146A:3181-3185.
162. Blake KD, Davenport SL, Hall BD, et al. CHARGE association: an update and review for the primary pediatrician. Clin Pediatr (Phila). 1998;37:159-173.
163. Davenport SL, Hefner MA, Mitchell JA. The spectrum of clinical features in CHARGE syndrome. Clin Genet. 1986;29:298-310.
164. Vissers LE, van Ravenswaaij CM, Admiraal R, et al. Mutations in a new member of the chromodomain gene family cause CHARGE syndrome. Nat Genet. 2004;36:955-957.
165. Lalani SR, Safiullah AM, Fernbach SD, et al. Spectrum of CHD7 mutations in 110 individuals with CHARGE syndrome and genotype-phenotype correlation. Am J Hum Genet. 2006;78:303-314.
166. Niikawa N, Matsuura N, Fukushima Y, et al. Kabuki make-up syndrome: a syndrome of mental retardation, unusual facies, large and protruding ears, and postnatal growth deficiency. J Pediatr. 1981;99:565-569.
167. Matsumoto N, Niikawa N. Kabuki make-up syndrome: a review. Am J Med Genet C Semin Med Genet. 2003;117C:57-65.
168. Ng SB, Bigham AW, Buckingham KJ, et al. Exome sequencing identifies MLL2 mutations as a cause of Kabuki syndrome. Nat Genet. 2010;9:790-793.
169. Korbel JO, Tirosh-Wagner T, Urban AE, et al. The genetic architecture of Down syndrome phenotypes revealed by high-resolution analysis of human segmental trisomies. Proc Natl Acad Sci U S A. 2009;106:12031-12036.
170. Lyle R, Bena F, Gagos S, et al. Genotype-phenotype correlations in Down syndrome identified by array CGH in 30 cases of partial trisomy and partial monosomy chromosome 21. Eur J Hum Genet. 2009;17:454-466.
171. Delabar JM, Theophile D, Rahmani Z, et al. Molecular mapping of twenty-four features of Down syndrome on chromosome 21. Eur J Hum Genet. 1993;1:114-124.
172. Rani S, Jyothi A, Reddy PP, et al. Reproduction in Down's syndrome. Int J Gynaecol Obstet`. 1990;31:81-86.
173. Sheridan R, Llerena J Jr, Matkins S, et al. Fertility in a male with trisomy 21. J Med Genet. 1989;26(5):294-298.
174. Gotzsche CO, Krag-Olsen B, Nielsen J, et al. Prevalence of cardiovascular malformations and association with karyotypes in Turner's syndrome. Arch Dis Child. 1994;71:433-436.
175. Rao E, Weiss B, Fukami M, et al. Pseudoautosomal deletions encompassing a novel homeobox gene cause growth failure in idiopathic short stature and Turner syndrome. Nat Genet. 1997;16:54-63.
176. Bondy CA. Aortic dissection in Turner syndrome. Curr Opin Cardiol. 2008;23:519-526.
177. Matura LA, Ho VB, Rosing DR, et al. Aortic dilatation and dissection in Turner syndrome. Circulation. 2007;116:1663-167.
178. Shprintzen RJ. Velo-cardio-facial syndrome: 30 years of study. Dev Disabil Res Rev. 2008;14: 3-10.
179. Oskarsdottir S, Persson C, Eriksson BO, et al. Presenting phenotype in 100 children with the 22q11 deletion syndrome. Eur J Pediatr. 2005;164:146-153.
180. McDonald-McGinn DM, Tonnesen MK, Laufer-Cahana A, et al. Phenotype of the 22q11.2 deletion in individuals identified through an affected relative: cast a wide FISHing net! Genet Med. 2001;3: 23-29.
181. Driscoll DA, Budarf ML, Emanuel BS. A genetic etiology for DiGeorge syndrome: consistent deletions and microdeletions of 22q11. Am J Hum Genet. 1992;50:924-933.
182. Gong W, Gottlieb S, Collins J, et al. Mutation analysis of TBX1 in non-deleted patients with features of DGS/VCFS or isolated cardiovascular defects. J Med Genet. 2001;38:E45.
183. Yagi H, Furutani Y, Hamada H, et al. Role of TBX1 in human del22q11.2 syndrome. Lancet. 2003;362:1366-1373.
184. Preus M. The Williams syndrome: objective definition and diagnosis. Clin Genet. 1984;25: 422-428.
185. Morris CA, Demsey SA, Leonard CO, et al. Natural history of Williams syndrome: physical characteristics. J Pediatr. 1988;113:318-326.
186. Ewart AK, Morris CA, Atkinson D, et al. Hemizygosity at the elastin locus in a developmental disorder, Williams syndrome. Nat Genet. 1993;5:11-16.
187. Morris CA, Thomas IT, Greenberg F. Williams syndrome: autosomal dominant inheritance. Am J Med Genet. 1993;47:478-481.
188. Cohen MS, Anderson MH, Cohen MI, et al. Controversies, genetics, diagnostic assessment, and outcomes relating to the heterotaxy syndrome. Cardiol Young. 2007;17(suppl 2):29-43.
189. Sutherland MJ, Ware SM. Disorders of left-right asymmetry: heterotaxy and situs inversus. Am J Med Genet C Semin Med Genet. 2009;151C(4):307-317.
190. Belmont JW, Mohapatra B, Towbin JA, et al. Molecular genetics of heterotaxy syndromes. Curr Opin Cardiol`. 2004;19(3):216-220.

CHAPTER 18

Human Cardiac Development in the First Trimester

Preeta Dhanantwari, MD, Linda Leatherbury, MD,
Cecilia W. Lo, PhD, Mary T. Donofrio, MD, FAAP, FACC, FASE

18

In current clinical practice of fetal cardiology, rapid advances in medical imaging have opened the door to the diagnosis of human congenital heart disease (CHD) in the first trimester. It is within the first trimester that all of the major cardiac developmental processes that impact CHD occur, and yet much of our current knowledge of these cardiac developmental events has been extrapolated from research studies in animal models. Given differences in developmental timing and cardiovascular anatomy, data documenting normal first trimester human cardiac development is essential. Data on human cardiac development for accurate fetal diagnosis in the clinical setting is of particular importance given increasing feasibility for in utero surgical intervention. A large dataset was obtained from imaging human embryos donated from the Kyoto collection to the Carnegie collection. The complex morphogenetic changes occurring during human heart development were examined using magnetic resonance imaging (MRI) and episcopic fluorescence image capture (EFIC). This analysis included 52 human embryos and spanned 6⅔-9³⁄₇ weeks estimated gestational age (EGA), corresponding to Carnegie stages (CS) 13-23. Serial 2D image stacks and 3D reconstructions allowed analysis of external morphology and internal structures of the heart. The developmental timeline of all the major events in human cardiac morphogenesis from 6 to 10 weeks of gestation was constructed, including the temporal profile of atrial and ventricular septation, outflow septation, and valvular morphogenesis. A reference guide for these developmental milestones was generated to aid clinical practice. This analysis and its results are the source of the information presented in this chapter. Gaining an understanding of heart development in the first trimester is critically important for appropriate counseling of families, and for the development of in utero therapy and intervention to improve the prognosis of fetuses with CHD.

Background

With rapid advances in medical imaging, fetal diagnosis of human CHD is now technically feasible in the first trimester. Although the first human embryologic studies were recorded by Hippocrates in 300-400 BC, present day knowledge of normal human cardiac development in the first trimester is still limited. In 1886, two papers by Dr. His described development of the heart based on dissections of young human embryos. Free hand wax models were made that illustrated the external developmental anatomy. These wax plate reconstruction methods were used by many other investigators until the early 1900s.[1] Subsequently serial histological sections of human embryos have been used to further investigate human cardiac development.[2-6] Based on analysis of histological sections and scaled reproductions of human embryos, Grant showed a large cushion in the developing heart at $6\frac{5}{7}$ weeks (CS 14) and separate atrioventricular valves at $9\frac{1}{7}$ weeks (CS 22).[2] At the end of the eighth week (CS 8), separate aortic and pulmonary outflows were observed. Orts-Llorca and colleagues used 3D reconstructions of transverse sections of human embryos to define development of the truncus arteriosus and described completion of septation of the truncus arteriosus in 14- to 16-mm embryos, equivalent to EGA 8 weeks (CS 18).[5]

Given the complex tissue remodeling associated with cardiac chamber formation and inflow/outflow tract and valvular morphogenesis, the plane of sectioning often limited the information that can be gathered on developing structures in the embryonic heart. These technical limitations, along with limited access to human embryo specimens, have meant that much of our understanding of early cardiac development in the human embryo is largely extrapolated from studies in model organisms.[7-10] With possible species differences in developmental timing and variation in cardiovascular anatomy, characterization of normal cardiac development in human embryos is necessary for clinical evaluation and diagnosis of CHD in the first trimester. This will be increasingly important as improvements in medical technology allow earlier access to first trimester human fetal cardiac imaging and in utero intervention.

Recent studies have shown the feasibility of using MRI to obtain information on human embryo tissue structure.[11,12] MRI data can be digitally resectioned for viewing of the specimen in any orientation, and 3D renderings can be obtained with ease. Similarly, EFIC, a novel histological imaging technique, provides registered 2D image stacks that can be resectioned in arbitrary planes and also rapidly 3D rendered.[10] With EFIC imaging, tissue is embedded in paraffin and cut with a sledge microtome. Tissue autofluorescence at the block face is captured and used to generate registered serial 2D images of the specimen with image resolution better than MRI. Data obtained by MRI or EFIC imaging can be easily resectioned digitally or reconstructed in 3D to facilitate the analysis of complex morphological changes in the developing embryonic heart. In this manner, the developing heart in every embryo can be analyzed in its entirety with no loss of information due to the plane of sectioning.

Using MRI and EFIC imaging, the research group at the National Institutes of Health conducted a systematic analysis of human cardiovascular development in the first trimester. Two-dimensional image stacks and 3D volumes were generated from 52 human embryos from $6\frac{4}{7}$ to $9\frac{3}{7}$ weeks EGA, equivalent to CS 13-23. These stages encompass the developmental window during which all of the major milestones of cardiac morphogenesis can be observed. Using the MRI and EFIC imaging data, a digital atlas of human heart development was constructed. Data from the atlas were used to generate charts summarizing the major milestones of normal human heart development through the first trimester. MRI and EFIC images obtained as part of this study can be viewed as part of an online Human Embryo Atlas. To view the Human Embryo Atlas content, visit http://apps.devbio.pitt.edu/HumanAtlas; guest login ID Human, password Embryo. This chapter highlights the findings of this landmark evaluation (original article published in Circulation 2009;120;343-351). Permission for reproduction of that original work was obtained from Lippincott Williams & Wilkins (http://lww.com).

Table 18-1 HUMAN EMBRYO IMAGING BY MRI AND EPISCOPIC FLUORESCENCE IMAGE CAPTURE

Estimated Gestational Age (weeks)	Carnegie Stage	Total Number Embryos Imaged	Imaging by MRI*	Imaging by EFIC*	EFIC and MRI
6⁴⁄₇	13	3	2 (2)	1 (1)	
6⁶⁄₇	14	4	3 (3)	2 (1)	1
7¹⁄₇	15	3	1 (1)	2 (2)	
7³⁄₇	16	8	6 (6)	4 (3)	2
7⁵⁄₇	17	4	2 (2)	2 (2)	1
8	18	6	4 (3)	2 (1)	
8²⁄₇	19	5	3 (3)	2 (0)	
8⁴⁄₇	20	5	3 (3)	1 (0)	
8⁶⁄₇	21	4	2 (2)	2 (0)	
9¹⁄₇	22	6	5 (3)	1 (0)	
9³⁄₇	23	4	3 (3)	3 (1)	2
Totals		52 (42)	34 (31)	22 (11)	

*Number of specimens yielding good imaging data indicated in parentheses.

Specimens

Embryos from the Kyoto collection at the Congenital Anomaly Research Center at the Kyoto University in Japan were collected after termination of pregnancies for socioeconomic reasons under the Maternity Protection Law of Japan. Embryos were derived from normal pregnancies without any clinical presentations. The specimens were in fixative for an estimated duration of 30 to more than 40 years, making them unsuitable for immunohistochemistry or any molecular/cellular analysis. This collection represents a random sample of the total intrauterine population of Japan.[13-16] During accessioning into the Kyoto collection, the embryos were examined and staged according to the criteria of CS proposed by O'Rahilly.[17] For this study, 52 embryos from the Kyoto collection (Table 18-1) were donated to the Carnegie collection of normal human embryos archived at the National Museum of Health and Medicine of the Armed Forces Institute of Pathology (http://nmhm.washingtondc.museum/collections/hdac/Carnegie_collection.htm). Each embryo's age was determined using postconceptional ages previously reported, which were then converted to estimated gestational age or menstrual age by adding 14 days, and reported in weeks.[14]

Magnetic Resonance Imaging, Episcopic Fluorescence Image Capture, Processing, and Analysis

High-resolution MRI and EFIC images were obtained during preparation for accessioning of the embryos into the Carnegie collection. MRI was performed at the NIH Mouse Imaging Facility. Over the collection, MRI resolution ranged from $29 \times 35 \times 35$ to $117 \times 105 \times 105$ μm^3. Resolution was proportionate to the sample size with the smallest embryos having the highest resolution datasets.

Embryos were prepared for EFIC imaging using techniques previously described.[10,18] They were sectioned and sequentially photographed using an ORCA-ER digital camera (Hamamatsu, Hamamatsu, Japan).

Both the EFIC and MRI data were processed using OpenLab (Improvision Inc., Waltham, Mass.). Three-dimensional reconstructions and Quicktime virtual reality (QTVR) movies were generated using Volocity (Improvision Inc.). The 2D image stacks also were digitally resectioned using Volocity (Improvision Inc.) to view internal and external cardiac structures in planes similar to standard echocardiographic imaging planes used clinically. For each embryo, we generated serial 2D image stacks and 3D reconstructions. From this analysis, we were able to delineate all of the major milestones of human heart development, including chamber formation, septation of the atria, ventricles, and truncus arteriosus, and valvular morphogenesis.

Cardiac Looping

The cardiac loop or looped heart tube is observed from EGA $6\frac{4}{7}$ to $7\frac{5}{7}$ weeks (CS 13 to CS 17). Three-dimensional reconstruction of the heart at $7\frac{5}{7}$ weeks (CS 17) reveals internal structures of the cardiac loop in Figure 18-1. The only exit for blood from the left-sided inflow limb, consisting of the atrial cavity, atrioventricular junction, and the presumptive left ventricle, is the interventricular foramen (also known as primary foramen, primary interventricular foramen, bulboventricular foramen, or embryonic interventricular foramen) (double arrow in Fig. 18-1); the only exit for blood from the right-sided outflow limb, consisting of the presumptive right ventricle, is the truncus arteriosus (arrowhead in Fig. 18-1). Also of note, the atrioventricular junction (AV in Fig. 18-1) is surrounded by endocardial cushion tissue, which is contiguous with the truncus arteriosus.

The developmental changes seen in the cardiac loop are shown in more detail in Figure 18-2, with images from embryos at $6\frac{4}{7}$ (CS 13) (Fig. 18-2A-E) and $7\frac{5}{7}$ weeks (CS 17) (Fig. 18-2F-I). As the looped heart tube matures, the atrial and ventricular chambers expand in size, giving rise to distinct subdivisions recognizable as the primitive left and right atria and presumptive left and right ventricles

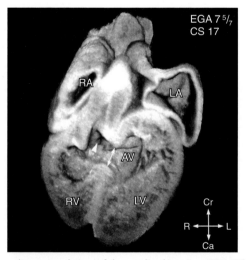

Figure 18-1   Three-dimensional view of the cardiac loop in a EGA $7\frac{5}{7}$ weeks (CS 17) embryo. Two-dimensional EFIC image stacks were reconstructed in 3D to show the looped heart tube in an EGA $7\frac{5}{7}$-week (CS 17) embryo. The double-headed arrow indicates the interventricular foramen. The orifice of the developing atrioventricular junction is seen as a horizontal line above the label AV. The truncus arteriosus (*arrowhead*) is also seen. Endocardial cushion tissue surrounding the atrioventricular junction is adjacent to the truncus arteriosus. LA, left atrium; LV, presumptive left ventricle; RV, presumptive right ventricle; Scale bar = 0.6 mm. Compass: A, anterior; Ca, caudal; Cr, cranial; L, left; P, posterior; R, right; RA, right atrium.

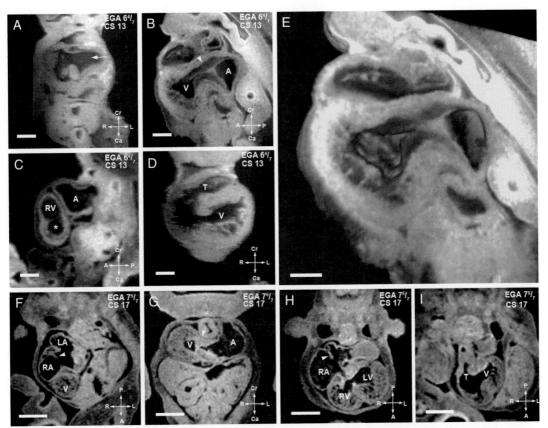

Figure 18-2 Defining structures of the cardiac loop. **A-E**, EFIC and MRI images of EGA 6⁴/₇-week (CS 13) embryos shown in various imaging planes. Imaging in the frontal plane **(A)** shows the common cardinal veins or the open venous confluence (*arrow*), while sagittal view **(B)** shows primitive endocardial cushions at the atrioventricular junction (*arrowhead*). A 3D model of the same embryo **(E)** shows the extent of the interventricular foramen as well as the contour of the endocardial cushions. MRI image of another embryo in the sagittal plane **(C)** shows the presumptive right ventricle (RV), atrial chamber (A), and a nondistinct interventricular foramen (*), while the ventricular chamber (V) and a single, undivided truncus arteriosus (T) can be seen in a frontal section of a third embryo **(D)**. Scale bars: **A-D** = 0.4 mm, **E** = 0.25 mm. **F-I**, MRI images of EGA 7⁵/₇-week (CS 17) embryo. Image from an oblique transverse plane **(F)** shows the right and left atrial (RA, LA) chambers as septation is progressing (*arrowhead*). The developing ventricle (V) is seen. Viewed in the transverse plane in **G**, well-formed dense endocardial cushion tissue is seen at the atrioventricular junction (*arrowhead*). Another section in the transverse plane in **H** shows the right and left ventricular cavities with a more distinct interventricular foramen (*). Septum primum can be seen as atrial septation progresses (*arrowhead*). The single undivided truncus arteriosus (T) and interventricular foramen communicating with the presumptive left ventricle (V) can be seen in an oblique transverse plane **I**. Scale bar: **E-H** = 1.250 mm. LV, presumptive left ventricular chamber; T, truncus arteriosus. Compass: A, anterior; Ca, caudal; Cr, cranial; L, left; P, posterior; R, right.

(Fig. 18-2H). At 6⁴/₇ weeks (CS 13), the endocardial cushions seen lining the atrioventricular junction appear thin with little apparent cellular content. As development progresses, they become filled with dense material (Fig. 18-2B, E, G). The interventricular foramen also shows striking changes during this developmental period. It is a wide and open communication at 6⁴/₇ weeks (CS 13) (asterisk in Fig. 18-2C), but as the chambers grow, it becomes a narrow and more distinct opening (foramen) by 7³/₇-7⁵/₇ weeks (CS 16-17) (asterisk in Figs. 18-2H and 18-3C). The superior atrioventricular cushion can be seen (Fig. 18-2G). The inflow consisting of the venous confluence or primitive atrium (Fig. 18-2A) is observed to communicate with the ventricular chamber via the atrioventricular junction (Fig. 18-2B, E, G). The presumptive left ventricle communicates with the presumptive right ventricle

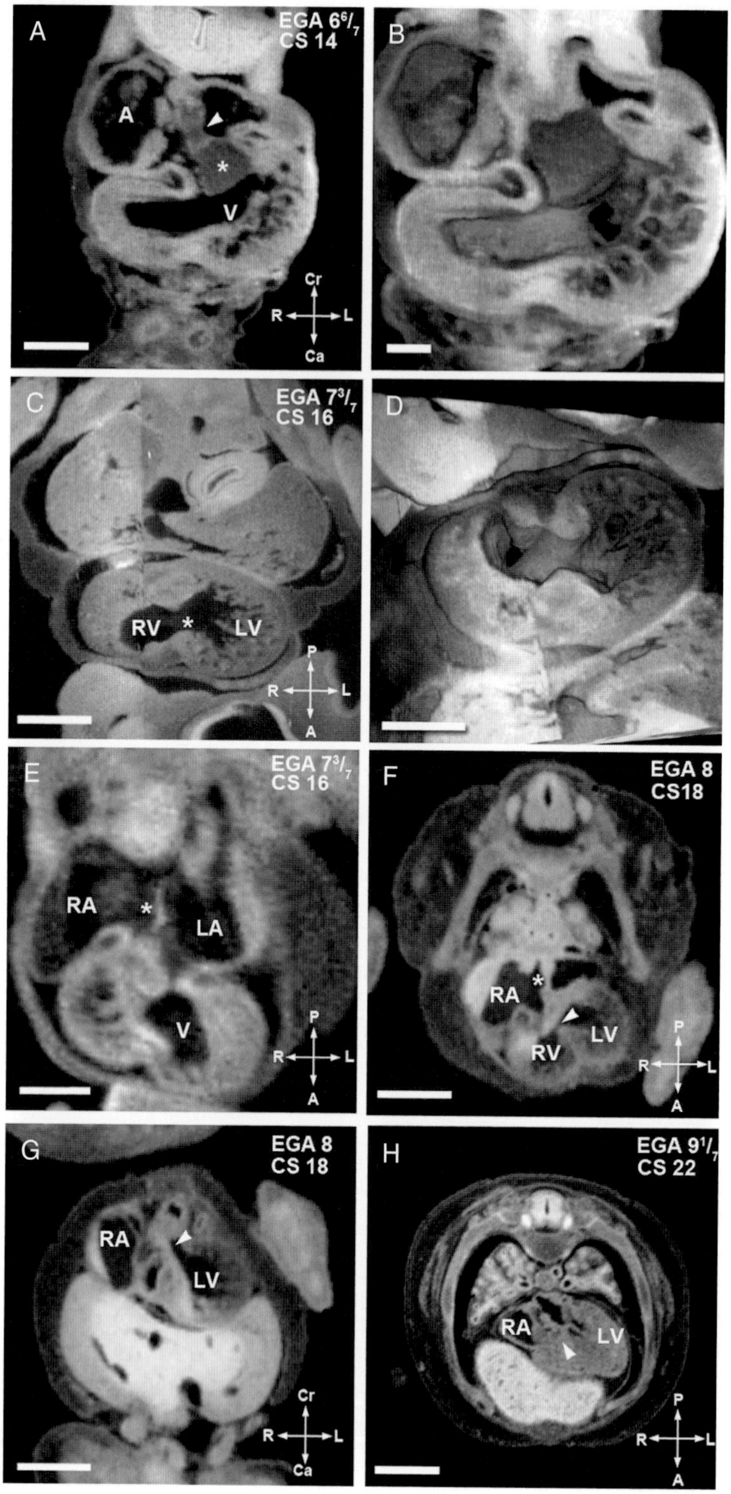

Figure 18-3 Major events of atrial and ventricular septation. **A-B,** EFIC image of EGA 6⅚-week (CS 14) embryo in the transverse plane **(A)** shows the atrial spine (*arrowhead*) attached to the inferior cushion (*asterisks*). Three-dimensional reconstruction **(B)** highlights the endocardial cushions and trabeculation in the ventricular chamber. Scale bar = 0.515 mm in **A**, 0.272 mm in **B**. **C-D,** An EFIC image of EGA 7⅗-week (CS 16) embryo in the oblique plane **(C)** showing right and left ventricular chambers connected by an interventricular foramen (*). Three-dimensional reconstruction of the same embryo **(D)** delineates the contour of the interventricular foramen and the orifices of the atrioventricular canal and the truncus arteriosus. Scale bar = 0.5 mm for **C** and 0.900 mm for **D**. **E,** MRI image of an embryo at EGA 7⅗ weeks (CS 16) also in the transverse plane. It shows the formation of septum primum (*) between the right and left atria (RA, LA). Scale bar = 0.5 mm. **F-G,** MRI image of an EGA 8-week (CS 18) embryo in an oblique transverse plane **(F)** shows a complete atrial septum (*). The most caudal portion of the septum primum, the mesenchymal cap, has fused to the superior cushion. The growth of the muscular ventricular septum into the ventricular cavity is also shown. The crest of the muscular interventricular septum is present with an incomplete inlet ventricular septum (*arrowhead*) immediately above it. Panel **G,** another MRI image of the same embryo in an oblique coronal plane, shows the formed outlet ventricular septum (*arrowhead*). Together these two images show that outlet ventricular septation is completed before inlet ventricular septation. Scale bars in **F** and **G** = 1.5 mm. **H,** MRI image of embryo at EGA 9⅐ weeks (CS 22) in an oblique coronal plane shows a completed inlet ventricular septum (*arrowhead*). Scale bar = 2 mm. A, primitive atrium/venous confluence; LA, left atrium; LV, left ventricular chamber; RA, right atrium; RV, right ventricular chamber; V, ventricular chamber. Compass: A, anterior; Ca, caudal; Cr, cranial; L, left; P, posterior; R, right.

via the interventricular foramen (asterisk in Fig. 18-2C, H). The outflow from the cardiac loop comprises the yet undivided truncus arteriosus (T in Fig. 18-2D, I) arising from the presumptive right ventricle.

Atrial Septation (Estimated Gestational Age 6⁶/₇-8 Weeks)

The process of atrial septation is thought to begin with a thin septum primum growing from the posterior wall of the atrium, from a location cranial to the pulmonary vein orifice. It grows toward and eventually fuses with the endocardial cushions.[19] At 6⁶/₇ weeks gestation (CS 14), the mesenchymal cap of the primary atrial septum could be seen in contact with the superior atrioventricular cushion. The atrial spine, a mesenchymal structure, was also observed. The atrial spine fuses with the inferior atrioventricular cushion (6⁶/₇ weeks; CS 14) (Fig. 18-3A, B), and plays an important role in closure of the primary foramen. Although the pulmonary vein orifice was not seen by our imaging, it can be inferred from previous studies that it lies to the left of the atrial spine.[20] Septum primum can be observed at 6⁶/₇ weeks of gestation and its developmental progression through 7³/₇ weeks can be seen in Figures 18-2H, 3A, B, and E. Later, septum secundum develops as an infolding of the dorsal wall of the right atrium, completing atrial septation with fenestrations forming the foramen ovale. Both atrial septum primum and secundum were present by 8 weeks (CS 18). At this stage, the mesenchymal cap can be seen fused with the now divided superior atrioventricular cushion (Fig. 18-3F). This is consistent with developmental timing suggested by others.[21,22]

Ventricular Septation (Estimated Gestational Age 7³/₇-9¹/₇ Weeks)

Toward the end of the looped heart tube stages of development (7²/₇ and 7³/₇ weeks, CS 16, 17), distinct separation of presumptive left ventricular (LV) and right ventricular (RV) chambers is evident. The beginning of the muscular interventricular septum can be seen at these stages, but ventricular septation is not yet complete (Figs. 18-2H, 3C, D). By 8 weeks (CS 18), the muscular ventricular septum can be seen extending from the floor of the ventricular chamber towards the crux of the heart (Fig. 18-3F). This leaves open a relatively large interventricular foramen which allows communication between the ventricles. Recent lineage tracing experiments in mice have suggested that closure of the interventricular septum is mediated by migration of a subpopulation of cells derived from the secondary heart field.[23] Immunohistochemical analysis of human fetal cardiac tissue showed myocytes expressing G1N2 antigen localized around the junction between the future right and left ventricles.[24] In later developmental stages, G1N2 expressing cells are found in the area clinically termed the inlet ventricular septum, but not in the subaortic outflow septum.

At 8 weeks (CS 18), the ventricular septum at the level of the left ventricular outflow is closed (Fig. 18-3G), but part of the inlet ventricular septum at the level of the atrioventricular valves remains open (arrowhead in Fig. 18-3F). The inlet and membranous portions of the ventricular septum are fully closed at 9¹/₇ weeks (CS 18), completing ventricular septation (Fig. 18-3H). The area clinically termed the inlet ventricular septum has been shown in prior studies to originate from the embryonic right ventricle.[25] In agreement with previous reports on human development, the data showed that the final portion of the ventricular septum to close included what likely comprises portions of both the membranous and inlet ventricular septa. These findings suggest that an arrest in development of the ventricular septum could result in ventricular septal defects similar to those observed clinically.

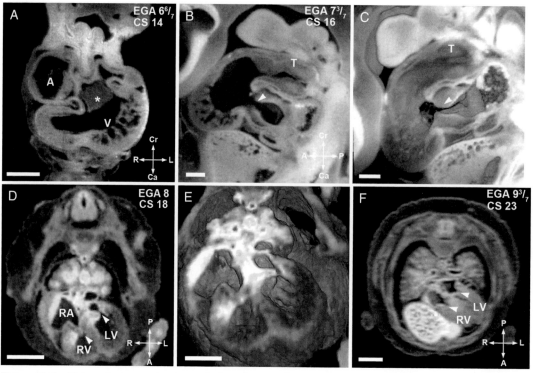

Figure 18-4   Major milestones of atrioventricular valve morphogenesis. **A,** EFIC image of an embryo at EGA 6⁶/₇ weeks (CS 14) in the transverse plane shows a large endocardial cushion (*) in the center of the cardiac loop. Scale bar = 0.515 mm. **B-C,** EFIC image of an embryo at EGA 7³/₇ weeks (CS 16) in a sagittal plane **(B)** shows a tight, well-formed atrioventricular junction (*arrowhead*) and the truncus arteriosus (T). Three-dimensional volume of the same embryo **(C)** shows exquisite detail of the contour and shape of the endocardial cushions and the truncus arteriosus (T). Scale bar in **B-C** = 0.389 mm. **D-E,** MRI image in an oblique transverse plane **(D)** of an embryo at EGA 8 weeks (CS 18) shows separate atrioventricular valves. The valve leaflets appear thick at this stage. Note right and left atrioventricular valves denoted by arrowheads. Three-dimensional volume of the same embryo **(E)** shows indentation associated with the opening in the inlet ventricular septum. Scale bar for **D** = 1.5 mm and for **E** = 1.1 mm. **F,** MRI image in an oblique transverse plane of a more mature EGA 9³/₇-week (CS 23) embryo. It shows separate atrioventricular valves with thinner valve leaflets (*arrowheads*). The inlet septum is closed. Scale bar = 2 mm. A, primitive atrium; LV, left ventricular chamber; RA, right atrium; RV, right ventricular chamber; V, ventricular chamber. Compass: A, anterior; Ca, caudal; Cr, cranial; L, left; P, posterior; R, right.

Formation of the Atrioventricular Valves (Estimated Gestational Age 7³/₇-8weeks)

Atrioventricular valve morphogenesis begins at the looped heart tube stages, with large endocardial cushions prominently seen at the center of the cardiac loop (asterisks in Fig. 18-3A, 4A). The atrioventricular canal is divided by the endocardial cushions, which form on the posterior (dorsal) and anterior (ventral) walls of the atrioventricular canal. These cushions eventually divide the atrioventricular canal into right and left atrioventricular orifices.[2,19] A well-delineated atrioventricular junction can be seen at 7³/₇ weeks' gestation (CS 16) (Fig. 18-4B, C). At 7³/₇ and 7⁵/₇ weeks (CS 16 and CS 17), the atrioventricular junction was still undivided. A few days later, by 8 weeks' gestation (CS 18), separate atrioventricular valves can be seen (arrowheads in Fig. 18-4D, E), with left-sided mitral and right-sided tricuspid valves forming. An embryo at 8 weeks (CS 18) is approximately 10 mm in size, correlating well with the embryonic stage at which fusion of the endocardial cushions is thought to occur.[26] The valve leaflets however appear thick at this stage. By 9¹/₇ weeks (CS 22), the atrioventricular valve leaflets are thinner and more mature

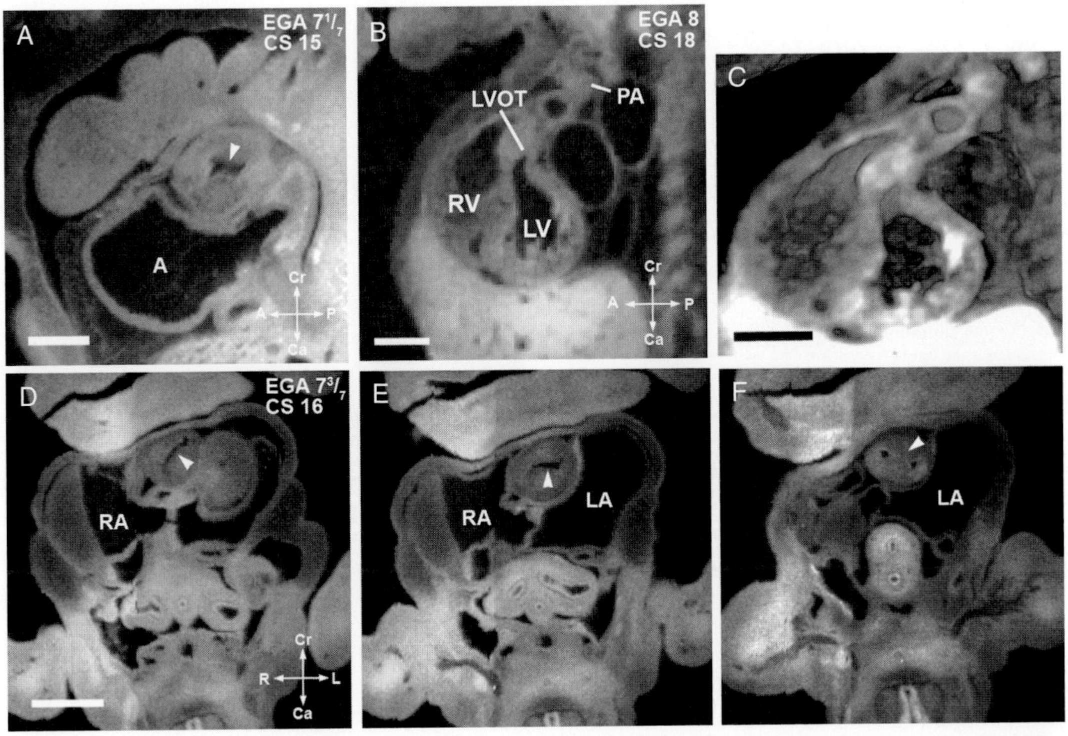

Figure 18-5 Septation of the truncus arteriosus. **A,** EFIC image of an embryo at EGA 7$\frac{1}{7}$ weeks (CS 15) in the sagittal plane shows a single orifice of the truncus arteriosus with inward swelling of the aorticopulmonary septum (*arrowhead*), which precedes septation of the truncus arteriosus. Scale bar = 0.622 mm. **B-C,** EFIC image of an EGA 8-week (CS 18) embryo **(B)** shows a distinct pulmonary artery (PA) emerging from the right ventricle (RV) and a left ventricular outflow tract (LVOT) or aorta emerging from the left ventricle (LV). Three-dimensional volume of the same embryo **(C)** shows crossing of the great arteries. Scale bar for **B-C** = 1.35 mm. **D-F,** EFIC images of an embryo at EGA 7$\frac{3}{7}$ weeks (CS 16) in oblique transverse planes showing the truncus arteriosus. Note changing orientation of the lumen **(D, E)** indicative of spiraling of the cushions (see arrowheads). **F,** The aorticopulmonary septum (*arrowhead*) has divided the distal portion of the truncus arteriosus into two separate arterial channels to the right and left of the aorticopulmonary septum. Scale bar = 0.9 mm. A, primitive atrium; LA, left atrium; LV, left ventricle; RA, right atrium; RV, right ventricle. Compass: A, anterior; Ca, caudal; Cr, cranial; L, left; P, posterior; R, right.

in appearance (Fig. 18-3H). At 7$\frac{3}{7}$ weeks (CS 16), distinct posterior and anterior cushions are not observed, the inferior atrioventricular cushion is observed. This timing is consistent with previous reports of human embryonic development.[22]

Outflow Septation and Semilunar Valve Morphogenesis (Estimated Gestational Age 7$\frac{3}{7}$-8 Weeks)

The major developmental processes occurring at the level of the truncus arteriosus consist of septation into two separate arterial channels and semilunar valve morphogenesis. The truncus arteriosus is formed largely from cells derived from the secondary heart field.[27] Septation of the truncus arteriosus is dependent on activity of the secondary heart field and migrating neural crest cells, and is achieved with ingrowth of ridges.[28,29] In the proximal truncus arteriosus, truncal cushions in the form of swellings at 7$\frac{1}{7}$ weeks (CS 15) (arrowhead in Fig. 18-5A) were observed. This forming aorticopulmonary septum undergoes a gradual spiraling course that ultimately completes truncus arteriosus septation into separate aorta and pulmonary arteries.[28] At 7$\frac{3}{7}$ weeks (CS 16), this spiraling course of the

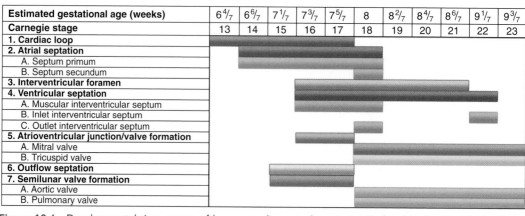

Estimated gestational age (weeks)	$6^4/_7$	$6^6/_7$	$7^1/_7$	$7^3/_7$	$7^5/_7$	8	$8^2/_7$	$8^4/_7$	$8^6/_7$	$9^1/_7$	$9^3/_7$
Carnegie stage	13	14	15	16	17	18	19	20	21	22	23
1. Cardiac loop											
2. Atrial septation											
A. Septum primum											
B. Septum secundum											
3. Interventricular foramen											
4. Ventricular septation											
A. Muscular interventricular septum											
B. Inlet interventricular septum											
C. Outlet interventricular septum											
5. Atrioventricular junction/valve formation											
A. Mitral valve											
B. Tricuspid valve											
6. Outflow septation											
7. Semilunar valve formation											
A. Aortic valve											
B. Pulmonary valve											

Figure 18-6 Developmental time course of human cardiac morphogenesis. Outlined in the chart is the timing for major cardiac morphogenetic events and the presence of various cardiac structures in the human embryo. The timeline indicated for atrioventricular junction/valve formation refers to when a distinct atrioventricular junction is observed before atrioventricular valve leaflets are evident. The timeline indicated for semilunar valve formation refers to when distinct truncal cushion tissue is observed and before semilunar valve leaflets are evident. The demarcation of mitral valve, tricuspid valve, aortic valve, and pulmonary valve delineates the developmental stages when distinct valve leaflets are observed and the stages when the valve leaflets continue to undergo maturation and thinning. The timeline indicated for interventricular foramen refers to when any communication is present between the right and left ventricular chambers. (See Expert Consult site for color image.)

forming aorticopulmonary septum is evident as a spiraling in the orientation of the lumen along the proximodistal axis of the truncus arteriosus (Fig. 18-5D-F). The truncus arteriosus remains as a single channel proximally (Fig. 18-5D-E), but distally, it divides into two separate channels (Fig. 18-5F). Smooth muscle derived from the secondary heart field and from cardiac neural crest cells plays a crucial role in the septation and alignment of the truncus arteriosus.[28]

Bartelings and Gittenberger-de Groot suggested that in $7^3/_7$ week (CS 16), embryos septation begins at the ventriculoarterial junction and progresses proximal to distal in the truncus arteriosus.[6] However, findings from these images show septation of the truncus arteriosus occurring in the opposite direction, being complete distally in the $7^3/_7$-week (CS 16) embryo, at a time when the proximal truncus arteriosus is still undivided. This would suggest that the direction of septation is distal to proximal. This is supported by Kirby's work, who described the proximal truncus arteriosus closing zipper-like from distal to proximal toward the ventricles.[28] Our data also support both the timing and direction of septation proposed by Anderson and colleagues.[29] They described septation of the truncus arteriosus initiating distally and progressing proximally with the presence of distal septation and the absence of proximal septation at $7^3/_7$ weeks (CS 16). Moore described bulbar ridges at the fifth week postconception, equivalent to 7 weeks gestation.[19] Assuming the bulbar and truncal cushions are forming at the same time, the finding of truncal cushions in the outflow at $7^1/_7$ weeks (CS 15) also corroborates these investigators' timeframe.

The process of semilunar valve morphogenesis, similar to atrioventricular valve morphogenesis, began earlier with the formation of truncal cushion tissue, which was observed in the outflow starting at $7^1/_7$ weeks (CS 15). At 8 weeks (CS 18), distinct pulmonary and aortic valves can be seen (Fig. 18-5B, C). These valve leaflets, as well as atrioventricular valve leaflets, are initially thick. They undergo a process of thinning as the valve leaflets continue to form and mature; a process that continues well after the formation of distinct valve leaflets (Fig. 18-6). By $9^1/_7$ weeks (CS 22), all of the major structures of the heart are formed, with the last developmental milestone being completion of the inlet ventricular septum.

Carnegie stage	13	14	15	16	17
Estimated gestational age (weeks)	$6\frac{4}{7}$	$6\frac{6}{7}$	$7\frac{1}{7}$	$7\frac{3}{7}$	$7\frac{5}{7}$
Scale bars	0.40 mm	0.515 mm	0.622 mm	0.90 mm	1.25 mm
Inflow					
Atrioventricular junction					
Ventricular mass					
Outflow					

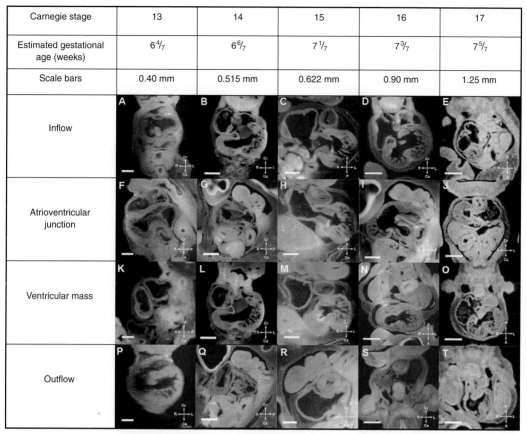

Figure 18-7 Summary of human cardiac developmental milestones. Major cardiac developmental structures present in EGA $6\frac{4}{7}$-$7\frac{5}{7}$-week (CS 13-17) embryos. The compass orients the observer to the plane of section. **F-J,** Atrioventricular junction. **K-O,** Ventricular mass. **P-T,** Outflow.

Conclusion

As rapid advances in technology provide first trimester human fetal cardiac imaging and opportunities for in utero intervention continue to advance, there is increasing need for data documenting human cardiac development in the first trimester. Using a large dataset generated by MRI and EFIC imaging, the major developmental milestones of human cardiac morphogenesis were delineated spanning EGA $6\frac{4}{7}$-$9\frac{3}{7}$ weeks. A summary timeline is provided in Figure 18-6 for the temporal profile of atrial and ventricular septation, outflow septation, and valvular morphogenesis. In addition, Figures 18-7 and 18-8 are intended as reference guides to aid clinical practice. They contain thumbnail images of cardiac structures seen at each developmental milestone of cardiac morphogenesis. Full-size images and Quicktime movies of the 2D serial image stacks of these embryos can be viewed in the web-based Human Embryo Atlas (http://apps.devbio.pitt.edu/HumanAtlas) using guest login *Human* and password *Embryo*. A deeper understanding of human cardiovascular development, including this large dataset and the reference guides generated, may ultimately aid in clinical practice and facilitate prenatal diagnosis of CHD and appropriate counseling of families.

Acknowledgments

This work was supported by NIH grant ZO1-HL005701. The Kyoto collection was supported by Japanese Ministry of Education, Culture, Sports, Science and Technology (Grant 19390050); Japanese Ministry of Health, Labor and Welfare (Grant: 17A-6), and Japan Science Technology Agency (BIRD grant). We would like to thank the research team at the National Institutes of Health. Their contribution was essential to

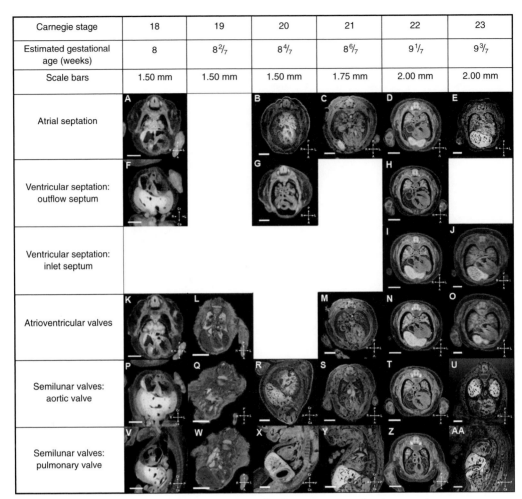

Carnegie stage	18	19	20	21	22	23
Estimated gestational age (weeks)	8	$8^2/_7$	$8^4/_7$	$8^6/_7$	$9^1/_7$	$9^3/_7$
Scale bars	1.50 mm	1.50 mm	1.50 mm	1.75 mm	2.00 mm	2.00 mm
Atrial septation	A		B	C	D	E
Ventricular septation: outflow septum	F		G		H	
Ventricular septation: inlet septum					I	J
Atrioventricular valves	K	L		M	N	O
Semilunar valves: aortic valve	P	Q	R	S	T	U
Semilunar valves: pulmonary valve	V	W	X	Y	Z	AA

Figure 18-8 Summary of human cardiac developmental milestones. Major developmental structures present in EGA 8- to 9⅗-week (CS 18-23) embryos. One can look at a developmental structure at a specific estimated gestational age to determine what normal development is for that structure at that age in human cardiac development. The compass orients the observer to the plane of section. **A-E,** Atrial septation. **F-H,** Ventricular septation: outflow septum. **I-J,** Ventricular septation: inlet septum. **K-O,** Atrioventricular valves. **P-U,** Semilunar valves: aortic valves. **V-AA,** Semilunar valves: pulmonary valve.

the original work. Members of the team include Elaine Lee, BA, Anita Krishnan, MD, Rajeev Samtani, Shigehito Yamada, MD, PhD , Stasia Anderson, PhD, and Elizabeth Lockett, MA. Shigehito.Yamada was supported by Kyoto University Foundation

References

1. Kramer T. The partitioning of the truncus and conus and the formation of the membranous portion of the interventricular septum in the human heart. Am J Anat. 1942;71:343-370.
2. Grant RP. The embryology of ventricular flow pathways in man. Circulation. 1962;25:756-779.
3. Goor DA, Edwards JE, Lillehei CW. The development of the interventricular septum of the human heart; correlative morphogenetic study. Chest. 1970;58(5):453-467.
4. Anderson RH, Wilkinson JL, Arnold R, et al. Morphogenesis of bulboventricular malformations. I. Consideration of embryogenesis in the normal heart. Br Heart J. 1974;36(3):242-255.
5. Orts-Llorca F, Puerta Fonolla J, Sobrado J. The formation, septation and fate of the truncus arteriosus in man. J Anat. 1982;134(Pt 1):41-56.
6. Bartelings MM, Gittenberger-de Groot AC. The outflow tract of the heart–embryologic and morphologic correlations. Int J Cardiol. 1989;22(3):289-300.
7. Tonge M. Observations on the development of the semilunar valves of the aorta and pulmonary artery of the heart of the chick. Phil Trans Roy Soc (London). 1869;159:387-411.
8. Hamburger VHH. A series of normal stages in the development of the chick embryo. J Morphol. 1951;88:49-92.

9. DeHaan RL. Development of form in the embryonic heart. An experimental approach. Circulation. 1967;35(5):821-833.

10. Rosenthal J, Mangal V, Walker D, et al. Rapid high resolution three dimensional reconstruction of embryos with episcopic fluorescence image capture. Birth Defects Res C Embryo Today. 2004;72(3):213-223.

11. Smith BR, Linney E, Huff DS, et al. Magnetic resonance microscopy of embryos. Comput Med Imaging Graph. 1996;20(6):483-490.

12. Shiota K, Yamada S, Nakatsu-Komatsu T, et al. Visualization of human prenatal development by magnetic resonance imaging (MRI). Am J Med Genet A. 2007;143A(24):3121-3126.

13. Nishimura H. Prenatal versus postnatal malformations based on the Japanese experience on induced abortions in the human being. In: Blandau RJ, ed. Aging gametes: their biology and pathology. Basel: Karger AG; 1975.

14. Nishimura H, Takano K, Tanimura T, et al. Normal and abnormal development of human embryos: first report of the analysis of 1,213 intact embryos. Teratology. 1968;1(3):281-290.

15. Shiota K. Development and intrauterine fate of normal and abnormal human conceptuses. Congenit Anom Kyoto. 1991;31:67-80.

16. Yamada S, Uwabe C, Fujii S, et al. Phenotypic variability in human embryonic holoprosencephaly in the Kyoto Collection. Birth Defects Res A Clin Mol Teratol. 2004;70(8):495-508.

17. O'Rahilly RMF. Developmental stages in human embryos: including a revision of Streeter's "Horizons" and a survey of the Carnegie collection. Washington, DC: Carnegie Institution of Washington; 1987.

18. Weninger WJ, Mohun T. Phenotyping transgenic embryos: a rapid 3-D screening method based on episcopic fluorescence image capturing. Nat Genet. 2002;30(1):59-65.

19. Moore K, Persaud T. The developing human clinically oriented embryology, 8th ed. Philadelphia: WB Saunders; 2007.

20. Lamers WH, Moorman AF. Cardiac septation: a late contribution of the embryonic primary myocardium to heart morphogenesis. Circ Res. 2002;91(2):93-103.

21. Wessels A, Anderson RH, Markwald RR, et al. Atrial development in the human heart: an immuno-histochemical study with emphasis on the role of mesenchymal tissues. Anat Rec. 2000;259(3): 288-300.

22. Anderson RH, Webb S, Brown NA, et al. Development of the heart: (2) Septation of the atriums and ventricles. Heart. 2003;89(8):949-958.

23. Stadtfeld M, Ye M, Graf T. Identification of interventricular septum precursor cells in the mouse embryo. Dev Biol. 2007;302(1):195-207.

24. Wessels A, Vermeulen JL, Verbeek FJ, et al. Spatial distribution of "tissue-specific" antigens in the developing human heart and skeletal muscle. III. An immunohistochemical analysis of the distribution of the neural tissue antigen G1N2 in the embryonic heart; implications for the development of the atrioventricular conduction system. Anat Rec. 1992;232(1):97-111.

25. Lamers WH, Wessels A, Verbeek FJ, et al. New findings concerning ventricular septation in the human heart. Implications for maldevelopment. Circulation. 1992;86(4):1194-1205.

26. Van Mierop LH, Kutsche LM. Development of the ventricular septum of the heart. Heart Vessels. 1985;1(2):114-119.

27. Waldo KL, Hutson MR, Ward CC, et al. Secondary heart field contributes myocardium and smooth muscle to the arterial pole of the developing heart. Dev Biol. 2005;281(1):78-90.

28. Kirby M. Cardiac development. New York: Oxford University Press; 2007.

29. Anderson RH, Webb S, Brown NA, et al. Development of the heart: (3) formation of the ventricular outflow tracts, arterial valves, and intrapericardial arterial trunks. Heart. 2003;89(9): 1110-1118.

18

CHAPTER 19

The Reappraisal of Normal and Abnormal Cardiac Development

Robert H. Anderson, MD, FRCPath, Nigel A. Brown, PhD,
Bill Chaudhry, MB, ChB, PhD, Deborah J. Henderson, PhD,
Simon D. Bamforth, PhD, Timothy J. Mohun, PhD,
Antoon F. M. Moorman, PhD

19

Those interested in congenital cardiac malformations have always shown a remarkable fascination for their presumed morphogenesis. Maude Abbott, the doyenne of cardiac morphologists, in her superb atlas, wrote as long ago as the 1930s: "An understanding of the elementary facts of human and comparative embryology is essential to an intelligent grasp of the ontogenetic problems of congenital cardiac disease."[1] When the most senior of the authors of this paper began his career, some of his first papers were devoted to descriptions of cardiac development.[2,3] When assessed in retrospect, they left much to be desired, so much so that, a few years later, he collaborated in casting doubt on the role cardiac embryology might play in improving the understanding of the morphology of congenital cardiac malformations.[4] In response to the provocative statement that embryology might have been a hindrance rather than a help, another of the current authors pointed out that the issues might better be clarified when molecular approaches are combined with appropriate anatomic understanding.[5] Even in the short period that has elapsed since the time of this response, huge strides have been made in understanding the molecular basis of cardiac development. The progress achieved fully justifies the premise but, as was emphasized, the molecular findings need to be assessed on the basis of appropriate anatomic understanding.

Such a need for a combination of molecular and morphological approaches is nowhere more evident than when we consider recent findings relative to normal and abnormal cardiac development, such as the role of the so-called second heart field. It was long since recognized that material was added to the poles of the heart subsequent to the appearance of the linear heart tube.[6,7] Until relatively recently, however, development was interpreted on the basis that the initial linear heart tube contained the primordia of all the so-called cardiac segments, these being the presumed precursors for the compartments as seen in the formed heart. The appearance of three publications in the same year, just after the turn of the century, then confirmed that the initial linear heart tube produced little more than the left ventricle of the definitive heart, or even just the left ventricular apex and the left half of the muscular ventricular septum.[8-11] In the decade that has elapsed since the appearance of those works, a bewildering number of genes have been associated with the components added to the venous and arterial poles of the developing heart.[12] Currently, nonetheless, there is no consensus as to whether the so-called second field is a true field of gene expression or morphogenetic signaling, in the sense that it contains all the cells with the potential to contribute to the myocardium, nor whether it is appropriate to recognize two, as opposed to one, or even more, such field or fields.[13,14] In this chapter, we reappraise knowledge of normal and abnormal cardiac development, explaining our own preference for considering the appearance of the structures added to the heart at its arterial and venous poles as representing no more than temporal steps in the movement and programming of tissues from the heart-forming regions of the developing embryo.[14] We then suggest that understanding of these developmental processes can, indeed, help in understanding the morphology, and potentially the morphogenesis, of the normal and malformed heart.

How Does the Heart Develop?

Subsequent to gastrulation, the developing embryo possesses three germ layers, the ectoderm, the endoderm, and an intermediate mesodermal layer. The layers are found within the embryonic disc, which merges at its margins with the extraembryonic tissues formed by the amnion and yolk sac (Fig. 19-1). The subsequent extensive growth of the disc relative to the surrounding extraembryonic tissues produces folding, which gives the embryo its characteristic shape. Subsequent to the completion of the folding, the original junction between the disc and the extraembryonic tissues is no more than the navel of the embryo (Fig. 19-2). In consequence, the parts of the disc initially positioned peripherally become positioned ventrally within the body of the developing embryo. The orifice of the developing mouth is initially closed by the stomatopharyngeal membrane, itself flanked caudally and centrally by pharyngeal mesoderm. This pharyngeal area is then bordered peripherally by the cardiogenic mesoderm. The overall cardiac area is contiguous with the hepatogenic mesoderm, which develops in the transverse septum, in which will develop the liver.

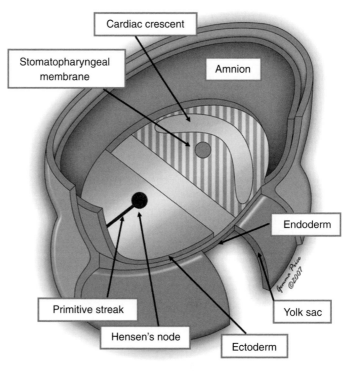

Figure 19-1   The cartoon shows the embryonic disc in conjunction with the amniotic cavity and the yolk sac. Note that, subsequent to its folding, the edges of the embryonic disc form the navel.

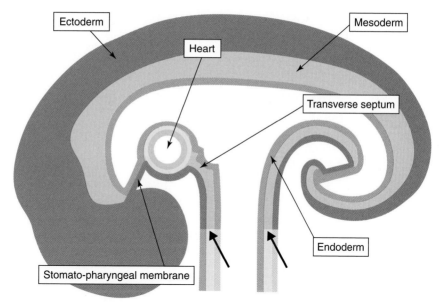

Figure 19-2 The cartoon shows how, subsequent to folding of the embryonic disc, the margins of the disc are no more than the surrounds of the navel (*black arrows*).

During the stage at which the embryo is a disc, this transverse septum is located at its upper edge, but subsequent to the completion of folding, it is located cranial to the navel (Fig. 19-2).

When the developing embryo is no more than a disc, the division between its right and left sides is marked by the primitive streak, with the node at its cranial end. The cells that will form the heart migrate from the anterior part of the primitive streak during the process of gastrulation, producing the right- and left-sided heart-forming regions within the mesodermal layer.[15-17] With continuing development, these two areas fuse across the midline, thus forming the cardiac crescent (Fig. 19-3). As the disc folds, the crescent also undergoes folding, forming a trough that starts

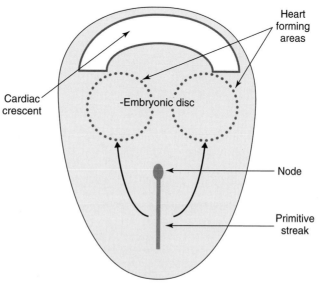

Figure 19-3 The cartoon shows an idealized view from above of the embryonic disc, indicating how migrations of cells from the primitive streak between the ectodermal and endodermal layers form initially the heart-forming areas, and then coalesce to form the cardiac crescent.

to close dorsally. The part of the trough that closes first produces the initial linear heart tube, which eventually becomes the left ventricular apex and septum.[11] Closure of the trough then proceeds in both cranial and caudal directions. With folding of the embryo, the part of the crescent that was initially positioned centrally becomes located mediodorsally relative to the developing body of the embryo. The initially peripheral margin of the crescent, in contrast, becomes the ventrocaudal part of the definitive heart tube. It is the part of the heart-forming area initially located centro-medially that has been nominated as the second heart field, with this part itself now further described in terms of its cranial and caudal components.[18,19] From its central position, this area is able to add material to both the arterial and venous poles of the developing heart tube, and through the dorsal mesocardium when that portal still exists.

Molecular analyses of cell lineage have now demonstrated in unambiguous fashion that new myocardium is added to both ends of the initial linear myocardial heart tube.[19,20] The techniques have revealed a similar developmental programme to that observed in the differentiation of the primary heart field, involving the transcription factors Nkx2-5, Gata4, and Mef2c, as well as fibroblast growth factors and bone morphogenetic proteins.[12] Differences in opinion remain, nonetheless, as to the origin of the cardiac components formed at the arterial pole. Some suggest that the so-called second field, previously considered simply as visceral mesoderm, forms only the myocardial components of the trunks.[10] Genetic lineage studies show that, whatever it is called, the area makes contributions to both the inflow and outflow region of the heart.[19,20] These findings have led to suggestions that malformations involving the two poles are a common phenomenon.[21] The suggested differences between the so-called fields, however, may be more apparent than real, since morphological boundaries are not themselves necessarily static. The changes seen are probably no more than the consequence of complex temporal patterning of the initial heart-forming area. Experimental studies in chicken suggest that the cells initially present within this area, depending on their position, have the capacity to form all parts of the heart.[22] Such a notion is in keeping with current views on cellular diversity, since differences in the concentration of diffusing morphogens can create a number of different fates for a given cell, promoting diversity within a field that was initially homogeneous.

We suggest, therefore, that differences between the so-called first and second heart fields are temporal rather than morphological. Indeed, recent findings have pointed to the importance of ongoing movement of tissues into the venous pole of the heart via a protrusion of the dorsal pharyngeal mesenchyme.[23] As we will explain, a similar protrusion is to be found at the arterial pole, which is populated by cells derived from neural crest.

Along with others, we believe that the changes recapitulate the evolutionary development of the cardiovascular system.[24] In the lower vertebrates, the heart contains no more than the components of the systemic circulation, namely an atrium, a ventricle, and a myocardial outflow tract. It is much later in evolutionary development that we see the appearance of the pulmonary circulation, represented by the right ventricle and the dorsal atrial wall, including the atrial septum. Within the evolutionary tree, pulmonary veins are first seen in lungfish, uniting to drain to a left atrium that was initially present as part of a common chamber, but which has now become separated from its right atrial counterpart by the atrial septum. This sets the scene for a separate pulmonary circulation, and also for the appearance of the atrial septum. As we will show, the mammalian atrial septum, along with the dorsal atrial wall, are formed from mediastinal myocardium.[25] Along with the outflow tract and the right ventricle, this mediastinal myocardium is derived from the tissues currently described as the second heart field, with the atrial components being added through the venous pole. We would suggest that patterning of a single heart-forming area, albeit with different temporal sequences, is sufficient to provide all the material needed to construct the four-chambered heart. The crucial point underscoring our current reappraisal is that not all precursors are present within the initial linear myocardial heart tube.

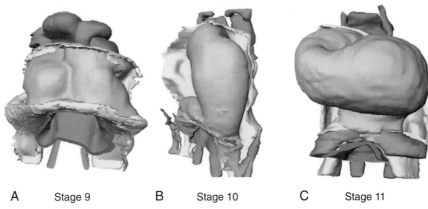

A   Stage 9   B   Stage 10   C   Stage 11

Figure 19-4   These reconstructions of the developing heart show the changes that take place in Carnegie stages 9 through 11 in the human heart. The myocardium is shown in gray, the margins of the pericardial cavity in yellow, and the pharyngeal mesenchyme in green. (See Expert Consult site for color image.) (Modified from Sizarov A, Ya J, de Boer BA, et al. Development of the building plan of the human heart: morphogenesis, growth and differentiation. Circulation 2011;123:1125-1135.)

Cardiac Looping

The first signs of the developing human heart become apparent at stage 9 in the Carnegie series of stages, equivalent to about 20 days of development.[26] When first seen, the myocardial component is a ventral strip that plasters the two bilateral vascular channels against the developing foregut, the endocardial jelly separating the myocardial and endothelial layers (Fig. 19-4A). By stage 10, the strip of myocardium has folded around the fused vascular channels, which now exist as a solitary lumen within the heart tube, the tube itself enclosed within the pericardial cavity in the cervical region of the developing embryo (Fig. 19-4B). At its cranial end, the vascular channel contained within the myocardial tube divides to pass in symmetrical fashion through the pharyngeal mesenchyme as the first aortic arches. The caudal part of the tube, which receives the systemic venous tributaries, dilates and constitutes the primordium of the developing atrial components. By stage 11, equivalent to about 25 days of development, the tube becomes S-shaped in the process of so-called looping (Fig. 19-4C). The changes producing the looping itself were initially thought to be the consequence of rapid growth of the tube within a pericardial cavity, the pericardial covering expanding much more slowly.[27] The tube continues to loop, however, even when deprived of its normal arterial and venous attachments, and also loops when no longer beating, ruling out the role of hemodynamics as a morphogenetic factor.[28,29] Looping, therefore, is an intrinsic feature of the heart itself, albeit that the exact cause has still to be determined. Be that as it may, the tube usually curves to the right. This rightward turning is part of the breaking of symmetry within the developing embryo, but is independent of rightness or leftness within the heart. As we will describe, the ventricles form in series from the looping tube, rather than being derived in parallel, as is the case for the atrial appendages. Rightward looping has frequently been considered to represent the first morphological evidence of the breaking of cardiac symmetry. This is incorrect. Asymmetry is already evident in the position of the atrioventricular canal when it is first seen, and in the formation of the atrial primordium at the linear heart-tube stage (Fig. 19-4B).[26,30]

Formation of the Cardiac Chambers

When first formed as a tube, the myocardial layer has particular features that permit its description as primary myocardium. The cardiomyocytes making up the myocardial layer express neither atrial natriuretic factor nor connexin40.[26,31] During

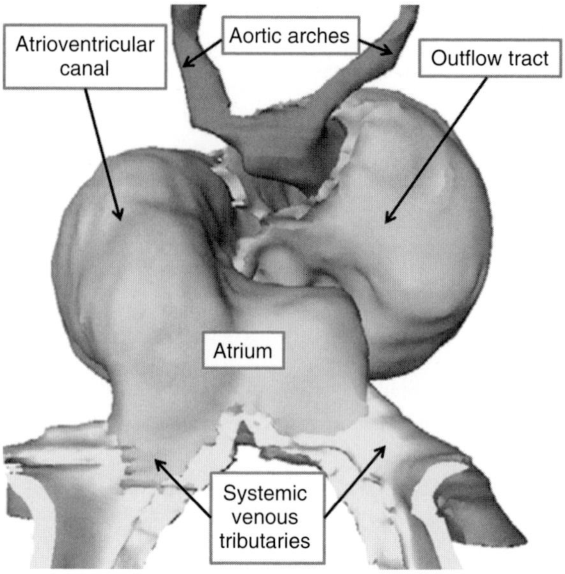

Figure 19-5   The reconstruction shows a stage 11 human heart viewed from behind. It shows the leftward location of the atrioventricular canal relative to the atrial component of the heart tube. The systemic venous tributaries are relatively symmetrical at this stage. (See Expert Consult site for color image.) (Modified from Sizarov A, Ya J, de Boer BA, et al. Development of the building plan of the human heart: morphogenesis, growth and differentiation. Circulation 2011;123:1125-1135.)

stages 12 through 16, representing around 26 through 38 days of development, the changes are seen that, by a process of ballooning, produce the so-called chamber myocardium.[26,31] This chamber myocardium expresses both atrial natriuretic factor and connexin40.[26,31,32] Subsequent to looping, it is possible to recognize the embryonic atrial and ventricular components of the heart tube, with the systemic venous tributaries draining in relatively symmetrical fashion to the atrial part, and the atrioventricular canal joining the atrial and ventricular components in left-sided position (Fig. 19-5). The ventricular component of the tube, at this stage, continues as the myocardial outflow tract, which continues extrapericardially at the cranial margin of the pericardial cavity to give rise to the arteries of the developing first pharyngeal arches. The atrial appendages grow in parallel from the common atrial component of the tube (Fig. 19-6A), developing their definitive rightward and leftward positions (Fig. 19-6B). The apical parts of the ventricular chambers, in contrast, balloon from the proximal leftward and distal rightward parts of the ventricular loop (Fig. 19-7). As the apical parts of the developing ventricles become apparent, the luminal parts are filled by numerous trabeculations, seen first in the developing left ventricle (Fig. 19-7). The circumference of the atrioventricular canal is supported exclusively by the myocardial walls of the developing left ventricle. With increasing ballooning of the apical components, the cavity of the right side of the atrial component effectively shifts rightward, with the direct right-sided atrioventricular connection having become evident by Carnegie stage 16 (Fig. 19-8). The changes in formation of the chamber myocardium are accompanied by addition of still more myocardial tissue to the heart through the venous pole. This takes place through the relatively small dorsal area, known as the dorsal mesocardium, where the myocardial atrial walls retain their continuity with the pharyngeal mesenchyme, and also at the sites of junction with the developing systemic venous tributaries. The new myocardium added to the heart through the dorsal mesocardium is positive for connexin40, but negative for atrial natriuretic factor, thus distinguishing it from both the primary and chamber myocardial components. This third component is mediastinal myocardium.[25] It forms the smooth-walled dorsal wall of the developing left atrium, as well as providing the site of formation of the primary atrial septum.

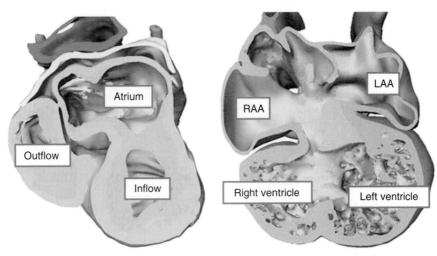

Figure 19-6   These reconstructions, showing four-chamber sections through the developing human heart at Carnegie stages 12 and 14, reveal how the atrial appendages balloon from the same atrial component of the heart tube, whereas the ventricular apical components balloon in series from the ventricular part of the tube. Note also the rightward shift of the atrioventricular canal concomitant with formation of the right atrioventricular junction. Note also how the endocardial jelly, shown in yellow, has compacted to form the cushions. (See Expert Consult site for color image.) (Modified from Sizarov A, Ya J, de Boer BA, et al. Development of the building plan of the human heart: morphogenesis, growth and differentiation. Circulation 2011;123:1125-1135.)

Subsequent to the process of ballooning, and with the addition of the mediastinal myocardium, it is possible to recognize the primordiums of the right and left atrial and ventricular chambers. Concomitant with this growth, important changes have taken place with regard to the alignment of the systemic venous tributaries. At stage 11, the systemic venous tributaries open in relatively symmetrical fashion to the developing atrial component, albeit that the union of the atrial component with the atrioventricular canal is remarkably eccentric (Fig. 19-5). By stage 12, there is still relative symmetry in terms of the developing right- and left-sided systemic venoatrial connections, but by stage 14 there has been a marked right-sided shift of the sinuatrial junction. With this shift, the junction itself becomes recognizable anatomically, being guarded by the venous valves (Fig. 19-9). As the venoatrial

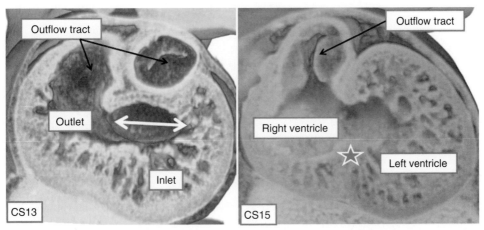

Figure 19-7   These images are sections taken from reconstructed episcopic datasets from human embryos at Carnegie stages 13 (*left panel*) and 15 (*right panel*). They show how the ventricular apical components balloon from the inlet and outlet components of the ventricular loop. Note that the overall circumference of the atrioventricular canal (*double-headed arrow*) is initially committed almost exclusively to the inlet of the tube. The primary ventricular septum (*star*) appears concomitant with the process of ballooning. (See Expert Consult site for color image.)

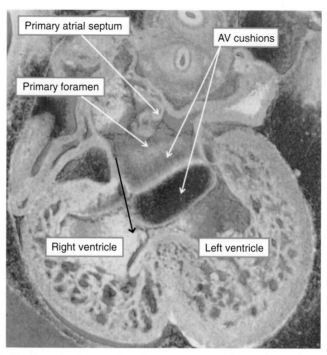

Figure 19-8 This four-chamber section, from an episcopic dataset from a human embryo at Carnegie stage 16, shows how, with continued growth, the atrioventricular canal, occupied by the atrioventricular (AV) endocardial cushions, has expanded rightward to achieve direct access to the developing right ventricle (*black arrow*). Note that the primary foramen remains patent at this stage of development.

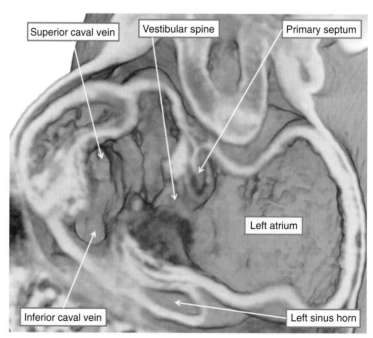

Figure 19-9 This section, showing a cross-section of the developing atrial chambers, is from an episcopic dataset from a human embryo at Carnegie stage 14. It shows how the systemic venous tributaries have moved rightward so as to open into the developing right atrium, with the sinuatrial junction now marked by the venous valves. Note the primary atrial septum growing from the atrial roof, with a mesenchymal cap on its leading edge.

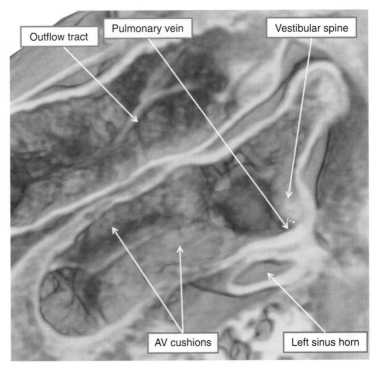

Figure 19-10 The image is a long axis section through the developing human heart at Carnegie stage 14. It shows the left atrium, the atrioventricular canal, and the outflow tract. Note that the opening of the pulmonary vein is a solitary orifice adjacent to the developing left atrioventricular junction, which contains the left sinus horn, the latter having its own discrete walls. The bulge made by the ventral protrusion from the pharyngeal mesenchyme is seen to the right of the pulmonary venous orifice.

junction effectively moves rightward, so the left-sided venous tributary bringing blood from the embryo back to the heart, the left superior cardinal vein, becomes incorporated into the left side of the developing left atrioventricular junction, albeit draining into the right atrium. Throughout this process, the vein retains its own discrete walls. Once incorporated into the junction, it passes dorsal and caudal relative to the persisting dorsal mesocardium. Important changes also occur in this mesocardial connection during this crucial period, corresponding with initial formation of the lungbuds at the terminations of the dividing tracheal diverticulum of the foregut. As the lungs begin to form, vessels appear around them, and channels begin to canalize within the mesenchyme of the dorsal mesocardium. This canalization produces the extensive splanchnic capillary network, where pulmonary veins are developing. Later, pulmonary venous capillaries are joining to form one single venous channel, which initially opens to the left atrium through a solitary orifice adjacent to the atrioventricular canal. The communication with the atrium is first seen in embryos at Carnegie stages 13 to 14, and is bordered at its right margin by a marked protrusion (Fig. 19-10). Initially described by Wilhelm His the Elder in the nineteenth century as the *spina vestibuli*,[34] this ventral protrusion of the dorsal pharyngeal mesenchyme is now known to be key to the completion of atrial and atrioventricular septation. It interposes at all times between the systemic and pulmonary venous orifices. Thus at no stage is the pulmonary venous channel in continuity with the lumens of the systemic venous tributaries.[35] As in the mouse, its opening to the atrium in man is through the mediastinal myocardium.[22,36]

Cardiac Septation

Much has been learned of the mechanisms of cardiac septation over the last 2 decades, with the findings largely confirming classic accounts, but revealing new features that are particularly pertinent to considerations of the new contributions made at the venous and arterial poles. Both muscular and mesenchymal components contribute to the definitive septal components, although some parts described as septums are folds and sandwiches rather than discrete solitary separating walls.[37] The mesenchymal components are largely derived from the endocardial cells undergoing endothelial-to-mesenchymal transformation and invading the cardiac jelly, which initially lines the entirety of the heart tube, separating its myocardial and endothelial layers. Key mesenchymal structures, nonetheless, are incorporated from extrapericardial sources to complete the division of the atrioventricular canal and the intrapericardial arterial trunks. Between Carnegie stages 10 and 14, the endocardial jelly changes its shape so that it is seen as facing cushions within the atrioventricular canal (Fig. 19-6) and the cushions that extend throughout the outflow tract (Figs. 19-7, 19-10). As the endocardial layer becomes mesenchymalized to form the cushions in the atrioventricular canal, the jelly disappears from the larger parts of the atrial lumen. A strip of jelly remains, however, in the atrial roof and can be seen at Carnegie stage 12, marking the site of formation of the muscular primary atrial septum (Fig. 19-6A). As the muscular primary septum grows from the atrial roof, it carries a mesenchymal cap on its leading edge (Fig. 19-9). The caudal growth carries the edge of the developing septum toward the atrioventricular cushions, which are themselves growing toward each other from the superior and inferior margins of the atrioventricular canal to divide it into right and left orifices (Fig. 19-8). The gap between the mesenchymal cap and the atrial surface of the endocardial cushions is the primary atrial foramen, which closes by merging and fusion of the mesenchymal tissues. By the time the primary foramen has closed, the primary atrial septum has become interrupted, thus forming the secondary foramen, which permits the richly oxygenated blood entering the heart through the inferior caval vein to reach the left side of the heart. We now know that the final separation of the atrioventricular canal into its right and left junctions requires the contribution from an additional mesenchymal structure, the so-called vestibular spine, or dorsal mesenchymal protrusion.[34,37] We also now believe that it is deficiency of this developmental component, rather than failure of fusion of the endocardial cushions, that is the essential abnormality underscoring the appearance of atrioventricular septal defects with common atrioventricular junction.[38] The protrusion enters the heart from the visceral mesenchyme through the right pulmonary ridge (Fig. 19-11), reinforcing the right side of the zone of fusion between the mesenchymal cap carried on the primary atrial septum and the atrioventricular cushions. We now know that the tissue within the protrusion shows no evidence of cellular proliferation once it has formed within the right pulmonary ridge.[26] The inference, therefore, is that the right and left atrioventricular junctions expand caudally relative to the spine once the primary foramen has been closed. Such an event correlates well with the formation of the so-called muscular atrioventricular septum, which in reality is a sandwich between the vestibular myocardium of the right atrium and the crest of the muscular ventricular septum.[38] The secondary interatrial foramen does not become converted into the oval foramen until much later development. The so-called atrial septum secundum is no more than a deep fold between the attachments of the caval veins to the right atrium and the pulmonary veins to the left atrium. The fold does not achieve its definitive form until the pulmonary venoatrial junction is positioned at the roof of the left atrium.[33] By the time the veins have achieved their location in the atrial roof, there are usually four venous orifices. The superior rim of the oval foramen is then formed by the deep fold between the connections of the right pulmonary veins to the left atrium and the superior caval vein to the right atrium. The fold overlaps the upper edge of the primary atrial septum, which is then able to oppose the fold and closes the oval foramen once the left atrial pressure exceeds right atrial pressure in postnatal life (Fig. 19-12). By the time of formation of the superior interatrial fold, the tissue derived from the ventral protrusion of the dorsal pharyngeal mesenchyme will have muscularized to form the anteroinferior muscular buttress of the oval foramen.

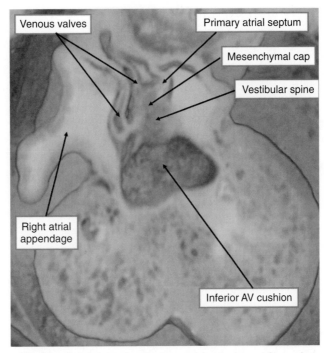

Figure 19-11 The four-chamber section from an episcopic dataset from a human embryo at Carnegie stage 17 shows how the mesenchymal cap on the primary atrail septum, the vestibular spine, and the inferior endocardial cushion have fused together to close the primary atrial foramen. A section taken further cranially showed that the upper margin of the primary septum had broken down to form the secondary atrial foramen.

Figure 19-12 The cartoons show the steps in formation of the atrial septum. Panel A shows how the primary atrial septum grows from the atrial roof towards the atrioventricular endocardial cushions, carrying a mesenchymal cap on its leading edge. The gap between the cap and the cushions is the primary atrial foramen (bracket). Panel B shows how fusion of the cap with the cushions, reinforced by growth of the vestibular spine from the visceral mesenchyme, or so-called second heart field, obliterates the primary foramen, but by this time the cranial edge of the primary septum has broken down to form the secondary interatrial foramen (bracket). At this stage, the pulmonary veins are still positioned caudally within the developing left atrium, and the atrial roof is flat. It is only subsequent to movement of the pulmonary veins to the atrial roof, as shown in panel C, that there is formation of the so-called septum secundum, which in reality is the superior interatrial fold. At the same time, there is muscularization of the vestibular spine to form the anteroinferior buttress of the septum. The flap valve, formed from the primary septum, then abuts against the superior interatrial fold, with the space between now forming the oval foramen (bracket).

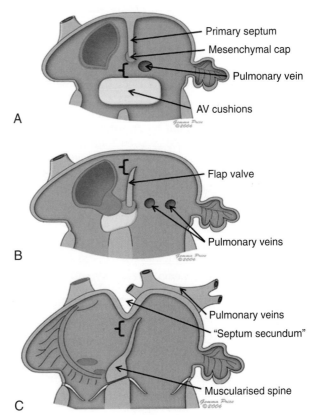

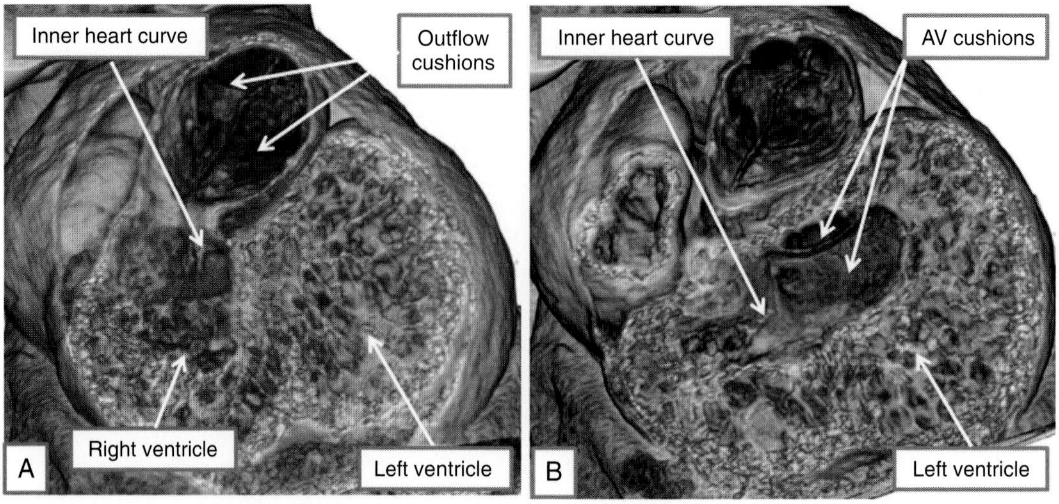

Figure 19-13 These four-chamber sections are from an episcopic dataset from a human embryo at Carnegie stage 14. They confirm that, at this early stage, and as shown in Figure 19-8, the outflow tract arises exclusively from the developing right ventricle (panel A), while the atrioventricular canal opens predominantly into the developing left ventricle (panel B), even though the wall is already in continuity with the right ventricle through the inner heart curvature.

Ventricular septation is also dependent on new contributions to the heart from heart-forming areas, with studies in the mouse showing that the so-called primary heart field forms little more than the apex of the left ventricle and the left side of the muscular ventricular septum.[12] The entirety of the musculature of the right ventricle and the right side of the septum is derived by the addition of further tissues to the developing heart tube. The muscular septum itself is formed concomitant with the ballooning of the apical ventricular components, with the septum appearing as the apical cavities expand caudally to either side of the initial septal crest (compare Figs. 19-7 and 19-8). In the chicken heart, the septum itself is formed by conglomeration of multiple trabecular layers.[39] The finding of multiple apical ventricular septal defects in the setting of so-called ventricular noncompaction in the human suggests that formation of the muscular septum in man may also require the compaction of multiple trabeculations, although there is no evidence of such individual components seen during normal development (Fig. 19-9). When the muscular septum is first formed, the circumference of the atrioventricular canal is confined almost exclusively to its left side, while the orifice of the common lumen of the outflow tract is to its right side (Fig. 19-13). There is, therefore, considerable remolding of the initial interventricular foramen during growth and its eventual closure. This process was clarified by study of the positional changes of the margins of the embryonic interventricular communication made possible by the serendipitous staining of these components by an antibody to the nodose ganglion of the chick.[40] The original margins of the ventricular communication eventually surround the orifices of the tricuspid valve and the aortic root. Subsequent to these realignments, the persisting interventricular communication is closed by adherence of the proximal outflow cushions with the crest of the muscular septum, with the mesenchymal tissues becoming transformed with time into the membranous septum. Closure of the embryonic interventricular foramen occurs at about 8 weeks of development in the human, but only much later in development does the developing membranous part of the septum become divided into its atrioventricular and interventricular components, occurring concomitant with delamination of the septal leaflet of the tricuspid valve from the surface of the muscular septum.[41]

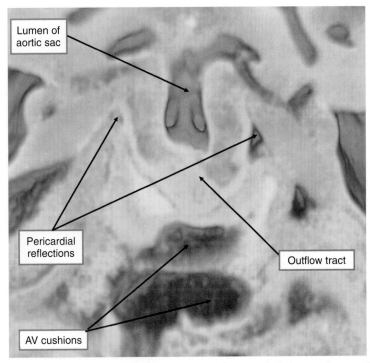

Figure 19-14   The frontal section from an episcopic dataset of a human embryo at Carnegie stage 13 shows how the cavity of the outflow tract becomes continuous with that of the aortic sac at the margins of the pericardial cavity. The orifices of the arteries running through the third, fourth, and sixth aortic arches are seen taking their origin from the dorsal wall of the aortic sac.

Development and Separation of the Outflow Tract

We do not include septation of the outflow tract as part of the overall process of cardiac septation because, in the normally formed postnatal heart, there are virtually no septal structures interposing between the separate pulmonary and systemic outflow channels. As we will show, septal structures certainly exist in the developing heart, but they subsequently disappear concomitant with maturation of the discrete walls of the pulmonary and systemic outflow channels. The outflow tract itself initially arises exclusively from the outlet of the developing right ventricle (Fig. 19-13), then extending in serpentine fashion to the margins of the pericardial cavity, where its lumen becomes continuous with the cavity of the aortic sac, a manifold embedded within the pharyngeal mesenchyme (Fig. 19-14). By Carnegie stage 13, the arteries of the third, fourth, and sixth branchial arches have developed within the pharyngeal mesenchyme, and at this stage are bilaterally symmetrical (Fig. 19-15). Initially, the walls of the intrapericardial outflow tract are exclusively muscular, and the solitary lumen is lined circumferentially by a layer of endocardial jelly. With development, the outflow tract becomes less serpentine. By Carnegie stage 14, it is possible to recognize its proximal and distal components, with a marked bend at their junction (Fig. 19-16). As in the mouse heart, all the myocardial walls of the outflow tract at this stage, along with the walls of the right ventricle, are known to have been newly added to the heart from the heart-forming areas.[26] With ongoing development, there is still further addition of new cells to the distal outflow tract, combined with invasion of the endocardial jelly by cells migrating from the neural crest.

These changes produce marked remolding of the distal part of the outflow tract. The new material added from the heart-forming areas initially occupies the parietal

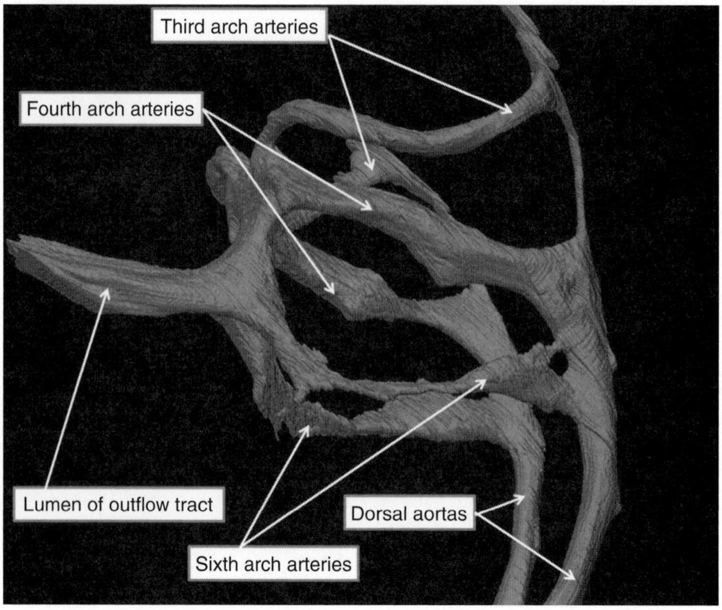

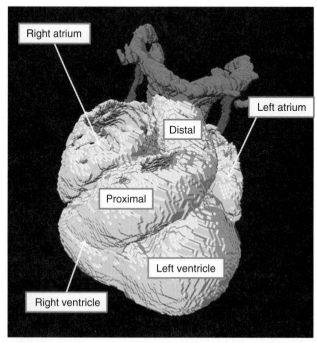

Figure 19-15 The image shows the arteries running through the branchial arches in a human embryo at Carnegie stage 13. The arteries were reconstructed from an episcopic dataset, and the reconstruction is shown from the left side. It can be seen that the arteries are bilaterally symmetrical at this early stage of development and that there is a solitary lumen within the distal outflow tract. (See Expert Consult site for color image.)

Figure 19-16 The image shows a frontal view of a reconstructed heart from an optical tomographic dataset from a human embryo at Carnegie stage 13. The myocardial walls have been shown in silver. At this stage, the entire outflow tract has myocardial walls, and an obvious dogleg bend permits recognition of proximal and distal components. (See Expert Consult site for color image.)

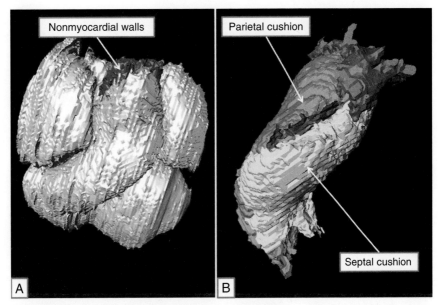

Figure 19-17 The images are reconstructions made from an optical tomographic dataset from a human embryo at Carnegie stage 15. The green areas in panels A and B show the nonmyocardial walls that have grown into the pericardial cavity at the distal margins of the outflow tract, producing a fishmouth appearance to the distal myocardial border, shown in silver in panel A. Panel B shows a reconstruction of the cushions that have developed from the cardiac jelly, viewed from the left side. The spiraling nature of the cushions is well seen, along with their interdigitation with the nonmyocardial walls, again shown in green. (See Expert Consult site for color image.)

parts of the outflow tract, with the myocardial border regressing from the margins of the pericardial cavity on the right and left sides concomitant with the addition of the nonmyocardial material. The effect is to produce a fishmouth appearance to the distal myocardial border.[42] As the myocardial border has regressed from the pericardial margins parietally, so have changes occurred in the morphology of the endocardial jelly. Initially forming a circumferential lining, the jelly becomes compacted into cushions, which face each other in spiraling fashion as they extend from positions cranially and caudally in the distal outflow tract to become septally and parietally located at the junction of the outflow tract with the right ventricle (Fig. 19-17). The distal ends of the cushions extend into the jaws of the myocardial fishmouth, with the angles of the jaws filled by the newly formed nonmyocardial walls. At this stage, the space between the distal margins of the outflow cushions and the dorsal wall of the aortic sac represents an aortopulmonary foramen, since it produces continuity between the cranial origins of the third and fourth arch arteries and the caudal origins of the arteries percolating through the sixth pharyngeal arches (Fig. 19-18). The pulmonary arteries themselves have begun to appear by this stage and take their origin from the midportions of the arteries running through the sixth arches. Major remodeling then takes place rapidly within the pharyngeal mesenchyme, resulting in obliteration of the right-sided fourth and sixth arch arteries. Once these arteries are obliterated, the union of the back wall of the aortic sac with the distal ends of the outflow cushions has placed the arteries of the third and fourth arches in continuity with the right-sided channel produced in the distal outflow tract by fusion of the outflow cushions themselves, and the pulmonary arteries, now being fed from the floor of the aortic sac, with the left-sided channel in the distal outflow tract. This process is achieved by ventral protrusion of the dorsal wall of the aortic sac into the pericardial cavity. The protrusion is populated by cells migrating centrally into the pharyngeal mesenchyme from the neural crest. It is the eventual fusion of the ventral protrusion with the ends of the distal outflow cushions that obliterates the

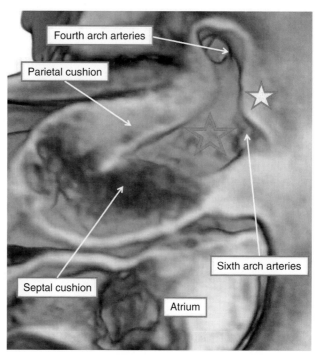

Figure 19-18   The image shows a sagittal section through the distal part of the outflow tract in a human embryo at Carnegie stage 14. The open red star shows the aortopulmonary foramen between the distal ends of the cushions and the back wall of the aortic sac (*white star*). The dorsal wall of the sac, separating the arteries of the fourth and sixth arches, is an effective aortopulmonary septum at this stage of development. (See Expert Consult site for color image.)

aortopulmonary foramen initially present in the lumen of the distal outflow tract (Fig. 19-19).

Fusion of the protrusion with the distal ends of the outflow cushions divides the distal outflow tract into right-sided and left-sided channels, with the right-sided channel now feeding the systemic circulation, and the left-sided channel in communication with the floor of the aortic sac, which now gives rise to the right and left pulmonary arteries. The caudal part of the aortic sac also continues through the left-sided artery of the sixth pharyngeal arch, which itself joins the dorsal aorta as the arterial duct. We have already explained how, within the distal part of the outflow tract, the growth into the pericardial cavity of nonmyocardial tissues derived from the initial heart-forming areas has produced the parietal walls of the intrapericardial components of the aorta and pulmonary trunk (Fig. 19-20), with the wall of the aorta extending craniocaudally, while that of the pulmonary trunk extends ventrodorsally (Fig. 19-21). The adjacent walls of the intrapericardial trunks are now formed by arterialization of the fused ventral protrusion and distal cushions, a process that occurs with great rapidity. At the same time, new intercalated cushions are formed parietally at the right and left borders of the middle part of outflow tract. With the appearance of these intercalated cushions, it is possible to recognize the outflow tract as having proximal, intermediate, and distal components (Fig. 19-22). The intercalated cushions lie edge to edge with the unfused margins of the major outflow cushions in the middle part of the developing aortic and pulmonary channels (Fig. 19-23). These cushions located within the intermediate part of the outflow tract provide the scaffolding for formation of the arterial valves. Evidence from genetically engineered mice has shown that the major cushions themselves are filled with cells derived from the neural crest. These cells also contribute to the walls of the intrapericardial aorta and pulmonary trunk. The central part of the fused cushion mass, however, ameliorates in subsequent development, being converted into the

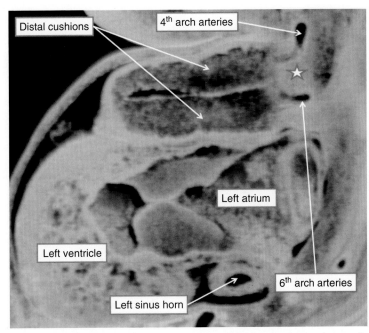

Figure 19-19   The image is a long axis section through the developing heart of a human embryo at Carnegie stage 15. It shows fusion of the ventral protrusion of the dorsal wall of the aortic sac (*star*) with the distal ends of the outflow cushions, obliterating the aortopulmonary foramen shown in Figure 19-18. Note the separate walls of the left sinus horn in the left atrioventricular junction. (See Expert Consult site for color image.)

extramural connective tissue separating the intrapericardial arterial trunks and the arterial roots. The changes within the middle part of the outflow tract, leading to the formation of the arterial valvar sinuses and leaflets, take place within a persisting sleeve of outflow musculature, which subsequently disappears by a process of apoptosis, with apoptosis also removing the central part of the fused cushion mass.[43-45] The end result is that, by excavation of the cushions and by conversion of the central part of the fused cushions to extraluminal connective tissue, the aortic

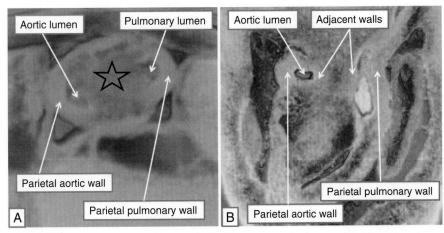

Figure 19-20   These images are both derived from episcopic datasets from human embryos at Carnegie stage 16. They show the rapidity with which the surfaces of the fused distal cushions and the ventral protrusion become converted into the adjacent walls of the intrapericardial aorta and pulmonary trunk. In the heart shown in panel A, cut in the frontal plane, the fused cushion mass (star) is still mesenchymal, whereas in the heart shown in panel B, cut in short axis plane, the adjacent walls of the arterial trunks have begun to arterialize.

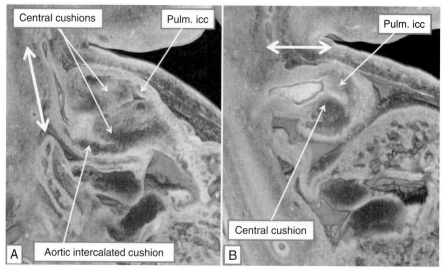

Figure 19-21   The images are taken through an episcopic dataset from a human embryo at Carnegie stage 16. Panel A shows how the intrapericardial aorta extends cranially to caudally, while panel B, sectioned to show the long axis of the pulmonary (pulm.) trunk, shows that this runs ventrally to dorsally (*double headed arrows*). Note also that the intercalated cushions (icc) are now seen in the middle part of the developing outflow tract.

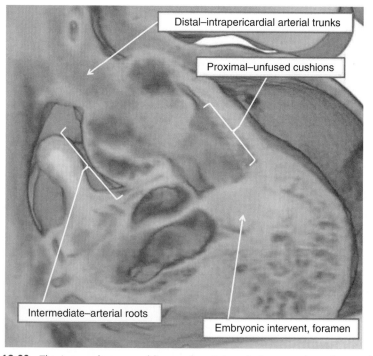

Figure 19-22   The image shows an oblique subcostal equivalent cut through an episcopic dataset from a human embryo at Carnegie stage 17. It shows well the three parts of the developing outflow tract, albeit the intrapericardial arterial component is cut through its central portion, which will become an extraluminal tissue plane.

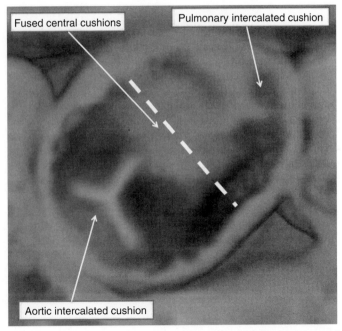

Fused central cushions

Pulmonary intercalated cushion

Aortic intercalated cushion

Figure 19-23 The image shows a short axis cut across the developing intermediate part of the outflow tract in a human embryo at Carnegie stage 16. It shows the primordia of the developing arterial roots, and reveals how the margins of the central cushions remain unfused, interdigitating with the intercalated cushions to provide the templates for formation of the arterial valves. The central part will subsequently separate along the plane of the dotted line.

and pulmonary roots are produced as separate structures in the middle part of the developing outflow tracts.

The parts of the central outflow cushions occupying the proximal regions of the outflow tract are the last to fuse. As these cushions fuse, they also muscularize. The muscularized intracardiac shelf thus produced then fuses with the crest of the primary muscular interventricular septum so as to wall the caudal lumen of the proximal outflow tract into the developing left ventricle. Because of the spiral arrangement of the cushions within the entire length of the outflow tract, this caudal proximal channel is continuous with the right-sided channel produced by fusion of the cushions in the distal outflow tract. Thus fusion of the muscularized proximal cushions with the crest of the muscular interventricular septum places the left ventricle in direct continuity with the intrapericardial aorta and leaves the right ventricle in continuity with the cranial proximal channel in the outflow tract, which continues dorsally as the pulmonary trunk (Fig. 19-24). The process of apoptosis occurring within the central part of the fused cushion mass continues proximally. The removal of the central part of the fused proximal cushion mass then leaves the muscularized surface of the cushions as part of the muscular subpulmonary infundibulum, the apoptosed central part becoming the extramural tissue plane interposed between the subpulmonary infundibulum and the aortic root. Even after the muscularized cushions have fused with the crest of the muscular ventricular septum to wall the aorta into the left ventricle, there remains a small persisting interventricular communication. This hole (Fig. 19-25) is closed by fusion of the muscularizing outflow cushions with the atrioventricular cushions, the mesenchymal tissues eventually remolding to become the fibrous membranous septum. As already emphasized, at the stage of closure of the embryonic interventricular communication, the septal leaflet of the tricuspid valve has still to delaminate from the surface of the muscular ventricular septum.[41] It is only at a later stage, therefore, that the membranous septum is divided into its atrioventricular and interventricular components.[46] It is also only at a later stage that the musculature of the inner heart curvature, which initially separated the

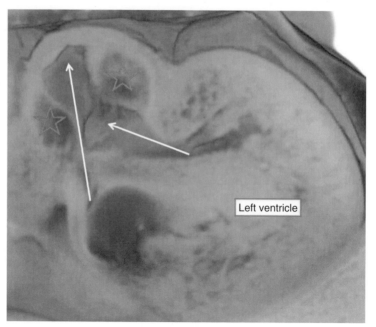

Figure 19-24   The image shows a short axis cut across the developing atrioventricular and ventriculoarterial junctions in a human embryo at Carnegie stage 16. When the proximal cushions (*stars*) fuse with each other, and also with the crest of the muscular ventricular septum, the caudal channel of the outflow tract, feeding the aorta, will arise from the left ventricle, while the cranial pulmonary channel will continue to be fed from the right ventricle, as shown by the arrows.

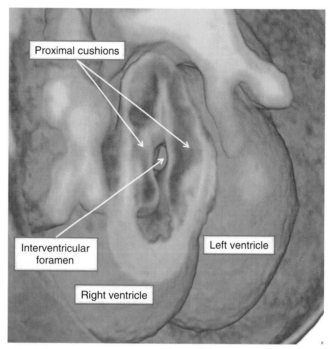

Figure 19-25   The image shows the developing pulmonary outflow tract seen from above, having removed its parietal wall, in a human embryo at Carnegie stage 17. It shows the persisting embryonic interventricular foramen, which will close by apposition of the proximal outflow cushions with the right margins of the atrioventricular cushions.

developing leaflets of the aortic and mitral valves, becomes converted into fibrous tissue, thus producing the area of aortic-to-mitral fibrous continuity that is one of the morphological features of the definitive left ventricle.

Relationship to Congenital Cardiac Malformations

Since the entirety of the right ventricle and outflow tract, along with the atrial chambers, is added to the developing heart subsequent to formation of the initial linear heart tube, it is hardly surprising that abnormal migration of the new tissues from the heart-forming areas is being related to the morphogenesis of congenital cardiac malformations. As already discussed, it has now been suggested that the contributions made at both the venous and arterial poles implies that the malformations should involve both ends of the heart.[21] The malformations seen in the human heart typically involving both the arterial and venous structures are those associated with so-called visceral heterotaxy. The essential feature of this so-called heterotaxy as now defined clinically, despite some early skepticism, is now known to be isomeric, rather than lateralized, formation of the atrial appendages and the lungs.[47-49] It has been analysis of genetically modified mice that has shown unequivocally that isomerism is a real thing in the setting of the congenitally malformed heart, even though the only structures that are recognizably isomeric are the atrial appendages and the sinus nodes.[50,51] Proper analysis of so-called heterotaxy by fetal cardiologists, furthermore, requires its separation into the two isomeric variants, more so since left isomerism is now known to carry a bad prognosis when diagnosed during fetal life because of its association with congenitally complete heart block.[52] In this light, therefore, the finding that the contributions from the caudal region of the heart-forming areas to the atrial myocardium is conditioned in the mouse by the acquisition of left-right identity subsequent to the expression of PitX2 is of obvious importance. It is also well established that the majority of patients seen in postnatal life with either right or left isomerism have common atrioventricular junctions, and it is now known that failure of formation of the dorsal mesenchymal protrusion is the likely morphogenetic factor underscoring the formation of the common junction as opposed to the separate right and left atrioventricular junctions. For many years, those investigating the causes of atrioventricular septal defect with common atrioventricular junction concentrated their attention on the development of the atrioventricular cushions, with the lesion often described in terms of endocardial cushion defects.[53] The very fact that hearts could be found with a common atrioventricular junction even in the setting of separate valvar orifices for the right and left ventricles should have pointed to the potential difficulties in expecting nonfusion of the cushions to be the causative feature.[38] With attention now being focused on the formation of the mesenchymal protrusion, as well as the potential lack of contributions from the heart-forming areas, it is likely that more light will be shed on the appropriate morphogenesis.

It is in lesions involving the outflow tracts, however, that most light is likely to emerge concerning morphogenesis when attention is directed toward the new contributions made by the heart-forming areas at the arterial pole. As we have shown, when assessing the development of the outflow tract, analysis is greatly facilitated by recognition of its distal, intermediate, and proximal components. Such analysis has much to commend it when compared to division into the so-called conus and truncus, since there is no consensus on the boundaries of these latter components, nor the structures to which they give rise in the postnatal heart. There are similar problems with so-called conotruncal defects, since there is no agreement as to which lesions should or should not be placed in this category.

The situation becomes much clearer when lesions involving the outflow tract are considered in terms of those involving the extrapericardial arterial channels, the intrapericardial arterial trunks, the arterial roots, and the ventricular outflow tracts. Such an approach will permit more accurate correlation with the account of cardiac development as presented in this chapter. Note also needs to be taken when considering morphogenesis that contributions from the heart-forming areas are supplemented by the migration into the heart from the neural crest, since it is the so-called crestopathies that have received most attention in recent years.[53] It should now be possible, however, to separate the contributions made by the neural crest as opposed to the new additions from the heart-forming areas when we correlate the developmental with the morphological changes. For example, the ventral arterial protrusion has as its core the visceral mesoderm, but carries on its surface cells derived from the neural crest.

Morphological evidence points very strongly to aortopulmonary window representing failure of closure of the embryonic aortopulmonary window, and hence to a likely failure of contribution from the central migration from the neural crest.[54] Failure of migration of cells from the neural crest, nonetheless, is also well established as being the substrate for production of common arterial trunk.[55] The pathognomonic feature of common trunk, however, is the commonality of the ventriculoarterial junction, resulting from failure of fusion of the major outflow cushions. Clinical subdivision of the lesion depends on the nature of the intrapericardial arterial pathways, and these depend anatomically on formation of the ventral arterial protrusion. Thus the contributions made by separate migrations from the neural crest, coupled with those made from the heart-forming areas, are likely to be of major importance when seeking to establish the morphogenesis of the various forms of common arterial trunk. At the same time, the morphological evidence shows clearly that the doubly committed and subarterial ventricular septal defect is more closely related to common arterial trunk than the other types of interventricular communication, since its pathognomonic feature, as with common arterial trunk, is the commonality of the ventriculoarterial junction.

There are manifold lesions involving the outflow tract and the right ventricle. Surely the ever-expanding body of knowledge concerning the molecular mechanisms underscoring cardiac development will elucidate the morphogenesis of congenital cardiac malformations, providing it is interpreted in the light of the appropriate cardiac morphology.

Acknowledgment

We are indebted to Aleksander Sizarov for his critical reading of earlier versions of the manuscript.

References

1. Abbott ME. Atlas of congenital cardiac disease. New York: American Heart Association; 1936:2.
2. Anderson RH, Wilkinson JL, Arnold R, et al. Morphogenesis of bulboventricular malformations. 1: Consideration of embryogenesis in the normal heart. Br Heart J. 1974;36:242-255.
3. Anderson RH, Wilkinson JL, Arnold R, et al. Morphogenesis of bulboventricular malformations. II. Observations on malformed hearts. Br Heart J. 1974;36:948-970.
4. Becker AE, Anderson RH. Cardiac embryology: a help or hindrance in understanding congenital heart disease? In: Nora JJ, Takao A, eds. Congenital heart disease: causes and processes. Mount Kisco, NY: Futura Publishing; 1984:339-358.
5. Moorman AFM. Cardiac anatomy: a help or a hindrance in understanding cardiac embryology. In: Anderson RH, Moorman AFM, Piek JJ, et al, eds. 35 Years cardiovascular pathology in Amsterdam. Ridderkerk: Ridderprint; 2004:91-100.
6. Viragh S, Challice CE. Origin and differentiation of cardiac muscle cells in the mouse. J Ultrastruct Res. 1973;42:1-24.
7. Arguello C, De la Cruz MV, Gomez CS. Experimental study of the formation of the heart tube in the chick embryo. J Embryol Exp Morphol. 1975:33;1-11.
8. Kelly RG, Brown NA, Buckingham ME. The arterial pole of the mouse heart forms from Fgf10-expressing cells in pharyngeal mesoderm. Dev Cell. 2001;1:435-440.
9. Mjaatvedt CH, Nakaoka T, Moreno-Rodriguez R, et al. The outflow tract of the heart is recruited from a novel heart-forming field. Dev Biol. 2001;238:97-109.
10. Waldo KL, Kumiski DH, Wallis KT, et al. Conotruncal myocardium arises from a secondary heart field. Development. 2001;128:3179-3188.
11. Aanhaanen WT, Brons JF, Dominguez JN, et al. The Tbx2+ primary myocardium of the atrioventricular canal forms the atrioventricular node and the base of the left ventricle. Circ Res. 2009;104:1267-1274.
12. Kelly RG, Evans SM. The second heart field. In: Rosenthal N, Harvey RP, eds. Heart development and regeneration. Amsterdam: Academic Press; 2010:143-170.
13. Abu-Issa R, Waldo K, Kirby ML. Heart fields: one, two or more? Dev Biol. 2004;272:281-285.
14. Moorman AFM, Christoffels VM, Anderson RH, et al. The heart-forming fields—one or multiple? Phil Trans R Soc B. 2007;362:1257-1265.

15. Rawles ME. The heart-forming regions of the early chick blastoderm. Physiol Zool. 1943;16:22-42.
16. Rosenquist GC. Location and movements of cardiogenic cells in the chick embryo: the heart forming portion of the primitive streak. Dev Biol. 1970;22:461-475.
17. Garcia-Martinez V, Schoenwolf GC. Primitive streak origin of the cardiovascular system in avian embryos. Dev Biol. 1993;159:706-719.
18. Cai CL, Liang X, Shi Y, et al. Isl1 identifies a cardiac progenitor population that proliferates prior to differentiation and contributes a majority of cells to the heart. Dev Cell. 2003;5:877-889.
19. Galli D, Dominguez JN, Zaffran S, et al. Atrial myocardium derives from the posterior region of the second heart field, which acquires left-right identity as Pitx2 is expressed. Development. 2008;135:1157-1167.
20. Zaffran S, Kelly RG, Meilhac SM, et al. Right ventricular myocardium derives from the anterior heart field. Circ Res. 2004;95:261-268.
21. Epstein JA. Cardiac development and implications for heart disease. NEJM. 2010;363:1638-1647.
22. Rosenquist GC, de Haan RL. Migration of precardiac cells in the chick embryo: a radioautographic study. In: Publication 625 Contributions to embryology. 263rd ed. Washington, DC: Carnegie Inst; 1966:111-121.
23. Snarr BS, O'Neal JL, Chintalapudi MR, et al. Isl1 expression at the venous pole identifies a novel role for the second heart field in cardiac development. Circ Res. 2007;101:971-974.
24. Grimes A, Duran AC, Sans-Coma V, et al. Phylogeny informs ontogeny: a proposed common theme in the arterial pole of the vertebrate heart. Evolution Dev. 2010;12:552-567.
25. Soufan AT, van den Hoff MJB, Ruijter JM, et al. Reconstruction of the patterns of gene expression in the developing mouse heart reveals an architectural arrangement that facilitates the understanding of atrial malformations and arrhythmias. Circ Res. 2004;95:1207-1215.
26. Sizarov A, Ya J, de Boer BA, et al. Development of the building plan of the human heart: morphogenesis, growth and differentiation. Circulation. 2011;123:1125-1135.
27. Patten BM. The development of the heart. In: Gould SE, ed. Pathology of the heart and blood vessels, 3rd ed. Charles. C. Thomas: Springfield, IL: 1968:20-90.
28. Orts Llorca F, Ruano Gil D. A causal analysis of the heart curvatures in the chicken embryo. Roux Archiv für Entwicklungsmechanik der Organismen. 1967;158:52-63.
29. Manasek FJ, Monroe RG. Early cardiac morphogenesis is independent of function. Dev Biol. 1972;27:584-588.
30. Brown NA, Anderson RH. Symmetry and laterality in the human heart: developmental implications. In: Harvey RP, Rosenthal N, eds. Heart development. San Diego: Academic Press; 1999:447-462.
31. Moorman AFM, Christoffels VM. Cardiac chamber formation: development, genes, and evolution. Physiol Rev. 2003;83:1223-1267.
32. Soufan AT, van den Hoff MJ, Ruijter JM, et al. Reconstruction of the patterns of gene expression in the developing mouse heart reveals an architectural arrangement that facilitates the understanding of atrial malformations and arrhythmias. Circ Res. 2004;95:1207-1215.
33. Webb S, Kanani M, Anderson RH, et al. Development of the human pulmonary vein and its incorporation in the morphologically left atrium. Cardiol Young. 2001;11:632-642.
34. His W. Das Herz. In: His W, ed. Anatomie menschlicher Embryonen, vol 3. Zür Geschichte der Organe. Leipzig, Vogel; 1885:129-184.
35. Webb S, Brown NA, Wessels A, et al. Development of the murine pulmonary vein and its relationship to the embryonic venous sinus. Anat Rec. 1998;250:325-334.
36. Anderson RH, Brown NA. The anatomy of the heart revisited. Anat Rec. 1996;246:1-7.
37. Webb S, Brown NA, Anderson RH. Formation of the atrioventricular septal structures in the normal mouse. Circ Res. 1998;82:645-656.
38. Anderson RH, Wessels A, Vettukattil JJ. Morphology and morphogenesis of atrioventricular septal defect with common atrioventricular junction. World J Ped Cong Heart Surg. 2010;1:59-67.
39. Ben-Shachar G, Arcilla RA, Lucas RV, et al. Ventricular trabeculations in the chick embryo heart and their contribution to ventricular and muscular septal development. Circ Res. 1985;57:759-766.
40. Lamers WH, Wessels A, Verbeek FJ, et al. New findings concerning ventricular septation in the human heart. Implications for maldevelopment. Circulation. 1992;86:1194-1205.
41. Lamers WH, Virááh S, Wessels A, et al. Formation of the tricuspid valve in the human heart. Circulation. 1995;91:111-121.
42. Bartelings MM, Gittenberger-de Groot AC. The outflow tract of the heart- embryologic and morphologic correlations. Int J Cardiol. 1989;22:289-300.
43. Ya J, van den Hoff MJB, de Boer PAJ, et al. The normal development of the outflow tract in the rat. Circ Res. 1998;82:464-472.
44. Sharma PR, Anderson RH, Copp AJ, et al. Spatiotemporal analysis of programmed cell death during mouse cardiac septation. Anat Rec Part A. 2004;277:355-369.
45. Webb S, Qayyum SR, Anderson RH, et al. Septation and separation within the outflow tract of the developing heart. J Anat. 2003;202:327-342.
46. Allwork SP, Anderson RH. Developmental anatomy of the membranous part of the ventricular septum in the human heart. Br Heart J. 1979;41:275-280.
47. Jacobs JP, Anderson RH, Weinberg P, et al. The nomenclature, definition and classification of cardiac structures in the setting of heterotaxy. Cardiol Young. 2007;17(Suppl 2):1-28.
48. Van Praagh R, Van Praagh S. Atrial isomerism in the heterotaxy syndromes with asplenia, or polysplenia, or normally formed spleen: an erroneous concept. Am J Cardiol. 1990;66:1504-1506.

19

49. Uemura H, Ho SY, Devine WA, et al. Atrial appendages and venoatrial connections in hearts from patients with visceral heterotaxy. Ann Thorac Surg. 1995;60:561-569.
50. Bamforth SD, Bragança J, Farthing CR, et al. Cited2 controls left-right patterning and heart development through a Nodal-Pitx2c pathway. Nat Genet. 2004;36:1189-1196.
51. Hildreth V, Webb S, Chaudhry B, et al. Left cardiac isomerism in the Sonic hedgehog null mouse. J Anat. 2009;214:894-904.
52. Cohen MS, Anderson RH, Cohen MI, et al. Controversies, genetics, diagnostic assessment, and outcomes relating to the heterotaxy syndromes. Cardiol Young. 2007;17(Suppl 2):29-43.
53. Brown CB, Baldwin HS. Neural crest contribution to the cardiovascular system. Adv Exp Med Biol. 2006;589:134-154.
54. Anderson RH, Cook A, Brown NA, et al. Development of the outflow tracts with reference to aorto-pulmonary windows and aortoventricular tunnels. Cardiol Young. 2010;20(Suppl 3):1-8.
55. Gittenberger-de Groot AC, Bartelings MM, Bogers AJJC, et al. The embryology of the common arterial trunk. Prog Ped Cardiol. 2002;15:1-8.

Fetal and Neonatal Cardiology

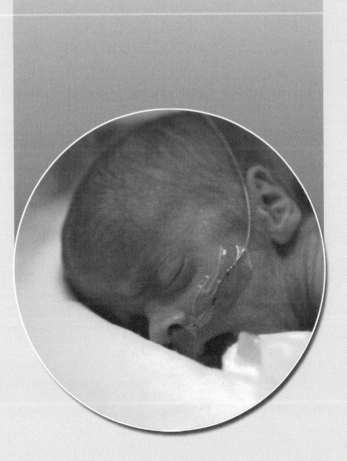

CHAPTER 20

New Concepts for Training the Pediatric Cardiology Workforce of the Future

Arthur Garson, Jr., MD, MPH

Background and Significance

The world's population is aging with high rates of chronic disease leading to increased demand for and utilization of health services. Currently, almost 50% of Americans have one or more chronic conditions and caring for them consumes 85% of the nation's health care dollars.[1] Despite the increased demand for health services, the supply of physicians and nurses is shrinking and is projected to decrease even more over the next 10 years, worsening the mismatch of supply and demand for access to care. This mismatch is, or shortly will be, manifested by longer waits to see physicians in emergency departments and clinics, lack of available timely follow-up for chronic diseases, and a shortage of practitioners in underserved areas, both rural and urban. This trend can be seen in the supply of pediatric cardiologists as well. According to the American Board of Pediatrics, there is a nationwide shortage of pediatric subspecialists, particularly in rural areas.[2] A 2009 report of the American College of Cardiology Workforce Task Force indicated that cardiology faces decades of workforce shortages including a shortage of pediatric cardiologists.[3]

In the United States, even if insurance coverage is made available to every citizen, access to care—being able to receive care in a timely manner—will continue to be of paramount importance. The state of Massachusetts reduced its population of uninsured by 75% and found that the time to see a primary care physician increased from 33 to 52 days.[4] These trends will continue if we continue to deliver medicine in the same way.

We must identify new team-based models of health care delivery and change the paradigm of care to reflect the needs of the population over the entire health care continuum. These new models will support a redesigned health system that provides a conduit to proper care, which recognizes the need for alternative ways to provide health care yet also efficiently allocates scarce professional resources to improve health, and health care, across all, but particularly underserved, populations.

This redesigned health system is based on care teams that begin with the patient, progressing to community health workers, nurses, advanced practice nurses, primary care physicians, and specialists. Point-of-care devices linked to an interoperable electronic health record tie the team together and promise coordinated care for the patient. The point of care devices will provide the community health worker with protocols and decision support tools created for these workers. Nurse leaders are the vital link in this chain of care in that they provide essential oversight and communication between physicians and nurses and between nurses and community health workers.

Implementing true team-based care requires a fresh look at how we train physicians and nurses and realizes the importance of incorporating trusted members of the community to serve as the liaison between patient and health professionals. Models for training caring community members have worked well serving Native American populations and in Alaska through the community health aide program. These programs have provided outstanding care to those who lack it. Only by expanding our thinking beyond traditional training and medical practice models and embracing the potential of a team-based model over a continuum of patient care needs will we, as a nation, be ready to address the health care and workforce challenges of tomorrow.

Challenges Facing the Health Workforce Today

If you want to see the future of access to primary care today, look at Massachusetts, the state with almost universal health insurance coverage resulting from the 2006 legislation that required all residents to have health insurance. Although Massachusetts has the highest ratio of physicians per capita in the country, finding a primary care physician has proved difficult, leading to decreased access to health care. Last year only 60% of family medicine practices—and only 44% of internal medicine practices—were accepting new patients, down from 70% in 2007 for family physicians and 64% in 2005 for general internists. Not surprisingly, this reduction in access had led to an increased volume in preventable trips to hospital emergency departments; in 2008, nearly half of outpatient emergency visits were considered avoidable.[5]

Primary and preventive care are important for improving and maintaining health, and form the point of entry into a larger continuum of patient care. Having access to basic health services is particularly important now, as 133 million Americans have at least one chronic illness with the number expected to grow to 157 million by 2020.[6] Despite this worrisome trend, 65 million people live in regions without adequate primary care. According to the federal Health Resources and Services Administration (HRSA), more than 16,000 additional primary care providers would be required today just to meet the need of those in underserved regions, a need that would still not be met even if all medical school graduates in 2008 had become primary care providers.[7] There is an equal problem (sometimes worse) with access to specialists in medically underserved areas. Outside of medically underserved regions, the doctor shortage problem extends to the health system as a whole and affects many medical specialties as well as primary care. The federal government estimates that the demand for overall physician services will increase 22% over the next 15 years while the number of primary care physicians will only increase 18%.[8]

With the passage of the Patient Protection and Affordable Care Act (PPACA) in March 2010, tens of millions of currently uninsured Americans are expected to have health coverage over the next 10 years. Combined with the aging of the 76 million baby boomers there will be an unprecedented demand for health care professionals to provide medical services, yet by all accounts there will not be enough physicians and nurses to meet the need. According to the Association of American Medical Colleges (AAMC), there will be an overall shortage of 91,500 active patient care physicians in 2020, with a primary care shortage of 45,400 and the other half a shortage of specialists.[9] Thirty percent of pediatric cardiologists are expected to retire within the next 10 years, echoing previous studies that have suggested workforce shortages due to retirement will exacerbate the physician supply problem, particularly since the numbers of retiring physicians are generally underestimated.[3,10] This will further strain the need for the 1.1 million physicians that the federal government projects will be necessary to respond to the increased numbers of Americans needing care by 2020.[11]

The same is true for nurses. Concerns about nursing shortages have existed for years, and, moving into the future, projected shortages suggest there will be 300,000 to a million fewer nurses than needed.[12] This trend is exacerbated by the fact that nurses, on average, are older than other health professionals. By 2006, the average age of the nursing workforce was just under 44 years, with estimates that the average age of employed nurses will increase by a year—to almost 45 years—by 2012.[13] Like physicians, the projected shortage is partially driven by the number of older nurses retiring during the next decade who will be replaced by smaller numbers of nurses following them.[14]

Inadequacy of the Current Health Care Delivery System

The current health care delivery system in the United States cannot meet the complex needs of patients. On the front end of the health care delivery system, many patients report difficulties being seen by a primary care physician in a timely manner when ill,[15] with nearly half of adults in the United States reporting failures in the coordination of their medical care between primary care physicians and specialists.[16] Many physicians are overwhelmed by crowded schedules and inefficient work environments, leading to a less effective patient-physician relationship.[17,18]

The health care delivery system of today is ill equipped to transform itself into the electronically connected interdisciplinary health team of tomorrow as the vast majority of primary care is still delivered in small physician settings with one or two physicians, with little use of electronic medical records.[19] In a recent physician survey, only 4% of physicians reported having an extensive, fully functional electronic records system in the outpatient sector, and only a slightly larger percentage—13%—reported having even a basic system.[20]

Although primary care physicians represent 35% of the US physician workforce and 57% of all patient visits, only 6-7% of total health care spending in the Medicare program is for primary care.[21] It is important to have both a strong primary care foundation and a responsive, evidence-based specialty care system that refers from and integrates with primary care. When people have access to primary care there are fewer emergency department visits, fewer preventable hospitalizations, and early treatment prevents the onset of more serious complications. When physicians communicate across specialties it encourages a move toward clinical efficacy and improved effectiveness.[22] This is why it is important to transform today's medical practice environment into a true team-based model of patient-centered interdisciplinary care.

In recognition of the importance of moving toward a patient-centered model of care, experts and policy makers are recommending the use of patient-centered medical homes (PCMH), a more complete model of patient care. PCMH providers offer a broader scope of medical care through practice redesign in which teams of health professionals coordinate and monitor the care of a population of patients both in community and hospital settings. Currently, hundreds of PCMH demonstration projects—many focusing on chronic care management—are being conducted around the country, emphasizing team approaches to care, including whole person orientation, mechanisms (like information technology) to support the integration and measurement of care provided, and an enhanced payment for the added value.[23] Early PCMH successes include Geisinger Health System, an integrated system that employs salaried physicians and nurses in a team model of care with a particular focus on the chronically ill. Since the inception of the practice model three years ago, Geisinger has experienced an 18% drop in hospital admissions and a decrease in overall medical expenses of 7%. Geisinger now uses the PCMH model in 37 of its practices.[24]

The Health Care System of the Future

In order to transform the way care is delivered it will be necessary to move from the singular concept of a medical home, or from a model of primary care alone, to one of an integrated team-based system where care is delivered along a health maintenance and treatment continuum that begins with preventive services at the community level and follows the patient into the hospital.

The health care system of the future must have a continuum beginning with the patient as part of the workforce and then shifting to primary care and then to specialty care in a coordinated and collaborative system of care. The focus will include not only the individual patient but also the entire population so that health outcomes can be measured and improvements in care can be integrated into daily practices. This will require a paradigm shift in the provision of patient care, shifting the focus from solo practitioner or a group that shares ideas and discussions but produces individual work products to a true team model where members have a common commitment and purpose and a set of performance goals for the patient and the community for which they hold themselves mutually accountable.[25] In addition, the mode of caring for patients—face-to-face visits—will have to be supplanted with multiple types of modes of encounter, such as e-mail visits, home visits, and a greater emphasis on patient self-maintenance. This will allow physicians to concentrate on those patients with complex conditions that may be difficult to diagnose and treat, leaving nonacute, preventive, and chronic care services to other members of the care team.

The health care system of the future will require leveraging all health care team workers up one notch: patients, community health workers, nurses, and physicians.

Patients

Patients will become part of the health care workforce. Under a renewed team-based care model, patients will have to become more interested in and responsible for their health. This will not be easy, as less than half of the adult population is actively engaged in their health and health care.[26] A range of tools can be employed to increase patient engagement, from educational interventions geared to appeal to individualized information that leads to healthier behaviors to more explicit financial incentives that reward or punish certain behaviors such as taking medications as prescribed. Currently, one third to one half of all patients do not take medication as prescribed, and up to one fourth never fill prescriptions at all, eventually costing the health care system $100 billion because those patients often get sicker. Recent pilot programs have shown that patients do respond to financial incentives offered to increase adherence to medication regimens, and some low-income Medicaid beneficiaries with low literacy skills are responding to financial "credits" given to reward healthy behaviors.[27,28] Alternatively, patients who are able to care for themselves could be compelled, via a financial penalty or increased insurance premiums, to take medications, enter wellness programs such as nutrition education or tobacco cessation, or receive recommended vaccines. This "beneficent coercion" could be justified, in part, by the growing health problems like obesity and increased medical care expenditures brought on by lack of medication adherence and healthy lifestyle changes, and as a component of individual responsibility.[29]

However, to justify such levels of enforcement we need to have a much better understanding of how individuals perceive health risks and how best to promote positive health-seeking behaviors using educational tools. It is important to remember that 50% of the population has an IQ under 100.[30] Strategies specific to each patient could be employed to tailor educational materials in order to promote health maintenance and individual health responsibility. This has been tested in a pilot program at the University of Virginia looking at tailored educational approaches for consumer health. We found that understanding individual preferences can promote the design of appropriate materials or programs that support patient education, treatment adherence, and an improved sense of personal responsibility regarding one's health and health care.[31]

Community Health Workers and Grand-Aides

According to the federal Bureau of Health Professions, community health workers (CWHs) are "lay members of communities who work either for pay or as volunteers in association with the local health care system in both urban and rural environments and usually share ethnicity, language, socioeconomic status, and life experiences with the community members they serve."[32] Recognized as improving health care access in communities, CHWs nevertheless have had limited demonstrated effectiveness in improving a population's overall health status because of lack of standardized training and reproducible patient care outcome measures.[33] Although some states sponsor training or certificate programs for CHWs, few have passed legislation to require workers to obtain specific training or certification.[34]

A revised patient-centered team model would rely on a new model of the CHW, one that builds on the traditional peer-to-peer relationships of trust with patients but also requires formal training to ensure knowledge of primary chronic and palliative care and skills alongside patient advocacy and cultural competency. The new CHW model would offer state-level credentialing within a set of core courses and standardized curricula. This would professionalize CHWs, provide them with their own scope of practice, and allow them to be compensated as part of an integrated health care team. Several sections of the PPACA include references to the community engagement and training needs of CHWs as members of the health care workforce.[35] Federal and state policy initiatives can support CHWs, blending the traditional role of improving patients' access to care with a more professionalized role that offers additional services in a greater scope of care that can also improve patient outcomes.[36]

One model of an "advanced" CHW is in place in several communities in the worldwide: a corps of trained grandparents acting as CHWs called "Grand-Aides." Grandparents have cared for two generations of their own children and grandchildren and are well suited to act as trusted health care agents in a community. The Grand-Aide model includes 6 months of intense training on how to use protocols to treat the 28 most common conditions in children and adults, e.g. colds, vomiting, fever, and rash. They are trained on how to use a mini-computer with an electronic medical record as well as telephone and video for communication to the supervisory nurse team member. After training, Grand-Aides are assigned 25 families in their own underserved area, and they provide home visits in follow-up of calls as necessary and teach about healthy self-care. With more training, they will be able to help physicians and nurses improve medication compliance for chronic diseases such as heart failure and provide support for palliative care. The Grand-Aides program currently has US demonstrations in Houston, Texas, and rural Virginia with future programs planned for Boston and Southern California.

Nurses

Nurses outnumber all other health professionals, spend the most time with patients, and play a key role in promoting patient care quality and safety.[37,38] For years, nurses have been playing a greater role in the nation's health care, especially in regions with few doctors, a trend that will continue into the future. Because of the physician shortage and because advanced practice nurse practitioners provide primary care in a cost-effective way, 28 states are currently considering actions to expand what nurse practitioners can do.[39]

Studies report higher levels of patient satisfaction in care encounters with nurse practitioners.[40,41,42] Glenn Steele, MD, president and chief executive officer of Geisinger Health System in Pennsylvania, echoes the belief in the quality and value of nurse practitioner health care providers as part of a medical team. In a recent interview in the journal *Health Affairs*, Dr. Steele notes, "We have more than 1000 nurse practitioners, physician assistants, pharmacists, and other so-called physician extenders. What we're trying to do is have folks work up to the limit of their license and really do things to see if redistributing caregiving work can increase quality and decrease cost."[43] Similarly, the American College of Cardiology (ACC) has developed an educational program to assist nurse practitioners gain more proficiency specific to cardiology care. This will accelerate the availability of cardiology-trained nonphysician practitioners.[3]

Physicians

In today's medical practice world, physicians "work nonstop with patients and have little direct interaction with others in their clinical team."[44] For the health care system to meet the growing demands of comprehensively managing patient care, the culture of physician-centered practice will have to change. Increased coordination achieved by integrated health care teams leads to improved clinical performance, effective care, patient satisfaction, and reduced workloads for individual clinicians.[45] In recognition of the value of team-based care, numerous organizations and payers have called for a changed role of physicians in a model of care, which begins with patient need at the point of care and coordinates that care within an interactive, collaborative team-based model that encompasses all workforce levels from the patient, through the lay health worker, to the generalist nurse and physician, to the specialist nurse and physician.[46] The highest quality workforce, which is equally valued, will provide the highest quality patient-centered care that is effective, efficient, timely, and safe. Physicians will have new roles since advanced practice nurses will care for the routinely ill patient and primary care physicians will need to care for more complex patients. The same will be true for specialists as specialty advanced practice nurses will care for routinely ill specialty patients, leaving the more complex patients to the specialty physician.

The health care model of the future is seamless, beginning with the patient, and extending to community health workers, grand-aides, nurses, and physicians connected by technology—an interoperable electronic health record as well as telecommunications, e-mail and text—and incorporating whatever newer ways to communicate are developed in the future.

Training the New Health Professionals: Questioning Assumptions

Training all members of a high-quality patient-centered team of care will require many changes in the training environment, from the community to the classroom to the examination room. Medical and nursing curricula change like clockwork every 5-10 years, but rarely, if ever, have the underlying assumptions of educating health care professionals been questioned. It is worth recalling the Cardiac Arrhythmia Suppression Trial in which the underlying assumption was that suppression of premature ventricular beats would prevent sudden death. Imagine everyone's surprise when the patients receiving the "antiarrhythmic" drugs had worse outcomes.[47] The assumption was wrong. Likewise, we have a number of assumptions underlying the education requirements of health professionals over the entire health care continuum. It is time to question those assumptions and find answers to questions. These answers are available—but must be sought with rigorous experimentation in education research. Examples of answerable questions follow.

How Much Do Patients Want to Know?

This process of examination begins with the patient. We know that consumers seek and receive health information based on their health status and information-seeking preferences, but there is evidence that there is a wide gap in perception when it comes to patient knowledge and understanding of their diagnosis and treatment when under the care of physicians. Understanding how patients seek and understand care information in order to be more self-directed in their care will mean rethinking our current curricula in health professionals' training. This will require moving from the professional isolation of today's medical and nursing school curricula grounded in basic science didactic lectures to a model that educates and trains health professionals to be able to communicate effectively and collaboratively for team-based care. Advancing these changes will touch every element of professional training: admissions, accreditation, organizational structures, clinical partnerships, funding models, and, perhaps the most difficult, professional cultures.[48]

Are We Training for Teamwork?

Working in teams moves patient care forward because the care is built on a model of mutual responsibility and accountability. As the provision of patient care is distributed to health professionals in the team other than just the physician (e.g., the patient, community health worker, and nurse—as well as several physicians per patient), the need for communication is ever more important. Effective teams provide the foundation for outstanding communication and trust among team members as both are required for outstanding care. Unlike a group that merely shares ideas, an effective team produces work products that reflect contributions from all team members. Morrison and colleagues have distinguished teams from working groups by comparing various traits[49]: whereas working groups have a strong, focused leader, teams have shared leadership roles; working groups stress individual accountability, while teams have individual and mutual accountability; working groups value efficient meetings, where teams value open-ended discussion and active problem solving. Perhaps the most important difference is that working groups discuss, decide, and delegate while teams discuss, decide, and work together. The "team" interdependence, with the patient outcome as the shared responsibility, is the goal, rather than the productive assembly of individuals found in the working group.

A team member must be able to demonstrate competencies in conflict resolution, give direct and timely feedback, and be flexible and adaptable. As such, new training models will have to be developed that broaden the development of these types of competencies across the continuum. Presently, the education of medical students is not geared toward true team-based learning: a model in which students work together toward a common goal with each student contributing toward that goal. Similarly, most medical schools do not have faculty that have expertise in team-based learning.[48] To prepare students to be accountable, team members in the service of patient care will require medical schools to assess the competency of a student as she or he functions as a team member, and to emphasize a different set of curriculum-related skills and experiences such as management and communication courses alongside expanded service-learning and community-service exposures.[50]

Do Physicians Need to Be Well Rounded? How Much Education Is Necessary?

The shortage of primary care and specialist physicians, the geographic maldistribution of health care professionals, and the growing need for a more ethnically diverse health care workforce to care for an aging, chronically ill population is forcing medical schools to rethink the structure, content, and length of their curricula. There are calls for reform at all levels of physician education, from premedical through medical and residency education. While medical schools all around the country have modernized teaching methods and developed innovative curricula, the content of physician education has remained largely unchanged for decades. In general, the 4-year curriculum continues to have 18 months to 2 years of basic science with the remainder as clinical work or electives. Despite efforts to repackage basic science into organ systems taught alongside the integration with clinical work, too often it represents little more than "rearranging the deck chairs."[51]

What may be needed is a reexamination of medical training based on what makes a good physician from a patient's viewpoint. A patient might want to choose a physician who, after a decade out of medical school, exhibits the following traits: works well with and is appreciated by patients; provides appropriate care when needed in a safe and timely way; and is happy and content both inside and outside his/her career. If we looked at medical training through that lens, we might want to redesign medical education so that we first attract students who have a service ethic alongside the ability to think critically and assimilate new information. Second, we would want to concentrate within the curriculum the further development of communication, compassion, empathy, and judgment. These types of admission standards and curriculum priorities would turn on its head the classic premedical science-based curriculum requirements and may question the need for the traditional premedical liberal arts education. Indeed, in Donald Barr's recent essay in *The Lancet*, he contends that that the premedical sciences "diet" abundant in chemistry, biology, and physics but lacking in essential psychological "nutrients" has weakened the ability to practice the "art of medicine."[52] Barr calls for challenging the "superstition" that scientific knowledge is the most important metric for the study of medicine, and asks us to consider, through empirical examination and measurement, whether cognitive characteristics might ultimately be more predictive of professional success in providing topnotch patient-centered care.

Changing a medical school's curriculum is a herculean task because, even in collaborative environments, faculty, students, and administrators may espouse very different goals for medical education and disagree about how best to achieve these goals. In less favorable environments, curriculum reformers no doubt will encounter stiff resistance from faculty, students, and administrators if the reforms challenge entrenched interests, traditions, and institutional cultures.[53] We need better research and outcome data before we can begin to change the prevailing culture in medical education and determine a more relevant curriculum.

The increasingly complex roles physicians play in health care delivery require new skills and fundamental knowledge in addition to a foundation in essential biomedical and clinical science. On a broader level, the influence of medical graduates' educational debt may exacerbate physician workforce issues such as diversity and specialty choice. Rethinking the nature and structure of physician education is a necessary step in addressing the nation's health care needs in the coming decades, beginning with a new curriculum that recognizes the impending shortage of physicians and fosters team-based care. As such, educational institutions will have to consider shortening the training time from premedical through medical training, perhaps looking at the viability of the European model of six years as opposed to the US model of 8 years. To that end, some leaders in medical education are currently calling for a shortened curriculum.[54]

The ACC has initiated several educational programs to alleviate workforce issues and accelerate the development of team-based education. In addition to the aforementioned educational program to assist nurse practitioners to gain more proficiency in cardiology care, the ACC has established a work group to develop recommendations for the redesign of fellowship training to include a pilot proposal for a paradigm that would permit completion of internal medicine and cardiovascular fellowship training in 5 rather than the current 6 years.[3]

Shortening the training period and increasing the effectiveness and relevancy of a medical education is the desired goal within a transformed medical education system. Currently, a shortened and more integrated premedical through medical curriculum initiative is under review between the general academic and health-related institutions of the University of Texas System.[55] Operating in partnership to offer joint pilot programs between undergraduate and medical campuses, educators from the health-related and academic institutions are developing a framework for collaborative generation of pilot project ideas that serve undergraduate and medical school components. Programs will address physician education comprehensively, including integration both across disciplines (e.g., nursing and medicine school as well as other health professions) and across traditional educational boundaries. The Texas innovative initiative will examine the evolution of health care delivery and of physician competencies, the use of optimal educational methods, the duration of physician education, the selection and professional growth of student-physicians, and the need for support of faculty educators. This enterprise, and others like it around the country, will provide the model of the future for the training of a true team-based physician.

Interprofessional Education?

Collaborative, or interprofessional, education occurs when students from the health professions and related disciplines learn together about the concepts of health care and the provision of health care services toward the goal of providing more effective and higher quality health care. Interprofessional education generally involves the following elements: collaboration, respectful communication, reflection, application of knowledge and skills, and experience in interprofessional teams.[56] One good example of interprofessional education in performing community research and service as teams is the Dreyfus Foundation's program, "Problem Solving for Better Health" (PSBH), a process that begins with a training workshop that helps participants define a problem, identify a solution, create a good plan of action, and take that action. The PSBH program utilizes the potential within individuals to enact change in their communities, emphasizing responsibility, commitment, and action, all in the service of promoting better health.[57]

As interprofessional education promotes improved communication skills, it also provides students with an understanding of the roles and responsibilities of other health professionals, essential for working in patient-centered care teams. However, entrenched cultures in medical and nursing education are barriers to collaborative education, as is a lack of explicit funding for interprofessional education in primary care training. With varying approaches, a few colleges and universities around the country have successfully implemented interprofessional education programs in the health professions, and, as mentioned earlier, the University of Texas System is embarking upon a multiinstitutional initiative to transform medical education.

Although there is expert consensus regarding the value of collaborative education in the service of promoting team-based care, there is little scientific research or evidence to verify the successful outcomes. Therefore, in each of these pilots and demonstrations it will be necessary to conduct robust evaluations as to how collaborative educational training models relates to students' abilities to be successful team members.[48]

The Ideal Team

As we move forward to design the integrated patient-centered health care teams of tomorrow, we need to examine the various roles for the different team members (patient, community-health worker, generalist nurse/specialist nurse, generalist physician/specialist physician) as well as the capabilities within each of the roles. We know that patients are interested in seeking medical information and respond to incentives to practice healthier behaviors and so tailoring information and education to them will encourage their partnership in the team. This is especially important as anecdotal recommendations from family and friends are more highly valued and used than evidence-based consumer information.[58] As the first contact with patients, community health workers have been shown to be effective in increasing health access in vulnerable communities but a redesigned lay health worker in the future will require formal, standardized training and professional certification in order for them to be fully functioning and electronically savvy team partners. Likewise, generalist and specialist nurses and physicians will have to sort out their roles, dismantling the professional "silos" that prevent them currently from sharing information and being fully accountable team members. In their new roles, physicians and nurses will need to be dependent upon and accountable to each other in the service of appropriate patient care. Only in this way will the attributes of the team be realized: excellent communication with patients and other providers, the provision of 24-hour access to care so that it will not be necessary for patients to go to the emergency department, and collaborative relationships among health professionals and patients in order to manage complex conditions and provide continuous improvement. The new health care reform law reinforces these requirements.[59]

A Futuristic Ideal: The College for Health

How will we train these health professionals in the future? What might the structure be of the college of the future that promotes health and medicine along the continuum of care? A hypothetical model might include:

- **A College for Health** as part of a major university in which there are different schools that support true learning across disciplines: patients, as well as physician and nurse faculty members teach nursing and medical students. Courses and exercises for all learners are the cornerstones of the common themes for the college. In the college, the coursework is based upon data that shows that the various courses and parts of the curriculum are essential for the education of future members of the health care team.

- **A School for the Public** with teachers who develop curricula for the public by asking how to incentivize healthy behavior and how to deliver health information in a meaningful and effective way. The School for the Public would educate lay practitioners who, with 1 year of training, can provide front-line outpatient and inpatient team-based services such as preventive care, chronic care management, surgical aid, and discharge planning.

- **In the School of Nursing,** nurses, trained for 3 years after high school plus 1-year required service "residency" in needed areas, taking science and nonscience courses as shown by research to be most relevant to education of the nurse of the future. Nurses are paid during their residency, beginning to defray the cost of loans that might be incurred over the maximum of 3 years in the college.

- **Advanced practice nurses** (e.g., nurse-practitioners) have one additional year of training (or 6 months for those showing special competency after at least 5 years of experience).

- **In the School of Medicine,** physicians are educated for 4 years after high school in nonmedical, science, clinical (including learning about important skills such as communication and professionalism), as well as community (such as public health) coursework as dictated by research findings as to the best way of translating coursework and experience into team-based competencies. The curricula will include earlier exposure to specialties so that the traditional fourth year in medical school is no longer necessary, followed by the completion of a 2-year practical generalist "residency" in a primary care discipline in needed parts of the country. During this generalist residency, the physicians are paid, which will begin to defray the cost of loans that might be incurred over the maximum of 4 years in the college. The 2 years of residency would be credited toward a 3-year residency in a primary care discipline, but would not be counted toward specialty training, thus helping to stimulate physicians to pursue primary care.

In this revised structure of nursing and medical education, physicians and nurses are the same age during training, thus bolstering the value of interprofessional education, and also addressing the deficiencies and "silo" mentality in today's health professions education. The required internships will help the health provider shortage, particularly in rural and inner city areas. Physicians and nurses who desire academic careers will have two additional years of education involving such subjects as methods of teaching and research, as well as management and leadership.

To get to the ideal training model of tomorrow, we must begin today to design and implement demonstration projects. We could begin the demonstrations in five academic health centers, with pilots that will require sophisticated educational research and therefore close collaboration with schools of education. At the same time, we would need to work with state and federal health care workforce commissions to recommend such changes and also with the accrediting and certifying bodies charged with the authority to change certain scopes of practice and to provide professional certifications. This is especially important in order to certify Community Health Workers across the United States.

Final Thoughts

There are many challenges facing health care today as the increasing demand for health services coexists within a diminishing health practitioner supply. This is exemplified in the area of pediatric cardiology where the emergence of fetal cardiology services over the past 20 years has dramatically increased the number of patients with chronic heart disease and created access concerns, particularly in geographically underserved areas.[3] Current health professionals' education and training models do not serve the needs of a society that is increasingly aging and chronically ill, and more accelerated training programs like the ones proposed through the University of Texas System and the ACC will be necessary to align medical education with the need for more physicians practicing in a team-based care model. Despite these challenges, policy makers, patients, and experts believe that the ability to provide a continuum of appropriate patient-centered care is "too important to fail."[60] A new health system, made up of teams of patients, lay health workers, nurses, and physicians will help move us toward a more effective, equitable, efficient, safe, and affordable health system for all Americans.

References

1. Anderson G. Chronic Care: making the case for ongoing care. Robert Wood Johnson Foundation, February 2010, accessed 18 August 2010 at: http://www.rwjf.org/pr/product.jsp?id=50968.
2. U.S. faces shortage of pediatric subspecialists. Medical News Today September 28, 2007, accessed 8 November 2010 at: http://www.medicalnewstoday.com/articles/83798.php.
3. Rodgers GP, et al. ACC 2009 survey results and recommendations: addressing the cardiology workforce crisis. J Am Coll Cardiol. 2009;54:1195-1208.
4. Sack K. In Massachusetts, universal coverage strains care. New York Times 2008, accessed 4 August 2010 at: http://www.nytimes.com/2008/04/05/us/05doctors.html?pagewanted=print.
5. Cooney E. Access to primary care physicians getting tougher, report finds. Boston Globe July 26, 2010, accessed 4 August 2010 at: http://www.boston.com/news/health/articles/2010/07/26/access_to_primary_care_physicians_getting_tougher_report_finds/?rss_id=Boston.com+-+Health+news.
6. Bodenheimer T, Chen E, Bennett HD. Confronting the growing burden of chronic disease: can the U.S. health care workforce do the job? Health Affairs. 2009;28(1):64-74.
7. Commonwealth Fund. State and federal efforts to enhance access to basic health care. 2009, accessed 4 August 2010 at: http://www.commonwealthfund.org/Content/Newsletters/States-in-Action/2010/Mar/March-April-2010/Feature/Feature.aspx.
8. Kirch DG. How to fix the doctor shortage. The Wall Street Journal January 5, 2010, accessed 4 August 2010 at: http://online.wsj.com/article/NA_WSJ_PUB:SB10001424052748703483604574630321885059520.html.
9. AAMC. The impact of health care reform on the future supply and demand for physicians updated projections through 2025, accessed 4 August 2010 at: http://www.aamc.org/workforce/impactofhrconprojections.pdf.
10. Staiger DO, Auerbach DI, Buerhous PI. Comparison of physician workforce estimates and supply projections. JAMA. 2009;302(15):1674-1680.
11. DHHS, HRSA. The physician workforce: projections and research into current issues affecting supply and demand. 2008, accessed 4 August 2010 at: ftp://ftp.hrsa.gov/bhpr/workforce/physicianworkforce.pdf.
12. Bovbjerg R, Ormond BA, Pindus N. The nursing workforce challenge: public policy for a dynamic and complex market. The Urban Institute, 2009, accessed 4 August 2010 at: http://www.urban.org/publications/411933.html.
13. Buerhaus PI. Current and future state of the U.S. nursing workforce. JAMA. 2008;300(20):2422-2424.
14. Buerhaus PI, Auerbach DI, Staiger DO. The recent surge in nurse employment: causes and implications. Health Affairs Web Exclusive. 12 June 2009:w657-668.
15. Murray M, Berwick DM. Advanced access: reducing waiting and delays in primary care. JAMA. 2003;289(8):1035-1040.
16. How SK, Shih A, Lau J, Schoen C. Public views on U.S. health system organization: a call for new directions. The Commonwealth Fund, 2008, accessed 22 August, 2010 at: http://www.commonwealthfund.org/Content/Publications/Data-Briefs/2008/Aug/Public-Views-on-U-S–Health-System-Organization–A-Call-for-New-Directions.aspx.
17. Grumbach K, Bodenheimer T. A primary care home for Americans: putting the house in order. JAMA. 2002;288:889-893.
18. Montgomery JE, Irish JT, Wilson IB, et al. Primary care experiences of Medicare beneficiaries, 1998-2000. J Gen Intern Med. 2004;19(10):991-998.

19. Bodenheimer T, Pham HH. Primary care: proposed problems and proposed solutions. Health Affairs. 2010;29(5):799-805.

20. DesRoches CM, Campbell EG, Rao SR, et al. Electronic health records in ambulatory care—a national survey of physicians. N Engl J Med. 2008;359(1):50-60.

21. Phillips RL, Bazemore AW. Primary care and why it matters for U.S. health system reform. Health Affairs. 2010;29(5):806-810.

22. Hanauer SB. A poor view from specialty silos. Nat Rev Gastroenterol Hepatol. 2010;7:1-2.

23. Crabtree BF, Nutting PA, Miller WL, et al. Summary of the National Demonstration Project and recommendations for the patient-centered medical home. Ann Fam Med. 2010;8(Suppl 1): S80-S90.

24. Abelson R. A health insurer pays more to save. New York Times, June 21, 2010, accessed 11 August 2010 at: http://www.nytimes.com/2010/06/22/business/22geisinger.html.

25. Katzenbach J, Smith D. The discipline of teams. Harvard Business Review. 2005;83:162-171.

26. Hibbard J, Cunningham P. How engaged are consumers in their health and health care, and why does it matter? Center for Studying Health System Change, No. 8, October 2008, accessed 14 August 2010 at: http://www.hschange.org/CONTENT/1019/1019.pdf.

27. Belluck P. For forgetful, cash helps the medicine go down. New York Times June 13, 2010, accessed 14 August 2010 at http://www.nytimes.com/2010/06/14/health/14meds.html.

28. Barth J, Greene J. Encouraging healthy behaviors in Medicaid: early lessons from Florida and Idaho. Center for Health Care Strategies, Inc., Issue Brief, 2007, accessed August 20, 2010 at: http://www.chcs.org/usr_doc/Encouraging_Healthy_Behaviors_in_Medicaid.pdf.

29. Brook RH. Rights and responsibilities in health care: striking a balance. JAMA. 2010;303(22): 2289-2290.

30. http://hiqnews.megafoundation.org/Definition_of_IQ1.html.

31. Cohn W, Pannone A, Schubart J, et al. Tailored reducational approaches for consumer health (TEACH): a model system for addressing health communication. AMIA. 2006 Symposium Proceedings, page 894, accessed 14 August 2010 at: http://www.ncbi.nlm.nih.gov/pmc/articles/PMC1839357/pdf/AMIA2006_0894.pdf.

32. U.S. Health Resources and Services Administration, Bureau of Health Professions. Community health workers national workforce study. Rockville, Md: HRSA; 2007.

33. Swider SM. Outcome effectiveness of community health workers: an integrative literature review. Public Health Nursing. 2002;19(1):11-20.

34. Goodwin K, Tobler L. Community health workers: expanding the scope of the health care delivery system. National Conference of State Legislatures, Issue Brief, 2008, accessed 14 August 2010 at: http://www.ncsl.org/print/health/CHWBrief.pdf.

35. Patient Protection and Affordable Care Act of 2010. PL 111-148, secs. 5101, 5102, 5313, 5403, and 3509, accessed 14 August 2010 at: http://www.gpo.gov/fdsys/pkg/PLAW-111publ148/content-detail.html.

36. Rosenthal EL, Brownstein JN, Rush CH, et al. Community health workers: part of the solution. Health Affairs. 2010;29(7):1338-1342.

37. Bureau of Labor Statistics, U.S. Department of Labor. Occupational employment statistics: occupational employment and wages, May 2007—29-1111 registered nurses. Washington, DC: BLS, 2008. accessed 14 August 2008 at: http://stats.bls.gov/oes/current/oes291111.htm.

38. Rother J, Lavizzo-Mourney R. Addressing the nursing workforce: a critical element for health reform. Health Affairs Web Exclusive. 12 June 2009:w620-w624.

39. Johnson C. Doctor shortage? 28 States may expand nurses' role, 2010. Physorg.com, April 13, 2010, accessed 30 August 2010 at: http://www.physorg.com/news190391761.html.

40. U.S. Office of Technology Assessment. Nurse practitioners, physician assistants, and certified nurse-midwives: a policy analysis, OTA-HCS-37, December 1986, available at: www.fas.org/ota/reports/8615.pdf.

41. Naylor M, Kurtzman E. "The role of nurse practitioners in reinventing primary care." Health Affairs. 2010;29(5):893-899.

42. Mehrotra A, et al. "Comparing costs and quality of care at retail clinics with that of other medical settings for 3 common illnesses." Annals of Internal Medicine. 2009;151(5):321-328, available at www.annals.org/content/151/5/321.full.pdf+html.

43. Dentzer S. Geisinger Chief Glenn Steele: seizing health reform's potential to build a superior system. Health Affairs. 2010;29(6):1200-1207.

44. Chesluk BJ, Holmboe ES. How teams work—or don't—in primary care: a field study on internal medicine practices. Health Affairs. 2010;29(5):874-879.

45. Bodenheimer T. (2007). Building teams in primary care: lessons learned. California Healthcare Foundation Report, accessed 17 August 2010 at: http://www.chcf.org/~/media/Files/PDF/B/Building-TeamsInPrimaryCareLessons.pdf.

46. O'Malley AS, Tynan A, Cohen GR, et al. Coordination of care by primary care practices: strategies, lessons, and implications. Center for Studying Health System Change Research Brief No. 12, April 2009, accessed 16 August 2010 at: http://www.hschange.org/CONTENT/1058/.

47. Echt DS, Liebson PR, Mitchell LB, et al. Cardiac arrhythmia suppression trial August 22, 1991. N Engl J Med. 1991;324:781-788.

48. Schuetz B, Mann E, Everett W. Educating health professionals collaboratively for team-based primary care. Health Affairs. 2010;29(8):1476-1480.

49. Morrison G, Goldfarb S, Lanken PN. Team training of medical students in the 21st century: Would Flexner approve? Acad Med. 2010;85(2):254-259.

50. Lianov L, Johnson M. Physician competencies for prescribing lifestyle medicine. JAMA. 2010; 304(2):202-203.
51. A situation when someone tries to futilely reform the way things are done in a failing system. Definition accessed The Urban Dictionary 27 August 2010 at: http://www.urbandictionary.com/define.php?term=Rearranging%20the%20deck%20chairs%20on%20the%20titanic&defid=944126.
52. Barr DA. The art of medicine. Lancet. 2010;376:678-679.
53. Fetterman DM, Deitz J, Gesundheit N. Empowerment evaluation: a collaborative approach to evaluating and transforming a medical school curriculum. Acad Med. 2010;85(5):813-931.
54. Whitcomb ME. Who will study medicine in the future? Acad Med. 2006;81(3):205-206.
55. Personal communication and draft document, Transformation in medical education (TIME): A multi-institutional initiative within the University of Texas System, and message from the Dean of the School of Medicine, accessed 22 August 2010 at: http://som.utmb.edu/news/081610Med_Ed_Initiative.pdf.
56. University of Minnesota, Center for Interprofessional Education, accessed 17 August 2010 at: http://www.ipe.umn.edu/what/index.shtml.
57. Dreyfus Health Foundation, accessed 23 August 2010 at: http://www.dhfglobal.org/who/methodology.html.
58. Huppertz JW, Carlson JP. Consumers' use of HCAHPS ratings and word-of-mouth in hospital choice. Health Services Research, prepublication on-line, accessed 24 August 2010 at: http://onlinelibrary.wiley.com/doi/10.1111/j.1475-6773.2010.01153.x/pdf.
59. Abrams M, Schor EL, Schoenbaum S. How physician practices could share personnel and resources to support a medical home. Health Affairs. 2010;29(6):1194-1199.
60. Meyers DS, Clancy CM. Primary care: too important to fail. Ann Intern Med. 2009;150(4):272-273.

20

CHAPTER 21

The Current Role of Fetal Echocardiography

†Charles S. Kleinman, MD, Julie S. Glickstein, MD,
Ganga Krishnamurthy, MD, Jodie K. Votava-Smith, MD

21

Fetal echocardiography and fetal cardiology have been incorporated into many pediatric cardiology programs during the past 2 decades, and the role of fetal cardiology varies considerably from location to location. In many cases the role of fetal cardiology is dependent upon the relationship that exists between maternal-fetal-medicine and pediatric cardiology in the institution, and whether individual institutions have obstetrical and neonatal services housed under the same roof.

We have reviewed the role that prenatal cardiac diagnosis has had over 4 calendar years (2007-2010) at the Morgan Stanley Children's Hospital of the Columbia University Medical Center campus of New York- Presbyterian Hospital. This service represents a highly evolved fetal cardiology service, with an extremely active Department of Obstetrics and Gynecology, with a Maternal-Fetal-Medicine Division that has been actively involved in the performance of detailed fetal echocardiography for many years. Similarly, the Pediatric Echocardiography service of the Morgan Stanley Children's Hospital has been extremely aggressive in its approach to fetal cardiology, and the integration of these patients into the neonatal cardiology and cardiovascular surgery service.

Unlike at many centers, where the pediatric cardiology service provides "screening" services for fetal congenital heart disease, the service at our hospital is based on a model in which the pregnant woman is seen, almost exclusively, by the obstetrical service, until a high-risk indication for a targeted fetal echocardiogram is identified. While services that perform screening studies usually find evidence of fetal cardiovascular disease in ~10% of scans, with the predominant indication for scan being a previous family history of congenital heart disease, we have a very different experience (Table 21-1).

In 2007-2010, our laboratory detected 615 fetuses with congenital cardiovascular abnormalities among 2828 fetuses (including 27 sets of twins) undergoing fetal echocardiography (yield 22%) (Table 21-2). There were 31 false-positive results (cases of relative right heart enlargement and suspected coarctation of the aorta, including six fetuses with left-sided congenital diaphragmatic hernia with rightward deviation of the heart and mediastinum). Fourteen false-negative cases were documented, including three small ventricular septal defects (VSDs) that did not require surgical or medical management and three moderate-to-large VSDs that required surgery in the first months of life.

Of the 615 patients with congenital heart disease, follow-up is complete for 90%. Sixty patients (10%) have been lost to follow-up and an additional 15 of those are known to have been liveborn at outside hospitals. Of 396 babies known to have been liveborn 64% (252) underwent surgery during the first 6 months of life (249 at Columbia University Medical Center and three at outside hospitals). Ten additional babies underwent interventional catheterization procedures at Columbia. Of these babies, 88 (33%) have undergone additional surgery within the first 6 months of life and nine are less than 6 months of age as of the time of writing this chapter.

---

†Deceased.

Table 21-1 REASONS FOR REFERRAL FOR FETAL ECHO, 2007-2010
(N = 2542 PREGNANCIES)

Reason for Referral	No. of Pregnancies	Percentage of Pregnancies
Suspected CHD	965	38
Subgroup of arrhythmia	129	
Other fetal indications:	692	27
Extracardiac anomaly	495	
Chromosomal anomaly, quad screen, or nuchal thickness	124	
Two-vessel cord	55	
Multiple gestation (not mono-di)	18	
Family history	367	14
Maternal indication	323	13
Maternal diabetes mellitus	236	
Maternal medical issue or medication	84	
Advanced maternal age	3	
Mono-di twins or TTTS	139	5
Other	56	2
Poor visualization of heart	38	
In vitro fertilization	7	
Unknown	7	
Research	4	

CHD, congenital heart disease; TTTS, twin-twin transfusion syndrome.

Table 21-2 CONGENITAL CARDIAC MALFORMATIONS DIAGNOSED IN
UTERO (2007-2010) (N = 615)

Diagnosis	2007	2008	2009	2010	Total
Conotruncal malformations					
d-Transposition/IVS	11	12	8	5	36
d-Transposition + VSD/PS/or CoA	6	1	11	3	21
Double-outlet RV (± malposition)	12	16	8	9	45
Tetralogy of Fallot	9	15	11	20	55
Pulmonary atresia/VSD/PDA	5	4	3	6	18
Pulmonary Atresia/VSD /MAPCAs	3	3	2	2	10
Tetralogy with absent PV syndrome	0	2	3	0	5
Tetralogy of Fallot/AVC	1	1	4	1	7
L – TGA (± VSD)	3	1	0	1	5
Truncus arteriosus	3	2	2	4	11
Left heart obstructive lesions					
HLHS	15	22	16	16	69
HLHS variant	7	5	0	1	13
Shone's complex	10	10	6	6	32
Isolated mitral valve anomaly	0	2	0	0	2
Aortic stenosis	5	2	2	1	10

Table 21-2 CONGENITAL CARDIAC MALFORMATIONS DIAGNOSED IN UTERO (2007-2010) (N = 615)—cont'd

Diagnosis	2007	2008	2009	2010	Total
Left-to-right shunt lesions					
Atrioventricular septal defects					
Complete atrioventricular canal	9	10	4	6	29
Ostium primum ASD	1	3	3	1	8
Ventricular septal defect—mod to large	2	10	5	19	36
Ventricular septal defect—small	4	9	10	10	33
Right heart obstructive lesions					
Tricuspid atresia (± d-TGA)	1	6	4	6	16
Pulmonary atresia + IVS	6	3	5	3	17
Tricuspid stenosis	0	1	0	1	2
Pulmonary stenosis	2	4	6	4	16
Visceral heterotaxia	7	7	9	10	33
Double inlet left ventricle	5	3	5	5	18
Absent pulmonary valve/IVS	1	0	1	0	2
Aortic arch anomalies					
Isolated coarctation	1	1	2	0	4
Coarctation + VSD	1	4	4	4	13
Interrupted aortic arch + VSD	3	5	1	1	10
Ebstein's malformation of the TV	3	3	5	3	14
Single ventricle variants	3	5	6	3	17
Complex conjoined hearts	0	0	2	0	2
Other (1 of a kind)	1	1	2	2	6
Total	140	172	150	153	615

ASD, atrial septal defect; AVC, atrioventricular canal; CoA, coarctation of the aorta; HLHS, hypoplastic left heart syndrome; IVS, intact ventricular septum; MAPCAs, multiple aortopulmonary collateral arteries; PDA, patent ductus arteriosus; PS, pulmonary stenosis; PV, pulmonary valve; RV, right ventricle; TGA, transposition of the great arteries; TV, tricuspid valve; VSD, ventricular septal defect.

Of the 615 cases of correctly identified congenital heart disease (see Table 21-2), the categories of abnormality, in descending order of frequency, consisted of conotruncal malformations (213, 35%), obstructive lesions on the left side of the heart (126, 20%), left-to-right shunt lesions (106, 17%, including 29 complete atrioventricular canal defects), obstructions on the right side of the heart (51, 8%), visceral heterotaxia (33, 5%), double-inlet left ventricle (18, 3%), aortic arch anomalies (27, 4%), Ebstein's malformation of the tricuspid valve (14, 2%), single ventricle variants (17, 3%), absent pulmonary valve syndrome with intact ventricular septum (2, <1%), complex conjoined hearts in thoracopagus twins (2, <1%), and other, one-of-a-kind anomalies (6, 1%).

The single largest subgroup of patients undergoing prenatal diagnosis had some form of conotruncal malformation (Fig. 21-3) rather than an abnormality disrupting the integrity of the four-chamber screening view of the heart. This emphasizes the importance of including biventricular outflow views in screening programs for congenital heart disease.

One hundred and thirty-one (22%) patients either underwent termination of pregnancy (102) or chose nonintervention ("compassionate care") (28) for their offspring. The diagnoses of these fetuses, presented in Table 21-3, were weighted

Table 21-3 TERMINATIONS OF PREGNANCY (N = 102) OR COMPASSIONATE NONINTERVENTIONAL CARE (N = 28) FOR FETUSES WITH CONGENITAL HEART DISEASE 2007-2010 (N = 130)

Cardiac Lesion	No. of Cases	Genetic or Extracardiac Abnormality or Other Issues
Terminations of Pregnancy (N = 102)		
Hypoplastic left heart syndrome	13	None
Tetralogy of Fallot	13	22q11 deletion(1), Trisomy 21 (1), XYY (1)
VSD	11	Trisomy 18 (3), trisomy 13 (1), chromosome 13 deletion (1), cardiomyopathy (1), CDH (1), CNS (1), skeletal (2), renal (1)
Heterotaxy	9	CDH and renal (1)
DORV	6	Trisomy 13 (1)
AV canal	5	Trisomy 21 (4)
Complex single ventricle	4	CNS (1)
Tricuspid atresia	4	None
Pulmonary atresia/intact ventricular septum	4	Cleft lip palate (1)
Double inlet left ventricle	4	CDH (1)
Pulmonary atresia/VSD/PDA	4	None
Interrupted arch/VSD	3	22q11 deletion (1)
Truncus arteriosus	3	22q11 deletion (2)
Ebstein's anomaly	3	None
HLHS variant	3	CNS and renal (1)
Pulmonary atresia/VSD/MAPCAs	2	22q11 deletion (1)
Coarctation/VSD	2	Limb/body wall complex (1)
TOF/absent pulmonary valve syndrome	2	22q11 deletion (1)
d-TGA	1	None
Hypoplastic aortic arch	1	CNS and skeletal (1)
Aortic stenosis	1	Trisomy 18 (1)
TOF/AV Canal	1	Trisomy 21 (1)
Shone syndrome	1	CNS (1)
Absent pulmonary valve syndrome/IVS	1	None
Complex conjoined hearts	1	Conjoined twins (1)
Total	**102**	
Compassionate (hospice) care n = 28		
DORV	5	Trisomy 18 (2), CHARGE (1), CNS anomaly (1), Perinatal CNS insult (1)
VSD	4	Trisomy 18 (2), trisomy 21 with hydrops (1), abnormal head vessel anatomy (1)
HLHS variant	3	16q24 deletion (1), chromosome 8 deletion (1), abnormal head vessel anatomy
HLHS	3	Intact arterial septum/premature triplet (1), Poor RV function and TR (1), compassionate care given at outside hospital (1)

Table 21-3 TERMINATIONS OF PREGNANCY (N = 102) OR COMPASSIONATE NONINTERVENTIONAL CARE (N = 28) FOR FETUSES WITH CONGENITAL HEART DISEASE 2007-2010 (N = 130)—cont'd

Cardiac Lesion	No. of Cases	Genetic or Extracardiac Abnormality or Other Issues
Heterotaxy	3	Obstructive pulmonary venous return as component of cardiac lesion (2), hydrops and heart block (1)
Single ventricle variant	1	Chromosome 4 deletion
AV canal with coarctation of aorta	1	Trisomy 18
Pulmonary atresia/intact ventricular septum	1	Severe cardiomyopathy
PA/VSD/MAPCAs	1	22q11 deletion, premature twin
TOF	1	Renal disease, anhydramnios
Critical pulmonary stenosis	1	Congenital diaphragmatic hernia
Ebstein's anomaly	1	Hydrops
PA/VSD	1	Trisomy 13
Shone syndrome	1	Restrictive foramen ovale
Complex conjoined hearts	1	Thoracopagus twins
Total	28	

AV, atrioventricular; CDH, congenital diaphragmatic hernia; CNS, central nervous system; DORV, double-outlet right ventricle; HLHS, hypoplastic left heart syndrome; IVS, interventricular septum; MAPCAs, multiple aortopulmonary collateral arteries; PA, pulmonary atresia; PDA, patent ductus arteriosus; TGA, transposition of the great arteries; TOF, tetralogy of Fallot; VSD, ventricular septal defect.

toward severe anomalies such as hypoplastic left heart syndrome and visceral heterotaxia and those with chromosomal and severe extracardiac abnormalities.

Twenty-eight patients suffered intrauterine fetal demise (Table 21-4). These included 10 with documented chromosomal anomalies, including five fetuses with trisomy 18, three with trisomy 21, and two with trisomy 13. Two fetuses with demise had additional severe anomalies but no chromosomal study, including one with a complex single ventricle and absent kidneys, and one with double-outlet right ventricle and pentalogy of Cantrell. Four fetuses who suffered intrauterine demise had normal chromosomes with an extracardiac fetal anomaly or a maternal abnormality, including three fetuses with hypoplastic left heart variants (one with an absent stomach, one with prune belly syndrome, and one with maternal protein S deficiency), and one fetus with persistent truncus arteriosus and placental insufficiency. Three fetuses had intrauterine demise associated with complete atrioventricular block, including two with left atrial isomerism, and one with atrial and ventricular septal defects. The remaining nine fetuses with intrauterine demise had congenital heart disease but no additional anomalies, including four fetuses with Ebstein's malformation of the tricuspid valve (comprising 29% of fetuses with Ebstein's malformation seen), two fetuses with pulmonary atresia and intact ventricular septum (one of whom also had left ventricular outflow obstruction and no karyotype, the other with severe cardiomegaly and a normal karyotype), two fetuses with atrioventricular canal defects and hydrops fetalis (one complete atrioventricular canal defect with no chromosomal study and one unbalanced left ventricular–dominant canal with normal chromosomes), and one fetus with absent pulmonary valve syndrome and intact ventricular septum.

A review of the mode of delivery of the 410 fetuses with congenital heart disease (Table 21-5) who were liveborn at Columbia University Medical Center showed that there were 222 spontaneous vaginal deliveries and 188 (46%) cesarean deliveries.

Table 21-4 FETAL CONGENITAL HEART DISEASE WITH INTRAUTERINE FETAL DEMISE 2007-2010 (N = 28)

Cardiac Diagnosis	Other Findings	Karyotype
Absent PV Syndrome/ IVS	Hydrops fetalis	None
ASD and VSD	Complete heart block	None
AV Canal	Hydrops fetalis	None
AV Canal	None	Trisomy 21
AV Canal	None	Trisomy 21
AV Canal	Oligohydramnios	Trisomy 21
AV Canal, LV-dominant	Hydrops fetalis	Normal
AV Canal, LV-dominant with AS, Left atrial isomerism	Complete heart block	Normal
AV Canal/DORV/MGV, Left atrial isomerism	Complete heart block, renal anomaly, Hydrops fetalis	Normal
Complex single ventricle	Absent kidneys, anhydramnios	None
DORV	Duodenal atresia	Trisomy 18
DORV	CNS, renal, and skeletal anomalies	Trisomy 18
DORV	Arnold Chiari, neural tube defect, renal and skeletal anomalies, Hydrops fetalis	Trisomy 13
DORV/MA/AA	Absent stomach	Normal
DORV/MGV	Congenital diaphragmatic hernia, skeletal anomalies	Trisomy 18
DORV/PA with Ectopia Cordis	Pentalogy of Cantrell	None
Ebstein malformation	Hydrops fetalis	None
Ebstein malformation	Hydrops fetalis	None
Ebstein malformation	Hydrops fetalis	Normal
Ebstein malformation	None	None
HLHS (MS/AA)	Prune belly syndrome	Normal
HLHS (MA/AA)	Maternal Protein S deficiency, on Lovenox	Normal
Pulmonary atresia/IVS, also LVOT obstruction	Hydrops fetalis	None
Pulmonary atresia/IVS	Severe cardiomegaly	Normal
Pulmonary atresia/VSD	Cleft lip and palate, cerebral, and genital anomalies, Hydrops fetalis	Trisomy 13
Truncus arteriosus	Placental insufficiency	Normal
VSD (large inlet)	Skeletal anomalies	Trisomy 18
VSD (large inlet)	Congenital diagphragmatic hernia, Skeletal anomalies, hydrops	Trisomy 18

AA, aortic atresia; AS, aortic stenosis; ASD, atrial septal defect; AV, atrioventricular; CNS, central nervous system; DORV, double outlet right; IVS, intact ventricular septum; LV, left ventricle; LVOT, left ventricular outflow tract; MA, mitral atresia; MGV, malposed great vessels; PV, pulmonary valve; VSD, ventricular septal defect.

Table 21-5 METHOD OF DELIVERY OF INFANTS PRENATALLY DIAGNOSED WITH CONGENITAL HEART DISEASE 2007-2010*

Normal spontaneous vaginal delivery	222	
Unassisted	213	
Vacuum or forceps	9	
Cesarean section	**188**	46% of deliveries
Reasons for c-section		
Repeat	60	
Fetal distress or nonreassuring tracing	29	10% of attempted vaginal deliveries
Failure to progress	27	10% of attempted vaginal deliveries
Multiple gestation	22	
Breech presentation	19	
Maternal health issue	8	
Timed for CHD	8	2% of all CHD babies
TGA	5	14% of all TGA
HLHS	2	3% of all HLHS
Double inlet left ventricle	1	
Placental position	5	
Fetal health urgency	5	
Fetal anomaly precluding vaginal delivery	3	
Parental preference	2	

*410 patients born at MS-CHONY, including compassionate care patients.
CHD, congenital heart disease; HLHS, hypoplastic left heart syndrome; TGA, transposition of the great arteries.

Of the latter group, all but eight cesarean deliveries were performed for obstetrical reasons, including two cases in which the maternal preference was for cesarean delivery. In only eight cases (2% of all cases with congenital heart disease), cesarean delivery was performed to facilitate the timing of urgent neonatal intervention by neonatology and perinatal cardiology. Of these eight cases, seven involved situations in which premature or in utero closure of the foramen ovale was considered a critical issue, requiring urgent catheterization intervention. These included five cases of complete transposition of the great arteries (14% of all patients with transposition of the great arteries) and two cases of hypoplastic left heart syndrome (HLHS) (3% of all cases of HLHS) (Fig. 21-1). There was one case of tetralogy of Fallot with absent pulmonary valve syndrome in which massive pulmonary arterial dilation was considered likely to cause significant neonatal airway compression, and thus post-natal airway management was the indication for a timed delivery. (Fig. 21-2).

Of the 615 fetuses with suspected congenital cardiac malformations, 327 (53%) underwent prenatal karyotyping. Seventy (21%) of these fetuses had identifiable genetic syndromes while 169 patients underwent only postnatal genetic testing, of which 17 (10%) had an abnormality. Chromosomal abnormalities included 39 cases of trisomy 21 (including 15 with complete atrioventricular canal defect and 13 with tetralogy of Fallot), 13 with trisomy 18, (seven with VSD, four with double-outlet right ventricle, one with complete atrioventricular canal defect, six with trisomy 13 (three with pulmonary atresia with VSD and patent ductus arteriosus (PDA), two with double outlet right ventricle, and one with an isolated VSD), and four with

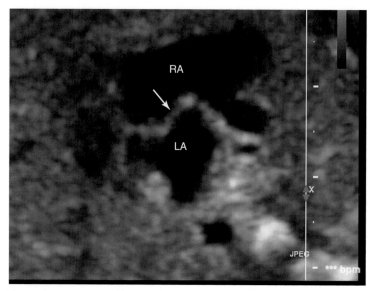

Figure 21-1 Atrial septal aneurysm in a fetus with hypoplastic left heart syndrome. The bulging atrial septum primum, in the center of the picture, imparts almost complete closure of the atrial septum prior to birth. This serves as an area of obstruction to the pulmonary venous pathway which, in turn, is associated with severe pulmonary venous obstruction that will result in severe pulmonary edema and critical cyanosis in the neonate. If this obstruction is not relieved in a neonate with absent atrioventricular valve egress to pulmonary venous return, the likelihood of short-term survival is almost nil. In such a case, one may consider the potential for in utero placement of a coronary arterial stent within the atrial septum or a planned delivery, timed to minimize the waiting period between cord clamping and catheterization to establish an adequate vent for pulmonary venous return. Two of the fetuses discussed in this cohort were delivered by planned cesarean delivery to facilitate the timely performance of interventional catheterization as part of the immediate postnatal resuscitation. In both cases the resuscitation was successful and the infants went on to survive first stage palliation by Norwood-Sano procedures.

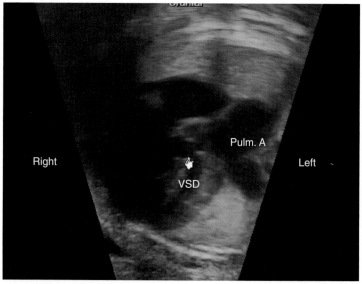

Figure 21-2 Heart and great arteries of fetus with the syndrome of tetralogy of Fallot with absent pulmonary valve. The hand is pointing to the malalignment ventricular septal defect, which defines this as a conotruncal malformation. While the genetic studies of this fetus were normal, this syndrome is associated with chromosome 22q11.2 microdeletions (DiGeorge or velocardiofacial syndrome) in 25-30% of affected fetuses. The finding of this conotruncal malformation should, therefore, engender a genetic evaluation to rule out this particular genetic abnormality. Note the aneurysm of the pulmonary arteries (Pulm A), with branch pulmonary arteries with diameters more than 7 standard deviations above the mean for gestational age. In motion it was possible to visualize the back and forth flow across the rudimentary, mildly stenotic, and severely regurgitant, pulmonary valve and the systolic ballooning of the aneurysmal pulmonary arteries. There was obvious compromise of the carinal region of the trachea and at least the initial portion of the right mainstem bronchus. Because of the likely association with tracheobronchomalacia, this fetus was delivered by elective cesarean delivery to ensure timely and efficient airway management. While tracheobronchomalacia proved to be a significant problem for this child, the airway obstruction was not fully manifest until several days after birth.

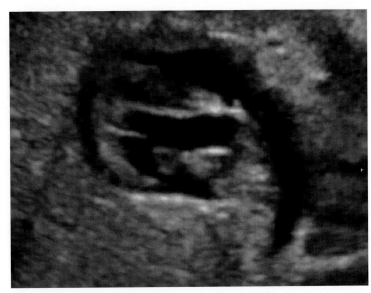

Figure 21-3 Typical long-axis view of the outflow tracts of a fetus with complete transposition of the great arteries. The aorta arises from above the subarterial conus of the right ventricle and is anterior and to the right of the outflow to the more posterior and leftward pulmonary artery, which arises in fibrous continuity with the ventricular septum. While the four-chamber anatomy of the fetal heart in such cases appears perfectly normal, inclusion of routine imaging of the ventricular outflow tracts in screening protocols has made the prenatal detection of this common and potentially deadly anomaly relatively commonplace. Such fetuses will depend upon mixing of saturated and desaturated atrial venous return in order to supply the body with adequate oxygen delivery and the lungs with desaturated blood for oxygenation. Prenatal suggestion of premature closure or stenosis of the foramen ovale necessitated cesarean delivery of 5 of the 36 (14%) fetuses with complete transposition of the great arteries with intact ventricular septum to facilitate timely balloon atrial septostomy at our center between 2007 and 2010.

Turner syndrome (two bicommissural aortic valves, one with hypoplastic left heart syndrome, and one with a small VSD). Eighteen patients were found to have chromosome 22q11.2 microdeletion (five with truncus arteriosus communis, four with tetralogy of Fallot with pulmonary atresia and major aortopulmonary collateral arteries, three with tetralogy of Fallot, three with interrupted aortic arch with VSD, one with hypoplastic left heart with a cervical aortic arch, one tetralogy of Fallot with absent pulmonary valve syndrome, and one with pulmonary atresia with VSD and PDA). An additional nine patients had unique abnormalities consisting of a chromosomal deletion, gain, inversion, or translocation. Two patients underwent prenatal karyotyping but were not diagnosed as having genetic syndromes until postnatal genetic testing took place (one with a 22q11.2 microdeletion and one with an XrX ring chromosome). Table 21-6 reviews the results of chromosomal testing on this cohort of patients.

One hundred and thirty-seven fetuses were identified who had congenital cardiac malformations and associated extracardiac malformations. The latter included 63 fetuses with multiple extracardiac anomalies and 74 with single extracardiac anomalies, including six with associated congenital diaphragmatic hernia, 18 with central nervous system anomalies, 15 with renal anomalies, 9 with gastrointestinal anomalies, 6 with skeletal anomalies, and 6 with abdominal wall defects (Table 21-6).

Indications for detailed fetal echocardiographic study are presented in Table 21-1. Note the marked predominance of "suspected congenital heart disease" in this list and the relative infrequency of "family history of congenital heart disease." We attribute this weight of referrals towards those with suspected cardiac disease, as well as the paucity of cases of associated chromosomal abnormalities, to the maturity of the screening program within maternal-fetal medicine at our hospital.

Table 21-6 CHROMOSOMAL ANOMALIES OF FETUSES WITH CONGENITAL HEART DISEASE 2007-2010 (N = 89)

Chromosomal Defect	No. of Fetuses
Trisomy 21	**39**
Complete AV Canal	**15**
TOF/AV Canal	7
VSD	7
TOF	6
Partial AV Canal	2
AV Canal-single ventricle variant	2
22q11 deletion	**18**
Truncus	5
PA/VSD/MAPCAs	4
TOF	3
IAA/VSD	3
Aortic atresia/cervical arch/VSD	1
TOF/absent pulmonary valve	1
Pulmonary atresia/VSD/PDA	1
Trisomy 18	**13**
VSD	7
DORV	4
AV Canal	1
Aortic Stenosis	1
Trisomy 13	**6**
Pulmonary atresia/VSD/PDA	3
DORV	2
VSD	1
Turner syndrome (and similar variants)	**4**
Bicuspid Aortic valve, mild AS	2
Small VSD	1
Hypoplastic left heart	1
Other	**9**
Total	**89**

AS, aortic stenosis; AV, atrioventricular; DORV, double outlet right ventricle; IAA, interrupted aortic arch; MAPCAs, multiple aortopulmonary collateral arteries; PA, pulmonary atresia; PDA, patent ductus arteriosus; TOF, tetralogy of Fallot; VSD, ventricular septal defect.

In a recent review of our experience, we gained important perspectives that have led us to reexamine our mission.[1] During the 4-year interval between 2004 and 2008, 439 neonates underwent cardiothoracic surgery at our institution. Of these, 294 (67%) were diagnosed prenatally. The majority underwent neonatal surgery with a surgical severity score of 3-6. Eighteen of these patients underwent emergency surgery and three required extracorporeal membrane oxygenatio (ECMO) support.

A detailed comparison between the prenatally and postnatally diagnosed infants was performed. Not surprisingly, single ventricle variants, including hypoplastic left heart syndrome, were significantly more likely to be diagnosed prenatally. This alone was responsible for the significantly higher surgical severity score among the neonates who were diagnosed prenatally. While double-outlet right ventricle was significantly more likely to be diagnosed prenatally, the same did not hold for tetralogy of Fallot. Transposition of the great arteries was significantly more likely to be diagnosed postnatally, and total anomalous pulmonary venous connection was, by far, more frequently a postnatal finding rather than a prenatal diagnosis.

Somewhat surprisingly, we found no difference between arterial pH or highest measured serum lactate between the prenatal and postnatal diagnosis groups. The prenatal diagnosis group was significantly more premature at birth (37.9 ± 2 weeks vs. 38.6 ± 2 weeks). This almost certainly reflects our policy of suggesting elective induction of labor for women who live at any significant distance from our center and whose fetuses have potential ductal dependency. This may have deleterious effects on the development of the brain, which has been found to lag in development in many fetuses with severe forms of congenital heart disease. We are reexamining this policy to avoid elective deliveries before 39 weeks' gestation. Another disturbing finding, which may be unique to our institution, is that the average age at surgery was 6-7 days, regardless of whether the infant was diagnosed prenatally or postnatally (in fact, the prenatal group always waited significantly longer for surgery (time of surgery on median day of life 7, interquartile range 5-8) than the postnatal diagnosis group (median day of life 6, interquartile range 5-9). This trend held, even when the groups were stratified according to cardiac diagnosis. This may be related to the much higher propensity for surgery to be postponed for the infants who were diagnosed prenatally (22.8% vs. 11.7%, $P = .006$). The latter is disturbing, and suggests that length of stay and total hospital costs could be impacted significantly for the prenatal group if we are more assiduous in scheduling surgery upon admission for delivery of the prenatal diagnosis group.

Conclusion

Fetal cardiology is a nascent field that over the past 30 years has evolved into a field with complex prenatal diagnoses. Advancements in medicine, surgery, and technology have made prenatal diagnosis part of the field of pediatric cardiology. The field of fetal cardiology owes its origins to the research studies of Dr. Abraham Rudolph and his colleagues, who used fetal lambs to understand cardiovascular development in the normal fetus and neonate and the adaptations in blood flow in the mammalian fetus during gestation, through transition to the neonatal circulation, in the presence of congenital heart disease. Dr. Charles Kleinman, the senior author on this chapter was one of the grandfathers of the field of fetal cardiology. Shortly after this chapter was written and submitted, he passed away. He left behind a legacy of patients, colleagues, and knowledge of a field that he helped to create. We at the Morgan Stanley Children's Hospital of New York Presbyterian are indebted to Dr. Charles Kleinman for his leadership, skills, and teaching. It has made us all better fetal cardiologists and physicans.

Reference

1. Levey A, Glickstein J, Kleinman CS, et al. The impact of prenatal diagnosis of complex congenital heart disease on neonatal outcomes. Pediatr Cardiol. 2010;31:587-597.

CHAPTER 22

Clinical Evaluation of Cardiovascular Function in the Human Fetus

James Huhta, MD

The Fetal Circulation

The fetal ventricles pump blood in parallel rather than in series: The left ventricle (LV) pumps to the aorta and upper body, and the right ventricle (RV) pumps to the ductus arteriosus and the lower body and placenta. The lungs have a high resistance in utero and the placenta fulfills the role of oxygenating the blood and ridding the body of wastes. Highly oxygenated blood from the placenta passes to the ductus venosus where a portion bypasses the liver and passes predominantly to the left atrium. Deoxygenated blood from the upper body passes to the tricuspid valve and then to both the ductus arteriosus and lungs. Deoxygenated blood from the inferior vena cava and the right hepatic veins is directed to the right atrium and predominantly to the tricuspid valve. Three shunts (ductus venosus, foramen ovale, and ductus arteriosus) allow the fetal heart to work with two parallel rather than one series circulation. Right and left atrial pressures are almost equal because of the presence of the foramen ovale and right and left ventricular end-diastolic pressures are equal due to the ductus arteriosus.

Factors Affecting Fetal Cardiac Output

The fetal myocardium develops less active tension than the adult at similar muscle lengths. Structural differences such as less T-tubular system and less organized myofibrils are observed but there are also differences in calcium uptake into the sarcoplasmic reticulum. There is decreased sympathetic innervation in the immature myocardium that could influence the stress response of the myocardium. Fetal myocytes are smaller in size, have less mitochondria, sarcoplasmic reticulum, myofilaments, alpha- and beta-adrenoceptors, and T-tubuli, and have higher concentrations of DNA, reflecting a larger number of nuclei. Growth or increased workload in the fetus results in hyperplasia of the myocardium with an increased number of cells, whereas growth of the myocardium after birth is only by increased cell size or hypertrophy (increased protein content of each cell). In the very immature heart, myofilaments are arranged in a more chaotic way, but they become better organized as gestation advances. The metabolic source of energy for the fetal myocardium is glucose almost exclusively. In adults, fatty acids are the major source of energy for the myocardium. The fetus has a range of heart rates between 55 and 200 at which the stroke volume of the ventricular chambers can adapt to maintain adequate cardiac output and tissue perfusion. Outside of this range, heart failure often results. In summary, the major determinant of cardiac output is the afterload of the fetal ventricle. It follows that any influence that raises the impedance to ejection will inversely lower the ventricular stroke volume by the effect on both the systolic and diastolic function of the heart.

The Transitional Circulation

After birth, the function of gas exchange is transferred from the placenta to the lungs. There is a decrease in pulmonary vascular resistance, and the closure of the ductus arteriosus within 2-3 days, and foramen ovale pressure gradient reverses.

The Etiology of Hydrops Fetalis

All of the following factors contribute to decreased cardiac reserve in response to stress and to a higher susceptibility of the fetus for the development of cardiac failure: the reduced ability of the fetal heart to contract and to generate force, the lower myocardial compliance, and the diminished Frank Starling mechanism, the higher dependence of cardiac output on heart rate, and the lack of adrenoceptors. All these factors favor fluid movement out of the capillary into tissue, causing fluid accumulation in fetal tissue. The younger the fetus, the higher its extracellular water content and the lower its tissue pressure. Fluid movement between intravascular and extravascular space is dependent on intravascular and extravascular hydrostatic and oncotic pressure and the fluid filtration coefficient, which is determined by the capillary membrane (in the fetus more permeable for fluid and protein). Albumin concentration, largely responsible for oncotic pressure, is lower in the fetus and increases with gestational age.

Faced with the fetus with hydrops fetalis, one must first determine if the hydrops is cardiac, inflammatory, or metabolic. There are several possibilities for the cause of heart failure in the fetus after ruling out fetal infection (Table 22-1).

Mechanisms of Fetal Congestive Heart Failure

Increased Afterload

Twin-Twin Transfusion

The recipient, the larger twin in twin-twin transfusion syndrome, can experience marked elevations in cardiac output and blood pressure. Typically, the larger twin maintains a high cardiac output due to the volume of transfusion plus a state of vasoconstriction due to vasoactive substances produced by the smaller twin. With slow increases in the workload of the RV, there is compensatory hypertrophy and systolic function and minimal signs of hemodynamic compensation. With more rapid onset of volume and pressure overload, the RV stretches and the tricuspid valve begins to leak. The coronary perfusion and subendocardial blood flow are progressively compromised by the hypertrophy and increased early systolic

Table 22-1 CAUSES OF FETAL CONGESTIVE HEART FAILURE

Fetal arrhythmias
Anemia
Congenital heart disease with valvular regurgitation
Primary myocardial disease
Noncardiac malformations such as diaphragmatic hernia or cystic hygroma
Twin-twin transfusion recipient volume and pressure overload

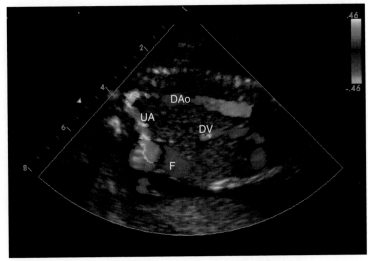

Figure 22-1   Arteriovenous fistula (F) with high cardiac output from an umbilical artery (UA) to umbilical vein connection. DAo, descending aorta; DV, ductus venosus.

workload. These signs are probably associated with increases in the end-diastolic pressure of the RV. This is reflected in the end-diastolic pressure of the right atrium which is elevated. These A-contractions against elevated pressure resistance produce retrograde flow during atrial systole in the hepatic and inferior caval veins. The ductus venosus is the earliest site to see altered flow patterns. With the onset of atrial reversal in this site or umbilical venous pulsations, the onset of metabolic acidosis is imminent. Although many factors influence this outcome, one of the most important is the RV myocardial reserve. A cardiovascular (CV) score has been developed to assess the severity of cardiac involvement.[1]

Increased Preload

Arteriovenous Fistula

A shunt from the arterial to the venous circulation in the human fetus will result in a large volume of blood returning to the right atrium. This results in dilated right heart structures and a high cardiac output. The fetal heart is well adapted to handle increasing volume loads if they are imposed gradually. If rapid increasing severity shunts occur as is sometimes seen in sacrococcygeal teratoma, then cardiac decompensation and the development of hydrops fetalis can occur quickly. Another common cause of heart failure is vein of Galen aneurysm, which is an arteriovenous (AV) fistula with increasing flow to the head. A relatively common AV fistula is one from the umbilical artery to the umbilical vein. This unilateral connection causes the umbilical vein "varix" referred to in early literature. It may cause cardiomegaly only or cause progression to severe congestive heart failure (CHF) and hydrops (Fig. 22-1).

Another defect causing high cardiac output is absent ductus venosus with direct connection of the umbilical vein to the heart or inferior vena cava (IVC). It is significantly associated with fetal cardiac and extracardiac anomalies, aneuploidies, and hydrops. Fetuses with liver bypass have an additional risk of developing congestive heart failure that significantly affects outcome, even if the fetal CV anatomy is otherwise normal.[2]

An important sign of RV decompensation in these scenarios is valvular regurgitation. Early signs of tricuspid regurgitation if only very mild should signal an increase in fetal surveillance. The subsequent development of mitral regurgitation is ominous and is a clear sign of a prehydropic state.

External Compression

The fetus with cystic adenomatoid malformation in the lung can present with cardiac external compression and a small heart size. Hydrops was noted in 15 of 41 fetuses (36.5%). The fetuses that developed hydrops had a lower cardiac/thoracic ratio than those that did not develop hydrops (0.18 vs. 0.23, P = .001). Those fetuses with hydrops also demonstrated an increase in early ventricular filling. The ratio of early ventricular filling to atrial contraction (E/A ratio) at both the tricuspid and mitral valves was significantly higher in the fetuses with hydrops (P = .005 and P = .03, respectively). Doppler interrogation of the inferior vena cava demonstrated a greater degree of reversal with atrial contraction in the hydrops group (29.7% vs. 15.1%, P = .003).

Prognosis of Fetal Heart Failure—Markers of Fetal Mortality

Introduction to the Use of the Cardiovascular Profile Score (Table 22-2)

Fetal echocardiographic approach to defining the prognosis of fetal CHF has been published over the past 20 years as individual studies correlating one variable to fetal outcome (survival).

- Cardiac size/thoracic size. Cardiac divided by thoracic area ratio (normal 0.25-0.35) or C/T circumference ratio (normal < 0.5).[3,4] In fetuses with cystic adenomatoid malformation, a small C/T ratio (<0.2) is associated with a poor prognosis.[5] Cardiomegaly is a heart-to-chest area ratio greater than 0.35 at any time in gestation.
- Venous Doppler. Inferior caval (or hepatic venous) (increased atrial reversal), ductus venosus (with a wave reversal) and umbilical cord vein (pulsations).[6,7]
- Four-valve Doppler (atrioventricular and semilunar). Any leak of the valve should be evaluated further.[8,9]

Ventricular Function in the Fetus

Cardiac function can be estimated using the Tei index or myocardial performance index. This is calculated using the filling time of the AV valve and the ejection time of the ventricle.[10]

Fetal Congestive Heart Failure

The diagnosis of fetal congestive heart failure therefore must be addressed in a clinical fashion similar to that after birth. The classical postnatal clinical tetrad of cardiomegaly, tachycardia, tachypnea, and hepatomegaly has been used in neonates and children. This clinical state in the fetus can be characterized by findings in at least five categories, which are obtained during the ultrasonographic examination. These five have been combined in a CV profile score.[11] The following five categories are each worth 2 points in a 10-point scoring system to assess the CV system. Abnormalities in the CV profile score may occur prior to the clinical state of hydrops fetalis. The five categories are hydrops, umbilical venous Doppler, heart size, abnormal myocardial function, and arterial Doppler. Within specific disease entities, more emphasis is placed on certain areas by the attending physician to predict the prognosis. As always, this information can only comprise a portion of the total picture and must be integrated by the attending physician into the diagnostic and treatment plan for the patient. The Cardiovascular Profile Score gives a semiquantitative score of the fetal cardiac well-being and uses known markers by ultrasound, which have been correlated with poor fetal outcome (Table 22-2). This profile is normal if the score is 10 and signs of cardiac abnormalities result in a decrease of the score from normal. For example, if there is hydrops with ascites and no other abnormalities, there would be a deduction of 1 point for hydrops (ascites but no skin edema) and no deductions for the other categories for a score of 9 out of 10.

Table 22-2 CARDIOVASCULAR PROFILE SCORE

	NORMAL	−1 POINT	−2 POINTS
		10 POINTS = NORMAL	
Hydrops	None (2 pts)	Ascites *or* Pleural effusion *or* Pericardial effusion	Skin edema
Venous Doppler (umbilical vein) (ductus venosus)	UV DV (2 pts)	UV DV	UV pulsations
Heart size (heart area/chest area)	>0.20 and ≤0.35 (2 pts)	0.35-0.50	>0.50 or <0.20
Cardiac function	Normal TV and MV RV/LV SF > 0.28 Biphasic diastolic filling (2 pts)	Holosystolic TR *or* RV/LV SF < 0.28	Holosystolic MR *or* TR dP/dt < 400 *or* Monophasic filling
Arterial Doppler (umbilical artery)	UA (2 pts)	UA (AEDV)	UA (REDV)

The heart failure score is 10 if there are no abnormal signs and reflects 2 points for each of five categories: hydrops, venous Doppler, heart size, cardiac function, and arterial Doppler. AEDV, absent end-diastolic velocity; dP/dt, change in pressure over time of TR jet; DV, ductus venosus; LV, left ventricle; MR, mitral valve regurgitation; MV, mitral valve; pts, points; REDV, reversed end-diastolic velocity; RV, right ventricle; SF, ventricular shortening fraction; TR, tricuspid valve regurgitation; TV, tricuspid valve; UA, umbilical artery; UV, umbilical vein.

The CV profile score comprises 2 points in each of the five categories used in serial studies to provide a method of uniform physiological assessment. By taking a multivariate approach, this type of multifactorial score can combine assessment of direct and indirect markers of CV function. Initial validation of the CV profile score in hydrops was shown by Falkensammer and colleagues.[10] Seven fetuses with hydrops including three with congenital heart disease had correlation of the CV profile score with the myocardial performance index (Tei index). RV and LV Tei indices were assessed in normal subjects and showed no change with gestational age. Hofstaetter and colleagues measured the CV profile score in 59 hydrops fetuses.[12] Mortality was 21/59. The median score in those who died pre- or postnatally was 5. The score was lower in those who died than in the survivors. Studying fetuses with congenital heart disease, there was an inverse correlation between 30-day mortality and the CV profile score.[13] In the work of Makikallio and colleagues studying 75 growth-restricted fetuses, there were seven deaths with a median CV profile score of 4-5 while those who survived had a median score of 8.[14]

Cardiovascular Profile Score in Ebstein's Anomaly

Chen and colleagues sought to determine whether cerebral vascular resistance and left ventricular myocardial performance (LV Tei) are abnormal in fetuses with Ebstein's anomaly.[15] The pulsatility index of the middle cerebral artery (MCAPI) and umbilical artery (UAPI), LV Tei, left ventricular ejection fraction (LVEF), and fetal CV profile score in 11 fetuses with Ebstein's anomaly were evaluated by fetal echocardiography. MCAPI/UAPI values were calculated for the Ebstein's anomaly group. The control group included 44 healthy fetuses of uncomplicated pregnancies matched for gestational age (according to 1:4). MCAPI and MCAPI/UAPI were significantly lower in fetuses with Ebstein's anomaly than in control subjects (all $P < .001$). UAPI and LV Tei were higher in fetuses with Ebstein's anomaly than in control fetuses ($P < .001$, $P < .05$, respectively). No significant between-group difference was observed for LVEF ($P > .05$). The median CV profile score (CVPS) for the fetuses with Ebstein's anomaly (median, 7.0; interquartile range [IQR], 5.-8.0) was a full point lower than for control subjects (median, 10.0; IQR 10.0-10.0). This difference was statistically significant ($P < .001$). MCAPI and LV Tei were both correlated with fetal CVPS in fetuses with Ebstein's anomaly (correlation coefficient 1 = 0.477, $P < .05$; correlation coefficient 2 = −0.602, $P < .05$). They concluded that in fetuses with Ebstein's anomaly in utero, cerebral vascular resistance is decreased and that global LV performance, as assessed by the Tei index, is abnormal.

Treatment of Fetal Heart Failure

Interventions aimed at improving the effective cardiac output are also aimed at prolonging the pregnancy and preventing prematurity and prenatal asphyxia.[16]

Treatment with digoxin for evidence of decreased ventricular shortening is controversial. Digoxin is known to decrease the catecholamine response to congestive heart failure and if there is diastolic dysfunction in the fetus, then this may improve filling and lower filling pressures. If the afterload is high, then an increase in oxygen consumption could result from increased inotropy without improved myocardial perfusion. Terbutaline appears to have promise as an inotropic and chronotropic agent but studies of the possible negative effects on the fetal myocardium are needed. At the present time, we use digoxin for fetal cardiac failure due to arrhythmias and high output states such as fistula and anemia. In a recent case of acardiac twinning where the normal fetuses were supporting two circulations, digoxin appeared to improve cardiac function and result in a prolonged and successful gestation for the normal twin.

Laser treatment of the twin-twin communications or cord ligation with acardiac twins can be applied to improve cardiac failure. Attempts have been made to occlude the feeding artery in AV fistulas with limited success. With anemia, it is possible to transfuse the fetus via the umbilical vein. The diagnosis of fetal anemia can be made using the middle cerebral artery peak velocity. With anemia, the cardiac output is increased with a reduced oxygen-carrying capacity. When there is cardiomegaly (see earlier for criteria), it is rational to use transplacental treatment of the fetus to support the myocardium if the pregnancy will be continuing long enough for medications to reach therapeutic levels.

Digoxin

Digoxin is widely used in perinatology for the transplacental treatment of fetal arrhythmias. To use it for heart failure in the fetus should not impose increased risks for the mother because the doses for CHF are lower than those for conversion of supraventricular tachycardia. In adult cardiology, it is known that therapeutic doses of digoxin associated with digoxin levels of 0.5 μg/nL in serum are associated with decreased mortality from CHF.

Digoxin has been used in such circumstances due to its antiadrenergic benefits and the significant experience that has been gained about its safety in pregnancy. We use Lanoxin (Lanoxicaps) 0.2 mg or generic digoxin 0.25 mg tablets, orally two to four times per day based on maternal serum levels. We use a trough level of 1.0-2.0 to avoid any maternal side effects. In fetuses with arteriovenous fistula and heart failure, we also use digoxin to support the heart.[17]

When fetal valvular regurgitation is present on a congenital basis, it could be useful to decrease the afterload of the fetal ventricles as is done in infants with a similar problem. However, medications that reduce the afterload such as angiotensin-converting enzyme inhibitors are known to be dangerous to the fetus in pregnancy. Reduction of catecholamine levels could have a similar effect and digoxin could be useful in this situation.

In pregnant mothers with significant levels of anti-Rho and anti-La antibodies, we recommend dexamethasone 4 mg daily by mouth if there are signs of valvular regurgitation, heart block, valvulitis, myocardial dysfunction, myocardial echogenicity, or effusion. Early use of this medication may prevent progression of heart block and heart failure.

When myocardial dysfunction is seen without obvious reasons and fetal infection has been excluded, we consider that an inherited form of cardiomyopathy of either the LV or RV can present in utero. We use digoxin for these patients as long as there is no sign of ventricular ectopy or tachycardia.

The basis for our practice of using digoxin is in the paper of Patel and colleagues.[17] We attempted first to evaluate the effects of digoxin treatment on the severity and progression of fetal CHF by comparing composite CVPS and its components (degree of hydrops, arterial and venous Doppler flow patterns, heart size, and presence of markers of cardiac dysfunction) before and after digoxin therapy, and second to determine which components of the CVPS were the best predictors of perinatal death.

Medical records and video tapes from three tertiary care perinatal centers were reviewed for subjects who received digoxin for the sole purpose of treating fetal congestive heart failure. In this retrospective case series, 28 fetuses with CHF presented to these centers between 2000 and 2006, and all were given transplacental digoxin. Fetuses with either structural cardiac defects or fetuses with noncardiac defects that imposed increased preload or afterload on a structurally normal heart were included, while fetuses with non-sinus rhythm, including supraventricular tachycardia, atrial flutter, or AV block treated with digoxin, were excluded. Outcome was defined either as live birth or perinatal death (in utero demise).

The degree of heart failure was quantified by the 10-point CV profile score (Table 22-2). The baseline CVPS was measured immediately before instituting digoxin therapy. Posttreatment CVPS was ascertained weekly until delivery or perinatal death. The last CVPS was that recorded before delivery or before perinatal death.

Ten mothers received a loading dosage of 0.375 mg every 8 hours for three doses; the remaining mothers were given maintenance dosages of 0.25-0.375 mg every 8 to 12 hours. Maternal levels of serum digoxin were determined 1 hour before a maintenance dose 5-7 days after therapy was initiated.

Nineteen fetuses had CHF secondary to structural cardiac defects, and nine fetuses had CHF due to noncardiac anomalies including sacrococcygeal or cervical teratoma, cerebral arteriovenous malformation, and cystic hygroma, and the recipient twin with twin-to-twin transfusion syndrome (TTS). Twelve of 28 (43%) were severely hydropic at the time of presentation.

Digoxin Treatment

All mothers tolerated the digoxin with no side effects except for nausea during the loading dose in one mother, which necessitated reducing the dose. Trough maternal digoxin levels ranged from 0.4 to 2.3 ng/mL. The median gestational age at the time that digoxin therapy commenced was 27 weeks, and the median time of treatment was 4.5 (3.5-6) weeks (range 1-15 weeks). There were no significant differences between survivors and nonsurvivors for the gestational ages at initiation of digoxin therapy or the duration of treatment.

Outcome

Twenty-four fetuses (79%) survived to be born alive; perinatal mortality was 21%. Of those 24, five died prior to 20 days of age (neonatal mortality 21%).

Effect of Digoxin on CVPS

After digoxin treatment, CVPS improved overall in 54%. There was no significant change in the component markers of the CVPS before and after therapy.

Differences in CVPS Between Survivors and Nonsurvivors

The median composite CVPS differed significantly between survivors and nonsurvivors at baseline and after digoxin therapy. The median baseline, final, and 1 week post-therapy CVPS scores differed significantly between survivors and the group that died ($P = .017$). The best predictor of survival was a CVPS greater than or equal to 6. This gave a sensitivity of 83% and specificity of 75% (odds ratio 2.1).

Abnormal venous Doppler in the ductus venosus and umbilical vein was seen in 100% of nonsurvivors.

The findings of this study suggest that the CVPS and especially the component variables of hydrops and notching in the ductus venosus can be helpful in predicting perinatal outcome. Furthermore, these data suggest that for the fetus with mild to moderate heart failure and sinus rhythm, digoxin is beneficial in improving cardiac dysfunction or preventing its progression. Finally, if transplacental treatment is not initiated until hydrops is severe, or if hydrops progresses despite treatment, there is a high likelihood of fetal demise.

In utero resolution of hydrops and improvement of cardiac systolic function has been reported in fetuses with aortic stenosis and Ebstein's anomaly of the tricuspid valve, in fetuses with structurally normal hearts and TTS (even after laser occlusion of the chorioangiopagus vessels, obstructive intracardiac rhabdomyoma and with idiopathic or infectious nonimmune hydrops).[18]

Because of its high lipid solubility and low molecular weight, digoxin passively diffuses across the placenta, reaching steady state in 8-10 days. Fetal digoxin levels range from 60% to 90% of maternal levels, but are significantly less, 11-26%, with hydrops. Nonetheless, resolution of hydrops has been reported with maternal digoxin levels as low as 0.5 ng/mL, a level attained by every mother in this study.

How digoxin improves fetal cardiac dysfunction with or without hydrops is not understood. Digoxin, when given at low doses over 2-8 weeks to humans in mild to moderate heart failure, has both hemodynamic and autonomic effects. It improves the stress-shortening relationship, a load independent index of systolic performance, and, by increasing arterial baroreceptor and cardiac receptor nerve discharge, increases efferent parasympathetic activity and reduces the outflow of sympathetic activity.[19] An increase in cardiac sympathetic activity, as is seen in heart failure, results in elevated central filling pressures. In response to increased central venous filling pressure, the secretion of atrial natriuretic peptide (ANP) increases. ANP enhances vascular permeability of albumin into fetal tissues to lower blood volume and reduce preload. Tissue edema is exacerbated by the imbalance between elevated filling pressures and low oncotic pressure secondary to hypoalbuminemia in the fetus with hydrops. By its autonomic effects—enhancing baroreceptor-mediated parasympathetic discharge and reducing sympathetic output—digoxin may decrease filling pressure and heighten the threshold for sudden arrhythmogenic cardiac death seen with excess catecholamines known to be toxic to cardiac tissue. We speculate that in some cases in which hydrops did not resolve, digoxin may have prevented or slowed the progression of heart failure. Alternatively, the levels achieved in the fetus were too low to alter the natural history of the disease.

Further insight into these questions may be answered by a multicenter randomized study of prophylactic treatment of fetal congestive heart failure. In addition, digoxin's method of action, including whether or not it enhances fetal parasympathetic activity, may be elucidated by heart rate variability assessed by fetal electrocardiography or magnetocardiography. In summary, after digoxin treatment, fetal CVPS improved in 41% and did not worsen in 35%. A composite CVPS of < 7, and component variables of abnormal flow in the ductus venosus and hydrops at baseline and after digoxin, differed significantly between perinatal survivors and nonsurvivors.

We surmised that CVPS would be helpful not only to assess if fetuses with cardiac dysfunction and sinus rhythm might benefit from transplacental digoxin, but when to initiate such treatment but in fetuses with combined anatomical and functional deficits. This complicated group of patients also suggests that fetuses with congenital cardiac anomalies usually associated with fetal demise may have multifactorial causes of heart failure.

Terbutaline has been used as a tocolytic agent in mothers with preterm labor and has been recognized to have potential benefits in increasing fetal cardiac function.[20] In the treatment of complete heart block, maternal administration of this sympathomimetic can increase cardiac contraction and stabilize or reverse impending hydrops. We consider adding this medication to digoxin as a second-line drug for fetal heart failure that is refractory to digoxin when the fetus is very premature and there is no maternal contraindication.

In summary, fetal CV profile scores for assessment of fetal wellness can complement the biophysical score and may be useful in guiding therapy. The goal is to detect and intervene during the prehydropic state of compromised fetuses.

References

1. Rychik J, Tian Z, Bebbington M, et al. The twin-twin transfusion syndrome: spectrum of cardiovascular abnormality and development of a cardiovascular score to assess severity of disease. Am J Obstet Gynecol. 2007;197(4):392.e1-e8.
2. Berg C, Kamil D, Geipel A, et al. Absence of ductus venosus-importance of umbilical venous drainage site. Ultrasound Obstet Gynecol. 2006;28(3):275-281.
3. Respondek M, Respondek A, Huhta JC, et al. 2D echocardiographic assessment of the fetal heart size in the 2nd and 3rd trimester of uncomplicated pregnancy. Eur J Ob Gyn Reprod Biol. 1992;44:185-188.
4. Johnson P, Sharland G, Allan LD, et al. Umbilical venous pressure in nonimmune hydrops fetalis: correlation with cardiac size. Am J Obstet Gynecol. 1992;167:1309-1313.
5. Mahle WT, Rychik J, Tian ZY, et al. Echocardiographic evaluation of the fetus with congenital cystic adenomatoid malformation. Ultrasound Obstet Gynecol. 2000;16(7):620-624.
6. Gudmundsson S, Huhta JC, Wood DC, et al. Venous Doppler ultrasonography in the fetus with non-immune hydrops. Am J Obstet Gynecol. 1991;164:33-37.
7. Tulzer G, Gudmundsson S, Wood DC, et al. Doppler in non-immune hydrops fetalis. Ultrasound Obstet Gynecol. 1994;4:279-283.
8. Tulzer G, Gudmundsson S, Rotondo KM, et al. Doppler in the evaluation and prognosis of fetuses with tricuspid regurgitation J Matern Fetal Invest. 1991;1:15-18.
9. Respondek M, Kammermeier M, Ludomirsky A, et al. The prevalence and clinical significance of fetal tricuspid valve regurgitation with normal heart anatomy. Am J Obstet Gynecol. 1994;171:1265-1270.
10. Falkensammer CB, Paul J, Huhta JC. Fetal congestive heart failure: correlation of the Tei-Index and Cardiovascular Score. J Perinat Med. 2001;29:390-398.
11. Huhta JC. Right ventricular function in the human fetus. J Perinat Med. 2001;29:381-389.

12. Hofstaetter C, Hansmann M, Eik-Nes SH, et al. A cardiovascular profile score in the surveillance of fetal hydrops. J Matern Fetal Neonatal Med. 2006;19(7):407-413.

13. Wieczorek A, Hernandez-Robles J, Ewing L, et al. Prediction of outcome of fetal congenital heart disease using a cardiovascular profile score. Ultrasound Obstet Gynecol. 2008;31(3):284-288.

14. Makikallio K, Vuolteenaho O, Jouppila P, et al. Association of severe placental insufficiency and systemic venous pressure rise in the fetus with increased neonatal cardiac troponin T levels. Am J Obstet Gynecol. 2000;183:726-731.

15. Chen Y, Lv G, Li B, Wang Z. Cerebral vascular resistance and left ventricular myocardial performance in fetuses with Ebstein's anomaly. Am J Perinat. 2009;26(4):253-258.

16. Huhta JC. Fetal congestive heart failure. Semin Fetal Neonatal Med. 2005;10:542-552.

17. Patel D, Cuneo B, Viesca R, et al. Digoxin for the treatment of fetal congestive heart failure with sinus rhythm assessed by cardiovascular profile score. J Matern Fetal Neonatal Med. 2008;21(7):477-482.

18. Koike T, Minakami H, Shiraishi H, et al. Digitalization of the mother in treating hydrops fetalis in monochorionic twin with Ebstein's anomaly. J Perinat Med. 1997;24:295-297.

19. Newton GE, Tong JH, Schofield AM, et al. Digoxin reduces cardiac sympathetic activity in severe congestive heart failure. J Am Coll Cardiol. 1996;28:155-161.

20. Sharif DS, Huhta JC, Moise KJ, et al. Changes in fetal hemodynamics with terbutaline treatment and premature labor. J Clin Ultrasound. 1990;18:85-89.

CHAPTER 23

Cardiac Surgery in the Neonate with Congenital Heart Disease

Emile Bacha, MD, FACS, Jonathan M. Chen, MD, and
Jan M. Quaegebeur, MD, PhD

23

- Palliative Operations
- Specific Lesions
- Mechanical Circulatory Support in the Neonate
- Conclusion
- References

In 1952, scarcely more than 60 years ago, the first operation on the open human heart under direct vision—repair of an atrial septal defect (ASD) in a 5-year-old girl—was performed at the University of Minnesota.[1] This operation was accomplished using inflow occlusion and moderate total body hypothermia. With the development of cardiopulmonary bypass over the course of the next decade, this success could be extended to a wider variety of more complex lesions. Refinements in surgical technique, medical technology, and perioperative care have since resulted in excellent survival after the repair of even the most complex types of congenital heart disease (CHD) in increasingly smaller children. Further, with the growing availability and accuracy of prenatal diagnosis by fetal echocardiography, the postnatal management of these complicated newborns can often be anticipated and planned. Except for single ventricle palliation during the newborn period, surgical mortality in the neonate has decreased to the point that future work will focus on improving the short- and long-term morbidity associated with neonatal repair of CHD, in particular with regard to long-term functional status, neurodevelopmental outcomes, and the need for ongoing follow-up and reintervention, with the attendant psychological and financial burden this imposes on both the patient and the patient's family.

Initially, most operations for CHD performed in the neonatal period were extracardiac palliative procedures. Despite initial success with repair of intracardiac lesions by use of cross-circulation, most early attempts to use mechanical cardiopulmonary bypass (CPB) could not duplicate these results: surgical equipment and technology were unrefined.[2,3] Thus palliative procedures not requiring CPB were used either permanently or to defer repair until children were older. These procedures are still employed, but since the 1980s there has been a growing trend toward primary repair of CHD early in life. This trend has been spurred on by the recognition of the potentially deleterious effects of palliation upon cardiac mechanics, pulmonary physiology, neurological development, and pulmonary artery anatomy, as well as by advancements in the technology and perioperative management of CPB. In this brief overview, we discuss those common congenital heart conditions for which surgical intervention in the neonatal period is most common. Emerging techniques, both catheter-based and surgical (or a hybrid thereof), continue to modify this list and improve the outcomes of these newborns.

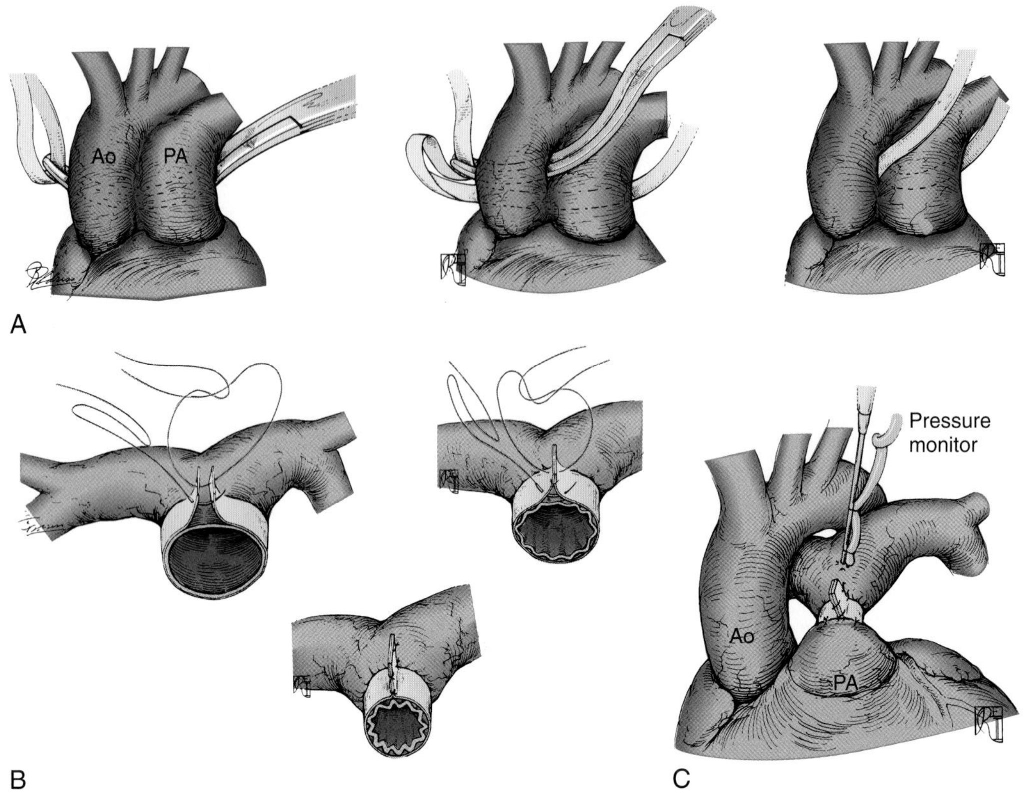

Figure 23-1   Placement of a pulmonary artery band. **A,** The pulmonary artery is encircled using the subtraction technique. **B,** Sutures are placed to tighten the band. **C,** Pressure measurement in the pulmonary artery distal to the site of band placement to assess band tightness. Ao, aorta; PA, pulmonary artery. (From Backer CL, Mavroudis C. Palliative operations. In: Mavroudis D, Backer CL, eds. Pediatric cardiac surgery, 3rd ed. Philadelphia: Mosby; 2003:160-170.)

Palliative Operations

Pulmonary Artery Banding

Historically, pulmonary artery banding was widely used in patients with large left-to-right shunts or single ventricle physiology, to limit pulmonary blood flow and pressure, and permit somatic growth and potential clinical improvement before subsequent staged repair. More recently, primary repair in the neonatal period has replaced staged surgery as the treatment of choice for many of these diagnoses. As a result, pulmonary artery banding is now performed infrequently.

Isolated pulmonary artery banding is best performed through a median sternotomy. In the procedure, a nonabsorbable material is used to surround the main pulmonary artery (Fig. 23-1). This "band" is secured gradually, either with sutures or clips, thereby limiting pulmonary blood flow so that the pulmonary artery pressures distal to the band range are between one third and one half of the systemic blood pressure; care is taken to avoid substantial arterial desaturation or impairment of cardiac output. The Trusler formula provides a guideline for the proper band circumference depending upon the patient's weight and physiology.[4] It is important to note that the Trusler formula was developed for high flow lesions such as ventricular septal defects (VSDs) and not for single ventricle palliation. Contraindications to pulmonary artery banding include significant atrioventricular valve regurgitation and a potential for significant subaortic obstruction with single-ventricle defects. Once optimal band tightness is achieved, the band is secured to the adventitia of the pulmonary artery to prevent movement, taking care not to impinge upon either branch of the pulmonary artery or the pulmonary valve.

Complications with pulmonary artery banding mostly relate to technical problems, including bands that are either too tight or too loose, or band migration. Permanent damage to the pulmonary valve may result from a band too close to the pulmonary valve, leading to impingement upon valve leaflet motion. Conversely, a band placed too far distally may produce branch pulmonary artery stenosis. At the subsequent staged procedure, band removal can be performed with facility for either reconstruction of the stenotic banding site or oversewing of the pulmonary outflow tract as indicated.

Aortopulmonary Shunts (Blalock-Taussig Shunt)

As with pulmonary artery banding, the increasing preference for primary repair of congenital cardiac defects in the neonatal period has led to a decrease in the use of isolated aortopulmonary shunts. First used in 1945 to augment pulmonary blood flow, the classic Blalock-Taussig (BT) shunt (creation of a subclavian artery-to-pulmonary artery anastomosis) was used as a palliative procedure for staged repair of several defects, including tetralogy of Fallot.[5]

Later modifications to the original technique of aortopulmonary shunting include the descending aorta-to-left pulmonary artery (Potts) shunt, the ascending aorta-to-right pulmonary anastomosis (Waterston shunt), the ascending aorta-to-main pulmonary artery ("central") shunt, and the use of prosthetic graft material such as Gore-tex (modified BT shunt). All these techniques aim to produce a controlled increase in pulmonary blood flow, which enables appropriate oxygenation in patients with cyanotic defects. Division of the main pulmonary artery in combination with a BT shunt may be used as an alternative to pulmonary artery banding in single-ventricle lesions to maintain oxygenation and limit pulmonary artery pressure.

The modified Blalock-Taussig shunt (Fig. 23-2) may be performed via thoracotomy or sternotomy. The benefits of thoracotomy include preservation of the median sternotomy approach for future repair and avoidance of cardiopulmonary bypass in the neonatal period, with its attendant risks. In contrast, the benefits of the sternotomy include access to the great vessels should emergent cardiopulmonary bypass prove necessary, the ability to ligate the ductus arteriosus at the time of shunt creation, and more proximal access to the branch pulmonary artery. In general, the shunt is performed on the side opposite to the insertion of the ductus arteriosus into the pulmonary artery. In doing so, the surgeon may clamp the branch pulmonary artery for the anastomosis, without affecting "antegrade" pulmonary blood flow via the ductus arteriosus. In the case of a right aortic arch, the shunt may still be performed from a right thoracotomy; however, if the origin is from the ascending aorta it may function more similarly to a central shunt than a modified Blalock-Taussig shunt from the subclavian artery (i.e., this location may mandate the use of a smaller shunt).

Complications of shunt insertion relate to: (1) the shunt material and operative technique (kinking, thrombosis); (2) anatomy (chylothorax, injury to the vagus or phrenic nerves); and (3) sequelae from the operation itself (e.g., branch pulmonary stenosis at the shunt insertion site). Acute shunt thrombosis in the first 24-48 hours postoperatively is a feared complication of shunt insertion. When shunts are "taken down" during the later staged procedure they are rarely completely removed, but, rather, are ligated and sometimes divided. Shunts may also be closed percutaneously in the catheterization laboratory with coils. Many surgeons prefer aspirin for anticoagulation in an effort to reduce platelet activation and shunt thrombosis.

Even though it is palliative and most frequently done off bypass, shunt insertion remains one of the highest mortality procedures in congenital heart surgery. A recent review[6] of 1273 cases from the Society of Thoracic Surgeons' (STS) database yielded a mortality of 7.2%. Weight less than 3 kg and diagnosis of pulmonary atresia with intact ventricular septum (PA/IVS) were significant risk factors for death.

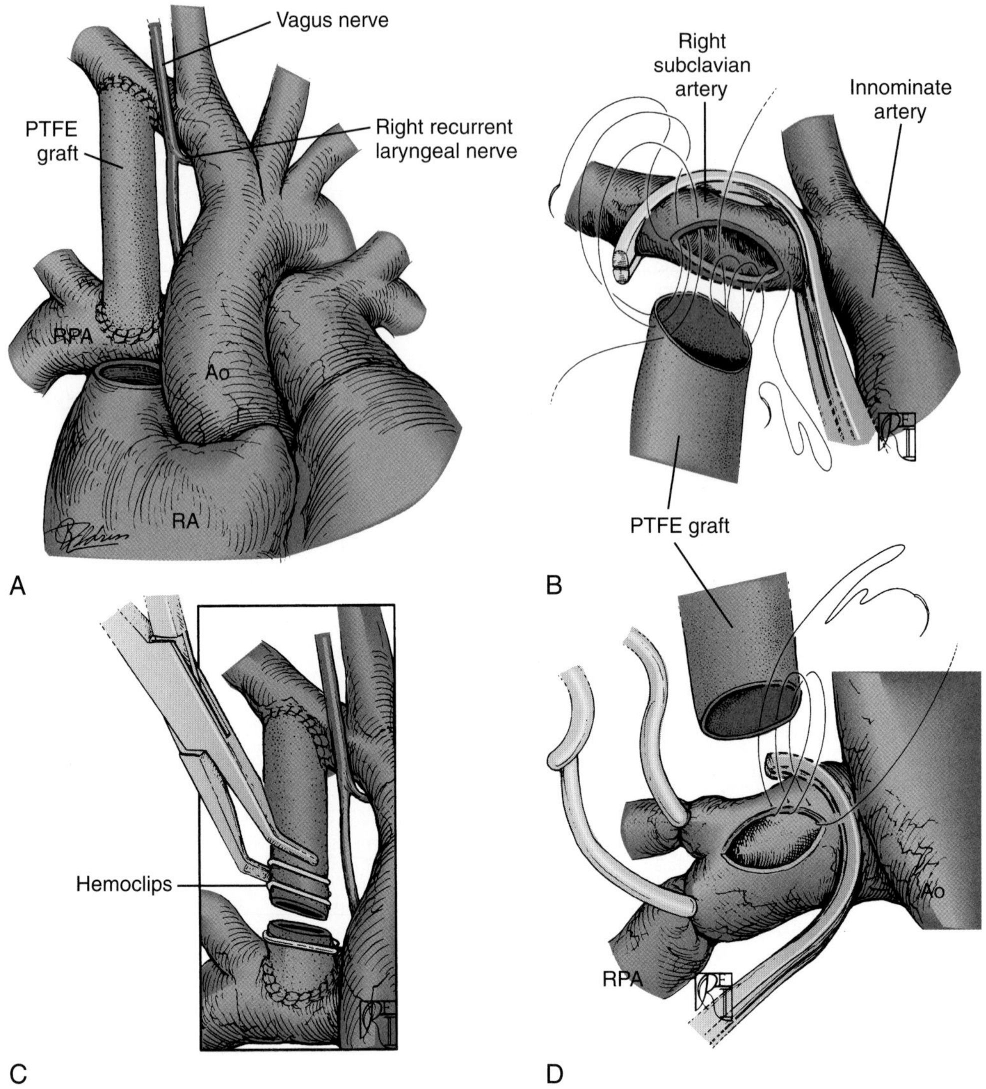

Figure 23-2 A, Modified Blalock-Taussig shunt (BTS) using a PTFE graft. Details of proximal **(B)** and distal **(C)** anastomosis for modified BTS. **D,** Take-down of modified BTS with hemoclips and shunt division. Ao, aorta; PTFE, polytetrafluoroethylene; RA, right atrium; RPA, right pulmonary artery. (From Backer CL, Mavroudis C. Palliative operations. In: Mavroudis D, Backer CL, eds. Pediatric cardiac surgery, 3rd ed. Philadelphia: Mosby; 2003:160-170.)

Specific Lesions

Left-to-Right Shunt Lesions

Ventricular Septal Defect

Infants with a large VSD and severe, intractable congestive heart failure may require surgical closure of the VSD during infancy; however, it is rare to require attention in the neonatal period. Occasionally, neonates born with so-called Swiss-cheese–like defects (multiple muscular VSDs that are poorly amenable to surgical repair but whose cumulative shunt fraction may be large) require pulmonary artery banding (see earlier) to limit pulmonary blood flow if they do not respond to aggressive medical management.

Patent Ductus Arteriosus of Botalli

The presence of a large patent ductus arteriosus (PDA) in an infant may be suspected whenever the clinical symptoms of a large left-to-right shunt are identified, including

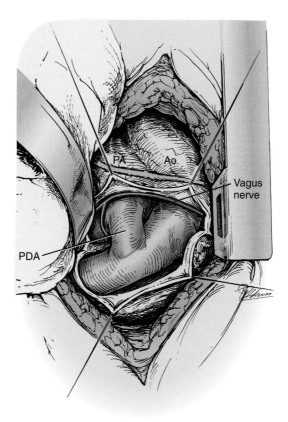

Figure 23-3 Operative exposure of a patent ductus arteriosus through a left thoracotomy. The mediastinal pleura is opened and reflected anteriorly and posteriorly. The vagus and recurrent laryngeal nerves are identified and preserved by retracting them medially. Ao, aorta; PA, pulmonary artery; PDA, patent ductus arteriosus. (From Hillman ND, Mavroudis C, Backer CL. Patent ductus arteriosus. In: Mavroudis C, Backer CL, eds. Pediatric cardiac surgery, 3rd ed. Philadelphia: Mosby; 2003:223-233.)

the presence of a heart murmur, bounding pulses, tachycardia, hyperdynamic precordial impulse, widened pulse pressure, and worsening respiratory status.[7] More common in premature infants, PDAs are unlikely to close spontaneously after the first few weeks of life. Where symptoms are present, closure should be performed immediately, but, in infants without symptoms, elective closure should be planned within three months.

In preterm infants, persistence of the PDA has been associated with increased mortality.[8] In general, initial medical therapy with a course (two to three doses) of indomethacin (ibuprofen) for PDA closure is preferred if the child exhibits no signs of renal insufficiency, necrotizing enterocolitis (NEC), or a bleeding diathesis. Contraindications to Indocin use or failure of this therapy is an indication for surgical ligation. Left-to-right shunting of a magnitude to cause abdominal end-organ hypoperfusion (renal failure, NEC) and insufficiency is not infrequent.

Ligation of the patent ductus is performed through a left-sided thoracotomy (Fig. 23-3). In most neonates, this may be achieved with the application of a permanent stainless steel hemoclip, which permits a minimally invasive incision and reduces both the need for manipulation of the fragile ductal tissue and the extent of surgical dissection required. In larger infants and children, a large PDA may require a double ligature, division, and oversewing. An echocardiogram performed as part of the preoperative analysis must demonstrate arch sidedness (which may dictate the side of the surgical incision), absence of other intracardiac lesions requiring surgical attention, and the directionality (left to right) of shunting across the ductus arteriosus. If the PDA is shunting from right to left this suggests either significant pulmonary hypertension or ductal dependency of the systemic circulation, each of which is a contraindication to closure. After the PDA is ligated the systemic diastolic pressure will often rise substantially. Complications of the procedure include damage to the recurrent laryngeal nerve, damage to the thoracic duct, ductal recanalization, and the possibility of significant hemorrhage.

Truncus Arteriosus

The primary abnormality of truncus arteriosus is the presence of a single arterial outflow from both ventricles (supplying the systemic, coronary, and pulmonary circulations) in association with a VSD. Physiologically, this results in a large left-to-right shunt that progressively worsens as pulmonary vascular resistance falls in the neonatal period. In addition, truncal valve insufficiency may exacerbate this volume load on the ventricles.

Although the occasional child may develop mild increases in pulmonary vascular resistance, which balance the pulmonary and systemic circulation enabling medium-term survival, most infants have a poor prognosis if left unrepaired. Untreated patients have 65% 1-month and 75% 1-year mortality, with early onset of severe congestive heart failure.[9] Consequently, repair is advocated in the neonatal period to prevent heart failure and myocardial ischemia, and to protect the lungs from accelerated pulmonary vascular obstructive disease. Repair at approximately 5-7 days of age as the pulmonary vascular resistance falls (heralded by tachypnea) is optimal.

Repair consists of separating ("septating") the great vessels, closing the VSD, and establishing right ventricle (RV) to pulmonary artery (PA) continuity with either a valved homograft or nonvalved conduit, or direct anastomosis of the RV to the PA confluence by use of a variety of materials (so-called direct connection).[10]

Several authors have reported excellent long-term survival in neonates frequently exceeding 90%.[10,11] Assiduous follow-up to assess for truncal valve insufficiency, ventricular failure, or the effects of somatic growth on conduit function and branch pulmonary growth is required, with early intervention (either operative or catheter-based), as indicated, to maintain function or to replace the conduit.

Aortopulmonary Window

A rare congenital defect, aortopulmonary window results from failure of complete septation of the truncus arteriosus into pulmonary artery and aorta. Repair is advocated upon diagnosis, except in very rare cases with a small, physiologically well-tolerated defect in which elective repair may be completed during infancy. In general, patch closure of the defect is performed, as the use of simple ligation is associated both with an increased risk of fatal postoperative bleeding and eventual recanalization of the defect. It can be easier sometimes to actually separate the pulmonary artery and the aorta and patch them separately, if a single patch is going to result in distortion of either vessel.

Obstructive Lesions

Pulmonary Stenosis or Pulmonary Atresia with Intact Ventricular Septum

A variety of congenital defects may coexist with some degree of right ventricular outflow tract obstruction. Patients with pulmonary atresia with intact ventricular septum have little or no connection between the right ventricle and the pulmonary artery, and are largely dependent on the left ventricle for both systemic and pulmonary blood flow (via the ductus or other aortopulmonary collateral vessels). Consequently, closure of the ductus arteriosus in these patients may result in rapid hemodynamic collapse. Without medical therapy and surgical intervention, mortality is high: 50% within 2 weeks of life and up to 85% at 6 months.[12]

For PA/IVS, initial medical therapy should be directed at maintaining ductal patency during the diagnostic workup, which always includes a diagnostic catheterization. The coronary anatomy needs to be defined, and the presence or absence of

RV-coronary fistulas as well as coronary stenoses documented. Depending on the right ventricular size and function (often best estimated by the relative size of the tricuspid valve annulus), and the presence of RV-dependent coronary vessels, appropriate surgical treatment may include decompression of the right ventricle via valvotomy or transannular patch, use of an aortopulmonary shunt to achieve pulmonary blood flow, or a combination of these two techniques. Strategies range from univentricular staged repair, or a so-called one-and-a-half ventricular repair, to a biventricular repair. RV dependent coronary blood flow as diagnosed by RV-coronary fistulas with proximal stenoses renders RV decompression by transannular patching absolutely contraindicated.

Isolated pulmonary stenosis may present at any age depending on the severity of the stenotic lesion. When it is manifest as cyanosis in the neonatal period, it is commonly referred to as "critical pulmonary stenosis."[12] Cardiac output is generally maintained through an atrial right-to-left shunt. If ductal closure occurs, progressive cyanosis and hemodynamic failure ensue. As with patients with pulmonary atresia, initial medical management should be directed at maintaining ductal patency. After the diagnosis of pulmonary stenosis, neonates may often be managed initially with transcatheter balloon valvuloplasty for right ventricular decompression. Four-year survival in the largest series is approximately 80%.[13] If the obstruction represents a composite of valvar and subvalvar (i.e., muscular or infundibular) obstruction, a further surgical procedure is often warranted. Surgery for this condition consists of placement of a patch across the annulus of the pulmonary valve and onto the right ventricular outflow tract (so-called transannular patch). Although this procedure creates obligate pulmonary insufficiency, it produces an unobstructed right ventricular outflow tract and represents the best chance for growth in right ventricular size (Fig. 23-4).

Aortic Stenosis

Valvar aortic stenosis is a common congenital cardiac defect with a wide range of morphologic and clinical variants, from bicuspid aortic valves which may be asymptomatic through adulthood to neonates with critical aortic stenosis requiring early operative intervention. When critical aortic stenosis presents in the neonate it is usually associated with severely dysmorphic aortic valve leaflets. As with right ventricular outflow tract obstruction, neonates with severe aortic stenosis may have ductal dependent cardiac output (PDA flow right-to-left to provide lower body perfusion).

In neonates, the onset of hemodynamic collapse with the advent of ductal closure signals the need for urgent intervention. During evaluation and planning, ductal patency should be maintained with prostaglandin E_1 (PGE$_1$) infusion. Additional preoperative interventions to optimize oxygenation and systemic perfusion include endotracheal intubation and mechanical ventilation, inotropic support, and management of fluid and electrolyte imbalances.

Appropriate intervention depends largely on the morphology of the left ventricle, mitral valve, and aortic valve: patients with a hypoplastic left heart may require a Norwood-type single ventricle repair or cardiac transplantation, whereas those with a ventricle likely to be able to support the systemic circulation may be treated with surgical or interventional aortic valvotomy.[14,15] Deciding whether a left ventricle is suitable for biventricular physiology can be very difficult. No definitive criteria exist. It is important to note that while the left ventricular outflow tract and aortic valve can be replaced if need be (Ross-Konno operation), a small and dysplastic mitral valve is typically beyond surgical enlargement and thus it is very important to pay attention to its anatomy during the initial assessment.

A variety of techniques are available for both surgical and balloon valvotomy (including recent attempts to mitigate the left ventricular changes associated with aortic stenosis through in utero interventional aortic valvotomy.[16] Recent series have reported operative survival of 90% or higher following valvotomy in patients with critical aortic stenosis in the absence of hypoplastic left heart (HLH) syndrome.[15] However, valvotomy should be considered a palliative procedure, as most patients

E

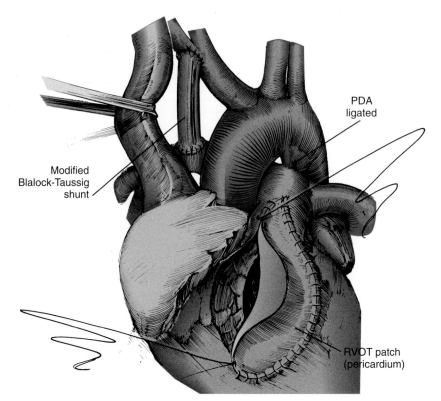

Figure 23-4 Placement of a transannular patch to enlarge the right ventricular outflow tract. The modified Blalock-Taussig shunt is also shown. PDA, patent ductus arteriosus; RVOT, right ventricular outflow tract. (From Castaneda A, Jonas RA, Mayer JE, et al. Pulmonary atresia with intact ventricular septum. In: Cardiac surgery of the infant and neonate. Philadelphia: WB Saunders; 1994:235-247.)

will need reoperation or reintervention for aortic valve insufficiency, stenosis, or both.[17,18] At present, for neonates in whom the aortic valve is irreparably dysmorphic, the Ross procedure is most commonly performed, in which the patient's pulmonary valve is used as an "autograft" to replace the aortic valve, and a cadaveric homograft is placed into the right ventricular outflow tract to establish right ventricle to pulmonary artery continuity. Because the pulmonary homograft is of a limited size, with no growth potential, it may necessitate several reoperations for homograft exchange throughout the lifetime of the patient.

Coarctation of the Aorta

Coarctation refers to a narrowing of the descending aorta adjacent to the insertion of the ductus arteriosus (so-called juxtaductal) and may represent the effect of fetal development and abnormal flow dynamics, or the presence of "extraanatomic" ductal tissue, which narrows abnormally with ductal closure (Fig. 23-5). Coarctation often coexists with generalized hypoplasia of the entire transverse aortic arch, the presence of which mandates a more complicated arch reconstruction at the time of repair.

As with other obstructive lesions, the natural history of aortic coarctation depends upon the degree to which systemic perfusion is dependent on a patent ductus arteriosus. In patients who tolerate closure of the ductus, symptoms generally develop later as a consequence of the proximal systemic hypertension. These patients are at risk for a significant number of complications, but unoperated survival can extend into adulthood.

In contrast, patients with severe aortic coarctation may present in the first week of life with the onset of cardiovascular collapse at the time of ductal closure. In this

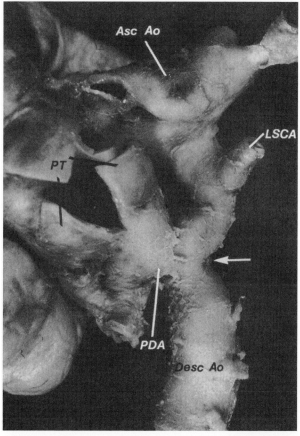

Figure 23-5 Autopsy specimen from a 6-week-old girl, showing juxtaductal coarctation by localized shelf with typical external deformity of the aorta at the site of narrowing. Asc Ao, ascending aorta; Desc Ao, descending aorta; LSCA, left subclavian artery; PDA, patent ductus arteriosus; PT, pulmonary trunk. (From Kouchoukos NT, Blackstone EH, Doty DB, et al. Cardiac surgery, 3rd ed. Philadelphia: Elsevier; 2003.)

population, collateral blood flow is insufficient to provide adequate perfusion to the abdominal organs and lower extremities, resulting in progressive organ ischemia and acidosis. Intravenous infusion of PGE_1 in these patients often maintains ductal patency, restoring perfusion of the lower body. In some cases, additional inotropic agents may be required to optimize perfusion and provide adequate resuscitation prior to operative repair.

Isolated coarctation of the aorta may be repaired through a left posterior-lateral thoracotomy, and involves mobilization of the descending aorta, resection of the coarctation segment, and end-to-end anastomosis. Because of problems with recurrence noted early in the history of this repair, currently a so-called extended end-to-end anastomosis (Fig. 23-6) is more commonly performed. Here, the proximal descending aortic segment is spatulated and anastomosed proximally to the underside of the mid-transverse aortic arch in an effort to remove all the abnormal ductal tissue thought to be a major contributor to recurrence.

For those neonates in whom the transverse aortic arch is also severely hypoplastic, the repair must be performed via median sternotomy using cardiopulmonary bypass. In particular, this aortic arch reconstruction and coarctation repair may require deep hypothermic circulatory arrest, in which the infants are cooled to 18°C and the circulation is discontinued for the duration of repair, or, alternatively, low-flow bypass with regional perfusion. Depending upon the degree and location of the hypoplastic transverse aortic arch, this reconstruction may or may not require

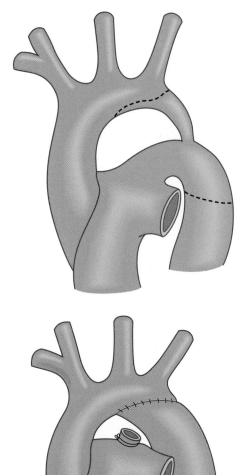

E

Figure 23-6 Extended resection and end-to-end anastomosis. Key technical points: (1) beveled anastomosis, brought up under the transverse arch; (2) extended as far proximally as deemed necessary to achieve relief of stenosis; (3) no prosthetic material used; (4) if the arch hypoplasia extends proximal to the left carotid artery and would require clamping of the innominate artery then the repair is approached through a median sternotomy and deep hypothermic circulatory arrest is used; otherwise, the repair is performed through a lateral thoracotomy. (From Wright GE, Nowak CA, Goldberg CS, et al. Extended resection and end-to-end anastomosis for aortic coarctation in infants: results of a tailored surgical approach. Am Thorac Surg. 2005;80:1453-1459.)

exogenous tissue (generally autologous pericardium or homograft tissue) for arch augmentation.

Risks of the coarctation repair either via thoracotomy or median sternotomy include infection, bleeding, death (one to three percent nationally), damage to the recurrent laryngeal nerve (which surrounds the ductus arteriosus and aorta) or the thoracic duct (less commonly), and paralysis (from spinal ischemia) during the time of aortic occlusion for the anastomosis. The latter complication is exceedingly rare. In all neonates undergoing coarctation repair there is a 5-15% likelihood of late recurrence requiring balloon dilatation.

Interrupted Aortic Arch

A condition similar to severe aortic coarctation is interrupted aortic arch, in which there is no continuity between the transverse and descending aorta; this may occur at different locations along the transverse aortic arch. The preferred surgical procedure is direct arch reconstruction and anastomosis, involving ligation and resection of the ductus arteriosus. Operative mortality from this procedure is low, and long-term mortality appears to be similarly low.[19-21] Because of the important association with DiGeorge syndrome, vigilance in the perioperative period and beyond for hypocalcemia or susceptibility to infection, or both, is important. Over the long term, approximately 20-30% of patients will require reintervention for left heart obstructive lesions, which may range from subaortic resection to more extensive procedures designed to expand the left ventricular outflow tract.[19,22]

Hypoplastic Left Heart Syndrome

Hypoplastic left heart syndrome (HLHS) consists of a range of congenital defects of the left ventricle, aorta, and associated valves, all resulting in a right ventricular-dependent systemic circulation (Fig. 23-7). In its most severe forms, HLHS exists in the context of critical aortic stenosis: left ventricular cardiac output is minimal or absent, and the entire arch and coronary vessels are perfused retrograde via the ductus arteriosus.

HLHS is invariably fatal without surgical repair, and before the 1980s, most infants would expire within the first month. In the modern era, after diagnosis of HLHS three options are available: the staged Norwood reconstruction, the staged hybrid approach, and cardiac transplantation. Transplantation has the advantage of restoring normal circulatory physiology, but the limited number of donor organs available precludes its use in all patients and represents a therapeutic strategy that is epidemiologically nonviable. In contrast, staged reconstruction requires multiple operations (usually three) and results in Fontan circulation, with the pulmonary and systemic circulations in series. Although perioperative survival following the Norwood procedure has improved, 1-year survival after stage I repair remains unsatisfactory. In the recently published Single Ventricle Reconstruction (SVR) Trial article,[23] transplantation-free survival 12 months after randomization was in the order of 70%.[24,25] Early postoperative survival after cardiac transplantation often approaches 90%; however, the complexities and outcomes of transplantation in the neonatal period are variable (and are discussed in a subsequent chapter).[26,27]

The Norwood reconstruction involves (1) augmentation of the hypoplastic aortic arch; (2) the creation of a common arterial outflow from the heart; (3) an atrial septectomy; and (4) the establishment of controlled pulmonary blood flow with either a modified BT shunt, or a so-called Sano RV-PA connection with a Gore-tex tube (Fig. 23-8). Specific technical difficulties of the procedure involve accurate arch reconstruction without twisting or kinking (with a native aorta that can be as small as 1-2 mm), residual distal arch obstruction, shunt-related problems, and, in the case of Sano patients, progressive stenosis at the distal pulmonary artery anastomosis requiring early advancement to the cavopulmonary shunt procedure. Both the RV-PA conduit and the modified BT shunt are acceptable options in the Norwood reconstruction. The SVR trial showed that although there was an early survival advantage for the RV-PA shunt patients, (transplantation-free survival 12 months after randomization was higher with the right ventricular to pulmonary artery shunt than with the modified BT shunt [74% vs. 64%, $P = .01$]), this survival benefit disappears over time with an increased need for heart transplantation for the RV-PA shunt patients.

Because HLHS includes a range of anatomical defects, attempts at improving outcomes with staged reconstruction have focused on improved patient selection and perioperative management based on preoperative anatomical and physiological factors predictive of poor outcomes after repair. Such research has identified several factors, which increase the risk to children undergoing the Norwood procedure. Patients aged more than 1 month have poor outcomes compared with those undergoing operation in the neonatal period.[25,28] Patients with increased pulmonary venous return (PVR) are prone to lethal pulmonary vascular crises.[29] A variety of other risk factors have been identified for poor outcomes after stage I reconstruction.[14,25,26,30-37] However, potentially correctable surgical technical problems resulted in a significant proportion of stage I mortality in early studies, accounting for the improved survival in the most recent series.[32]

Cyanotic Heart Lesions

Transposition of the Great Arteries

Transposition of the great arteries (TGA) consists of a reversal of the normal anatomical position of the great vessels so that the aorta represents the outflow of the right

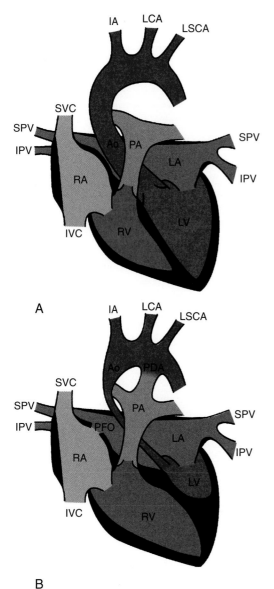

E

Figure 23-7 Schematic diagram of normal cardiac anatomy **(A)** and hypoplastic left heart (HLH) syndrome **(B).** Note the atretic aortic and hypoplastic left ventricle. Systemic blood flow is from the right ventricle through the patent ductus arteriosus into the aortic arch. Pulmonary venous return crosses from the left atrium to the right atrium through a patent foramen ovale. Ao, aorta; IA, innominate artery; IPV, inferior pulmonary vein; IVC, inferior vena cava; LA, left atrium; LCA, left carotid artery; LSCA, left subclavian artery; LV, left ventricle; PA, pulmonary artery; PDA, patent ductus arteriosus; PFO, patent foramen ovale; RA, right atrium; RV, right ventricle; SPV, superior pulmonary vein; SVC, superior vena cava.

ventricle and the pulmonary artery serves as the left ventricular outflow. This results in distinct and parallel systemic and pulmonary circulations connected through some form of obligate mixing between the circulations either via a VSD, a PDA, or, most often (and most effective), shunting through a patent foramen ovale (PFO). Patients with marginal systemic oxygenation and restrictive atrial communication may benefit from a bedside balloon atrial septostomy.

Depending on the degree of mixing and the associated cardiac anomalies, the degree of cyanosis in the neonate with TGA may vary widely. As with other congenital heart defects, initial medical management should be directed at optimizing acid-base, electrolyte, and oxygenation status. Early repair is advocated to enable development and growth of the cardiac chambers under the appropriate pressure loads: systemic pressure load on the left ventricle; pulmonary pressure load on the right ventricle. Prolonged "deconditioning" of the left ventricle may lead to muscular regression so that the left ventricle cannot support the systemic circulation and requires "training" before repair.

Figure 23-8 The Norwood reconstruction is shown using a modified Blalock-Taussig (BT) shunt **(A)** and the so-called Sano right ventricle-to-pulmonary artery connection **(B)**. Ao, aorta; IVC, inferior vena cava; LPA, left pulmonary artery; PA, pulmonary artery; PV, pulmonary veins; RV, right ventricle; SVC, superior vena cava; TV, tricuspid valve. (Reprinted from Griselli M, McGuirk SP, Stumper O, et al. Influence of surgical strategies on outcome after the Norwood procedure. J Thorac Cardiovasc Surg. 2006;131:418-426.)

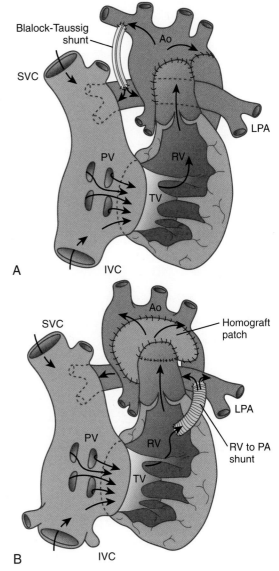

23

The procedure of choice in the current era is an arterial switch operation with concurrent coronary transfer (Fig. 23-9). In this operation, the great vessels are "switched" after the coronary arteries are implanted on the neoaorta, thus providing both an anatomical and physiological solution to the condition. Improvements in both operative technique and perioperative management have resulted in excellent short- and long-term outcomes with the arterial switch procedure.[38,39] Overall, 1-month, 1-year, and 5-year survival in patients undergoing arterial switch for TGA have been excellent, approaching 95% in most recent series.[40] Specific challenges to repair are generally related to anatomical variations of the coronary arteries, the geometric relationship of the great vessels and ventricles, and the integrity of the pulmonic (neoaortic) valve.

Total Anomalous Pulmonary Venous Connection

Disruption of any of the complex sequence of events in the development of the pulmonary venous system may result in significant abnormalities of pulmonary venous anatomy. Total anomalous pulmonary venous connection (TAPVC), also known as anomalous venous drainage or return, occurs when these abnormalities

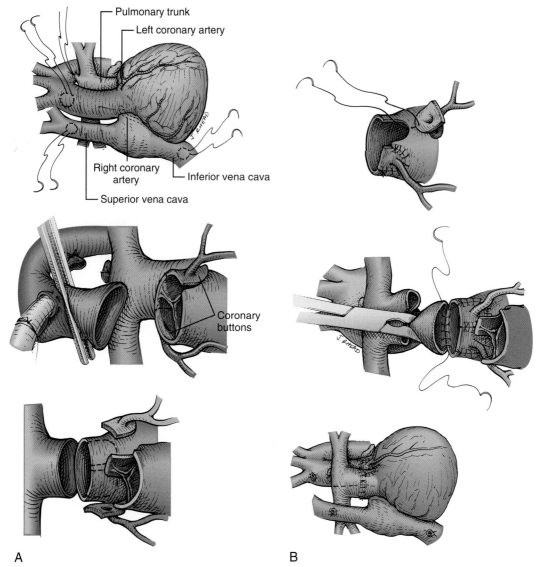

Figure 23-9   Arterial switch operation for transposition of the great arteries with the aorta anterior and rightward and usual coronary anatomy. (From Kouchoukos NT, Blackstone EH, Doty DB, et al. Cardiac surgery, 3rd ed. Philadelphia: Elsevier; 2003.)

result in return of oxygenated blood from the pulmonary circulation to the right side of the heart rather than the left atrium. An ASD or PFO is required in order for these infants to survive. The most common types of TAPVC include supracardiac connection with drainage into the left innominate vein, cardiac level connection to the coronary sinus, or infracardiac connection through the portal vein.

The clinical presentation of these patients is variable; many present with cyanosis, but the severity of the hemodynamic compromise depends not on the route of blood flow, but on the presence of other anomalies, the presence and severity of obstruction to pulmonary venous drainage, and the degree of obstruction across the atrial septum.[41] Patients without obstruction to pulmonary venous return and unrestricted atrial septal communication may develop symptoms during or after the neonatal period with progressive tachypnea, cyanosis, and right-sided heart failure caused by increased pulmonary blood flow and volume load on the right ventricle.

At the opposite end of the clinical spectrum are those patients with severe obstruction of PVR. These patients develop high pulmonary pressures early in the neonatal period in combination with elevated and labile pulmonary vascular resistance. Pulmonary edema combined with progressive decrease in pulmonary blood flow leads to severe hypoxemia and hemodynamic collapse. In these instances, extracorporeal membrane oxygenation (ECMO) or emergent intervention with surgery is often required.

Preoperative preparation of the neonate with TAPVC and pulmonary venous obstruction should be directed at resuscitation and expedited operative repair, and includes intubation with 100% oxygen, and inotropic support to assist the failing right ventricle. Inhaled nitric oxide should not be used in an attempt to augment systemic oxygen saturation, as this only provides for more pulmonary blood flow, thereby exacerbating pulmonary edema owing to the restriction to pulmonary venous drainage. Where these therapies are not successful, ECMO may be required in order to correct severe metabolic derangement prior to operative repair, often for as long as 48-72 hours.

Mortality without operative repair in TAPVC exceeds 80% at 1 year; therefore repair should be performed soon after diagnosis.[42] Patients without obstruction to pulmonary venous return may be managed with urgent rather than emergency surgery, but those with obstruction require either emergency surgery or rapid initiation of ECMO to support oxygenation and correct end-organ dysfunction prior to definitive repair.

Operative repair techniques vary depending on the anatomy of the venous connections, but all involve some connection of the pulmonary venous drainage into the left atrium and ligation of the anomalous connection ("vertical vein") to the systemic venous circulation. Usually, a single confluent vein drains all four anomalous pulmonary veins and this may be connected through as large an anastomosis as possible to the left atrium. More complex repairs may be required where anomalous pulmonary veins drain in pairs ("mixed"). Those infants with diffuse pulmonary venous atresia are generally considered inoperable. Recently, a so-called sutureless repair has been advocated for difficult cases, whereby no sutures are used on the veins themselves (hence the name), leaving the opened venous confluence to drain freely into a marsupialized left atrium and posterior pericardial well.[43]

Outcomes after repair are excellent, with operative mortality in the most recent series ranging from 5-9%.[44] Pulmonary hypertension in the immediate postoperative phase may require inhaled nitric oxide, and ECMO may be continued following surgical repair to maintain systemic oxygenation and allow for cardiac recovery. A subset of patients will require reoperation, often for pulmonary venous stenosis, which may occur in 6-11% of patients, most commonly those with infracardiac or mixed-type TAPVC. Long term, patients may be expected to grow normally with return of normal right ventricular function, resolution of right ventricular dilatation, and reversal of pulmonary vascular abnormalities.[44]

Mechanical Circulatory Support in the Neonate

Although mechanical circulatory support has been used with success in adults with cardiopulmonary heart failure, the extension of these successes to the neonatal population has been limited. Two factors in particular make mechanical support challenging in this population: small patient size requires devices designed specifically for a pediatric population, and congenital cardiac disease with abnormal anatomy (e.g., concurrent biventricular failure with or without pulmonary valvular issues) complicates the application of mechanical support. However, in patients with cardiac or pulmonary dysfunction refractory to maximal medical therapy, mechanical circulatory support may be beneficial in certain circumstances[45]:

- Preoperative stabilization before operative repair
- Postoperative support to allow for recovery of cardiac or pulmonary function, or both

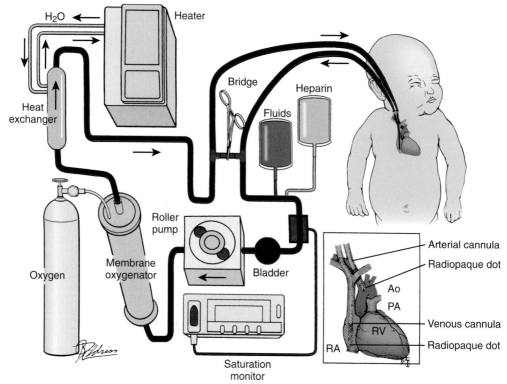

Figure 23-10 Extracorporeal membrane oxygenation (ECMO) uses venoarterial bypass with a membrane oxygenator. This technique allows both hemodynamic and pulmonary support. ECMO systems generally consist of a silicone membrane oxygenator, a heat exchanger, a bladder, and a roller pump. Ao, aorta; PA, pulmonary artery; RA, right atrium; RV, right ventricle. (From Jacobs JP. Pediatric mechanical circulatory support. In: Mavroudis C, Backler CL, eds. Pediatric cardiac surgery, 3rd ed. Philadelphia: Mosby; 2003:778-792.)

- Temporary support in patients not in need of cardiac repair whose cardiac or pulmonary function is expected to improve with time
- As a bridge to transplantation

Two forms of mechanical circulatory support are currently available to neonates: ECMO and ventricular assist device (VAD). Similar to cardiopulmonary bypass in the operating room, essentially, ECMO consists of venoarterial bypass with a membrane oxygenator (Fig. 23-10). In neonatal patients with respiratory failure, survival exceeds 80%.[46] Increasingly, ECMO has been used for postcardiotomy cardiopulmonary support in the pediatric cardiac surgical patient. However, in this application, survival in multicenter studies (of heterogeneous patient populations and indications) is only 32-44%, although some institutions have reported survival exceeding 50%.[45,47] Outcomes naturally vary depending upon the cardiac anatomy and the status of repair. Patients with biventricular physiology appear to have improved outcomes with ECMO when compared with those with single-ventricle physiology, and the management of aortopulmonary shunts (or patent ductus arteriosus) during ECMO remains controversial.[45]

Currently, few VAD options are available for neonates owing to their size constraints. Two devices have been used extensively in Europe for this indication, the MEDOS and Berlin Heart ventricular assist devices. The Berlin Heart (Berlin Heart AG) is a paracorporeal pulsatile, univentricular or biventricular assist device that is available across several different sizes of pumps (Fig. 23-11); for neonates, the 10-mL pumps are most often used. The pumps require inflow from the atrium (for right-sided assistance) or the ventricular apex (for left-sided support), as well as outflow (to either pulmonary artery, aorta, or both). Implantation requires cardiopulmonary bypass and often cardiac arrest. The cannulae for inflow and outflow exit the skin

Figure 23-11 **A,** The various pump sizes of the Berlin Heart EXCOR ventricular assist device. **B,** Correlation between patient size and pump size, based on the cardiac output delivered by each pump. (**A** and **B,** Courtesy of the Berlin Heart AG.)

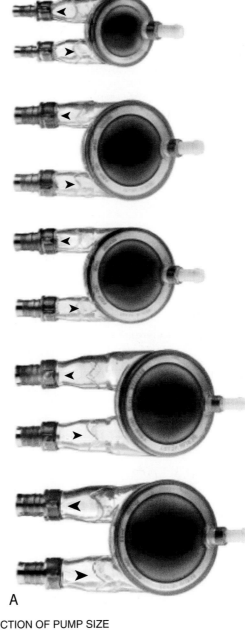

A

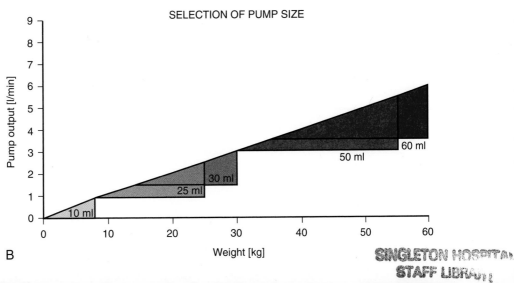

B

at the upper abdomen and are attached to two extracorporeal devices whose pumping mechanism is activated via pneumatic actuation from a separate console. The device requires systemic anticoagulation.

The device is currently allowed under a compassionate use protocol with the U.S. Food and Drug Administration. The time of device support is theoretically limitless; however, the ongoing risk of stroke or hemorrhage encourages weaning from device support (for reversible myocardial failure) or bridging to transplantation as soon as is physiologically possible. Several new devices are currently under development and investigation as part of an initiative by the National Heart, Lung and Blood Institute.

Conclusion

The 50 years since the inception of intracardiac repair of CHD have resulted in remarkable changes in operative techniques and the perioperative management of these patients. Consequently, the preferred age at definitive repair has steadily decreased, resulting in a parallel decrease in the need for palliative procedures in the neonatal period. The coming years should yield further advances, particularly with regard to the use of mechanical circulatory support in neonates, refinements in surgical repair techniques for both short-term outcomes and long-term durability, as well as the development of catheter-based solutions (isolated or in combination with open surgery) for early repair.

References

1. Lewis FJ, Taufic M. Closure of atrial septal defects with the aid of hypothermia: experimental accomplishments and the report of one successful case. Surgery. 1953;33:52-59.
2. Barrat-Boyes BG, Simpson M, Neutze JM. Intracardiac surgery in neonates and infants using deep hypothermia with surface cooling and limited cardiopulmonary bypass. Circulation. 1971;43:125-130.
3. Warden HE, Cohen M, Read RC, et al. Controlled cross circulation for open intracardiac surgery: physiologic studies and results of creation and closure of ventricular septal defects. J Thorac Surg. 1954;28:331-334, discussion 341-343.
4. Albus RA, Trusler GA, Izukawa T, et al. Pulmonary artery banding. J Thorac Cardiovasc Surg. 1984;88:645-653.
5. Blalock A, Taussig H. The surgical treatment of malformations of the heart in which there is pulmonary stenosis or pulmonary atresia. JAMA. 1984;251:2123-2138.
6. Petrucci O, O'Brien SM, Jacobs ML, et al. Risk factors for mortality and morbidity after the neonatal Blalock-Taussig shunt procedure. Ann Thorac Surg. 2011;92:642-651.
7. Davis P, Turner-Gomes S, Cunningham K, et al. Precision and accuracy of clinical and radiological signs in premature infants at risk of patent ductus arteriosus. Arch Pediatr Adolesc Med. 1995;149:1136-1141.
8. Gersony WM, Peckham GJ, Ellison RC, et al. Effects of indomethacin in premature infants with patent ductus arteriosus: results of a national collaborative study. J Pediatr. 1983;102:895-906.
9. Collett RW, Edwards JE. Persistent truncus arteriosus: a classification according to anatomic types. Surg Clin N Am. 1949;29:1245-1270.
10. Chen JM, Glickstein JS, Davis RR, et al. The effect of repair technique on postoperative right-sided obstruction in patients with truncus arteriosus. J Thorac Cardiovasc Surg. 2005;129:559-568.
11. Mavroudis C, Backer CL. Truncus arteriosus. In: Mavroudis C, Backler CL, eds. Pediatric cardiac surgery, 3rd ed. Philadelphia: Mosby; 2003:339-352.
12. Mitchell MB, Clarke DR. Isolated right ventricular outflow tract obstruction. In: Mavroudis C, Backler CL, eds. Pediatric cardiac surgery, 3rd ed. Philadelphia: Mosby; 2003:361-382.
13. Hanley FL, Sade RM, Freedom RM, et al. Outcomes in critically ill neonates with pulmonary stenosis and intact ventricular septum: a multiinstitutional study. Congenital Heart Surgeons Society. J Am Coll Cardiol. 1993;22:183-192.
14. Lofland GK, McCrindle BW, Williams WG, et al. Critical aortic stenosis in the neonate: a multi-institutional study of management outcomes, and risk factors. Congenital Heart Surgeons Society. J Thorac Cardiovasc Surg. 2001;121:10-27.
15. Tchervenkov CI, Chu VF, Shum-Tim D. Left ventricular outflow tract obstruction. In: Mavroudis C, Backler CL, eds. Pediatric cardiac surgery, 3rd ed. Philadelphia: Mosby; 2003:537-559.
16. Kohl T, Sharland G, Allan LD, et al. World experience of percutaneous ultrasound-guided balloon valvuloplasty in human fetuses with severe aortic value obstruction. Am J Cardiol. 2000;85:1230-1233.
17. Ettedgui JA, Tallman-Eddy T, Neches WH, et al. Long-term results of survivors of surgical valvotomy for severe aortic stenosis in early infancy. J Thorac Cardiovasc Surg. 1992;104:1714-1720.

18. Justo RN, McCrindle BW, Benson LN, et al. Aortic valve regurgitation after surgical versus percutaneous balloon valvotomy for congenital aortic valve stenosis. Am J Cardiol. 1996;77:1332-1338.
19. Jonas RA, Quaegebeur JM, Kirklin JW, et al. Outcomes in patients with interrupted aortic arch and ventricular septal defect. A multiinstitutional study. Congenital Heart Surgeons Society. J Thorac Cardiovasc Surg. 1994;107:1099-1113.
20. Sell JE, Jonas RA, Mayer JE, et al. The results of a surgical program for interrupted aortic arch. J Thorac Cardiovasc Surg. 1988;96:864-877.
21. Serraf A, Lacour-Gayet F, Robotin M, et al. Repair of interrupted aortic arch: a ten-year experience. J Thorac Cardiovasc Surg. 1996;112:1150-1160.
22. Jonas RA. Interrupted aortic arch. In: Mavroudis C, Backler CL, eds. Pediatric cardiac surgery, 3rd ed. Philadelphia: Mosby; 2003:273-282.
23. Ohye RG, Sleeper LA, Mahony L. Comparison of shunt types in the Norwood procedure for single-ventricle lesions. N Engl J Med. 2010;362:1980-1992.
24. Checcia PA, Larsen R, Sehra R, et al. Effect of a selection and postoperative care protocol on survival of infants with hypoplastic left heart syndrome. Ann Thorac Surg. 2004;77:477-483.
25. Mahle WT, Spray TL, Wernovsky G, et al. Survival after reconstructive surgery for hypoplastic left heart syndrome: a 15-year experience from a single institution. Circulation. 2001;102:136-141.
26. Bando K, Turrentine MW, Sun K, et al. Surgical management of hypoplastic left heart syndrome. Ann Thorac Surg. 1996;62:70-76.
27. Jenkins PC, Flanagan MF, Jenkins KJ, et al. Survival analysis and risk factors for mortality in transplantation and staged surgery for hypoplastic left heart syndrome. J Am Coll Cardiol. 2000;36:1178-1185.
28. Griselli M, McGuirk SP, Stumper O, et al. Influence of surgical strategies on outcome after the Norwood procedure. J Thorac Cardiovasc Surg. 2006;131:418-426.
29. Duncan BW, Rosenthal GL, Jones TK, et al. First-stage palliation of complex univentricular cardiac anomalies in older infants. Ann Thorac Surg. 2001;72:2077-2080.
30. Iannettoni MD, Bove EL, Mosca RS, et al. Improving results with first-stage palliation for hypoplastic left heart syndrome. J Thorac Cardiovasc Surg. 1994;107:934-940.
31. Andrews R, Tulloh R, Sharland G, et al. Outcome of staged reconstructive surgery for hypoplastic left heart syndrome following antenatal diagnosis. Arch Dis Child. 2001;85:474-477.
32. Bartram U, Grunenfelder J, Van Praagh R. Causes of death after the modified Norwood procedure: a study of 122 postmortem cases. Ann Thorac Surg. 1997;64:1795-1802.
33. Bove EL, Lloyd TR. Staged reconstruction for hypoplastic left heart syndrome. Contemporary results. Ann Surg. 1996;224:387-395.
34. Forbess JM, Cook N, Roth SJ, et al. Ten-year institutional experience with palliative surgery for hypoplastic left heart syndrome. Risk factors related to stage I mortality. Circulation. 1995;92:262-266.
35. Graziano JN, Heidelberger KP, Ensing GJ, et al. The influence of a restrictive atrial septal defect on pulmonary vascular morphology in patients with hypoplastic left heart syndrome. Pediatr Cardiol. 2002;23:146-151.
36. Jenkins PC, Flanagan MF, Sargent JD, et al. A comparison of treatment strategies for hypoplastic left heart syndrome using decision analysis. J Am Coll Cardiol. 2001;38:1181-1187.
37. Chang RK, Chen AY, Klitzner TS. Clinical management of infants with hypoplastic left heart syndrome in the United States, 1988-1997. Pediatrics. 2002;110:292-298.
38. Backer CL, Ilbawi MN, Ohtake S, et al. Transposition of the great arteries: a comparison of the results of the mustard procedure versus the arterial switch. Ann Thorac Surg. 1989;48:10-14.
39. Laks H. The arterial switch procedure for the neonate: coming of age. Ann Thorac Surg. 1989;48:3-4.
40. Kirklin JW, Blackstone EH, Tchervenkov CI, et al. Clinical outcomes after the arterial switch operation for transposition. Patient, support, procedure, and institutional risk factors. Congenital Heart Surgeons Society. Circulation. 1992;86:1501-1515.
41. Yee ES, Turley K, Hsieh WR, Ebert PA. Infant total anomalous pulmonary venous connection: factors influencing timing of presentation and operative outcome. Circulation. 1987;76:83-87.
42. Burroughs JT, Edwards JE. Total anomalous pulmonary venous connection. Am Heart J. 1960;59:913-931.
43. Yanagawa B, Alghamdi AA, Dragulescu A. Primary sutureless repair for "simple" total anomalous pulmonary venous connection: midterm results in a single institution. J Thorac Cardiovasc Surg. 2011;141:1346-1354.
44. Kirschbolm PM, Jaggers J, Ungerleider R. Total anomalous pulmonary venous connection. In: Mavroudis C, Backler CL, eds. Pediatric cardiac surgery, 3rd ed. Philadelphia: Mosby; 2003:612-624.
45. Jacobs JP. Pediatric mechanical circulatory support. In: Mavroudis C, Backler CL, eds. Pediatric cardiac surgery, 3rd ed. Philadelphia: Mosby; 2003:778-792.
46. Ichiba S, Bartlett RH. Current status of extracorporeal membrane oxygenation for severe respiratory failure. Artif Organs. 1996;20:120-123.
47. Walters HL, Hakimi M, Rice MD, et al. Pediatric cardiac surgical ECMO: multivariate analysis of risk factors for hospital death. Ann Thorac Surg. 1954;60:329-336.

CHAPTER 24

Regional Blood Flow Monitoring in the Perioperative Period

George M. Hoffman, MD, and James S. Tweddell, MD

Neonates with significant congenital cardiac disease experience multiple threats to adequate cellular oxygen delivery, before, during, and after corrective or palliative surgery, with or without deliberate intraoperative alteration of blood flow required to complete the surgical procedure. Factors that can reduce whole-body systemic oxygen delivery include pulmonary systemic flow tradeoff that can occur in all neonates with ductal patency and which may be exaggerated with pharmacological maintenance of ductal patency beyond the first few days of life; inefficiency of unpalliated or partially corrected cardiac anatomy; functional myocardial limitation following hypoxia-ischemia; anemia; and altered hemoglobin-oxygen transport function from stored blood. Increased metabolic demand for oxygen can result from inefficient cardiac anatomy, inotropic support, pain, cold stress, respiratory disease, wound healing, infection, and the inflammatory state that often is exaggerated following surgery and cardiopulmonary bypass in neonates. Even when whole-body supply-demand relationships appear adequate, regional, organ-specific supply-demand relationships can be impaired. The increasing use of organ-specific regional blood flow monitoring can open a window on these vulnerabilities and guide interventions to maintain adequate organ blood flow and oxygenation, with evidence for improved function. This chapter reviews the use of regional blood flow monitoring, primarily via near-infrared spectroscopy (NIRS), related to management of neonates in the perioperative period.

Historical Perspective and Technologic Development

Organ-specific oxygen monitoring with NIRS in cardiac surgery became practical less that 2 decades ago with the development of reflectance devices that could estimate the ratio of oxygenated to total hemoglobin in the monitored tissue field, without reliance on complex calibration procedures necessary to derive absolute concentrations.[1] While reports of relationships of cerebral desaturation to neurological outcomes came early in adults and children, the lack of standardized technology limited generalization of these findings.[2,3] A large study showing a positive outcome impact of interventions to improve cerebral oxygenation based on multimodal neurological monitoring with NIRS, transcranial Doppler, and electroencephalography highlighted the potential to improve neurological outcomes in infants and children undergoing cardiac surgery.[4] The commercial availability of versatile NIRS devices (Somanetics 3100A through 5100C), opened the door to more widespread adoption of the technology, such that use of NIRS in the perioperative care of neonates and children undergoing cardiac surgery is the standard at many centers worldwide.[4-10] Devices with a 4-cm source-detector distance can monitor organ-specific oxygenation or brain, kidney, and mesentery particularly well in small subjects, thus being specially suited to monitoring regional circulation in neonates and infants.[11]

While the brain was the organ or interest driving development of clinical NIRS technology with devices offering two probes for bilateral cerebral monitoring, the clinical scope of monitoring has more recently been broadened to noncerebral, somatic fields including skeletal muscle, renal (flank region), and mesenteric (anterior abdominal wall) regions.[11] The utility of simultaneous multiple-site monitoring has been highlighted in reports of cerebral and somatic monitoring during selective perfusion of the cerebral bed in lieu of total circulatory arrest during profound hypothermia for complex neonatal arch reconstructions and during repair of aortic coarctation.[12-15] These descriptive studies revealed not only distinct patterns of regional oxygenation evident during selective perfusion of different regional beds in the intraoperative management sequence, but also the feasibility of a noninvasive device to function as a continuous monitor of organ blood flow and circulatory physiology. Although much of the published material is physiologically mechanistic or descriptive, increasing evidence reveals a relationship of both cerebral and somatic oxygenation to various outcomes.[8,10,16,17]

Descriptive Physiology of Multiple Site Near-Infrared Spectroscopy

The organ specificity of multiple regional NIRS monitoring sites has been described by vascular cannulation and occlusion procedures in piglet models and human neonates and infants, with good evidence that a large portion of the signal is organ-specific, especially in infants weighing less than 10 kg.[11,18-20] By comparing the change in regional rSO_2 during isolated renal or mesenteric artery occlusion with the change during global ischemia (cardiac arrest), we estimated that renal and mesenteric contributions to the optical rSO_2 signal were 51% and 65%, respectively, thus validating the organ-specificity of regional measures.[18] The observed changes in organ oxygenation during global ischemia were related to the described flow-metabolism ratios of organs in the resting anesthetized animal, with the most rapid desaturation occurring in the cerebral bed (Fig. 24-1).[19] These normothermic desaturation kinetics recapitulate the relative sensitivities of brain, intestine, and kidney to ischemia, and their contributions to long-term morbidity in the critically ill infant.

In normal newborns over the first 5 days of life, the average cerebral rSO_2 was 78% and average renal rSO_2 was 87%.[21] The cerebral and particularly somatic-renal rSO_2 show high short-term variability as dynamic measures, reflecting changes in blood flow related to activity, blood oxygen and carbon dioxide levels, and sympathetic tone (Fig. 24-2). The difference between somatic-renal and cerebral rSO_2 in this normal population was 9%, an index of the relative distribution of blood flow between cerebral and somatic beds. The renal rSO_2 exceeded the cerebral rSO_2 in 24 of 25 of these normal neonates, reflecting the relatively high blood flow to metabolism ratio in the kidney that renders it susceptible to injury when sympathetic tone is high.

This pattern of regional oxygenation was altered in neonates with hypoplastic left heart syndrome (HLHS), both before and after stage 1 palliation (S1P).[22,23] In unpalliated neonates maintained on prostaglandin infusion, a wide arterioregional difference across the renal bed (average 24%) provided evidence of somatic hypoperfusion and a goal for management.[22] Both the somatic and cerebral

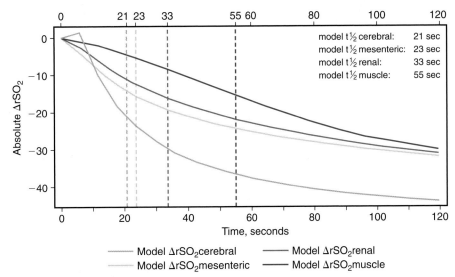

Figure 24-1 NIRS-derived desaturation curves from cerebral, mesenteric, renal, and skeletal muscle beds in isoflurane-anesthetized neonatal piglets during conditions of normothermic global ischemia induced by acute cardiac arrest. Data are expressed as the absolute change in regional saturation (rSO_2) from baseline, showing differential regional oxygen consumption across tissues. Cerebral tissue has the highest resting oxygen consumption and the most rapid desaturation. (From Hoffman GM, Wider MD. Changes in regional oxygenation by NIRS during global ischemia in piglets. Anesthesiology 2008;109:A1512, with permission.)

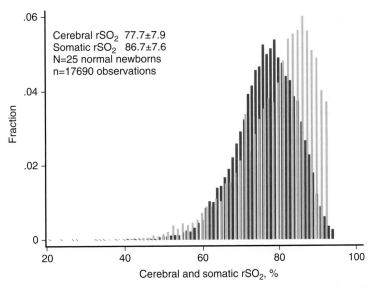

Figure 24-2 Cerebral and somatic (renal) regional saturation (rSO_2) measures from 25 normal newborns over the first 5 days of life. Individual measures were obtained at 10-second intervals over a 5-hour period that included resting and feeding. The cerebral extraction was 20%, and the somatic was 11%, with an average somatic-cerebral rSO_2 difference of 9%. Although highly dynamic in the short term, the pattern of average somatic rSO_2 exceeding average cerebral rSO_2 was observed in 24/25 neonates, and there were no consistent or important changes in either measure in the transition from resting to feeding. (From Bernal N, Hoffman G, Ghanayem N, Arca M. Cerebral and somatic near-infrared spectroscopy in normal newborns. J Pediatr Surg 2010;45:1306-1310, with permission.)

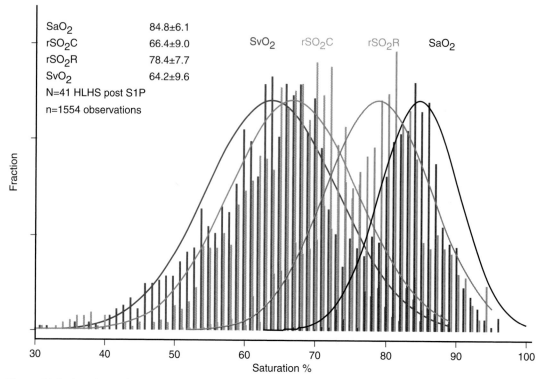

Figure 24-3 Invasive and noninvasive measures of systemic and regional oxygenation in neonates following stage one palliation of hypoplastic left heart syndrome while supported with mechanical ventilation and inotropic support. Although the arterial blood is desaturated, the relative profile of arterial, somatic, and cerebral saturations is close to that observed in normal newborns, with cerebral extraction of 18% and somatic extraction of 12%. (From Hoffman GM, Ghanayem NS, Stuth EA, et al. NIRS-derived somatic and cerebral saturation difference provides non-invasive real-time hemodynamic assessment of cardiogenic shock and risk of anaerobic metabolism. Anesthesiology 2004;99:A1448, with permission.)

arterioregional differences normalized after palliation, when the neonates were managed with inotropic and vasoactive agents targeting an SvO_2 greater than 50%, as previously described and with excellent outcome.[24] The pattern of arterial-cerebral, and arterial-somatic saturation differences, which are inversely proportional to regional blood flow, are remarkably similar in normal newborns and in our postoperative S1P population (Fig. 24-3). The observed regional oxygenation profile in normal newborns and in preoperative and postoperative HLHS are summarized in Table 24-1.

Goal-Directed Global Hemodynamic Management with Multisite Near-Infrared Spectroscopy

Evidence is strong for improved outcome in evolving shock states in adults and children by incorporation of global oxygen balance measures such as quasi-mixed venous saturation (SvO_2).[25,26] Because NIRS measures of hemoglobin saturation (rSO_2) are close to the regional venous saturation, a relationship between rSO_2 and SvO_2 is expected. Several studies have revealed that, under certain conditions, the cerebral rSO_2 and SvO_2 from the superior venal cava are correlated, since the cerebral venous drainage is the dominant contributor to SVC flow in the resting state.[27,28] Likewise, Doppler studies of the SVC are correlated with cerebral rSO_2.[29] However, the mixed SvO_2 is a flow-weighted average of all regional venous saturations, and thus multisite NIRS monitoring might reveal a more reliable indicator of changes in SvO_2. We found that a linear combination of cerebral and somatic rSO_2 best fit the changes in SvO_2 in the acute perioperative period (Fig. 24-4).[8,10,30]

Table 24-1 PROFILE OF ARTERIAL, VENOUS, AND REGIONAL NIRS (CEREBRAL AND SOMATIC) SATURATIONS IN NORMAL NEWBORNS AND NEONATES WITH HLHS

Regional oxygenation by pulse oximetry (SaO2), cerebral (rSO_2C) and renal somatic (rSO_2R) NIRS in normal newborns,[21] and patients with hypoplastic left heart syndrome before and after stage 1 palliation.[22,23] Derived parameters are somatic-cerebral rSO_2 difference (ΔrSO_2RC), arterial-cerebral difference ($\Delta arSO_2C$), and arterial-somatic difference ($\Delta a\ rSO_2R$). Somatic hypoperfusion is evident before palliation by a wide $\Delta arSO_2R$ and a narrow ΔrSO_2RC. Although the SaO_2 and regional rSO_2 after palliation is lower than normal newborns, the regional blood flow parameters are normalized.

Parameter	Normal (N = 25, n = 17690)	HLHS Pre-S1Pp (N = 47, n = 1831)	HLHS Post-S1P (N = 41, n = 1554)
SaO_2	98 ± 4	92.3 ± 5.4*	84.8 ± 6.1*
rSO_2C	77.7 ± 7.9	66.8 ± 8.5*	66.4 ± 9.0*
rSO_2R	86.7 ± 7.6	68.4 ± 8.8*	78.4 ± 7.7*
ΔrSO_2RC	9.0 ± 8.9	1.6 ± 9.4*#	11.9 ± 9.4
$\Delta arSO_2C$	20.3 ± 7.9	25.1 ± 9.0	18.2 ± 8.6
$\Delta arSO_2R$	11.2 ± 7.6	23.5 ± 9.1*#	6.3 ± 7.3
SvO_2			64.2 ± 9.6

*Different from normal neonates.
#Different from post-S1P.
HLHS, hypoplastic left heart syndrome; NIRS, near-infrared spectroscopy.

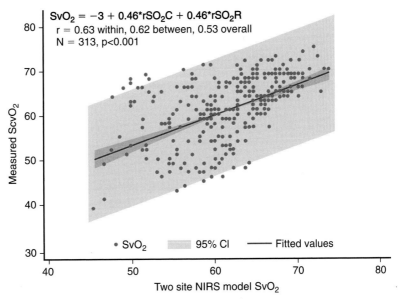

$$SvO_2 = -3 + 0.46*rSO_2C + 0.46*rSO_2R$$
r = 0.63 within, 0.62 between, 0.53 overall
N = 313, p<0.001

• SvO₂   95% CI   —— Fitted values

Measured ScvO₂ (y-axis)   Two site NIRS model SvO₂ (x-axis)

Figure 24-4 The risk of development of biochemical shock, defined by falling base excess of more than −4 mEq/L/hr, is highly related to somatic hypoperfusion as measured by the difference between somatic and cerebral rSO_2 in neonates following stage 1 palliation of hypoplastic left heart syndrome. The somatic-cerebral difference was a more reliable predictor of shock than the somatic measure alone; see text for details. (Adapted from Hoffman GM, Ghanayem NS, Mussatto KA, Berens RJ, Tweddell JS. Postoperative two-site NIRS predicts complications and mortality after stage 1 palliation of HLHS. Anesthesiology 2007;107:A234, with permission.)

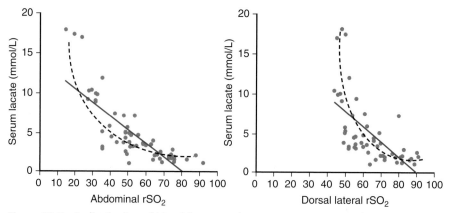

Figure 24-5   Redistribution of blood flow away from somatic regions results in a narrowing of the difference between somatic and cerebral rSO_2. This regional saturation pattern is predictive not only of biochemical shock, but of multiple organ dysfunction and death in neonates following stage 1 palliation of hypoplastic left heart syndrome. (From Hoffman GM, Ghanayem NS, Mussatto KA, Berens RJ, Tweddell JS. Postoperative two-site NIRS predicts complications and mortality after stage 1 palliation of HLHS. Anesthesiology 2007;107:A234, with permission.)

Monitoring multiple-site regional NIRS rSO_2 permits rapid, continuous, and noninvasive estimation of SvO_2, an indicator of whole-body oxygen economy that is consistently related to development of shock, and targeting of which can improve outcome.[24,31,32] This multiple-site NIRS approach can provide a similar predictor of biochemical shock as SvO_2. In the acute postoperative period following neonatal and infant cardiac repairs, somatic NIRS rSO_2, both from the anterior abdominal (mesenteric) and dorsolateral (renal) regions, was highly related to blood lactate levels.[33] Although those authors performed a linear fit between rSO_2 and biochemical indication of shock, the data observed have a curvilinear shape or breakpoint (Fig. 24-5). We found a similar relationship between renal-somatic rSO_2R and biochemical shock following stage 1 palliation of hypoplastic left heart syndrome, but a stronger, nonlinear relationship for the somatic-cerebral rSO_2 difference, ΔrSO_2RC (Fig. 24-6). This relationship indicates that the risk of biochemical shock in the early postoperative period rises as the renal-somatic bed becomes less well perfused compared to the brain, indicated by a fall in the ΔrSO_2RC from the normal value of about 10%. We postulate that contributions from arterial saturation and some patient-specific optical properties affecting NIRS rSO_2 are reduced when the difference between two sites is derived and that the altered somatic hypoperfusion that most frequently accompanies low cardiac output states is thus more accurately detected by signals that compare relative blood flow/metabolism relationships in different tissue regions. In a high-risk population of neonates following single ventricle palliation, the risk of biochemical shock, multiple organ dysfunction, and mortality were each related to reduction in the somatic-cerebral rSO_2 difference (Fig. 24-7).[34] The utility of cerebral and somatic NIRS to provide rapid, continuous, noninvasive hemodynamic assessment has been recommended as useful in the critically ill single ventricle infant at high risk for, or being resuscitated from, shock.[10,35,36]

Patients undergo a range of physiological stressors in the intraoperative period, including agitation and anxiety; drug-induced alterations in myocardial performance, vascular tone, and autonomic balance; changes in venous return with blood loss, positive pressure ventilation, positioning, and table tilting; changes in autonomic tone with surgical stimulation; direct manipulation of the lungs, heart, and blood vessels; interruption of blood flow by clamping the aorta to exclude the lower body during coarctation repair or the heart during procedures on cardiopulmonary bypass (CPB); and cardiac arrest either induced deliberately during deep hypothermic conditions (DHCA) or an unintended consequence of the convergence of the

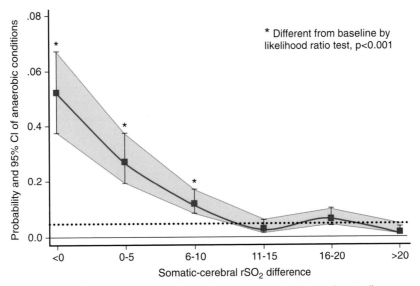

Figure 24-6 Simultaneous measures of cerebral and somatic rSO$_2$, and optically measured saturation from the superior vena cava, in neonates following stage one palliation of hypoplastic left heart syndrome. A linear combination of both cerebral and renal rSO$_2$ best fit the SvO2, with approximately equal weighting of cerebral and somatic sites. (Adapted from Hoffman GM, Ghanayem NS, Tweddell JS. Noninvasive assessment of cardiac output. Semin Thorac Cardiovasc Surg Pediatr Card Surg Annu 2005:12-21, with permission.)

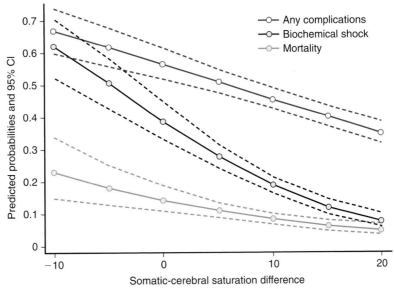

Figure 24-7 Relationship between somatic NIRS from the anterior abdominal wall (mesenteric) and flank (renal) and biochemical shock defined by blood lactate concentration in neonates and infants following one and two ventricle repairs. Although a linear relationship was depicted in the original publication, the data readily fit a curvilinear relationship with evidence for a threshold effect. (Modified from . Kaufman J, Almodovar MC, Zuk J, Friesen RH. Correlation of abdominal site near-infrared spectroscopy with gastric tonometry in infants following surgery for congenital heart disease. Pediatr Crit Care Med 2008;9:62-68, with permission.)

preceding factors. Although surgical procedures requiring anesthesia have relatively minor changes in standard parameters such as arterial saturation and blood pressure, blood pressure may be maintained at the expense of blood flow when autonomic activation or exogenous vasoactive drugs cause an increase in systemic vascular resistance and when intraoperative normalization of standard parameters does not adequately prevent complications.[37] The use of venous oximetric indicators, either directly by SvO_2 or indirectly by NIRS, provides a window on circulation by the continuous use of the Fick principle to estimate regional and whole-body blood flow/metabolism ratios. A basic premise of our perioperative strategy that has resulted in unsurpassed outcomes in complex neonatal surgery is that intraoperative hemodynamics are not spared from the requirement for goal-directed targets, such that all cardiac patients, and all neonates undergoing surgery, have NIRS monitoring to drive goal-directed approaches.[24,38]

Perioperative Cerebral Oxygenation and Function

Despite the induction of profound hypothermia to reduce metabolism, prolonged cardiac arrest during neonatal cardiac surgery is associated with higher likelihood of reduced neurodevelopmental performance.[39] A large body of literature is directed at characterizing the changes in cerebral oxygenation by NIRS during CPB, hypothermia, and DHCA to help identify risk conditions and drive treatment to improve outcome. Animal data clearly reveal a normothermic NIRS threshold for cerebral metabolism and cellular disruption that inflects sharply as cerebral oxygenation falls below 40%.[40] Cerebral injury following normothermic cerebral hypoxia to the 30-40% range by NIRS, shows a time-dose dependency that results in behavioral and histological abnormality when maintained for more than 1 hour.[41] The degree of hypothermia utilized on CPB may profoundly alter the relationship between cerebral saturation and injury, with competing effects on cerebral metabolism and oxygen availability, and the changes in pH, flow rate, and hemoglobin concentration introduce many interacting supply and demand side factors that threaten organ function.[42-45] In piglets undergoing CPB, NIRS could detect cerebral hypoxic conditions produced by alterations in cerebral blood flow, hemoglobin concentration, temperature, and pH management, and the degree of cerebral desaturation produced by combination of these conditions was directly related to cerebral injury, with a threshold near 55% at 26°C.[46-48]

During DHCA, the brain can continue to utilize oxygen that is present in stagnant blood in capillaries to meet metabolic demand. The rate of hemoglobin desaturation during DHCA will thus be related to continued utilization oxygen, and a reduction in the rate of desaturation would thus signal a decrease in brain oxygen uptake. Although an absolute rSO_2 threshold for injury during DHCA has not been identified, the duration of DHCA beyond the point at which oxygen uptake falls, a point termed the *nadir* even though it is not the lowest point, is highly related to injury.[47,49] Once the nadir has been identified by NIRS, preparations to reperfuse the brain can be planned to avoid conditions likely to cause injury.[50]

Curiously, the initial findings by Kurth and Austin of a relationship between intraoperative cerebral desaturation and postoperative neurological outcome have been difficult to characterize in more formal studies on humans.[3,4] Techniques for surgical repair, CPB, and physiological support have evolved over the past decade such that some of the conditions that can induce cerebral injury may have been reduced by programmatic, not patient-specific, strategies such as limitation of the duration of DHCA. However, evidence from the recent era again points to cerebral desaturation during normothermia immediately following CPB as a marker for, and potential cause of, cerebral injury, detected both by neuroimaging and neurodevelopmental testing during the second year of life.[16]

We had identified not only the period of DHCA but also the early postoperative period following it as a critical time for cerebral injury, showing a relationship between low superior vena cava SvO_2 in neonates and poor neurodevelopmental outcome at 4 years of age.[51] With hopes of reducing the occurrence of these bad

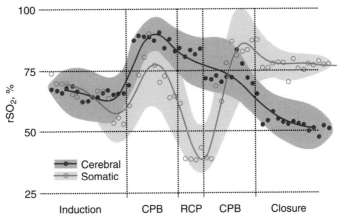

Figure 24-8   Cerebral and renal-somatic saturations (rSO$_2$) were measured during stage one palliation of hypoplastic left heart syndrome utilizing hypothermic cardiopulmonary bypass (CPB) and antegrade regional cerebral perfusion (RCP) for arch reconstruction. Cerebral rSO$_2$ was maintained during CPB and RCP, while somatic rSO$_2$ revealed the severe perfusion deficit during RCP. Following separation from cardiopulmonary bypass, cerebral rSO$_2$ was difficult to maintain above 50%. (From Hoffman GM, Stuth EA, Jaquiss RD, et al. Changes in cerebral and somatic oxygenation during stage 1 palliation of hypoplastic left heart syndrome using continuous regional cerebral perfusion. J Thorac Cardiovasc Surg 2004;127:223-233, with permission.)

outcomes, we avidly adopted a modified perfusion technique to avoid DHCA that had been demonstrated by Pigula and colleagues to maintain cerebral oxygenation at high levels by continuous direct perfusion of the innominate artery during repair of aortic arch abnormalities.[12] We profiled the changes in cerebral and somatic rSO$_2$ in neonates undergoing Norwood S1P for hypoplastic left heart syndrome utilizing this technique of hypothermic cardiopulmonary bypass and antegrade cerebral perfusion (Fig. 24-8).[14] Although cerebral rSO$_2$ was maintained above 80% by an average antegrade cerebral perfusion rate of 50 mL/minute, cerebral desaturation to less than 50% was disturbingly frequent in the post-CPB period. The physiological controls on cerebrovascular resistance appeared to be altered during the CPB period, with an increase in carbon dioxide reactivity but a decrease in pressure reactivity. These observations of altered hemodynamics and high risk of postoperative cerebral desaturation drove the utilization of NIRS in the postoperative period.

Following S1P, cerebral rSO$_2$ can remain low, showing little change in blood pressure over a normal range, moderate relationship to SaO$_2$, and stronger relationship to SvO$_2$ (Fig. 24-9).[6,50] This early postoperative cerebral desaturation occurs despite normalization of other hemodynamic parameters (Fig. 24-10).[52] We have preliminary work suggesting that prolonged profound hypothermia and pH-stat conditions, regardless of occurrence on CPB, antegrade perfusion, or DHCA, will alter cerebral autoregulation and vasoreactivity for many hours postoperatively, and that modification of pH conditions during antegrade perfusion might ameliorate this postoperative condition.[53] Prolonged cerebral desaturation following S1P for HLHS has been identified as a risk factor for both magnetic resonance imaging changes and reduced neurodevelopmental performance, with critical thresholds in the 45-55% range.[17,54]

Perioperative Somatic Oxygenation and Organ Function

The relationship between organ blood flow, oxygenation, function, and injury is complex, with disease-specific, pharmacologic, and autonomic influences, but hypoxic-ischemic injury remains a significant factor in renal and mesenteric injury in neonates.[8,34,55] Postoperative renal dysfunction, expressed as the ratio of current creatinine to the preoperative value, peaks on postoperative day 2 or 3. In the

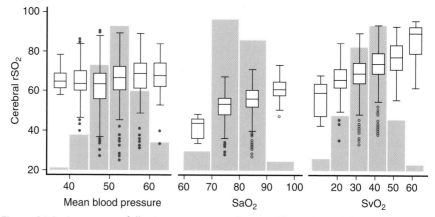

Figure 24-9 In neonates following stage one palliation of hypoplastic left heart syndrome, significant cerebral desaturation (less than 50%) occurred despite normal or acceptable levels of arterial saturation or blood pressure. Cerebral desaturation was frequent when SvO_2 was above 50%. (From Hoffman GM. Neurologic monitoring on cardiopulmonary bypass: what are we obligated to do? Ann Thorac Surg 2006;81:S2373-S2380, with permission.)

postoperative single-ventricle neonate, we found that renal-somatic rSO_2 on the first postoperative day to be the best predictor of the peak in creatinine rise on postoperative day 3 (Fig. 24-11).[56] In this patient population, with low systemic perfusion on the basis of myocardial dysfunction and aortopulmonary runoff, blood pressure had no relationship to the creatinine peak. In sepsis, there is evidence for both hypoperfusion and hyperperfusion as components of renal injury, and potentially protective renal vasodilatation is prostacyclin-dependent and impaired by indomethacin and related drugs.[57] Future studies might seek evidence for an optimal arterial-renal saturation function relationship, to help guide individual

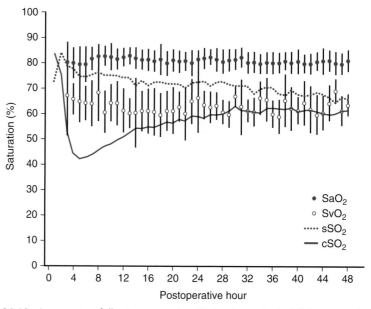

Figure 24-10 In neonates following stage 1 palliation hypoplastic left heart syndrome, an early postoperative period of cerebral desaturation was observed despite improving global hemodynamic measures, emphasizing the vulnerability of the cerebral circulation. (From Uebing A, Furck AK, Hansen JH, et al. Perioperative cerebral and somatic oxygenation in neonates with hypoplastic left heart syndrome or transposition of the great arteries. J Thorac Cardiovasc Surg 2011;142(3):523-530, with permission.)

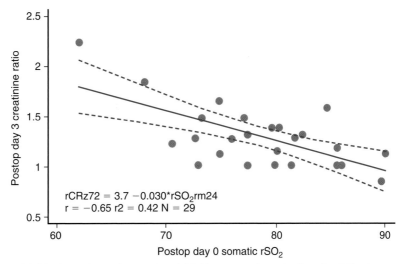

Figure 24-11 Somatic-renal saturation (rSO_2R) measured on the first day following stage 1 palliation of hypoplastic left heart syndrome was predictive of the peak creatinine observed 2 days later. (From Hoffman GM, Ghanayem NS, Mussatto KA, Musa N. Perioperative perfusion assessed by somatic NIRS predicts postoperative renal dysfunction. Anesthesiology 2005; 103:A1327, with permission.)

patient-specific vasoactive drug therapy to optimize renal function. Clinically, we do use a very low somatic extraction ratio as evidence for the need to increase systemic vascular resistance and a high extraction ratio as evidence for increasing cardiac output and reducing systemic vascular resistance.

Vascular resistance in the mesenteric vascular bed, as in the renal circulation, is under intense control by the sympathetic nervous system, and mesenteric ischemia is a source of potentially catastrophic injury in newborns. Animal data suggest that both mesenteric and renal circulations show similar responses to low cardiac output as monitored by NIRS, and the specific choice of somatic probe site is perhaps less important for monitoring global hemodynamics.[19] We observe frequent renal-somatic desaturation in newborns who have feeding difficulties, as distinct from normal newborns who do not demonstrate renal-somatic desaturation with feeding.[21] Placement of an NIRS probe on the lower anterior abdominal wall provides a window on the mesenteric circulation specifically and reveals an increased risk for necrotizing enterocolitis in premature infants and a close relationship to lactate and SvO_2 in the postcardiac surgical neonate.[33,58] In premature infants with large persistent patent ductus arteriosus (PDA), the mesenteric circulation may be at particular risk, and in this population the abdominal NIRS saturation was lower than in preterm infants without a large PDA.[59]

The distribution of blood flow between pulmonary (Qp) and systemic circulations (Qs) in the newborn with transitional circulation, large PDA, or complex congenital heart disease is dynamic. Just as the presence of a right-to-left shunt can be diagnosed by arterial desaturation, a left-to-right shunt can be detected by somatic desaturation. Modulation of pulmonary vascular resistance by manipulation of blood gas parameters is a frequent intervention strategy, but the arterial saturation alone is an inadequate determinant of Qp/Qs.[32] With estimation of SvO_2 by two-site NIRS, a continuous estimate of Qp/Qs can aid in the assessment and treatment of newborns with complex anatomy and physiology. Although pulmonary vascular resistance can be increased by hypoxic gas mixtures and hypercapnia, only the latter intervention increases systemic and cerebral oxygenation.[60,61]

While the effect of hypercapnia to evoke cerebral vasodilatation is well established, the effects on other aspects of regional perfusion are less clear. In single-ventricle neonates, with potential for carbon dioxide–induced changes in both Qp/

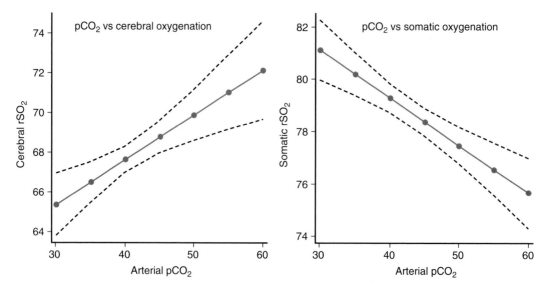

Figure 24-12 Changes in arterial carbon dioxide tension (pCO_2) can alter the distribution of regional vascular resistance and blood flow. In neonates following stage 1 palliation of hypoplastic left heart syndrome, an increase in pCO_2 causes an increase in cerebral blood flow and oxygenation, but this is mirrored by a reduction in renal-somatic blood flow and oxygenation. (From Hoffman GM, Ghanayem NS, Musa N, Mussatto KA, Berens RJ. Differential effects of carbon dioxide tension on cerebral and somatic oxygenation assessed by near infrared spectroscopy in postoperative neonates. Anesthesiology 2005;103:A1374, with permission.)

Qs and cerebrovascular resistance, we found evidence for a tradeoff of cerebral and renal circulation, such that hypercapnia resulted in a reduction in renal blood flow that mirrored the cerebral increase (Fig. 24-12).[62] Monitoring cerebral and somatic NIRS provides insight into potential changes in cardiac output distribution with changing ventilator strategy or other conditions that affect gas exchange.

Interstage and Home Monitoring

The "interstage" single ventricle patient, following S1P but before bidirectional Glenn, remains at substantial risk for mortality, due to shunt thrombosis and progressive systemic hypoperfusion. We continue regional NIRS monitoring for the duration of the cardiac neonatal intensive care unit stay, with improved outcome even in high-risk patients.[63] Patients who do not demonstrate severe or prolonged somatic desaturation during feeding, bathing, and physiological stress are transitioned to a less intense monitoring strategy for discharge to home. To enhance detection of physiological derangement before irreversible events after discharge, most high-risk patients are enrolled in a program of home monitoring that includes pulse oximetry when asleep and daily weight checks, resulting in nearly complete elimination of interstage mortality.[64] The interpretation of this monitoring information requires nuance and judgment, but the observations of poor weight gain or falling arterial saturation were indications for return appointment, with a high rate of subsequent intervention to improve hemodynamics (Fig. 24-13).

Conclusion

Our improved outcomes have paralleled the use of venous-side physiological measures of oxygen economy. Increasing evidence supports the validity of regional NIRS measures of oxygen saturation as estimates of organ-specific blood flow in the monitored field, with relationship to organ-specific and global hemodynamic state and outcomes. This information can also provide continuous diagnostic information in the cardiac neonate, with complex blood flow patterns, myocardial performance

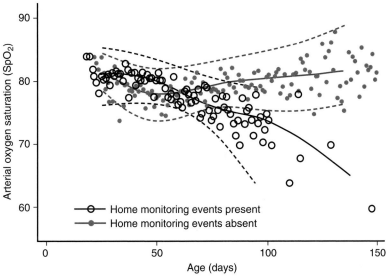

Figure 24-13 In infants with hypoplastic left heart syndrome enrolled in a program of home arterial saturation (SpO₂) monitoring, the finding of progressive reduction in SpO₂ identified patients likely to benefit from intervention, such that interstage death was virtually eliminated. (From Ghanayem NS, Hoffman GM, Mussatto KA, et al. Home surveillance program prevents interstage mortality after the Norwood procedure. J Thorac Cardiovasc Surg 2003;126:1367-1377, with permission.)

issues, and variable and bidirectional shunting. The venous-side information provided by NIRS is especially helpful during times of high-risk acute or complex physiological derangement, and its continuous noninvasive features will permit more longitudinal application in lieu of invasive monitoring.

References

1. Boushel R, Langberg H, Olesen J, et al. Monitoring tissue oxygen availability with near infrared spectroscopy (NIRS) in health and disease. Scand J Med Sci Sports. 2001;11:213-222.
2. Nollert G, Mohnle P, Tassani-Prell P, et al. Postoperative neuropsychological dysfunction and cerebral oxygenation during cardiac surgery. Thorac Cardiovasc Surg. 1995;43:260-264.
3. Kurth CD, Steven JM, Nicolson SC. Cerebral oxygenation during pediatric cardiac surgery using deep hypothermic circulatory arrest. Anesthesiology. 1995;82:74-82.
4. Austin EH 3rd, Edmonds HL Jr, Auden SM, et al. Benefit of neurophysiologic monitoring for pediatric cardiac surgery. J Thorac Cardiovasc Surg. 1997;114:707-717.
5. Andropoulos DB, Stayer SA, Diaz LK, et al. Neurological monitoring for congenital heart surgery. Anesth Analg. 2004;99:1365-1375.
6. Hoffman GM. Neurologic monitoring on cardiopulmonary bypass: what are we obligated to do? Ann Thorac Surg. 2006;81:S2373-S2380.
7. Wernovsky G, Ghanayem N, Ohye RG, et al. Hypoplastic left heart syndrome: consensus and controversies in 2007. Cardiol Young. 2007;17(Suppl 2):75-86.
8. Tweddell JS, Ghanayem NS, Hoffman GM. Pro: NIRS is "standard of care" for postoperative management. Semin Thorac Cardiovasc Surg Pediatr Card Surg Annu. 2010;13:44-50.
9. Hirsch JC, Charpie JR, Ohye RG, et al. Near infrared spectroscopy (NIRS) should not be standard of care for postoperative management. Semin Thorac Cardiovasc Surg Pediatr Card Surg Annu. 2010;13:51-54.
10. Ghanayem NS, Wernovsky G, Hoffman GM. Near-infrared spectroscopy as a hemodynamic monitor in critical illness. Pediatr Crit Care Med. 2011;12(Suppl 4):S27-S32.
11. Booth EA, Dukatz C, Ausman J, et al. Cerebral and somatic venous oximetry in adults and infants. Surg Neurol Int. 2010;1:75.
12. Pigula FA, Nemoto EM, Griffith BP, et al. Regional low-flow perfusion provides cerebral circulatory support during neonatal aortic arch reconstruction. J Thorac Cardiovasc Surg. 2000;119:331-339.
13. Pigula FA, Gandhi SK, Siewers RD, et al. Regional low-flow perfusion provides somatic circulatory support during neonatal aortic arch surgery. Ann Thorac Surg. 2001;72:401-407.
14. Hoffman GM, Stuth EA, Jaquiss RD, et al. Changes in cerebral and somatic oxygenation during stage 1 palliation of hypoplastic left heart syndrome using continuous regional cerebral perfusion. J Thorac Cardiovasc Surg. 2004;127:223-233.
15. Berens RJ, Stuth EA, Robertson FA, et al. Near infrared spectroscopy monitoring during pediatric aortic coarctation repair. Paediatr Anaesth. 2006;16:777-781.

16. Kussman BD, Wypij D, Laussen PC, et al. Relationship of intraoperative cerebral oxygen saturation to neurodevelopmental outcome and brain magnetic resonance imaging at 1 year of age in infants undergoing biventricular repair. Circulation. 2010;122:245-254.

17. Hoffman GM, Mussatto KA, Brosig CL, et al. Cerebral oxygenation and neurodevelopmental outcome in hypoplastic left heart syndrome. Available from: http://www.asaabstracts.com/strands/asaabstracts/abstract.htm?year=2008&index=16&absnum=1990. Accessed 09.02.12.

18. Hoffman GM, Wider MD. Organ specificity of rSO2 Measurements during regional ischemia in piglets. Anesthesiology [Internet]. 2008;109:[A1512]. Available from: http://www.asaabstracts.com/strands/asaabstracts/abstract.htm?year=2008&index=9&absnum=1984. Accessed 09.02.12.

19. Hoffman GM, Wider MD. Changes in regional oxygenation by NIRS during global ischemia in piglets. Anesthesiology. 2008;109:A1512.

20. Ortmann LA, Fontenot EE, Seib PM, et al. Use of near-infrared spectroscopy for estimation of renal oxygenation in children with heart disease. Pediatr Cardiol. 2011;32:748-753.

21. Bernal N, Hoffman G, Ghanayem N, et al. Cerebral and somatic near-infrared spectroscopy in normal newborns. J Pediatr Surg. 2010;45:1306-1310.

22. Johnson BA, Hoffman GM, Tweddell JS, et al. Near-infrared spectroscopy in neonates before palliation of hypoplastic left heart syndrome. Ann Thorac Surg. 2009;87:571-579.

23. Hoffman GM, Ghanayem NS, Stuth EA, et al. NIRS-derived somatic and cerebral saturation difference provides non-invasive real-time hemodynamic assessment of cardiogenic shock and risk of anaerobic metabolism. Anesthesiology [Internet]. 2004;99:[A1448]. Available from: http://www.asaabstracts.com/strands/asaabstracts/abstract.htm?year=2004&index=16&absnum=2206. Accessed 09.02.12.

24. Tweddell JS, Ghanayem NS, Mussatto KA, et al. Mixed venous oxygen saturation monitoring after stage 1 palliation for hypoplastic left heart syndrome. Ann Thorac Surg. 2007;84:1301-1311.

25. Rivers E, Nguyen B, Havstad S, et al. Early goal-directed therapy in the treatment of severe sepsis and septic shock. N Engl J Med. 2001;345:1368-1377.

26. de Oliveira CF, de Oliveira DS, Gottschald AF, et al. ACCM/PALS haemodynamic support guidelines for paediatric septic shock: an outcomes comparison with and without monitoring central venous oxygen saturation. Intensive Care Med. 2008;34:1065-1075.

27. Tortoriello TA, Stayer SA, Mott AR, et al. A noninvasive estimation of mixed venous oxygen saturation using near-infrared spectroscopy by cerebral oximetry in pediatric cardiac surgery patients. Paediatr Anaesth. 2005;15:495-503.

28. Li J, Van Arsdell GS, Zhang G, et al. Assessment of the relationship between cerebral and splanchnic oxygen saturations measured by near-infrared spectroscopy and direct measurements of systemic haemodynamic variables and oxygen transport after the Norwood procedure. Heart. 2006;92:1678-1685.

29. Moran M, Miletin J, Pichova K, et al. Cerebral tissue oxygenation index and superior vena cava blood flow in the very low birth weight infant. Acta Paediatr. 2009;98:43-46.

30. Hoffman GM, Ghanayem NS, Tweddell JS. Noninvasive assessment of cardiac output. Semin Thorac Cardiovasc Surg Pediatr Card Surg Annu 2005:12-21.

31. Hoffman GM, Ghanayem NS, Kampine JM, et al. Venous saturation and the anaerobic threshold in neonates after the Norwood procedure for hypoplastic left heart syndrome. Ann Thorac Surg. 2000;70:1515-1521.

32. Tweddell JS, Hoffman GM, Fedderly RT, et al. Phenoxybenzamine improves systemic oxygen delivery after the Norwood procedure. Ann Thorac Surg. 1999;67:161-168.

33. Kaufman J, Almodovar MC, Zuk J, et al. Correlation of abdominal site near-infrared spectroscopy with gastric tonometry in infants following surgery for congenital heart disease. Pediatr Crit Care Med. 2008;9:62-68.

34. Hoffman GM, Ghanayem NS, Mussatto KA, et al. Postoperative two-site NIRS predicts complications and mortality after stage 1 palliation of HLHS. Anesthesiology [Internet]. 2007;107:[A234]. Available from: http://www.asaabstracts.com/strands/asaabstracts/abstract.htm?year=2007&index=16&absnum=1585. Accessed 09.02.12.

35. Kleinman ME, Chameides L, Schexnayder SM, et al. Pediatric advanced life support: 2010 American Heart Association guidelines for cardiopulmonary resuscitation and emergency cardiovascular care. Pediatrics. 2010;126:e1361-e1399.

36. Tibby S, Hoffman GM. Resuscitation of the patient with single ventricle.Peds-059b. Worksheet for Evidence-Based Review of Science for Emergency Cardiac Care. International Liaison Committee on Resuscitation. 2010. Accessed 1 May 2011 at: http://circ.ahajournals.org/site/C2010/Peds-059.pdf.

37. Green D, Paklet L. Latest developments in peri-operative monitoring of the high-risk major surgery patient. Int J Surg. 2010;8:90-99.

38. Tweddell JS, Hoffman GM, Mussatto KA, et al. Improved survival of patients undergoing palliation of hypoplastic left heart syndrome: lessons learned from 115 consecutive patients. Circulation. 2002;106:I82-I89.

39. Wypij D, Newburger JW, Rappaport LA, et al. The effect of duration of deep hypothermic circulatory arrest in infant heart surgery on late neurodevelopment: the Boston Circulatory Arrest Trial. J Thorac Cardiovasc Surg. 2003;126:1397-1403.

40. Kurth CD, Levy WJ, McCann J. Near-infrared spectroscopy cerebral oxygen saturation thresholds for hypoxia-ischemia in piglets. J Cereb Blood Flow Metab. 2002;22:335-341.

41. Kurth CD, McCann JC, Wu J, et al. Cerebral oxygen saturation-time threshold for hypoxic-ischemic injury in piglets. Anesth Analg. 2009;108:1268-1277.

42. Greeley WJ, Ungerleider RM, Kern FH, et al. Effects of cardiopulmonary bypass on cerebral blood flow in neonates, infants, and children. Circulation. 1989;80:I209-I215.

43. Greeley WJ, Kern FH, Meliones JN, et al. Effect of deep hypothermia and circulatory arrest on cerebral blood flow and metabolism. Ann Thorac Surg. 1993;56:1464-1466.

44. Dexter F, Hindman BJ. Theoretical analysis of cerebral venous blood hemoglobin oxygen saturation as an index of cerebral oxygenation during hypothermic cardiopulmonary bypass. A counterproposal to the "luxury perfusion" hypothesis. Anesthesiology. 1995;83:405-412.

45. Dexter F, Kern FH, Hindman BJ, Greeley WJ. The brain uses mostly dissolved oxygen during profoundly hypothermic cardiopulmonary bypass. Ann Thorac Surg. 1997;63:1725-1729.

46. Kadoi Y, Kawahara F, Saito S, et al. Effects of hypothermic and normothermic cardiopulmonary bypass on brain oxygenation. Ann Thorac Surg. 1999;68:34-39.

47. Sakamoto T, Zurakowski D, Duebener LF, et al. Interaction of temperature with hematocrit level and pH determines safe duration of hypothermic circulatory arrest. J Thorac Cardiovasc Surg. 2004; 128:220-232.

48. Hagino I, Anttila V, Zurakowski D, et al. Tissue oxygenation index is a useful monitor of histologic and neurologic outcome after cardiopulmonary bypass in piglets. J Thorac Cardiovasc Surg. 2005; 130:384-392.

49. Sakamoto T, Hatsuoka S, Stock UA, et al. Prediction of safe duration of hypothermic circulatory arrest by near-infrared spectroscopy. J Thorac Cardiovasc Surg. 2001;122:339-350.

50. Hoffman GM, Ghanayem NS. Perioperative neuromonitoring in pediatric cardiac surgery: techniques and targets. Progress in Pediatric Cardiology. 2010;29:123-130.

51. Hoffman GM, Mussatto KA, Brosig CL, et al. Systemic venous oxygen saturation after the Norwood procedure and childhood neurodevelopmental outcome. J Thorac Cardiovasc Surg. 2005;130: 1094-1100.

52. Uebing A, Furck AK, Hansen JH, et al. Perioperative cerebral and somatic oxygenation in neonates with hypoplastic left heart syndrome or transposition of the great arteries. J Thorac Cardiovasc Surg. 2011 Sep;142(3):523-530.

53. Hoffman G, Groneck J, Mussatto K, et al. Modified pH strategy during antegrade cerebral perfusion improves cerebral hemodynamics. Anesthesiology 2009:A687.

54. Dent CL, Spaeth JP, Jones BV, et al. Brain magnetic resonance imaging abnormalities after the Norwood procedure using regional cerebral perfusion. J Thorac Cardiovasc Surg. 2006;131: 190-197.

55. Owens GE, King K, Gurney JG, et al. Low renal oximetry correlates with acute kidney injury after infant cardiac surgery. Pediatr Cardiol. 2011;32:183-188.

56. Hoffman GM, Ghanayem NS, Mussatto KA, et al. Perioperative perfusion assessed by somatic NIRS predicts postoperative renal dysfunction. Anesthesiology [Internet]. 2005;103:[A1327]. Available from: http://www.asaabstracts.com/strands/asaabstracts/abstract.htm?year=2005&index=15&absnum=1769. Accessed 09.02.12.

57. Furtado N, Beier UH, Gorla SR, et al. The effect of indomethacin on systemic and renal hemodynamics in neonatal piglets during experimental endotoxemia. Pediatr Surg Int. 2008;24:907-911.

58. Fortune PM, Wagstaff M, Petros AJ. Cerebro-splanchnic oxygenation ratio (CSOR) using near infrared spectroscopy may be able to predict splanchnic ischaemia in neonates. Intensive Care Med. 2001;27:1401-1407.

59. Petrova A, Bhatt M, Mehta R. Regional tissue oxygenation in preterm born infants in association with echocardiographically significant patent ductus arteriosus. J Perinatol. 2011;31(7):460-466.

60. Tabbutt S, Ramamoorthy C, Montenegro LM, et al. Impact of inspired gas mixtures on preoperative infants with hypoplastic left heart syndrome during controlled ventilation. Circulation. 2001;104: I159-I164.

61. Ramamoorthy C, Tabbutt S, Kurth CD, et al. Effects of inspired hypoxic and hypercapnic gas mixtures on cerebral oxygen saturation in neonates with univentricular heart defects. Anesthesiology. 2002;96:283-288.

62. Hoffman GM, Ghanayem NS, Musa N, et al. Differential effects of carbon dioxide tension on cerebral and somatic oxygenation assessed by near infrared spectroscopy in postoperative neonates. Anesthesiology [Internet]. 2005;103:[A1374]. Available from: http://www.asaabstracts.com/strands/asaabstracts/abstract.htm?year=2005&index=15&absnum=1852. Accessed 09.02.12.

63. Ghanayem NS, Hoffman GM, Mussatto KA, et al. Perioperative monitoring in high-risk infants after stage 1 palliation of univentricular congenital heart disease. J Thorac Cardiovasc Surg. 2010;140: 857-863.

64. Ghanayem NS, Hoffman GM, Mussatto KA, et al. Home surveillance program prevents interstage mortality after the Norwood procedure. J Thorac Cardiovasc Surg. 2003;126:1367-1377.

24

CHAPTER 25

Mechanical Pump Support and Cardiac Transplant in the Neonate

Marc E. Richmond, MD

Orthotopic heart transplantation remains the only definitive therapy for infants and children suffering from end-stage heart failure from a variety of causes including cardiomyopathy, myocarditis, and inoperable structural congenital heart disease. Despite the overall excellent short- and long-term outcomes in infants, heart transplantation has many limitations, not the least of which is the high mortality experienced in infants while on the waitlist for transplantation.

Neonatal Heart Transplantation

History

The history of neonatal and infant heart transplantation very much parallels that of heart transplantation in adults. Only 3 days after the first successful adult heart transplant by Dr. Christian Barnard in Capetown, South Africa, Dr. Adrian Kantrowitz performed the first, albeit unsuccessful, infant heart transplant in a 19-day-old infant with severe Ebstein's anomaly, an otherwise lethal condition at the time.[1] Modern pediatric heart transplantation began again in 1984 with the successful transplantation of a 4-year-boy by a team at Columbia University Medical Center, followed rapidly with similar successes at other institutions.[2] Shortly thereafter, infant transplantation was proven to be successful, and currently infants younger than 1 year of age account for approximately one fourth of all pediatric heart transplant recipients. Due to significant advances in both surgical and medical management, infants now have excellent survival with greater than 50% overall survival at 15 years, and more than 90% of survivors have no activity limitations 5 years after transplantation (Fig. 25-1).[3,4] Despite the high costs associated with heart transplantation and the large use of resources, analysis has put pediatric heart transplantation well within societal limits on cost per quality-adjusted life-years; in fact the financial costs per quality-adjusted life-years are significantly less than that associated with universal meningococcal vaccination of adolescents.[5] Furthermore, as long-term survival after infant heart transplantation continues to improve, these costs will necessarily decrease. Even so, heart transplantation has a well-defined role in the care of infants suffering from end-stage heart failure or inoperable congenital heart disease, and the barriers to successful transplantation in all infants who require such therapy must continually be pushed for the benefit of these children.

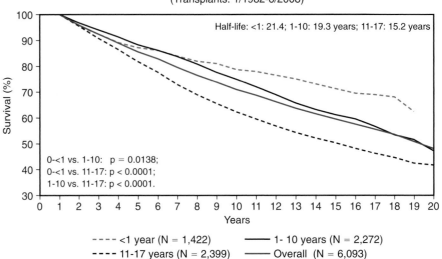

ONE-YEAR CONDITIONAL KAPLAN-MEIER SURVIVAL BY
AGE AT TRANSPLANT
(Transplants: 1/1982-6/2008)

Half-life: <1: 21.4; 1-10: 19.3 years; 11-17: 15.2 years

0-<1 vs. 1-10: p = 0.0138;
0-<1 vs. 11-17: p < 0.0001;
1-10 vs. 11-17: p < 0.0001.

- - - - <1 year (N = 1,422)   ——— 1- 10 years (N = 2,272)
- - - - 11-17 years (N = 2,399)   ——— Overall (N = 6,093)

Figure 25-1   Kaplan-Meier survival curves showing overall survival conditional on survival to 1-year posttransplantation separated by age at transplant. Infants younger than 1 year at the time of transplant have significantly better conditional survival than older children. (Adapted from Kirk R, Edwards LB, Kucheryavaya AY, et al. The registry of the International Society for Heart and Lung Transplantation: Thirteenth Official Pediatric Heart Transplantation Report—2010. J Heart Lung Transplant 2010;29:1119-1128.)

Indication for Transplant

Congenital heart disease remains the most common indication for heart transplant in recipients younger than 1 year of age, representing the indication for transplant in approximately 60% of patients in this age group, with only a third of infants requiring transplantation for cardiomyopathy. This is in stark contrast to older children in whom cardiomyopathy accounts for two thirds of all children requiring heart transplant.[3] Within congenital heart disease, hypoplastic left heart and other univentricular hearts comprise the most common anatomies and physiologies requiring transplant as an infant.

Until the mid- to late-1990s, many institutions, most notably Loma Linda University, performed heart transplantation as the procedure of choice for infants suffering from hypoplastic left heart syndrome (HLHS) and complex univentricular structural congenital heart disease.[6] This strategy was limited by the scarcity of donor organs, and the success of staged palliations by the end of the 1990s shifted the focus away from transplantation as the primary therapeutic option for these infants; in the years since, the number of infants undergoing transplantation for HLHS without prior surgical intervention has decreased dramatically.[7] With continual improvements in palliative surgery, it is now only the most complex and critically ill infants who require transplantation as their primary surgical therapy.[8-10] As such, waitlist mortality for infants with congenital heart disease remains extremely high, with one third of infants suffering from non-HLHS congenital heart disease dying before a donor heart is found.[7]

Unique Aspects of Heart Transplantation in Infants

Waitlist Mortality

The largest barrier to survival for infants who require heart transplantation may be waitlist mortality. Approximately 20% of all infant and pediatric patients listed for

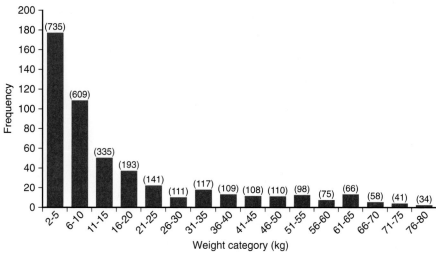

Figure 25-2 Graph depicting distribution of pediatric waitlist deaths over a 6-year period from January 1999 to July 2006. A total of 533 deaths occurred with 54% of deaths in children weighing less than 10 kg. (Adapted from Almond CSD, Thiagarajan RR, Piercey GE, et al. Waiting list mortality among children listed for heart transplantation in the United States. Circulation 2009;119:717-727.)

heart transplant died while on the waitlist, with the majority of deaths occurring in children weighing less than 10 kg (Fig. 25-2).[11,12] This is the highest waitlist mortality in all of solid organ transplantation. Infants are at an even greater risk for waitlist mortality, as common factors such as the presence of congenital heart disease and the need for mechanical support can worsen waitlist outcomes. For example, almost one third of infants with congenital heart disease who require mechanical ventilation will die before a suitable donor organ is available.[12] To combat this extremely high mortality, many centers have relied on the newest therapies available to prevent waitlist deaths in infants. Listing across ABO blood groups (discussed later), accepting donor hearts traditionally believed to be too large for an infant, and accepting longer ischemic times are all routinely employed to hasten the time between listing and finding a suitable donor organ. Furthermore, the use of extracorporeal membrane oxygenation (ECMO) and ventricular assist devices (VADs) has become more common to maintain end-organ function in infants awaiting heart transplantation. In infants with congenital heart disease, transcatheter and so-called hybrid approaches have been used to stabilize hemodynamics via stenting of the ductus arteriosus and/or placing pulmonary artery bands in patients with HLHS and other univentricular anatomies.[8,13] Despite these advances, it is likely that an increase in the available donor pool will be needed to counteract infant waitlist mortality. Heart transplantation in infants has been performed successfully with organs obtained from donors who have died of cardiocirculatory causes, but the many ethical and pragmatic questions surrounding these donors has prevented this method from being more widely implemented.[14,15]

ABO Incompatible Transplants

As discussed, a major limitation to successful transplantation in infants is the lack of available donors and subsequent high waitlist mortality. One successful attempt to increase suitable donors for infants awaiting heart transplantation has been to utilize donors with incompatible blood groups. The ability to successfully perform ABO-incompatible transplants takes advantage of the infant's immature immune system, as infants are not born with isohemagglutinins and typically do not develop anti-A or anti-B antibody titers until around 6 months. Even if present, these antibody titers usually remain low enough to permit cross-ABO blood group transplants until at least 12 months of age. Pioneered at the Hospital for Sick Children in

Toronto, ABO-incompatible heart transplantation has been shown to have similar outcomes in infants as ABO-compatible transplants, without any significant risk of hyperacute rejection.[16] In a recently presented review of all ABO-incompatible transplants in the Pediatric Heart Transplant Study Group database, 85 infants who had undergone ABO-incompatible transplantation were compared with infants with ABO-compatible donor hearts. Despite being younger and more likely to require pretransplant respiratory or circulatory support, there was no difference in survival or rejection outcomes between infants who received a compatible and those who received an incompatible donor heart.[17] In addition to equivocal survival, patients listed across ABO blood groups may have shorter waitlist times and decreased waitlist death, especially infants with blood type O.[18,19] Despite these encouraging data and the increasing use of this strategy, only about half of all infants listed for heart transplantation in the United States are currently listed across all ABO blood groups, and only about half of US centers have performed an ABO-incompatible heart transplant.[17-19]

Surgical Approach and Mortality

While heart transplantation surgical techniques have improved significantly over the past decades, infants undergoing transplant still have higher perioperative mortality than do older children. In analysis of the International Society for Heart and Lung Transplantation Registry data, the risk for death was highest in the first year for recipients younger than 1 year of age compared with all other age groups, a finding mimicked in other registries.[3,20] This increased risk may be related to the complexity of surgical repair required in transplantation of an infant with complex congenital heart disease, combined with other risk factors, including the need for ECMO support pretransplantation, and prior cardiac surgeries.[3,10,21,22] Additional repair at the time of transplantation, such as aortic arch reconstruction, pulmonary artery enlargement, and anomalous venous connections, is often required, increasing the complexity of the surgery and the duration of cardiopulmonary bypass, sometimes even requiring circulatory arrest—all known risk factors for poorer surgical outcomes. Some of this increased risk is likely unavoidable, but as nonsurgical techniques to stabilize infants with inoperable congenital heart disease improve and become more widely used, the hope is that some of this risk can be mitigated. Additionally, improvements in mechanical circulatory support may allow for many of these infants to be bridged to transplant outside the neonatal period without end-organ dysfunction, hopefully allowing for improved short-term outcomes.

Currently, a bicaval anastomosis, whereby the superior vena cava and inferior vena cava are independently sutured to the donor structures, is the preferred surgical technique for orthotopic heart transplantation in older children and adults. However, given the frequency of complex congenital heart lesions, including anomalous venous return, combined with the small size of the inferior and superior vena cavae, this approach is not always practical, nor is it advisable in neonates. Often the older-style, biatrial anastomosis is necessary to ensure appropriate venous drainage without obstruction. While data support worse long-term outcomes in adults, specifically with regard to atrial arrhythmias, the biatrial technique does not appear to hamper long-term outcomes in neonates, with conditional survival that surpasses other age groups.[23]

Immunosuppression and Rejection

Neonates and infants have by definition an immature immune system, with decreased cellular immunity exhibited by decreased T-cell number and function. Likely as a consequence of this immaturity, it has been well documented that children who undergo heart transplantation as infants have less frequent and potentially less aggressive rejection.[4,24] As such, it is possible to use less maintenance immunosuppression after heart transplantation in infants, and many of these children are now being maintained on a steroid-free regimen and sometimes even a single-drug regimen.[4,25,26] It has been hypothesized that the immaturity of the cellular immune system allows for this relative tolerance of the donor organ, and as such, the younger the infant, the less likely rejection will occur; however, this has not been definitively shown in the data. It is also possible that decreased immunity may also play a role in the lower rates of coronary graft vasculopathy seen in infant and neonate recipients, although the causes of graft vasculopathy remain elusive and likely are multifactorial.[27] Nonetheless, infants, once they survive the perioperative risk period, have the best survival curve and long-term outcomes of all age groups, perhaps due to their better graft tolerance.[3,28]

Mechanical Circulatory Support in the Infant

As the success of infant heart transplantation has been mostly limited by the availability of donor organs and subsequent high waitlist mortality, there has been a renewed focus on maintaining infants (and older children) alive until a suitable donor is identified. The use of well-designed, easy-to-implement VADs with relatively low complications rates, such as the HeartMate II (Thoratec Corp., Pleasanton, CA) has radically changed waitlist times and mortality for adults requiring heart transplantation. Unfortunately, no similar device is currently available for infants requiring mechanical circulatory support, as current options carry unacceptably high complication and mortality rates. Devices designed for adult use have been placed in adolescents and older children with increasing frequency and success.[29] Despite inherent limitations in adapting adult pumps for children, many pediatric centers have been able to achieve improved outcomes for these critically ill children. However, with fewer and less appropriate choices, infants requiring support have fared much worse than older children who are more likely to survive on adult-sized VADs.[29] In addition to providing support for infants awaiting heart transplantation, mechanical circulatory support devices can be used to support infants in whom recovery of cardiac function is likely, such as those with postoperative ventricular dysfunction or with acute heart failure from neonatal myocardial infarction or myocarditis. In such cases, successful explantation is often dependent upon early implementation of support and minimizing complications, allowing for recovery of myocardial function before other organ systems are in decline. When choosing to place an infant on support, anticipating the duration of support, estimating the likelihood of cardiac recovery, and an intimate understanding of the devices available are all paramount to choosing the most appropriate device for each patient.

Indications for Support

There are classically three potential goals for mechanical circulatory support: bridge-to-transplantation, bridge-to-recovery, and destination therapy. Destination therapy, the concept of sending a patient home on a VAD indefinitely, has been used in adult medicine to support patients who are otherwise not transplant candidates or for those who do not wish to be transplanted. This concept has no place in neonatal medicine given the limitations of current devices, but perhaps in the future, a suitable artificial heart could be placed in an infant that would allow discharge home and long-term survival with adequate quality of life. Until then, all infants placed on support are removed when there is sufficient recovery of cardiac function, a donor heart is identified, or death occurs. Recently a fourth goal has been espoused, bridge-to-decision. This is the concept by which an infant is placed on a short-term mechanical device (typically ECMO) until it can be determined what caused the hemodynamic decline, whether the patient is a transplant candidate, and whether or not recovery of cardiac function is likely. If the patient then requires bridge-to-transplantation, the patient is changed to support with a long-term device (VAD). While this concept is appealing, it does lead to difficult discussions and decisions regarding withdrawal of care in patients who are not transplant candidates and for whom cardiac recovery is unlikely. The path to decision and the possible outcomes should be fully discussed among the clinical care team and the family prior to initiation of support, with full agreement and understanding of the decision algorithm among all parties involved.

E

The key to placing an infant on mechanical circulatory support is to anticipate and preempt an irreversible decline in hemodynamics and subsequent end-organ damage. Typically these infants have severe cardiac dysfunction, are on high-dose inotropic support, and possibly suffer from intractable cardiac arrhythmias. If escalation of therapy (i.e., increasing inotropes/vasoconstrictors, mechanical ventilation, sedation, and/or paralysis) cannot stop the progression of renal and liver failure, mechanical support of circulation may be the only option to prevent multisystem organ failure and death. It is ideal to initiate mechanical support before irreversible renal failure and/or liver failure as either of those may make the infant unsuitable for transplant. Additionally, initiation prior to cardiopulmonary arrest is preferable as patients who are placed on mechanical support after arrest have very poor outcomes.[30]

Extracorporeal Membrane Oxygenation

Until recently, the only option for infant mechanical circulatory support was extracorporeal membrane oxygenation (ECMO). While highly successful for respiratory indications, cardiac ECMO is much less successful with less than 40% survival to discharge in infants.[31] Yet ECMO still remains the most common mechanical circulatory device for infants suffering from severe cardiac dysfunction with approximately 500 infants in the United States placed on cardiac ECMO annually.[31] As ECMO circuits always contain an oxygenator, the typical cannulation strategy for cardiac ECMO involves a venous inflow cannula and an arterial outflow cannula. This cannulation can occur centrally, as in surgical patients requiring postoperative support, or can be performed (at least in neonates) via the internal jugular vein and carotid artery, avoiding the need for sternotomy. In addition to its ability to provide full cardiac output support, ECMO also provides full oxygenation and respiratory gas exchange, which is useful in patients in whom there is the additional component of respiratory failure. However, many of the limitations of ECMO are related to the presence of the circuit oxygenator, including the need for aggressive anticoagulation, usually via systemic heparinization. Inadequate anticoagulation can lead to clot formation in the circuit or oxygenator and possibly oxygenator failure, complications that more often than not lead to death. The need for anticoagulation, and the risk of overanticoagulation, can result in the not infrequent development of intracranial, gastrointestinal, surgical site, and/or other hemorrhage.[31] Additionally, patients on ECMO are typically immobile, less of a concern for neonates than older children, and some may need to remain on a paralytic to ensure stability of the circuit.

Ideally, ECMO is used for short-term support while the heart recovers, and the average duration of support is approximately 1 week. However, ECMO support durations longer than a month have been used successfully, albeit with higher incidences of complications, including multiorgan system failure.[31] Therefore, as a short-term bridge to myocardial recovery in the postoperative patient, fulminant myocarditis, myocardial infarction, or acute cardiac allograft rejection, ECMO is often the device of choice. However, for infants who are awaiting heart transplantation, ECMO is decidedly less successful as wait times often exceed that of a successful ECMO run. In fact, in some studies, over half of children placed on ECMO as a bridge-to-transplant do not survive.[32,33] Given the limitations of long-term ECMO support, one common approach to the infant with acute cardiac decompensation is to initiate support with ECMO as a "bridge-to-a-bridge" and if myocardial recovery appears unlikely (usually determined by 5-7 days), transitioning of child to VAD support while awaiting transplantation can occur.[34]

It is important to note that ECMO, while providing full cardiac output, is essentially a right heart assist device, and in the absence of an adequate atrial or ventricular septal defect, does not decompress the left ventricle. In the severely dysfunctional left ventricle (i.e., one that cannot eject antegrade across the aortic valve when on ECMO), this results in left atrial hypertension and pulmonary congestion. This "white out" appearance on chest radiograph can significantly impact the ability to wean a patient from ECMO due to compromised pulmonary gas exchange. In such cases, an atrial septostomy should be performed to allow for decompression of the left heart and may be performed bedside or in the cardiac catheterization suite.[32]

Classically, an ECMO circuit uses a roller pump and membrane oxygenator; however, in adult medicine, there has been a move toward using centrifugal pumps and newer fiber oxygenators as this combination appears to be more successful in adult ECMO candidates.[35] Recent advances in both centrifugal pump design and newer fiber oxygenators have made them now appropriate for use in infants. In particular the Thoratec PediMag (Thoratec Corp., Pleasanton, CA) in tandem with the QUADROX-iD Pediatric Oxygenator (Maquet GmbH & Co. KG, Rastatt, Germany) can be used to support infants requiring cardiovascular and respiratory support.[36] Such systems are attractive, in that the oxygenator can be spliced into or out of the circuit if oxygenation needs change, but the need for circulatory support does not.[37] Additionally these newer systems may have an advantage with longer-term use than traditional ECMO circuits, although that remains to be proven.

Ventricular Assist Device

VADs are mechanical pumps designed to provide cardiac output when the patient's native heart cannot. While some VADs can be placed percutaneously, those devices and techniques are limited to larger children and adults. For neonates and infants, while ECMO can be placed via the neck, utilizing current technology a VAD must be implanted surgically. Ventricular support can be unilateral (right ventricular or more commonly left ventricular) or if needed, two pumps can be used to provide biventricular support. Because VADs are designed to only provide circulatory support, they do not include an oxygenator, and therefore require somewhat less anticoagulation than ECMO. The decreased anticoagulation requirement, along with other design factors improving durability, has allowed VADs to provide more long-term support, and VAD is the preferred method of supporting a patient until transplant. Additionally, unlike ECMO, being on a VAD at the time of transplant does not appear to have significant detrimental effects upon posttransplantation survival.[29,38,39] Assist devices can be categorized into two distinct design categories: continuous flow and pulsatile flow, both of which are able to provide left ventricular (LVAD), right ventricular (RVAD), or biventricular (BiVAD) support.[40] Each design carries its own unique aspects and the management of these patients varies from center to center. Currently there is no single device that is clearly best for supporting an infant as a bridge-to-transplantation, and no device is approved by the U.S. Food and Drug Administration (FDA) for this use either, although the Berlin Heart Excor VAD (Berlin Heart AG, Berlin, Germany) is currently under review for FDA approval. Even so, the number of children being placed on VADs is increasing, most rapidly in patients younger than 5 years of age, including infants.[34] Given the difficulties of supporting children on VADs, it is perhaps not surprising that most often implantation occurs at large, high-volume teaching hospitals and that these centers also have higher survival rates than centers that perform pediatric VAD implantations infrequently.[34] The degree of knowledge and expertise required of the entire medical team including surgeons, cardiologists, intensivists, neonatologists, clinical perfusionists, and nurses is quite high and very specialized. Furthermore, as no standard care protocols exist, each center must rely on its own experience to best tailor clinical care such as anticoagulation and prevention of infections.

Pulsatile Flow Devices

The first generation of VADs approved in the early 1990s all utilized a pulsatile pump design. Although they have somewhat fallen out of favor, there are currently many such devices designed for use in adults, including the Thoratec PVAD, iVAD, and HeartMate XVE (Thoratec Corp., Pleasanton, CA), and Toyobo VAD (Toyobo-National Cardiovascular Center, Osaka, Japan), but only the Berlin Heart Excor VAD has been designed for pediatric use. All pulsatile devices have the same basic design scheme (Fig. 25-3A). All contain an internal bladder which fills with blood during VAD diastole and is then compressed, pneumatically or otherwise, causing ejection of blood and VAD systole. These devices typically have one-way valves in both the

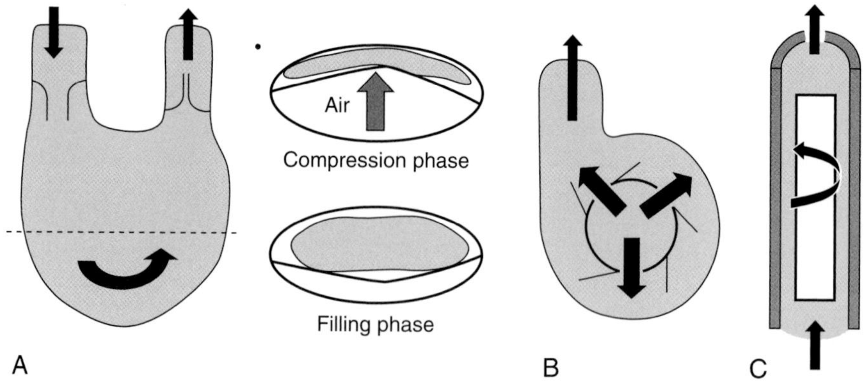

Figure 25-3 Schematics of three current VAD designs. Solid arrows represent the flow of blood into, within, and out of the pump. **A,** Pulsatile pump with an internal bladder that fills with blood during VAD diastole (filling phase) and blood is ejected during VAD systole (compression phase). Note the presence of one-way valves allowing for inflow and outflow of blood from the bladder without regurgitant flow. **B,** Centrifugal continuous flow pump with a central rotor that creates blood acceleration and flow via the outflow cannulas. **C,** Axial flow pump with an in-line impeller creating acceleration of blood through the device and in a parallel fashion. (Adapted from Pauliks LB, Undar A. New devices for pediatric mechanical circulatory support. Curr Opin Cardiol 2008;23:91-96.)

inflow and outflow cannulas of the pump to prevent regurgitant flow of blood. By design, the stroke volume of these pumps is essentially fixed, excluding all but the Berlin Heart Excor from use in small children and infants. Subsequently, with almost 1000 children supported worldwide, the Berlin Heart Excor is probably the most common device used to support infants and children as a bridge to transplantation. The Berlin Heart Excor is a paracorporeal device with the bladder situated just outside the infant's body and connected via a drive line to the controller console. A single pump can be implanted as an LVAD or RVAD, or two pumps can be implanted for BiVAD support. The uniqueness of the Berlin Heart Excor is that multiple sized pumps and cannulas are available, from a stroke volume of 10 to 60 mL, allowing implantation in a wide range of patients from infants as small as 3 kg to adults (Fig. 25-4).[41,42] Cannulation typically occurs via the left ventricular apex and aorta for LVAD support and the right atrium and pulmonary artery for RVAD support. Patients must be anticoagulated when on the device and although the ideal anticoagulation regimen is unknown and varies by center, it typically involves an antiplatelet agent as well as heparin and/or warfarin. With experience, some centers have reported as high as 60-70% survival rates using the Berlin Heart Excor in infants, significantly better than results typical of ECMO but still lower than current adult VAD survival numbers.[42-44] More concerning, higher on-device mortality has been associated with younger age, especially when requiring BiVAD, with over 60% mortality in that group.[41] Additionally, the rate of adverse events in infants supported with the Berlin Heart can be high, with 20-40% experiencing neurological complications and infections occurring in a third of infants.[44,45] Given the propensity for clot formation, many infants require pump exchanges at a rate higher than experienced by older children.[45] Despite the relatively wide use and successes of the Berlin Heart Excor, it remains an older design of VAD, belonging to the first generation of pulsatile devices. The vast majority of newer VADs designed for adults and even children have abandoned the pulsatile design in favor of continuous flow. As more data support adequate end-organ function with continuous flow devices, the mechanical and practical advantages of such devices are outweighing those of pulsatile design. It is entirely possible that the future of ventricular assist may not include pulsatile designs unless some of the inherent difficulties, such as the predisposition for valves to fail and/or develop thrombus, can be surmounted.

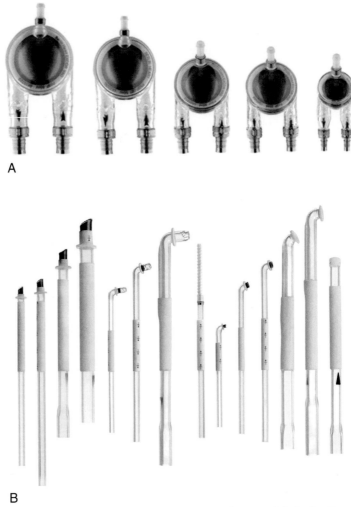

A

B

Figure 25-4 The Berlin Heart Excor Pediatric VAD (Berlin Heart AG, Berlin, Germany) has a variety of pump sizes **(A)** from a stroke volume of 10-60 mL and a variety of cannula sizes and configurations **(B)** to allow for implantation in infants as small as 3 kg and adult-sized patients as well. (Courtesy of Berlin Heart, EXCOR pediatric cannulae range.)

Continuous Flow Devices

Newer generations of VAD are mostly designed using continuous flow rotary pumps. All pumps of this classification utilize rotation of an impeller or rotor to create blood flow through the device and generate the required pressure gradient. Major differences within this class of pumps distinguish between those that use a centrifugal design, whereby the inflow and outflow of the pump are arranged perpendicular to each other, and those that use an axial flow design, whereby the impeller is in-line with the blood flow (see Fig. 25-3B, C). Pumps with continuous flow designs have some specific advantages over pulsatile design VADs, especially in relation to the use in infants and children. Because flow through the device is continuous, there is no need for valves within the pump, eliminating a potential area of thrombus formation and pump failure. Additionally, there are no areas of hemostasis as may be seen in the bladder of a pulsatile pump, theoretically decreasing the risk of thrombus formation within the pump. In adults supported by an axial flow pump (e.g., HeartMate II), this has resulted in lower anticoagulation requirements than pulsatile pumps. As experience with these designs in neonates is limited, whether infants receive the same benefit remains to be seen. Continuous flow devices and their controllers have also been somewhat easier to miniaturize with a number of implantable devices recently designed for adult use, some as small as a AAA battery. The removal of valves also decreases the number of moving parts and many rotary flow devices have excellent long-term use durability without experiencing significant device failure. Despite early concerns regarding the lack of pulsatile blood flow, with the exception of some minor biochemical changes overall end-organ function is very well preserved, and is similar to pulsatile flow devices.[46,47]

Adding to the appeal of continuous flow devices is their relative simplicity of use. Most devices essentially have one setting, speed of the impeller, usually set in revolutions per minute (RPM). The higher the RPM, the higher the blood flow. As many pumps allow for very small adjustments to the RPM, it is much easier to fine-tune the cardiac output provided by these devices for the individual patient. Once set, in the absence of pump failure, changes in cardiac output at a stable RPM can usually be explained and managed by patient factors such as preload, afterload, and clot formation in the circuit.

In pediatrics, most continuous flow VAD experience has been limited to relatively short-term use, most commonly in infants with a centrifugal pump.[29] One particular centrifugal device—the Thoratec PediMag (Thoratec Corp., Pleasanton, CA) (Fig. 25-5)—is designed specifically for use in infants and small children and has been used successfully for bridge-to-transplant and recovery as both a VAD and, when combined with an oxygenator, an ECMO circuit.[36,48,49] Based upon the Thoratec CentriMag adult-sized pump (Thoratec Corp., Pleasanton, CA), the PediMag pump decreases the prime volume to 14 mL and uses smaller ¼-inch tubing than its adult counterpart. This allows the pump to provide lower flows (less than 2.5 L/min) at higher RPMs than the CentriMag pump, resulting in less hemostasis, thrombosis, and pump failure.[50,51] This particular pump uses a centrifugal design with a magnetically levitated impeller, significantly decreasing friction, heat generation, and hemolysis and increasing longevity of the pump head, which are all advantages over other devices that use bearings to support the impeller. While currently approved for 30-day use in Europe, the PediMag system is not FDA approved, and even the adult CentriMag pump is only FDA approved for short-term (6-hour) use in adults. While the future of VADs in infants may indeed reside with rotary flow pumps, continuing improvements in design, miniaturization, and durability are needed before routine use of these pumps will occur.

Future

There are many barriers to designing and ultimately successfully implementing the "ideal" VAD for infants and children. The first and most obvious is the small size of infants relative to current technology. Any implantable device would have to be sufficiently small in total volume to be implantable in a 3-kg neonate. No current device even approximates this degree of miniaturization. Even for paracorporeal devices, the necessarily small diameter of the cannula imparts problems with fluid dynamics, including shear stress on red blood cells and resultant hemolysis. Furthermore, even with smaller caliber tubing and intrapump volumes, the ratio of circuit/pump surface area to patient body surface area is much larger than that with adults. This may result in increased inflammatory cascade activation and antibody presensitization, both concerning for long-term posttransplant outcomes. As has been seen with adult-sized pumps used in children, relative low-flow states associated with normal cardiac outputs in infants may predispose these miniaturized pumps to thrombosis. This major problem will need to be addressed with newer generations of infant VADs, as the consequences of needing aggressive anticoagulation are just as dire as those seen with thromboembolic events. Anatomical barriers related to structural congenital heart disease exist as well. One of the largest risk factors for poor outcome on ECMO or VAD support is the presence of congenital heart disease, which has been shown in many studies to be an independent risk factor for mortality in these patients, possibly in part due to inherent difficulties with supporting a child with abnormal cardiac and vascular anatomy.[29,34] Unique implantation techniques have

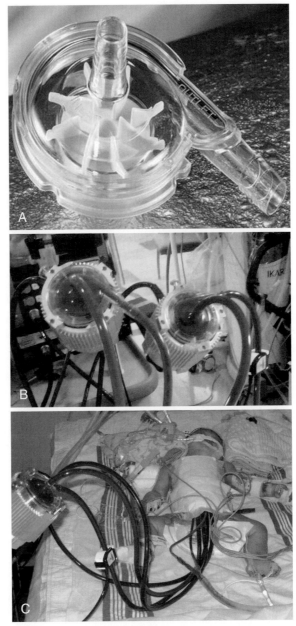

Figure 25-5   The Thoratec PediMag (Thoratec Corp., Pleasanton, CA) ventricular assist device consists of a 14-mL prime volume disposable centrifugal pump **(A)**, which is placed inside the motor housing **(B)** for LVAD, RVAD, or BiVAD (pictured) support. The PediMag provides blood flow up to 2.5 L/min, allowing for full support of infants and toddlers **(C)**. (Reprinted with permission of Thoratec Corp., Pleasanton, CA.)

been used in patients with congenital heart disease and will continue to evolve as the need and success of pediatric VADs increase. In addition to the aforementioned physiological barriers, the small numbers of patients who require cardiac support annually make infant VADs "small business" and further incentives beyond market share and profit will be needed for industry to devote the resources necessary to develop and market these products.

PumpKIN

Recognizing the difficulties of developing a pediatric-specific VAD, the National Heart, Lung and Blood Institute (NHLBI) created the Pediatric Support Program in

2004.[52] The goal of this preclinical program was to promote the development of novel circulatory support systems aimed at treating patients 2-25 kg in size. As part of this program, the NHLBI put forth criteria inherent in "ideal" devices, namely that they (1) may be deployed in under 1 hour, (2) minimize the prime volume of the pump, (3) have cannulation strategies appropriate for congenital heart disease, (4) minimize exposure to blood products, (5) minimize the risks for bleeding, thrombosis, hemolysis, and infection, and (6) may support a child for up to 6 months. Initial funding was awarded to five centers to develop ventricular assist devices specifically designed with these criteria in mind for use in pediatric patients.

As a follow-up to the Pediatric Support Program, the NHLBI announced the PumpKIN (Pumps for Kids, Infants and Neonates) program would begin clinical trials of four devices in 2012.[53] The four devices chosen include three pumps designed via the prior NHLBI Pediatric Support Program and one other device based upon Thoratec CentriMag and PediMag pumps. Two devices, the aforementioned Thoratec PediPL system (Thoratec Corp., Pleasanton, CA) and the Ension Pediatric Cardiopulmonary Support System (pCAS) (Ension Inc., Pittsburgh, PA), are designed as ECMO support systems, with integrated pump-oxygenators and the ability to support infants as small as 2 kg. The other two devices to be tested are pure ventricular support devices without oxygenators. Both the infant size Jarvik 2000 (Jarvik Heart) and the PediaFlow VAD (World Heart) are axial flow devices, intended for implantation as bridge-to-transplant in infants as small as 3 kg who may require intermediate (i.e., months) duration of support. Hopefully via the PumpKIN program and other initiatives, the options for infants and neonates who require cardiac support will become as varied and successful as that for adults, and will dramatically improve survival in this extremely fragile group of infants.

References

1. Kantrowitz A, Haller JD, Joos H, et al. Transplantation of the heart in an infant and an adult. Am J Cardiol. 1968;22:782-790.
2. Addonizio LJ, Rose EA. Cardiac transplantation in children and adolescents. J Pediatr. 1987;111:1034-1038.
3. Kirk R, Edwards LB, Kucheryavaya AY, et al. The registry of the international society for heart and lung transplantation: thirteenth official pediatric heart transplantation report—2010. J Heart Lung Transplant. 2010;29:1119-1128.
4. Dapper F, Bauer J, Kroll J, et al. Clinical experience with heart transplantation in infants. Eur J Cardiothorac Surg. 1998;14:1-6.
5. Dayton JD. Cost-effectiveness of pediatric heart transplantation. J Heart Lung Transplant. 2006; 25:409.
6. Bailey LL, Nehlsen-Cannarella SL, Doroshow RW, et al. Cardiac allotransplantation in newborns as therapy for hypoplastic left heart syndrome. N Engl J Med. 1986;315:949-951.
7. Guleserian KJ, Schechtman KB, Zheng J, et al. Outcomes after listing for primary transplantation for infants with unoperated-on non-hypoplastic left heart syndrome congenital heart disease: a multi-institutional study. J Heart Lung Transplant. 2011;30:1023-1032.
8. Gandhi R, Almond C, Singh TP, et al. Factors associated with in-hospital mortality in infants undergoing heart transplantation in the United States. J Thorac Cardiovasc Surg. 2011;141:531-536, 536.e1.
9. Huddleston CB. Indications for heart transplantation in children. Progr Pediatr Cardiol. 2009; 26:3-9.
10. Lamour JM, Kanter KR, Naftel DC, et al. The effect of age, diagnosis, and previous surgery in children and adults undergoing heart transplantation for congenital heart disease. J Am Coll Cardiol. 2009;54:160-165
11. Mah D. Incidence and risk factors for mortality in infants awaiting heart transplantation in the USA. J Heart Lung Transplant. 2009;28:1292.
12. Almond CS, Thiagarajan RR, Piercey GE, et al. Waiting list mortality among children listed for heart transplantation in the United States. Circulation. 2009;119:717-727.
13. Ruiz CE, Gamra H, Zhang HP, et al. Stenting of the ductus arteriosus as a bridge to cardiac transplantation in infants with the hypoplastic left-heart syndrome. N Engl J Med. 1993;328: 1605-1608.
14. Boucek MM, Mashburn C, Dunn SM, et al. Pediatric heart transplantation after declaration of cardiocirculatory death. N Engl J Med. 2008;359:709-714.
15. Curfman GD, Morrissey S, Drazen JM. Cardiac transplantation in infants. N Engl J Med. 2008;359:749-750.
16. West LJ. ABO-incompatible heart transplantation in infants. N Engl J Med. 2001;344:793-800.

17. Henderson HT. 261 ABO-incompatible heart transplantation in infants: analysis of the pediatric heart transplant study (PHTS) database. J Heart Lung Transplant. 2011;30:S92.
18. Almond CS, Gauvreau KS, Thiagarajan RR, et al. Impact of ABO-incompatible listing on wait-list outcomes among infants listed for heart transplantation in the United States: a propensity analysis. Circulation. 2010;121:1926-1933.
19. Everitt MD, Donaldson AE, Casper TC, et al. Effect of ABO-incompatible listing on infant heart transplant waitlist outcomes: analysis of the United Network for Organ Sharing (UNOS) database. J Heart Lung Transplant. 2009;28:1254-1260.
20. Canter C, Naftel D, Caldwell R, et al. Survival and risk factors for death after cardiac transplantation in infants : a multi-institutional study. Circulation. 1997;96:227-231.
21. Zuppan CW, Wells LM, Kerstetter JC, et al. Cause of death in pediatric and infant heart transplant recipients: review of a 20-year, single-institution cohort. J Heart Lung Transplant. 2009;28:579-584.
22. Morris MC, Wernovsky G, Nadkarni VM. Survival outcomes after extracorporeal cardiopulmonary resuscitation instituted during active chest compressions following refractory in-hospital pediatric cardiac arrest. Pediatr Crit Care Med. 2004;5:440-446.
23. Davies RR, Russo MJ, Morgan JA, et al. Standard versus bicaval techniques for orthotopic heart transplantation: an analysis of the United Network for Organ Sharing database. J Thorac Cardiovasc Surg. 2010;140:700-708.
24. Ibrahim JE, Sweet SC, Flippin M, et al. Rejection is reduced in thoracic organ recipients when transplanted in the first year of life. J Heart Lung Transplant. 2002;21:311-318.
25. Singh TP, Faber C, Blume ED, et al. Safety and early outcomes using a corticosteroid-avoidance immunosuppression protocol in pediatric heart transplant recipients. J Heart Lung Transplant. 2010;29:517-522.
26. Leonard H, Hornung T, Parry G, et al. Pediatric cardiac transplant: results using a steroid free maintenance regimen. Pediatric transplantation. 2003;7:59-63.
27. Nicolas RT, Kort HW, Balzer DT, et al. Surveillance for transplant coronary artery disease in infant, child and adolescent heart transplant recipients: an intravascular ultrasound study. J Heart Lung Transplant. 2006;25:921-927.
28. Morrow WR. Outcomes following heart transplantation in children. Progr Pediatr Cardiol. 2009;26:39-46.
29. Blume ED, Naftel DC, Bastardi HJ, et al. Outcomes of children bridged to heart transplantation with ventricular assist devices. Circulation. 2006;113:2313-2319.
30. DiBardino D, McElhinney D, Marshall A, et al. A review of ductal stenting in hypoplastic left heart syndrome: bridge to transplantation and hybrid stage I palliation. Pediatr Cardiol. 2008;29:251-257.
31. Haines NM. Extracorporeal life support registry report 2008: neonatal and pediatric cardiac cases. ASAIO J. 2009;55:111-116.
32. Bae J-O, Frischer JS, Waich M, et al. Extracorporeal membrane oxygenation in pediatric cardiac transplantation. J Pediatr Surg. 2005;40:1051-1057.
33. Almond CS. Extracorporeal membrane oxygenation for bridge to heart transplantation among children in the United States: analysis of data from the organ procurement and transplant network and extracorporeal life support organization registry. Circulation. 2011;123:2975-2984.
34. Morales DLS, Zafar F, Rossano JW, et al. Use of ventricular assist devices in children across the United States: analysis of 7.5 million pediatric hospitalizations. Ann Thorac Surg. 2010;90:1313-1319.
35. Aziz TA. Initial experience with CentriMag extracorporal membrane oxygenation for support of critically ill patients with refractory cardiogenic shock. J Heart Lung Transplant. 2010;29:66.
36. Gerrah R, Charette K, Chen JM. The first successful use of the Levitronix PediMag ventricular support device as a biventricular bridge to transplant in an infant. J Thorac Cardiovasc Surg. 2011;142:1282-1283.
37. Stiller B. Mechanical cardiovascular support in infants and children. Heart. 2011;97:596-602.
38. Gandhi SK. Ventricular assist devices in children. Progr Pediatr Cardiol. 2009;26:11-19.
39. Davies RR, Russo MJ, Hong KN, et al. The use of mechanical circulatory support as a bridge to transplantation in pediatric patients: an analysis of the United Network for Organ Sharing database. J Thorac Cardiovasc Surg. 2008;135:421-427.
40. Pauliks LB, Undar A, et al. New devices for pediatric mechanical circulatory support. Curr Opin Cardiol. 2008;23:91-96.
41. Morales DL, Almond CS, Jaquiss RD, et al. Bridging children of all sizes to cardiac transplantation: the initial multicenter North American experience with the Berlin Heart Excor ventricular assist device. J Heart Lung Transplant. 2011;30:1-8.
42. Hetzer R, Potapov EV, Stiller B, et al. Improvement in survival after mechanical circulatory support with pneumatic pulsatile ventricular assist devices in pediatric patients. Ann Thorac Surg. 2006;82:917-925.
43. Stiller B, Weng Y, Hübler M, et al. Pneumatic pulsatile ventricular assist devices in children under 1 year of age. Eur J Cardiothorac Surg. 2005;28:234-239.
44. Brancaccio G, Amodeo A, Ricci Z, et al. Mechanical assist device as a bridge to heart transplantation in children less than 10 kilograms. Ann Thorac Surg. 2010;90:58-62.
45. Karimova A, Van Doorn C, Brown K, et al. Mechanical bridging to orthotopic heart transplantation in children weighing less than 10 kg: feasibility and limitations. Eur J Cardiothorac Surg. 2011;39:304-309.

46. Sandner SE, Zimpfer D, Zrunek P, et al. Renal function after implantation of continuous versus pulsatile flow left ventricular assist devices. J Heart Lung Transplant. 2008;27:469-473.
47. Thalmann M, Schima H, Wieselthaler G, et al. Physiology of continuous blood flow in recipients of rotary cardiac assist devices. J Heart Lung Transplant. 2005;24:237-245.
48. Marks JD, Wearden P, Borovetz H, et al. Experience and lessons learned from the first 500 patients supported with the Levitronix Pedivas cardiopulmonary assist system; abstracts from the 18th congress of the international society for rotary blood pumps. Artif Organs. 2011;35:A43.
49. De Rita F, Barozzi L, Franchi G, et al. Rescue extracorporeal life support for acute verapamil and propranolol toxicity in a neonate. Artif Organs. 2011;35:416-420.
50. Dasse KA, Gellman B, Kameneva MV, et al. Assessment of hydraulic performance and biocompatibility of a Maglev centrifugal pump system designed for pediatric cardiac or cardiopulmonary support. ASAIO J. 2007;53:771-777.
51. Tuzun E, Harms K, Liu D, et al. Preclinical testing of the Levitronix UltraMag pediatric cardiac assist device in a lamb model. ASAIO J. 2007;53:392-396.
52. Baldwin JT. The national heart, lung, and blood institute pediatric circulatory support program. Circulation. 2005;113:147-155.
53. Baldwin JT. Introduction. ASAIO J. 2009;55:1-2.

CHAPTER 26

Catheter-Based Therapy in the Neonate with Congenital Heart Disease

Shabana Shahanavaz, MD, Ziyad M. Hijazi, MD, MPH, William E. Hellenbrand, MD, and Julie Anne Vincent, MD, FACC, FAAP

26

The first catheter-based therapeutic procedure was performed in 1966 when Drs. Rashkind and Miller performed a balloon atrial septostomy (BAS or Rashkind procedure) in an infant with transposition of the great arteries without a thoracotomy.[1] The success of this particular palliative, transcatheter procedure in an infant with congenital heart disease (CHD) has led to a multitude of advances in catheter-based technologies and techniques for both adults and children with congenital and acquired cardiovascular diseases over the past nearly 50 years. Further innovations and advances in noninvasive imaging as well as a trend toward procedural collaboration between cardiovascular surgeons and interventional cardiologists has significantly altered the role of the cardiac catheterization laboratory in the management of neonates with CHD as well as the indications for cardiac catheterization. In the current era, indications for catheterizations are more likely to be for catheter-based therapies rather than diagnostic purposes in patients with CHD. Neonatal interventions have also become more commonplace with further advances in catheter and device technologies with what has been an increased focus in congenital/structural heart disease on the part of industry and with multidisciplinary teams participating in what have been termed "hybrid" procedures, allowing transcatheter therapies on even the smallest patients. This chapter describes a variety of catheter-based therapies that are currently performed on neonates born with congenital heart disease.

Vascular Access

Complications of vascular access sites account for the majority of adverse events associated with neonatal cardiac catheterization.[2-4] Injury to the vessel and/or the surrounding area may occur with either venous or arterial access sites. Important acute and long-term sequelae are more often associated with arterial access sites in these small patients. Complications may include arterial spasm and/or thrombosis causing chronic occlusion, significant tearing or severing of the vessel with extravasation of blood into the surrounding tissue, hematoma, "false" or pseudoaneurysm formation, and creation of an arteriovenous fistula. The frequency of vascular complications has decreased with alterations in access techniques, improvements in availability of size-appropriate equipment for neonates, and meticulous management of the access site following the procedure. With the frequent use of indwelling central venous catheters and/or arterial cannulations and the need for repeated procedures in these small patients (and vessels), the incidence of chronic occlusion of these vessels has increased, necessitating the use of less "standard" access sites and approaches for catheter-based procedures in these patients. These include use of the umbilical vein (in the immediate newborn period), subclavian or jugular veins, or hepatic veins (transhepatic approach) for venous access or the umbilical artery, carotid artery (usually via a cutdown technique), or axillary artery for alternative arterial access.[4-10] In more recent years interventional cardiologists and cardiovascular surgeons have collaborated to obtain access to even larger, more central vessels or even direct access into the cardiac chambers for catheter-based therapies. Surgically obtained access in conjunction with transcatheter procedures have been called "hybrid" procedures.

Balloon Atrial Septostomy

Since Dr. Rashkind first performed BAS in an infant with transposition of the great arteries, the safety and efficacy of this procedure has been well established and has become a lifesaving procedure for patients with CHD who require improved atrial level mixing of blood or atrial decompression. Although initial procedures were performed using fluoroscopic guidance, it was Allan and colleagues who first described performing BAS under echocardiographic control in 1982.[11] Since then, improvements in echocardiographic imaging have allowed most neonatal BAS procedures to be performed at the bedside under echocardiographic guidance if the atrial septum anatomy is "straightforward" and the septum is not intact.[12] When an atrial communication is not present, most centers perform BAS in the catheterization laboratory using either fluoroscopic guidance with biplane imaging alone, or alternatively, fluoroscopy with transthoracic echocardiography (TTE) or transesophageal echocardiography (TEE) to better visualize the septum when septal perforation is required prior to creation of an atrial communication (see later). At the bedside, the baby is usually placed on the cardiac monitor (operators often make the heart rate audible during the procedure so that any arrhythmia may be quickly noted), intubated, and sedated. Vascular access is usually via either the umbilical or femoral vein. Once access has been obtained, a balloon septostomy catheter is advanced via an introducer sheath to the inferior vena cava and right atrium, across the patent foramen ovale (PFO) and into the left atrium under direct visualization using TTE imaging. Once the position of the catheter tip is confirmed to be in the body of the left atrium (and not in a pulmonary vein or across the mitral valve), the balloon at the tip of the catheter is slowly inflated with sterile saline while simultaneously pulling the balloon back against the left atrial side of the atrial septum. The amount of saline used to fill the balloon is dependent upon the type of septostomy catheter, the actual size of the left atrium, and the desired size of the resultant septal defect. Next, the balloon inflation lock is secured and the catheter is firmly and rapidly pulled into the right atrium aiming to produce a tear in the septum primum (Fig. 26-1). Once the balloon has been pulled across the septum, it is quickly deflated so as not to obstruct systemic venous inflow from the inferior vena cava. The procedure may be repeated using serial increases in the inflation volume to fill the balloon until an adequate defect is created or until the maximum volume of the septostomy catheter or the maximum balloon size the left atrium will accommodate have been reached. Once the septostomy procedure has been performed, 2-dimensional echocardiography as well as Doppler interrogation is performed to assess the resultant defect size and to determine presence and severity of any residual

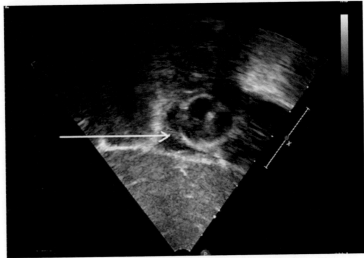

Figure 26-1   Two-dimensional echocardiographic image of an inflated septostomy catheter positioned in the left atrium. The arrow shows the septum.

atrial level restriction to blood flow or mixing (Fig. 26-2). Further echocardiographic assessment of the cardiac function, as well as for evidence of pericardial effusion or damage to any of the cardiac structures, is also recommended following BAS.

Although complications are not common, there have been reports of embolization of balloon fragments or air bubbles in the event of balloon rupture during the procedure (it should be noted here that careful de-airing of the balloon during preparation for BAS should take place to prevent air embolization if balloon rupture should occur). Other complications associated with BAS include heart block or other serious arrhythmias, mitral or tricuspid valve injury, thromboembolic events such as stroke, and inferior vena cava or pulmonary vein tear or rupture. Death has also occurred. Careful and appropriate echocardiographic imaging prior to and during balloon inflation can prevent valvular and/or vascular tears/ruptures from occurring. The success rate of BAS in newborns is over 98%, with a procedural mortality of

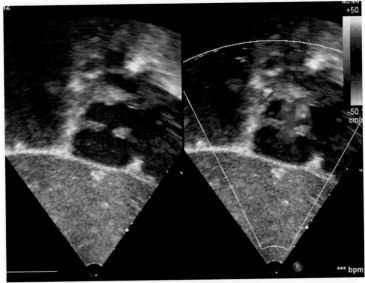

Figure 26-2   Two-dimensional and color Doppler images obtained in the subcostal longitudinal plane outlining the atrial septal defect post balloon septostomy. The color Doppler shows unrestricted flow across the atrial septal defect. (See Expert Consult site for color image.)

less than 1% and an incidence of major complications reported on the order of 0-3%.[13-15] Reports have suggested that there is an association between preoperative brain injury in neonates with transposition and performance of BAS.[15-17] Recently, Mukherjee and colleagues reported that there was a significant, positive association between Rashkind procedures and the diagnosis of stroke when comparing infants with transposition who either did or did not undergo a BAS procedure. However, lack of temporal data regarding timing of BAS and diagnosis of stroke limited the investigators' ability to prove causation.[15] In contrast, others have recently published reports that BAS was not associated with an increased risk of clinical stroke but that there was an increased incidence of preoperative periventricular leukomalacia (PVL) in neonates with transposition of the great arteries that had longer time to surgical repair and/or lower arterial oxygenation prior to intervention.[18-19] These authors further suggested that BAS was protective against PVL when the procedure resulted in timely improvement in arterial oxygenation.[18] Further studies are needed to better evaluate and define risk factors for preoperative brain injury in this patient population, which may include minimal oxygen saturation after birth and/or length of time from birth to BAS and improvement in systemic oxygenation.[20]

Atrial Septoplasty

Creation or enlargement of an atrial communication in neonates presenting after the immediate newborn period may be difficult due to the presence of a thick or intact atrial septum. Other infants, such as those with hypoplastic left heart syndrome (HLHS), may have malalignment of the atrial septum which is often associated with restriction of pulmonary venous return (Fig. 26-3). In patients such as these, standard BAS techniques may not be sufficient to create a nonrestrictive atrial communication and other "less standard" transcatheter techniques may be required. When the septum is intact, perforation of the septum to access the left atrium is required. Historically, this was and often still is performed by using a Brockenbrough needle to puncture the septum. In recent years, radiofrequency (RF)-assisted septal perforation has been reported using a 0.024-inch diameter wire with a 0.016-inch diameter metal tip (Baylis Medical, Montreal, Canada) attached to a dedicated RF generator

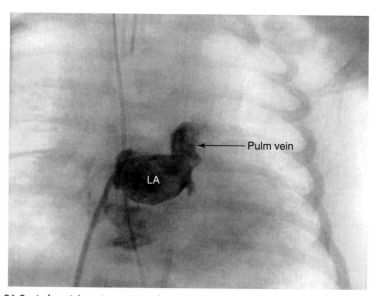

Figure 26-3 Left atrial angiogram in a hypoplastic left heart syndrome with restrictive atrial septum. Hand injection demonstrates complete filling of the left atrium with opacification of a left lower pulmonary vein which is dilated. The left atrium is small without much egress of dye into the right atrium.

(Baylis Radiofrequency Generator, Montreal, Canada). The wire is passed within a coaxial catheter that is, in turn, passed within a guide catheter or long introducer sheath/dilator, which has been placed with its tip adjacent to (and in contact with) the right atrial side of the septum. Perforation with this RF wire can be achieved with the application of 5-10 W of energy for 2-5 seconds.[21,22] Once mechanical or RF-assisted perforation of the septum and access into the left atrium is achieved, subsequent sequential static balloon dilation ("septoplasty") is performed, starting with small-diameter balloons, followed by serially larger diameter balloons to a maximum balloon diameter of typically 10-12 mm in neonates.[22] When there is a PFO but the septum is thick or malaligned, septal perforation is often performed in a more "favorable" position along the septum with subsequent septoplasty. In still other cases, standard septostomy or angioplasty catheters are not sufficient to create an adequate atrial communication. Use of coronary and peripheral cutting balloons (Boston Scientific, IVT, San Diego, CA) or high-pressure angioplasty balloons has been reported to be a safe and effective option for septoplasty in neonates (Fig. 26-4).[23-25] Finally in patients with difficult septal anatomy, an intravascular stent implantation at the atrial septum to maintain septal patency has provided effective palliation until surgical intervention or transplant can be achieved.[26-28]

Atrial perforations and septoplasties are performed in the cardiac catheterization laboratory using biplane fluoroscopic imaging. Many operators use either TTE or TEE imaging in the catheterization laboratory as adjunct to biplane fluoroscopic imaging to aid in proper positioning of the needle tip or RF wire along the septum prior to and during attempted perforation. When possible, TEE imaging is preferred as with TEE, the ultrasonographer's hand does not interfere with the fluoroscopic image during the procedure. In small infants in whom a pediatric/infant TEE probe may be too large, successful transesophageal imaging using an intracardiac echo (ICE) catheter (AcuNav, Acuson/Siemens, Mountain View, CA) has been reported.[29] Femoral venous access is preferred to umbilical vein access due to the complexity of the intervention and the more direct course from the femoral vein to the atrial septum.

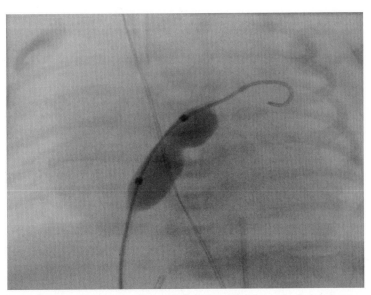

Figure 26-4 Balloon septoplasty of the atrial septum in a hypoplastic left heart syndrome with restrictive atrial septum. The balloon catheter is positioned in the mid-septum over a wire positioned with wire tip in the pulmonary vein. There is a discrete waist in the balloon seen in the region of the thick atrial septum.

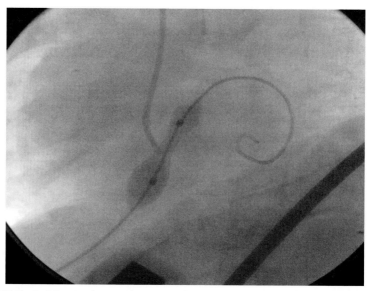

Figure 26-5 Atrial septoplasty with stent implantation in an infant with hypoplastic left heart syndrome and restrictive atrial septum. The premounted stent is implanted within the atrial septum under fluoroscopic guidance via a transhepatic sheath due to bilateral femoral vein obstruction.

Septoplasty with Interatrial Stent Placement

When balloon septoplasty is not sufficient to create or maintain an adequate atrial communication until surgical palliation can be achieved, implantation of an intravascular stent to maintain septal patency has been performed.[26-28] Although there are no available stents approved for this indication, previously approved balloon-expandable intravascular stents are used off label in these infants, often as a life-saving procedure. Prior to the advent of premounted noncoronary stents, stainless steel stents were hand-crimped on angioplasty balloons (usually 8-10 mm in diameter) and passed within long sheaths that had been positioned (often with much difficulty) in the left atrium or in a left-sided pulmonary vein. Premounted stainless steel stents are now available in appropriate lengths and diameters for this patient population and are currently used for interatrial stenting. These stents rarely require long sheaths for placement and risk of stent migration on the balloon during positioning or deployment is extremely rare. On occasion, techniques to cause the stent to flare at both ends ("dog-bone") during balloon inflation are performed to decrease the risk of stent embolization during deployment (Fig. 26-5).[26]

Complications of septoplasty techniques are similar to those of BAS and include vascular injury, perforation, significant bleeding or blood loss, thromboembolic events including stroke, heart block, or serious arrhythmias, and death. Atrial septoplasty has a published success rate of 73-90% in patients with HLHS. The mortality rate was higher in patients with restrictive atrial septum HLHS at 4.5% with overall adverse event rate of 8.9% when compared with patients with other cardiac diagnoses.[23,25]

Pulmonary Balloon Valvuloplasty in the Neonate

Neonates with critical pulmonary valvular stenosis usually present within the first 24-48 hours of life with progressive cyanosis as the ductus arteriosus closes. There is typically an outflow murmur from the stenotic valve. Cyanosis is due to persistent right to left shunting at the PFO in the presence of a hypertensive and hypertrophied noncompliant right ventricle. By definition, critical pulmonary valve stenosis is ductal-dependent as adequate pulmonary blood flow and oxygenation are dependent on systemic-to-pulmonary artery shunting via the ductus. Management of the infant who presents with critical pulmonary valve stenosis requires initiation of PGE-1 infusion to maintain ductal patency and augment pulmonary blood flow. In the current era, percutaneous balloon valvuloplasty is the initial procedure of choice for neonates with critical/severe pulmonary stenosis. These patients typically have a normal-sized tricuspid valve annulus, a tripartite right ventricle, and a normal pulmonary valve annulus. The right ventricle may be hypoplastic or the cavity may be relatively small due to the often severe right ventricular hypertrophy. The main pulmonary artery usually has evidence of poststenotic dilation from the spray of blood across the stenotic valve and there is almost always predominant right to left shunting at the atrial level (PFO) due to the stiff, noncompliant right ventricle (RV). Careful 2D echocardiographic and Doppler assessment of these patients prior to any interventions is of utmost importance. Echo evaluation should include measurements of the pulmonary valve annulus in preparation for catheter-based therapy.

Balloon valvuloplasty procedures for critical or severe pulmonary stenosis in the neonate are performed in the cardiac catheterization laboratory usually with the patient intubated and sedated or under general anesthesia. A femoral venous approach is typically utilized though this procedure has also been performed using umbilical venous access in very small neonates. After hemodynamic data are obtained, a right ventricular angiogram is performed to assess the size of the right ventricular cavity, the outflow tract, and the pulmonary valve annulus. The valve leaflets and annulus are best demonstrated on a straight lateral projection. This projection is also used for determining the annular diameter. An end-hole catheter is positioned with its tip in the RV outflow tract and a floppy-tipped torque wire is used to cross the stenotic orifice of the valve. When the ductus is patent, the wire is often able to be maneuvered across it into the descending aorta for more stable wire (and balloon position) during the procedure. On occasion it is not possible to pass the end-hole catheter across the stenotic valve and "predilation" using a very low profile, small diameter angioplasty balloon is necessary to dilate the valve orifice before an appropriate-sized balloon can be used for an effective valvuloplasty result. A balloon diameter to valve annulus diameter (balloon-annulus) ratio of 1-1.3 is used for pulmonary valvuloplasty. The balloon is inflated and deflated rapidly after having been positioned over the wire and across the valve. Inflation times are typically less than 10 seconds. The balloons may be inflated by hand or using an inflation device to measure inflation pressures. During inflation a waist is seen in the mid portion of the balloon at the level of the stenotic valve and this waist disappears with full inflation of the balloon. The balloon is removed over the wire and follow-up hemodynamic data is obtained to reassess the pulmonary valve gradient. With a patent ductus arteriosus the valve gradient may not accurately quantify the valve gradient that may persist. If the right ventricular pressure is still suprasystemic valvuloplasty may be repeated using a larger diameter balloon as long as a safe and appropriate balloon-annulus ratio is used. At the end of the procedure a final right ventricular angiogram is performed to assess for any damage to the right ventricle, tricuspid valve apparatus, and/or pulmonary artery and to assess location of any residual obstruction.

Following successful balloon valvuloplasty, most patients will have sufficient antegrade pulmonary blood flow so as to tolerate discontinuation of PGE-1 infusion and subsequent closure of the ductus. However, many will continue to have predominant right-to-left shunting at the atrial level until the right ventricular compliance improves. In some cases this may take 3-4 weeks with multiple attempts of trialing off and restarting PGE-1 infusion for systemic saturations that drop consistently to or below the 75-80% range due to decreased ductal level pulmonary blood flow in conjunction with a restricting or closing ductus. Most successful balloon valvuloplasty procedures result in some amount of pulmonary insufficiency. This is well tolerated in most infants and some have reported a beneficial effect of pulmonary insufficiency promoting right ventricular growth.[30,31] With regression of the right ventricular hypertrophy, improvement of the ventricular compliance, and growth of the right ventricle, the amount of right-to-left shunting at the atrial level decreases over time and adequate saturations are able to be maintained off PGE-1 infusion. Saturations continue to increase as these right ventricular changes continue or with spontaneous closure of the PFO. A small percentage of infants with critical pulmonary stenosis who have undergone a successful balloon valvuloplasty procedure may still be unable to maintain adequate pulmonary blood flow and systemic saturations off PGE-1 infusion greater than 4 weeks following valve dilation. In the past, these patients have undergone surgical placement of a Blalock-Taussig shunt to augment pulmonary blood flow. Some centers have gone on to perform ductal stenting in the catheterization laboratory to maintain ductal patency and augmented pulmonary blood flow off PGE-1 infusion. This is more commonly the case in patients with membranous pulmonary valve atresia following perforation of the valve with subsequent balloon valvuloplasty (see later).

Holzer and colleagues recently reported using a multicenter registry on 304 balloon pulmonary valvuloplasty procedures performed in eight institutions over a 34-month period. The median age at intervention was 2 months with 39% of procedures performed in the first month of life. Procedural success was achieved in 82% of all procedures, being defined as either a reduction in peak systolic valvar gradient to less than 25 mm Hg or greater than 50% reduction of the valve gradient or reduction of right ventricular systolic pressure ratio by 50%. There was a trend toward lower procedural success with moderate to severe thickening of the pulmonary valve (72%). Minor adverse events were documented in 10% of procedures, while moderate, major, or catastrophic adverse events were documented in 2% of procedures. There were no deaths.[32]

Perforation of Membranous Pulmonary Valve in Pulmonary Atresia and Intact Ventricular Septum

Pulmonary atresia with intact ventricular septum (PA IVS) is a complex disorder that is not only characterized by membranous or muscular atresia of the right ventricular outflow tract (RVOT) but also significant heterogeneity of the right ventricular morphology. The coronary artery anatomy may also be affected in this disorder with in utero development of connections between the right ventricle and the subepicardial coronary arteries (right ventricle to coronary artery sinusoids or fistulas) predisposing these patients to abnormal coronary circulations of various types and significance. Prognosis is related to the severity of the coronary circulation abnormalities as well as to tricuspid valve anatomy and function.[33,34] Prior to transcatheter or surgical intervention, careful assessment of the right heart and coronary anatomy must take place. Newborns with this disorder are obviously dependent on ductal flow and therefore PGE-1 infusion is initiated immediately after birth. TTE is performed for initial assessment. If it is clear that the tricuspid valve and/or right ventricle are severely hypoplastic and that biventricular repair will not be an option, then plans for a palliative shunt are made. In these patients, assessment of the atrial septum to determine adequacy of the atrial communication is made as restriction at the atrial level may lead to poor cardiac output and BAS should be considered. Cardiac catheterization with angiography to assess the coronary artery circulation is usually still performed in these patients even when there is no plan for right ventricular decompression as patients with severe coronary artery abnormalities may be ultimately managed with cardiac transplantation.[35] In patients where the echocardiographic assessment of right heart adequacy is less clear and/or when relief of the RVOT is considered, cardiac catheterization and angiography are performed to help characterize size of the right ventricular cavity and outflow tract as well as to define coronary artery anatomy and determine whether coronary circulation is dependent on high right ventricular pressures (right ventricular dependent coronary artery circulation or RVDCC). In patients with RVDCC, relief of the RVOT may result in a catastrophic event due to inadequate perfusion of the myocardium with a sudden drop in the systolic pressure of the right ventricle (i.e., coronary perfusion pressure in patients with RVDCC), resulting in myocardial ischemia, infarct, or death. If RVDCC is not present, then the decision to perform transcatheter relief of the RVOT with or without ductal stenting or surgical relief with placement of a systemic-to-pulmonary shunt is entertained.[36]

It is very important that procedures involving perforation of the membranous valve be performed using a high-quality, biplane x-ray imaging system. Infants should be intubated and sedated and/or paralyzed so that they do not move during the procedure. Historically, perforation of the atretic pulmonary valve was performed using the stiff end of a guidewire.[37,38] Use of a stiff wire tip in the RVOT of a neonate was often associated with significant and severe adverse events such as perforating the anterior part of the outflow tract, bleeding, need for emergent surgical procedures, and death.[38] Laser energy was the first energy source to be used for valvar perforations.[39,40] Unfortunately, the laser beam would perforate any tissue in its path beyond and/or adjacent to the valve as the depth of laser penetration is difficult to control.[39,40] RF energy is less powerful than laser energy but easier to control and has more recently been used to perforate atretic valve tissue.[36,41]

The development of a small, flexible coaxial catheter and wire system (Baylis Medical, Montreal, Canada) that could be advanced within small (4 French) catheters positioned with the tip in the RVOT just beneath the atretic pulmonary valve made it possible to deliver RF energy that was confined to the tip of the wire at the membranous valve for perforation. It is very important to clearly define the anatomy of the RVOT as well as the main pulmonary artery by angiography in preparation for this procedure. There is very little tactile feedback when RF energy is delivered and perforation is performed due to the ease in which this system moves through tissue. Operators often use permanent thoracic landmarks and image "roadmaps" in hopes of not inadvertently perforating outside the boundaries of the RVOT. Some advocate placing a retrograde catheter from the aorta across the ductus with its tip in the main pulmonary artery just above the atretic valve for something to aim at. Others have described passing a snare wire (Amplatz Gooseneck; Microvena, Vadnais Heights, MN) within the retrograde catheter and opening it within the main pulmonary artery to act as a "target" as well as to delineate the boundaries of the pulmonary artery lumen (Fig. 26-6).[42] Only 5-10 W of energy applied for 2 seconds is needed to perforate the tissue. Once perforation has been performed, the wire and coaxial catheter are advanced into the main pulmonary artery. The RF

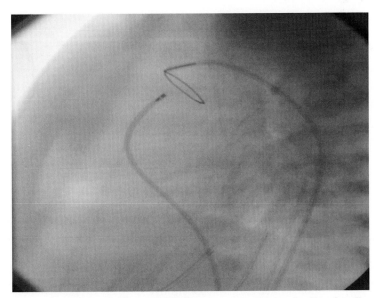

Figure 26-6 Lateral plane cinefluoroscopy demonstrating a snare wire (Amplatz Gooseneck; Microvena, Vadnais Heights, MN) passed retrograde from the aorta across the ductus to the main pulmonary artery to act as a "target" as well as to delineate the boundaries of the pulmonary artery lumen during RF perforation of an atretic pulmonary valve in this patient with pulmonary atresia with intact ventricular septum.

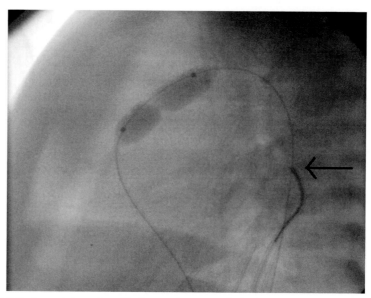

Figure 26-7   Lateral plane cine of balloon pulmonary valvuloplasty in an infant with pulmonary atresia with intact ventricular septum after successful RF perforation. The wire has been snared in the descending aorta (*arrow*) to gain wire stability for subsequent balloon valvuloplasty procedure.

wire can then be exchanged for a floppy-tipped guidewire that can be maneuvered across the ductus into the descending aorta. The snare may also be used to secure the wire tip in the descending aorta and provide maximum wire stability for tracking balloon catheters over it during subsequent valvuloplasty (Fig. 26-7). As described in patients with critical pulmonary stenosis, serial dilations with incremental balloon diameters may be necessary for successful valvuloplasty. Postprocedure angiography is performed to assess for any injury of the tricuspid valve apparatus, RV outflow tract, main pulmonary artery, or ductus. Due to the nature of the atretic valve, free pulmonary insufficiency is present following a successful procedure. Also, at this point consideration as to whether pulmonary blood flow will require augmentation by either ductal stenting or surgical shunt placement is made, although many centers may observe patients clinically following valvuloplasty and before implanting a stent or placing a shunt. It is possible that if the right ventricle is only mildly hypoplastic and if the tricuspid valve function is normal that adequate pulmonary blood flow will have been established by the perforation/valvuloplasty procedure and that the infant may tolerate cessation of the PGE-1 infusion and closure of the ductus without the need for further catheter-based or surgical procedures.

Success of this procedure has been reported by many centers.[43,44] Complications are similar to those associated with pulmonary balloon valvuloplasty for critical pulmonary valve stenosis. Due to the anatomical variability of this defect and the variability in management between centers, reports regarding factors that may be predictive of whether secondary intervention to increase pulmonary blood flow will be necessary and if so, that can aid in determining timing for such secondary interventions are lacking. Agnoletti and colleagues reported the long-term results in 33 newborns who underwent successful perforation/valvuloplasty procedures for PA IVS. Of these patients, 50% needed surgery in the neonatal period while an additional three patients had elective surgery beyond the neonatal period for augmentation of pulmonary blood flow.[43]

Similarly, Hirata and colleagues published an analysis of 17 patients who underwent initial catheter-based valvuloplasty procedures for PA IVS; only two did not have subsequent surgery to augment pulmonary blood flow in the neonatal period.[44]

Ductal Stenting

Stenting of the ductus arteriosus to augment or maintain adequate pulmonary blood flow in newborns with cyanotic heart defects was first attempted with the introduction of coronary artery stents in the early 1990s.[45,46] However, these early cases were complicated by use of delivery systems manufactured for adult procedures that were often too large and quite difficult to maneuver in small infants. Advances in stent and catheter technologies has allowed a wider variety of stent sizes, lower profile balloons, and more flexible delivery systems, making previously very difficult and risky catheter-based therapies an alternative to surgical interventions for neonates with CHD. In many centers throughout the world, ductal stenting is utilized as an alternative first-stage palliation to surgical placement of a systemic-to-pulmonary artery shunt in neonates with cyanotic CHD.[47-49] Reports have shown that in the current era, ductal stenting may be performed with relatively low risk, especially when performed in patients with restrictive but dual-sourced pulmonary blood flow.[50] Although in many centers surgically created systemic-to-pulmonary shunts are still the treatment of choice for neonates with cyanotic CHD, others consider ductal stenting as a way to delay or avoid the need for a surgical shunt and the associated postoperative morbidities and complications that may occur. There are no definite exclusion criteria in regard to ductal morphology although most feel that a very tortuous ductus (ones making a loop of greater than 270-degree curves) or those associated with significant pulmonary artery branch stenosis should be considered poor candidates.[45,50]

The acceptance of alternative vascular access sites has further decreased the procedure-related morbidity and vascular injuries. When performed in conjunction with perforation and/or valvuloplasty of the pulmonary valve, often ductal stenting may be performed via an antegrade approach using venous access. Femoral arterial access is often used, but may not allow the appropriate-sized delivery system necessary for this procedure in very small infants. Also, a typical ductus in patients with pulmonary atresia often arises off the underside from the transverse arch and may be difficult to access from a retrograde arterial approach. Alternative access sites may include a carotid artery (accessed via cutdown approach) or axillary artery using a percutaneous approach and are typically chosen based on ductal origin and shape as well as the site that favors the straightest or most direct course toward the ductal origin from the arch.[45,48]

These procedures are typically performed under general anesthesia or deep conscious sedation with assisted ventilation. There is no consensus as to when PGE-1 infusion should be discontinued prior to stent placement. Alwi and colleagues stopped PGE-1 infusion 6-12 hours before stent implantation except in those patients who remained PGE-1 dependent with a ductus being the sole source of pulmonary blood flow or when the ductus was significantly stenotic.[45,51] Angiography is performed to demonstrate aortic arch and head vessel anatomy, and the origin and course of the ductus, as well as to further assess pulmonary artery anatomy. This may be performed using an antegrade approach from venous access or from a retrograde arterial approach. Consideration is given as to the access site that would be the most straightforward route to the ductus and if an arterial cutdown (and repair) are considered, the surgical team is called. Once the introducer sheath is in place, an end-hole catheter with a preformed curve at the tip is used to access the origin of the PDA. A floppy-tipped, torque-controlled wire is used to cross the ductus and the tip is stabilized out distal in one of the branch pulmonary arteries. Premounted, either self-expanding or balloon-expandable, coronary stents are usually chosen for ductal stenting. With the wire in place, the coronary stent is passed over the wire and positioned in the ductus. Small hand injections of contrast are usually possible via the side arm of the delivery sheath to assess stent position prior to deployment. Follow-up angiography is performed to confirm satisfactory stent placement after deployment. Additional stents may be required to cover the full extent of the ductus. Any ductal tissue not stented will be at risk of early stenosis and therefore must be stented. Additional stents are telescoped one within another

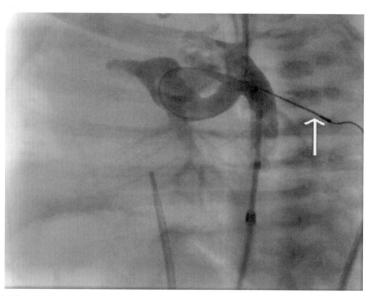

Figure 26-8 Angiography of a tortuous duct supplying the pulmonary artery. A floppy guidewire is positioned in a left lower lobe artery via the left axillary artery (*arrow*). Angiography was performed via a second catheter advanced from the right femoral artery to the proximal descending aorta.

at deployment (Figs. 26-8 through 26-11). Patients are heparinized at the beginning of the procedure once vascular access is obtained. Most continue heparin for 24-48 hours following the procedure. Long-term antiplatelet therapy with either aspirin (2-5 mg/kg/day) or clopidogrel (0.2 mg/kg/day) has been recommended.[50-52] Early restenosis of ductal stent(s) should be expected with patients presenting with a drop in systemic oxygen saturation at follow-up. Close surveillance and follow-up of these patients is imperative. Repeat cardiac catheterization is recommended when there has been a significant drop in the systemic saturations or prior to surgical intervention. In a recent report by Schranz and colleagues, ductal stenting was achieved in 58 newborns (27 of which were truly ductal-dependent) between 2003 and 2009

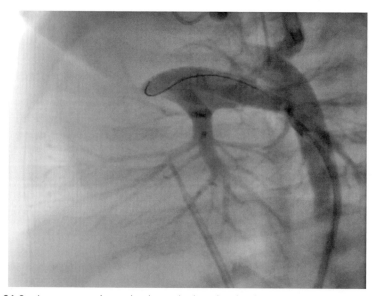

Figure 26-9 A premounted stent has been deployed in the ductus arteriosus via a retrograde approach from the femoral artery.

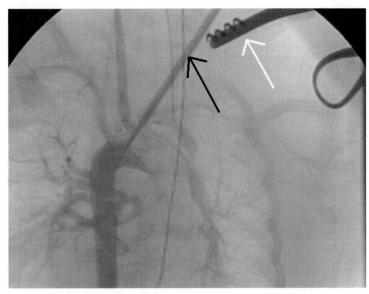

Figure 26-10 Transcarotid approach via surgical cutdown to the left common carotid in preparation for ductal stenting of a ductus off the left innominate artery in patient with tetralogy of Fallot with a right aortic arch and left pulmonary artery (LPA) arising from a left-sided patent ductus arteriosus. Black arrow points to sheath in left carotid and white arrow to surgical retractors used during carotid cutdown.

with no procedure-related mortality. Three of 27 required an acute surgical shunt and four of 24 required surgical shunts during midterm follow-up, with two others requiring stent redilation. Twenty-three patients went on to have surgical palliation or biventricular repair.[50] Similar results have been reported by others.[51,52]

Balloon Aortic Valvuloplasty in the Neonate

There is often considerable variability in the anatomy and morphology of infants born with aortic valve stenosis. Defects may range from isolated valvar stenosis with

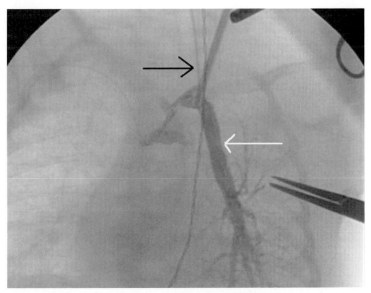

Figure 26-11 A premounted stent has been successfully deployed in the ductus arteriosus via the left carotid artery with resultant patency of the left pulmonary artery. Black arrow demonstrates carotid sheath and white arrow the stented ductus.

normal annulus size and variable valve morphologies to multiple associated left-sided obstructive lesions or variants of HLHS. When the left ventricle (LV) has been hypertensive in utero, endocardial scarring (fibrosis) may also be present, which has separate acute and long-term implications. In cases of small left heart structures associated with valvar stenosis, it is often difficult to decide on the most appropriate management plan. Decisions must first include whether the left heart structures will be able to sustain a biventricular circulation or whether univentricular palliation will be necessary. If biventricular circulation is considered, then one must decide whether to perform transcatheter balloon dilation of the valve versus surgical valvotomy. Most previous reports have shown comparable results between balloon aortic valvuloplasty (BAV) and surgical valvuloplasty with respect to primary outcomes of survival, efficacy at relieving aortic stenosis, and frequency of important complications, including aortic insufficiency (AI).[53-55] McElhinney also reported that those patients with initially small left heart structures were associated with worse subacute outcomes and that reinterventions for residual/recurrent aortic stenosis or iatrogenic AI was more common among early survivors of neonatal BAV, particularly in the first year after BAV.[53] Data obtained from the Congenital Heart Surgeons Society database showed a greater likelihood of important AI with BAV when compared with surgical valvuloplasty but residual stenosis was more often seen in the surgical group. However, mortality rate and risk of reintervention were similar.[54]

When the decision for transcatheter balloon valvuloplasty for severe or critical aortic stenosis in a neonate has been made, most procedures are performed in the cardiac catheterization laboratory under general anesthesia, although there have been reports of percutaneous aortic balloon valvuloplasty being performed at the bedside under echocardiographic guidance using a carotid artery approach.[56,57] Many of these infants present in cardiac failure and/or in a low output state, requiring mechanical ventilation, inotropic support, and PGE-1 infusion to augment systemic output via right-to-left shunting at the ductus. Aortic balloon dilation has been performed using both a prograde or retrograde approach using either venous or arterial access, respectively. Most commonly, a femoral or umbilical artery approach is utilized. Considerations regarding use of the umbilical artery include the tortuosity of the catheter course to the aortic valve compared with a more direct course from the femoral artery. However, use of the femoral artery increases risk of significant vascular injury and/or occlusion, especially in very small infants. Reports have suggested that the route from a carotid artery (retrograde) approach is most direct and improves ability (and therefore procedure time) to pass a wire across the stenotic valve orifice for subsequent balloon valvuloplasty; however, there is at least a theoretical increased risk of acute and long-term sequelae from carotid artery injury at the access site whether a percutaneous or surgical cutdown is used.[56-58] Once access has been obtained, the patient is heparinized and hemodynamic data are obtained. LV and ascending aortic angiography is performed for careful assessment of LV size and function, nature of LV outflow obstruction, aortic valve annulus size, coronary artery anatomy, and quantification of aortic insufficiency if present, and assessment of aortic arch anatomy. Next, wire position across the aortic valve is achieved, most often using a floppy-tipped, "torqueable" wire via an end-hole catheter from a retrograde approach. Once the wire is in place with the tip curled in the LV, the angioplasty catheter is passed over the wire and positioned across the valve. In contrast to the larger balloon-annulus ratios recommended for pulmonary valve dilations, a balloon-annulus ratio of 80-90% is recommended for aortic valve dilation to minimize risk of resultant AI.[59]

Recent studies report success rates for BAV of 87-97%.[60,61] A recent multicenter study by Torres and colleagues regarding aortic balloon valvuloplasty showed this procedure to be safe and effective at all ages with success rates of 87% in infants younger than 1 month of age.[62] In assessment for predictors of outcome, there were no significant predictors for patients younger than 1 month of age, although nonelective procedures and PGE-1 infusion at time of procedure tended to be associated with inadequate outcome (defined as residual gradient ≥ 45 mm Hg and ≥ 3 grade change in aortic insufficiency). For patients older than 1 month of age, a history of complex two-ventricle anatomy and prior transcatheter and/or surgical interventions was associated with inadequate outcome. In this report, high severity adverse events were more frequent in patients younger than 1 month of age (18%) versus those older than 1 month (5%) with no catastrophic events in either group. Most common severe adverse events were significant arrhythmias, pulse loss, and cardiac perforation in the neonates.[62]

Transcatheter Management for Neonatal Coarctation

Neonates with critical coarctation may present with circulatory collapse when the ductus closes. Less severe obstructions may present with congestive heart failure, systemic hypertension in the upper extremities, diminished lower extremity pulses, or symptoms secondary to other associated defects. Transcatheter therapies as primary treatment for native neonatal coarctation remain controversial. Historically, surgery has provided effective treatment for neonatal coarctation and with modifications in surgical techniques over the years; surgical treatment has been associated with low mortality and morbidity, relative freedom from aneurysm formation, and low incidence of recurrent coarctation in the neonatal population.[63] With the advent of low-profile/low pressure balloons that require smaller introducer sheaths, balloon angioplasty has been performed for both native and recurrent aortic coarctation in the neonate. In fact, many reports have concluded that balloon angioplasty should be considered as treatment of choice for all patients with postoperative recoarctation.[63-65] However, the role of balloon angioplasty for native coarctation in neonates remains controversial due to higher incidence of early restenosis, need for multiple interventions, potential serious vascular injury and limb ischemia, and incidence of aneurysm formation when compared with surgical treatment for the same diagnosis and patient population.[63-67] Furthermore, follow-up data comparing both groups up to 3 years postintervention are consistent with improved arch growth in neonates receiving surgical intervention.[63] Thus most often a primary balloon angioplasty procedure is only recommended under special circumstances and as palliative treatment for neonatal coarctation of the aorta.

Other Catheter-Based Therapies for Neonates with Congenital Heart Disease

Neonates with cyanotic heart disease who have undergone placement of aortopulmonary shunts may need emergent intervention for acute thrombosis of these shunts. Emergent balloon angioplasties of these obstructed shunts have been performed with success in reestablishing patency of the shunt.[68] There have been reports of successful stent placement in stenotic shunts to relieve life-threatening obstruction as well.[69]

Neonates with symptomatic anomalous vascular connections such as aortopulmonary collaterals, pulmonary sequestration, or congenital arteriovenous malformations often require intervention for interruption or occlusion of these connections. Historically most attempts involved surgical ligations when possible. Transcatheter occlusion is now frequently possible and can be performed safely with either coils or other vascular occlusion devices. The type of vascular connection, location, tortuosity, and flow dynamics help determine the specific technique and the type of device needed to embolize or occlude these vessels.[45]

Pulmonary arterial (PA) stenosis may occur as an isolated lesion or associated with other lesions or in conjunction with certain syndromes such as congenital rubella, Williams syndrome, and Alagille syndrome. Decisions to intervene as well as type of intervention are typically based on both echo and angiographic assessment. Often lung scintigraphy to assess relative perfusion to each lung is helpful in deciding when to intervene for isolated (one-sided) branch stenosis.[70,71] Balloon angioplasty using high-pressure angioplasty balloons in conjunction with cutting balloons is performed with variable success.[72] Stent implantation for neonates with branch pulmonary artery stenosis is typically not performed as available stents are not of appropriate size or length to be placed safely and effectively. Smaller, preloaded stents that may be technically able to be placed in neonatal PAs cannot be dilated to an appropriate adult size with somatic growth of the child and thus if implanted will require surgical intervention to treat the inevitable "restenosis" when the child is older.

Techniques on the Horizon

Biodegradable stents are definitely a much awaited technology due to the benefit of obviating surgical removal once placed. There is also the theoretical potential for subsequent growth of a vessel that has been previously stented with a biodegradable stent. These stents consist of an absorbable magnesium alloy with a novel design that allows for radial strength of the stent without measurable recoil after implantation. In animal studies complete degradation of the stents has been noted by 3 months post implantation.[73,74] There has been a case report of use of biodegradable stent in a 3-week-old with recurrent coarctation following surgical repair. Immediate relief of gradient was achieved; however, repeat intervention was required at 3 weeks after stent implant due to significant aortic obstruction at the level of the biodegradable stent.[75]

Conclusion

Therapeutic catheterization procedures are a major component in the treatment strategy for neonates with CHD. Long-term follow-up of these patients following such interventions will demonstrate the utility of these procedures in this patient population.

Acknowledgment

The author wishes to thank Dr. Qi-Ling Cao for his help with the figures.

References

1. Rashkind WJ, Miller WW. Creation of an atrial septal defect without thoracotomy: a palliative approach to complete transposition of the great arteries. JAMA. 1966;196:991.
2. Mehta R, Lee KJ, Chaturvedi R, et al. Complications of pediatric cardiac catheterization: a review in the current era. Catheter Cardiovasc Interv. 2008 1;72(2):278-285.
3. Agnolett G, Bonnet C, Boudjemline Y, et al. Complications of paediatric interventional catheterisation: an analysis of risk factors. Cardiol Young. 2005;15(4):402-408.
4. Cassidy SC, Schmidt KG, van Hare GF, et al. Complications of pediatric cardiac catheterization: a 3-year study. J Am Coll Cardiol. 1992;19:1285-1293.
5. Sapin SO, Linde LM, Emmanouilides GC. Umbilical vessel angiocardiography in the newborn infant. Pediatrics. 1963;31:946-951.
6. Giusti S, Borghi A, Redaelli S, et al. The carotid arterial approach for balloon dilation of critical aortic stenosis in neonates—immediate results and follow-up. Cardiol Young. 2008;2:155-160.
7. Schranz D, Michel-Behnke I. Axillary artery access for cardiac interventions in newborns. Ann Pediatr Cardiol. 2008;1(2):126-130.
8. Johnson JL, Fellows KE, Murphy JD. Transhepatic central venous access for cardiac catheterization and radiologic intervention. Cathet Cardiovasc Diagn. 1995;35(2):168-171.
9. Shim D, Lloyd TR, Beekman RH. Transhepatic therapeutic cardiac catheterization: a new option for the pediatric interventionalist. Catheter Cardiovasc Interv. 1999;47:41-45.
10. Davenport JJ, Lam L, Whalen-Glass R, et al. The successful use of alternative routes of vascular access for performing pediatric interventional cardiac catheterization. Catheter Cardiovasc Interv. 2008;1; 72(3):392-398.
11. Allan LD, Leanage R, Wainwright R, et al. Balloon atrial septostomy under two dimensional echocardiographic control. Br Heart J. 1982;47:41-43.
12. Zellers TM, Dixon K, Moake L, et al. Bedside balloon atrial septostomy is safe, efficacious, and cost-effective compared with septostomy performed in the cardiac catheterization laboratory. Am J Cardiol. 2002;1;89(5):613-615.
13. Mok Q, Darvell F, Mattos S, et al. Survival after balloon atrial septostomy for complete transposition of great arteries. Arch Dis Child. 1987;62:549-553.
14. Mullins CE. Balloon atrial septostomy. In: Mullins CE, ed. Cardiac catheterization in congenital heart disease: pediatric and adult. Malden, Mass: Blackwell Publishing; 2006:378-392.
15. Mukherjee D, Lindsay M, Zhang Y, et al. Analysis of 8681 neonates with transposition of the great arteries: outcomes with and without Rashkind balloon atrial septostomy. Cardiol Young. 2010;20(4): 373-380.
16. McQuillen PS, Hamrick SE, Perez MJ, et al. Balloon atrial septostomy is associated with preoperative stroke in neonates with transposition of the great arteries. Circulation. 2006;113(2):280-285.

17. McQuillen PS, Barkovich JA, Hamrick SEG, et al. Temporal and anatomic risk profile of brain injury with neonatal repair of congenital heart defects. Stroke. 2007;38:736-741.
18. Petit CJ, Rome JJ, Wernovsky G, et al. Preoperative brain injury in transposition of the great arteries is associated with oxygenation and time to surgery, not balloon atrial septostomy. Circulation. 2009;119(5):709-716.
19. Applegate SE, Lim DS. Incidence of stroke in patients with d-transposition of the great arteries that undergo balloon atrial septostomy in the University Healthsystem Consortium Clinical Data Base/Resource Manager. Catheter Cardiovasc Interv. 2010;76:129-131.
20. Beca J, Gunn J, Coleman L, et al. Pre-operative brain injury in newborn infants with transposition of the great arteries occurs at rates similar to other complex congenital heart disease and is not related to balloon atrial septostomy. J Am Coll Cardiol. 2009;53(19):1807-1811.
21. Justino H, Benson LN, Nykanen D. Transcatheter creation of an atrial septal defect using radiofrequency perforation. Cathet Cardiovasc Interv. 2001;54:83-87.
22. Du Marchie Sarvaas GJ, Trivedi KR, et al. Radiofrequency-assisted atrial septoplasty for an intact atrial septum in complex congenital heart disease. Catheter Cardiovasc Interv. 2002;56:412-415.
23. Holzer RJ, Wood A, Chisolm JL, et al. Atrial septal interventions in patients with hypoplastic left heart syndrome. Catheter Cardiovasc Interv. 2008;72(5):696-704.
24. Pedra CA, Neves JR, Pedra SR, et al. New transcatheter techniques for creation or enlargement of atrial septal defects in infants with complex congenital heart disease. Catheter Cardiovasc Interv. 2007;70:731-737.
25. Gossett J, Rocchini A, Lloyd T, et al. Catheter-based decompression of the left atrium in patients with hypoplastic left heart syndrome and restrictive atrial septum is safe and effective. Catheter Cardiovasc Interv. 2006;67:619-624.
26. Rupp S, Michel-Behnke I, Valeske K, et al. Implantation of stents to ensure an adequate interatrial communication in patients with hypoplastic left heart syndrome. Cardiol Young. 2007;17(5):535-540.
27. Leonard Jr GT, Justino H, Carlson KM, et al. Atrial septal stent implant: atrial septal defect creation in the management of complex congenital heart defects in infants. Congen Heart Dis. 2006;1(3):129-135.
28. Danon S, Levi D, Alejos J, et al. Reliable atrial septostomy by stenting of the atrial septum. Catheter Cardiovasc Interv. 2005;66:408-413.
29. Hill SL, Mizelle KM, Vellucci SM, et al. Radiofrequency perforation and cutting balloon septoplasty of intact atrial septum in a newborn with hypoplastic left heart syndrome using transesophageal ICE probe guidance. Cathet Cardiovasc Interv. 2005;64:214-217.
30. Berman W, Fripp RR, Raisher BD, et al. Significant pulmonary valve incompetence following oversize balloon pulmonary valveplasty in small infants: a long-term follow-up study. Cathet Cardiovasc Intervent. 1999;48(1):61-65.
31. Velvis H, Raines KH, Bensky AS, et al. Growth of the right heart after balloon valvuloplasty for critical pulmonary stenosis in the newborn. Am J Cardiol. 1997;79:982-984.
32. Holzer R, Kreutzer J, Hirsch R, et al. Balloon pulmonary valvuloplasty prospective analysis of procedure related adverse events and immediate outcome—results from a multicenter registry. Cathet Cardiovasc Intervent. 2010;76:S3-S36.
33. Akagi T, Benson LN, Williams WG, et al. Ventriculo-coronary arterial connections in pulmonary atresia with intact ventricular septum, and their influences on ventricular performance and clinical course. Am J Cardiol. 1993;72:586-590.
34. Hanley FL, Sade RM, Blackstone EH, et al. Outcomes in neonatal pulmonary atresia with intact ventricular septum: a multiinstitutional study. J Thorac Cardiovasc Surg. 1993;105:406-423.
35. Guleserian KJ, Armsby LB, Thiagarajan RR, et al. Natural history of pulmonary atresia with intact ventricular septum and right-ventricle-dependent coronary circulation managed by the single-ventricle approach. Ann Thorac Surg. 2006;81(6):2250-2257.
36. Walsh MA, Lee KJ, Chaturvedi R, et al. Radiofrequency perforation of the right ventricular outflow tract as a palliative strategy for pulmonary atresia with ventricular septal defect. Catheter Cardiovasc Interv. 2007;69(7):1015-1020.
37. Latson L. Nonsurgical treatment of a neonate with pulmonary atresia and intact ventricular septum by transcatheter puncture and balloon dilation of the atretic valve membrane. Am J Cardiol. 1991;68(2):277-279.
38. Gournay V, Piechaud JF, Delogu A, et al. Balloon valvotomy for critical stenosis or atresia of pulmonary valve in newborns. J Am Coll Cardiol. 1995;26:1725-1731.
39. Parsons JM, Rees MR, Gibbs JL. Percutaneous laser valvotomy with balloon dilatation of the pulmonary valve as primary treatment for pulmonary atresia. Br Heart J. 1991;66(1):36-38.
40. Qureshi SA, Rosenthal E, Tynan M, et al. Transcatheter laser-assisted balloon pulmonary valve dilation in pulmonic valve atresia. Am J Cardiol. 1991;67(5):428-431.
41. Hausdorf G, Schulze-Neick I, Lange PE. Radiofrequency-assisted "reconstruction" of the right ventricular outflow tract in muscular pulmonary atresia with ventricular septal defect. Br Heart J. 1993;69:343-346.
42. Asnes JD, Fahey JT. Novel catheter positioning technique for atretic pulmonary valve perforation. Cathet Cardiovasc Interv. 2008;71:850-852.
43. Agnoletti G, Piechaud JF, Bonhoeffer P, et al. Perforation of the atretic pulmonary valve. Long-term follow-up. J Am Coll Cardiol. 2003;41:1399-1403.
44. Hirata Y, Chen J, Quaegebeur J, et al. Pulmonary atresia with intact ventricular septum: limitations of catheter-based intervention. Ann Thorac Surg. 2007;84:574-580.

E

45. Kutty S, Zahn E. Interventional therapy for neonates with critical congenital heart disease. Cathet Cardiovasc Interv. 2008;72:663-674.

46. Coe JY, Olley PM. A novel method to maintain ductus arteriosus patency. J Am Coll Cardiol. 1991;18:837-841.

47. Santoro G, Gaio G, Palladino MT, Iacono C, et al. Stenting of the arterial duct in newborns with duct-dependent pulmonary circulation. Heart. 2008;94(7):925-929.

48. Mahesh K, Kannan BR, Vaidyanathan B, et al. Stenting the patent arterial duct to increase pulmonary blood flow. Indian Heart J. 2005;57(6):704-708.

49. Schneider M, Zartner P, Sidiropoulos A, et al. Stent implantation of the arterial duct in newborns with duct-dependent circulation. Eur Heart J. 1998;19(9):1401-1409.

50. Schranz, D, Michel-Behenke I, Heyer R, et al. Stent implantation of the arterial duct in newborns with a truly duct-dependent pulmonary circulation: a single-center experience with emphasis on aspects of the interventional technique. J Intervent Cardiol. 2010;23:581-588.

51. Alwi M, Choo KK, Latiff HA, et al. Initial results and medium-term follow-up of stent implantation of patent ductus arteriosus in duct-dependent pulmonary circulation. J Am Coll Cardiol. 2004;44:438-445.

52. Gibbs JL, Uzun O, Blackburn ME, et al. Fate of the stented arterial duct. Circulation. 1999;99: 1621-2625.

53. McElhinney D, Lock J, Keane J, et al. Left heart growth, function, and reintervention after balloon aortic valvuloplasty for neonatal aortic stenosis. Circulation. 2005;111;451-458.

54. McCrindle BW, Blackstone EH, Williams WG, et al. Are outcomes of surgical versus transcatheter balloon valvotomy equivalent in neonatal critical aortic stenosis? Circulation. 2001;104(suppl I):152-158.

55. Mosca RS, Iannettoni MD, Schwartz SM, et al. Critical aortic stenosis in the neonate: a comparison of balloon valvuloplasty and transventricular dilation. J Thorac Cardiovasc Surg. 1995;109:147-154.

56. Weber HS. Catheter management of aortic valve stenosis in neonates and children. Catheter Cardiovasc Interv. 2006;67(6):947-955.

57. Weber HS, Mart CR, Myers JL. Transcarotid balloon valvuloplasty for critical aortic valve stenosis at the bedside via continuous transesophageal echocardiographic guidance. Catheter Cardiovasc Interv. 2000;50(3):326-329.

58. Fischer DR, Ettedgui JA, Park SC, et al. Carotid artery approach for balloon dilation of aortic valve stenosis in the neonate: a preliminary report. J Am Coll Cardiol. 1990;15:1633-1636.

59. Sholler GF, Keane JF, Perry SB, et al. Balloon dilation of congenital aortic valve stenosis: results and influence of technical and morphological features on outcome. Circulation. 1988;78:351-360.

60. Lofland GK, McCrindle BW, Williams WG, et al. Critical aortic stenosis in the neonate: a multi-institutional study of management, outcomes, and risk factors; Congenital Heart Surgeons Society. J Thorac Cardiovasc Surg. 2001;121:10-27.

61. Han RK, Gurofsky RC, Lee KJ, et al. Outcome and growth potential of left heart structures after neonatal intervention for aortic valve stenosis. J Am Coll Cardiol. 2007;50(25):2406-2414.

62. Torres A, Bergersen L, Marshal AL, et al. Aortic balloon valvuloplasty in the 21st century: procedural success, efficacy and adverse events: results of a multicenter registry (C3PO). Circulation. 2010;122:A14392.

63. Fiore AC, Fischer LK, Schwartz T, et al. Comparison of angioplasty and surgery for neonatal aortic coarctation. Ann Thorac Surg. 2005;80(5):1659-1664.

64. Dilawar M, El Said H, El-Sisi A , et al. Safety and efficacy of low-profile balloons in native coarctation and recoarctation balloon angioplasty for infants. Pediatr Cardiol. 2009;30:404-408.

65. Früh S, Knirsch W, Dodge-Khatami A, et al. Comparison of surgical and interventional therapy of native and recurrent aortic coarctation regarding different age groups during childhood. Eur J Cardiothorac Surg. 2011;39:898-904.

66. Rodés-Cabau J, Miró J, Dancea A, et al. Comparison of surgical and transcatheter treatment for native coarctation of the aorta in patients > or = 1 year old. The Quebec Native Coarctation of the Aorta study. Am Heart J. 2007;154:186-192.

67. Cowley CG, Orsmond GS, Feola P, et al. Long-term randomized comparison of balloon angioplasty and surgery for native coarctation of the aorta in childhood. Circulation. 2005;111(25):3453-3456.

68. Sreeram N, Emmel M, Ben-Mime L, et al. Transcatheter recanalization of acutely occluded modified systemic to pulmonary artery shunts in infancy. Clin Res Cardiol. 2008;97(3):181-186.

69. Lee KJ, Humpl T, Hashmi A, et al. Restoration of aortopulmonary shunt patency. Am J Cardiol. 2001;88:325-328.

70. Geggel RL, Gauvreau K, Lock JE. Balloon dilation angioplasty of peripheral pulmonary stenosis associated with Williams syndrome. Circulation. 2001;103(17):2165-2170.

71. Kannan BRJ, Qureshi SA. Catheterisation laboratory is the place for rehabilitating the pulmonary arteries. Ann Pediatr Cardiol. 2008;1(2):107-113.

72. Gentles TL, Lock JE, Perry SB. High pressure balloon angioplasty for branch pulmonary artery stenosis: early experience. J Am Coll Cardiol. 1993;22:867-872.

73. Heublein B, Rohde R, Kaese V, et al. Biocorrosion of magnesium alloys: a new principle in cardiovascular implant technology. Heart. 2003;89:651-656.

74. Di Mario C, Griffiths H, Goktekin O, et al. Drug-eluting bioabsorbable magnesium stent. J Interv Cardiol. 2004;17:391-395.

75. Schranz D, Zartner P, Michel-Behnke I, et al. Bioabsorbable metal stents for percutaneous treatment of critical recoarctation of the aorta in a newborn. Catheter Cardiovasc Interv. 2006;67:671-673.

CHAPTER 27

Hybrid Management Techniques in the Treatment of the Neonate with Congenital Heart Disease

Damien Kenny, MD, Mark Galantowicz, MD,
John P. Cheatham, MD, and Ziyad M. Hijazi, MD, MPH

- **Hypoplastic Left Heart Syndrome**
- **Perventricular Ventricular Septal Defect Closure**
- **Adjustable Pulmonary Artery Bands**
- **Intraoperative Angiocardiography**
- **Conclusion**
- **References**

Management strategies for congenital heart disease in the neonate have evolved significantly over the last 3 decades. With advancement in both the technology and understanding of cardiopulmonary bypass, cardiac surgery is now routine in the neonatal period for conditions such as transposition of the great arteries, hypoplastic left heart syndrome, and total anomalous pulmonary venous drainage. Transcatheter interventional approaches have also grown exponentially with development of low-profile balloons for balloon valvuloplasty and radiofrequency energy for the intact atrial septum and the imperforate pulmonary valve. However, both surgery and transcatheter approaches have drawbacks. Surgery is maximally invasive, and cardiopulmonary bypass surgery in the neonatal period may have subtle effects on longer term neurodevelopmental outcomes. Transcatheter approaches are limited by access issues with delivery of occlusion devices or stents requiring relatively large delivery sheaths that are not maneuverable around small hearts. Thus increasingly the surgeon and the interventionalist are working together to maximize the benefits and minimize the limitations of each of their respective approaches. It is in this setting that the "hybrid" approach to congenital heart disease has evolved. These hybrid procedures include perventricular ventricular septal defect closure, and branch pulmonary artery banding with stenting of the arterial duct used to palliate neonates with hypoplastic left heart syndrome. Collaboration in this setting provides the interventionalist and surgeon with direct access to the heart and avoids the need for cardiopulmonary bypass. This chapter describes a number of these procedures, both established and evolving, and also diagnostic evaluation of immediate postoperative anatomy with intraoperative angiography. Such cooperation between surgeons and interventional cardiologists is likely to provide a cornerstone of patient management in the future of pediatric cardiology.

Hypoplastic Left Heart Syndrome

Historical Perspective

Wide anatomical variability is seen within hypoplastic left heart syndrome (HLHS); however, the condition is generally characterized by underdevelopment of the left heart rendering it unable to support the systemic circulation. Definitive treatment

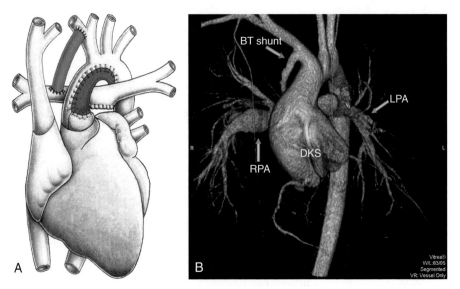

Figure 27-1 The Norwood procedure was proposed as a three-stage surgical palliation for newborns with hypoplastic left heart syndrome (HLHS) over 30 years ago. Stage 1 palliation is the most challenging and carries the greatest risk. **A,** The cartoon depicts the reconstructed aorta (blue), as well as the right modified Blalock–Taussig shunt (red) connecting the aorta to the right and left pulmonary arteries. **B,** A 3D rotational angiogram (3DRA) that has been reconstructed and nicely correlates these features. DKS, Damus-Kaye-Stansel; LPA, left pulmonary artery; RPA, right pulmonary artery. (See Expert Consult site for color image.)

strategies evolved with the introduction of the three-stage Norwood procedure in 1983 (Fig. 27-1); since then a plethora of surgical variations of, or alternatives to, the Norwood approach have been described, predominantly aimed at reducing the significant persistent mortality associated with stage 1 palliation and interstage follow-up that exists with this condition.[1-4] Despite many innovative approaches designed to address the major suspected culprits leading to mortality, namely inconsistent adequate coronary artery perfusion and right ventricle failure, survival is consistently reported between 65% and 70% at 5 years.[5,6] Even a modern day cohort of neonates with HLHS randomized into Norwood or Sano surgical palliation carries a heavy mortality burden at 2 years.[7] Within the cohort of survivors, concerns have been raised regarding longer term neurological developmental outcomes secondary to prolonged cardiopulmonary bypass with circulatory arrest in the neonatal period.[8] It is within this historical context that the hybrid approach to the treatment of HLHS evolved. The main caveats to this approach were to maintain adequate perfusion pressure to the systemic circulation across the arterial duct following the natural reduction in pulmonary vascular resistance after birth. The precursors to achieving this were supported by initial technical experience with stenting the arterial duct to maintain pulmonary circulation in the setting of pulmonary atresia.[9] Subsequently, this approach was employed in the setting of HLHS as a bridge to transplantation.[10] Although this strategy achieved its short-term goal, exclusive stenting of the arterial duct would eventually lead to pulmonary overflow and "steal" from the systemic circulation and thus further modifications were necessary for longer term palliation. The first complete hybrid palliative approach to HLHS was described in 1993 by Gibbs and colleagues, with surgical banding of the branch pulmonary arteries and percutaneous stenting of the arterial duct.[11] This was coupled with either surgical or percutaneous decompression of the left atrium by opening the atrial septum. Thus the three main physiological objectives of HLHS palliation, namely unobstructed systemic output, balanced pulmonary circulation, and an unrestrictive atrial communication, were addressed. Although there was no procedural mortality, two of the four patients died within 2 weeks due to excessive pulmonary blood flow and subsequent right ventricular failure, with prolonged hospitalization of the third patient due to similar concerns. Subsequent reports of extended experience with longer term follow-up from the same group confirmed these initial concerns, with no survivors beyond 30 months from all eight patients palliated with this approach.[12] The major cited reason for demise in five of the eight patients was pulmonary overcirculation with subsequent right ventricular failure. It was not clear from this report whether there were consistent targets for determining effective pulmonary artery banding; however, it was clear that pulmonary overcirculation was not tolerated in this group. Further experience with the hybrid approach was not described until 2002 when the group from Giessen reported clearer preprocedural targets for the tightness of the pulmonary artery band with the goal to achieve distal pulmonary artery pressures less than 50% of systemic pressures, confirmed by Doppler velocities of greater than 4 m/s across the bands and reduction in systemic oxygen saturations to approximately 80%.[13] Ten of the 11 patients survived to a stage 2 procedure, which was heart transplantation in two and a modified Norwood procedure in the remaining eight patients. There was one intraoperative death with overall survival through stage 2 of 82%. A further report from this group with experience in 58 patients confirmed these survival figures.[14] Interestingly the initial approach adopted by this group consisted of percutaneous ductal stenting followed by surgical pulmonary artery banding within 72 hours; however, stent dislodgment occurred in two patients due to manipulation at the time of surgery, and this approach was reversed so as to perform the pulmonary artery banding in the operating room followed by ductal stenting with either balloon-expandable or self-expanding stents depending on the duct morphology. During this same time period, other investigators (the Columbus group) were attempting to achieve pulmonary artery flow restriction and unobstructed flow to the systemic circulation exclusively via a transcatheter approach.[15] This involved deployment of custom-designed nitinol flow restrictors in the pulmonary arteries; however, delivery was associated with significant hemodynamic instability and this approach was abandoned. This group further evolved their practice to describe the first truly hybrid approach to HLHS with surgeon and interventionalist working side by side to band the pulmonary arteries and stent the arterial duct through the pulmonary artery with further transcatheter intervention to the atrial septum performed as a separate procedure if necessary (Fig. 27-2).[15] This group subsequently published their extended experience of 40 neonates with

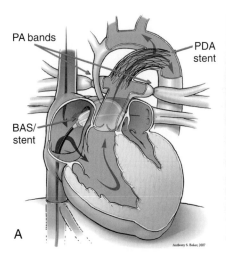
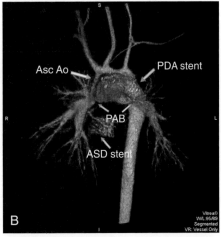

Figure 27-2 The hybrid stage 1 palliation. **A,** A cartoon demonstrates LPA and RPA bands, a PDA stent, and either balloon atrial septostomy (BAS) and/or stent implantation to create an unobstructed outlet from the left atrium. **B,** A reconstructed 3DRA demonstrating all of these components, including a stent in the atrial septum. 3DRA, three-dimensional rotational angiography; Asc Ao, ascending aorta; ASD, atrial septal defect; LPA, left pulmonary artery; PA, pulmonary artery; PAB, pulmonary artery bands; PDA, patent ductus arteriosus; RPA, right pulmonary artery. (See Expert Consult site for color image.)

Table 27-1 OUTLINES COMPARATIVE OUTCOMES OF PUBLISHED SERIES LOOKING AT HYBRID PALLIATION FOR HYPOPLASTIC LEFT HEART SYNDROME

Authors	Year	Patient Number	Predischarge Mortality	Interstage Mortality	Survival Post Stage 2*
Gibbs[12]	1999	8	63%	13%	0%
Akintuerk[13]	2002	11	0%	9%	82%
Galantowicz[15]	2005	29	17%	7%	59%
Bacha[21]	2006	14	23%	29%	50%
Akintuerk[14]	2007	58	3.4%	9%	83%
Caldarone[59]	2007	18	17%	0%	68%
Galantowicz[16]	2008	40	2.5%	5%	83%
Pizarro[60]	2008	14	21%	14%	43%
Pilla[61]	2008	15	60%	7%	7%
Venugopal[25]	2010	21	38%	5%	53%

*Includes comprehensive stage 2, heart transplant, or biventricular repair depending on the series.

this approach with 83% survival.[16] This included 15 patients through stage 3 palliation. Since this time, the hybrid approach to HLHS has evolved into a distinct management strategy with published reports on how to approach atrial septal interventions, the retrograde aortic arch, and anesthetic and enteral feeding management of these patients.[17-20] Controversy still exists whether this approach should be offered as an alternative to Norwood surgery or limited to neonates in whom surgery has proved to be substantially higher risk.[21]

Triumphs and Pitfalls

Although Honjo and colleagues reported a single-center nonrandomized series of neonatal Norwood (n = 39) and hybrid palliations (n = 19) with similar 1-year survival in both groups (70%), without definitive comparative trials, it is not possible to compare the longer-term outcomes of the hybrid approach with standard stage 1 surgery for HLHS.[22] Extensive experience now exists in many centers with surgical palliation whereas the hybrid approach represents a new endeavor and thus direct comparison is meaningless. Survival in the hybrid cohort varies significantly (Table 27-1) and operator experience and comorbidities of the neonates involved are undoubtedly contributory. However, certain cohorts (birthweight less than 2.5 kg, severe right ventricular dysfunction, intact or restrictive atrial septum, prematurity, associated severe noncardiac genetic abnormalities, intracerebral hemorrhage, and postnatal collapse with a pH less than 7) have been identified as high risk for surgical palliation with surgical stage 1 mortality rates of over 60% and the hybrid approach may represent a realistic alternative to cardiopulmonary bypass in these patients.[23,24] This initial approach was reported by Bacha and colleagues in 14 high-risk neonates with an overall post–stage 2 mortality of 50%.[21] A subsequent report from London mirrored these figures with nine of 16 "high-risk" infants surviving stage 2 surgery; thus it appears that mortality is significant in these high-risk infants regardless of approach.[25] The potential benefit of the hybrid approach on neurodevelopmental delay by avoiding the consequence of prolonged cardiopulmonary bypass and deep hypothermic circulatory arrest in neonatal life is unclear. However, studies are ongoing to assess transcranial Doppler flows and developmental outcomes in a cohort of infants following hybrid palliation (Personal communication with Sharon L. Hill, ACNP, PhDc, Nationwide Children's Hospital).

One of the potential benefits of the hybrid approach to HLHS is a less invasive strategy to assess potential growth of left heart structures in cases of borderline left ventricular size. This potential was initially reported by the group from Giessen with four of 18 patients demonstrating left ventricular growth after the hybrid procedure and subsequent biventricular repair.[15] A further small series from London demonstrated that three of seven patients achieved a functioning biventricular circulation following hybrid palliation.[26] Neither of these studies identified prospective indices predictive of left ventricular growth; however, the hybrid approach offers the opportunity for serial echocardiography and or magnetic resonance imaging to determine if left heart structures are growing. It is worth noting that a cohort of patients undergoing biventricular repair from both studies developed severe pulmonary hypertension as a consequence of poor left ventricular diastolic compliance and the longer term effects of this strategy require careful evaluation.

The hybrid approach to HLHS is fraught with potential complications and a steep learning curve has been reported. A successful approach must always focus intently on providing balanced pulmonary blood flow and must alleviate any obstruction across the aorta and atrial septum. One of the significant intraprocedural and interstage risks with the hybrid approach is obstruction to the retrograde aortic arch with ductal stenting. In cases of aortic atresia, both the coronary and cerebral circulations are dependent on retrograde aortic arch flow and supply may be through a diminutive ostium closure to the aortic end of the arterial duct (Fig. 27-3). The incidence of development of an interstage retrograde aortic arch obstruction has been reported at 24%.[18] Moreover, recent attempts at identifying echocardiographic/angiographic features of the angle of takeoff of the retrograde aortic arch from the patent ductus arteriosus (PDA) have been reported and may lead to better patient selection.[27] If retrograde flow obstruction is recognized before hybrid stage 1 palliation, a traditional surgical approach should be considered. However, an alternative approach has been described including a prophylactic main pulmonary artery to innominate artery shunt ("reverse Blalock-Taussig shunt") during stage 1 palliation (Fig. 27-4).[28] Indeed, stenting of the arterial duct in all cases requires accurate stent placement as undersizing of the stent length may lead to recoarctation of the aorta, also affecting retrograde as well as antegrade flow. Use of an open-cell self-expanding stent (SES) is now preferred by many centers, since obstruction of the aortic arch may be less likely with an open-cell design and also easier to treat. The use of balloon-expandable PDA (BES) stents are usually reserved when there is PDA stenosis and/or when the variable length of the BES is better suited to the PDA.

The final procedural objective is providing unrestrictive flow across the atrial septum (Fig. 27-5). Transcatheter fenestration of the septum may be challenging due to bowing of a thickened septum into the right atrium with a hypoplastic left atrium. Creation of an adequate opening may require initial transeptal or radiofrequency perforation (if intact), followed by static balloon and/or cutting balloon atrial septoplasty, or stenting of the thickened atrial septum. However, repeat interventions may be necessary in up to 20% of patients and major adverse events have been reported in 9% of cases.[17]

Further concerns with the hybrid approach relate to distortion of the pulmonary arteries following banding. If present this may impact upon the functionality of the eventual total cavopulmonary connection in which an unobstructed pulmonary circuit is essential to effective flow. However, angiographic and hemodynamic measurements have not demonstrated any difference in pulmonary artery growth when comparing the hybrid approach with standard Norwood stage 1.[22]

Future Potential

Significant variability exists in the pre-, peri- and postoperative management of HLHS, reflecting both the wide anatomical variations of the syndrome and the need to maximize adequate coronary perfusion and longer-term right ventricular function.[29] The hybrid approach is a relatively recent addition to these management strategies and in a short time has become a realistic alternative to stage 1 surgical palliation with at least comparable results in a similar cohort of patients. Technical refinements have been made and taught to others in an international forum of experts and attendees, which has shortened the natural learning curve expected in a new procedure or technique. With ongoing progress with early fetal recognition

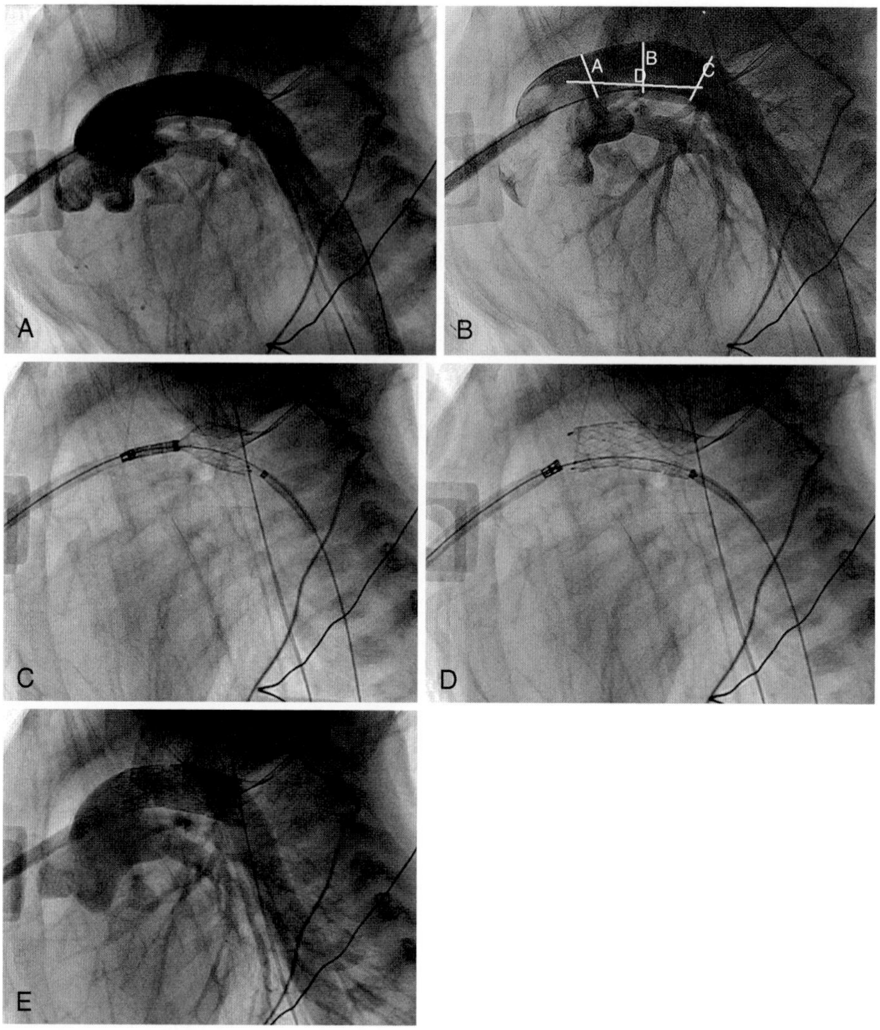

Figure 27-3 Either self-expandable (SES) or balloon-expandable stents (BES) can be used to maintain patency of the patent ductus arteriosus (PDA). In a hybrid setting and after the left pulmonary artery and right pulmonary artery bands have been placed via a small median sternotomy off cardiopulmonary bypass, an angiogram is performed through a short sheath placed directly into the main pulmonary artery above the valve and after a guidewire has been placed through the PDA into the descending aorta **(A).** Using a calibration tool, the PDA diameter is measured at the pulmonary entrance, the mid portion, at the aortic end, as well as the length required to cover the entire PDA **(B).** An SES was chosen because there was no evidence of PDA stenosis and is deployed **(C** and **D).** A final angiogram is performed after deployment to demonstrate the stent covering the entire length of the PDA, as well as the pulmonary artery bands and retrograde aortic flow **(E).**

and intervention for the borderline left ventricle, hybrid therapy may become part of this management strategy to strive for biventricular repair in these patients. In more severe forms of HLHS, achieving a fully palliated circulation requiring only one surgery bridged on either side with initial complete transcatheter neonatal management and following surgery, transcatheter completion of the total cavopulmonary circulation, is still a realistic goal. In the meantime meticulous attention to patient selection and preparation, with precise perioperative monitoring to ensure adequate organ perfusion, and frequent postprocedural follow-up to identify and intervene early on any hemodynamic obstruction are essential for progress. It is possible that with well designed collaborative studies a more patient-selective treatment strategy will emerge where the different subtypes of HLHS are better matched

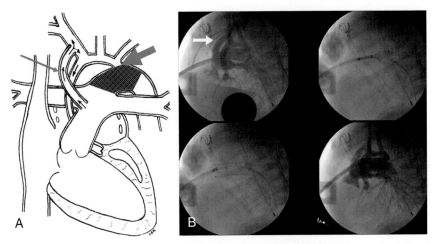

Figure 27-4 If aortic atresia is present and there is concern about adequacy of retrograde aortic arch flow through the stented patent ductus arteriosus (PDA) (*large red arrow*), a "reverse right modified BT shunt" (*smaller red arrow*) has been proposed by the team at Toronto Sick Children's Hospital. The pulmonary artery (PA) bands are not demonstrated in this image **(A)**. **B,** A series of four angiograms nicely demonstrate the PA bands, the PDA stent, and reverse BT shunt (*white arrow*). (See Expert Consult site for color image.)

with the interventional options (Hybrid, Norwood, Sano, or transplant) based on outcome measures.

Perventricluar Ventricular Septal Defect Closure

Ventricular septal defects (VSDs) account for 30% of all congenital heart disease. Larger defects require intervention in early infancy to prevent progressive congestive cardiac failure and eventual pulmonary vascular disease. Historically, intervention to close these lesions involved cardiopulmonary bypass and surgical patching of the

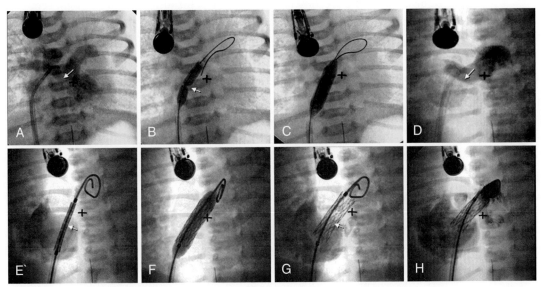

Figure 27-5 Series of images outlining balloon dilatation and stenting of the interatrial septum in the setting of hypoplastic left heart syndrome. **A,** Initial angiogram demonstrates a small left atrium with dilated pulmonary veins and a severely restricted atrial septum (white arrow). Balloon dilatation of this area **(B)** confirms the tiny communication with resolution of the waist following further dilatation with a cutting balloon **(C)**. The communication, however, remains restrictive **(D,** white arrow) and thus a balloon-expandable stent is placed across the atrial septum **(E-G)** with creation of unrestrictive flow from the left atrium on angiography **(H)**.

defect. However, with the introduction of the Amplatzer family of nitinol occlusion devices, transcatheter closure of ventricular septal defects has become an established therapeutic alternative to surgery.[30,31] The percutaneous approach, however, requires relatively large, stiff delivery sheaths and cables and is not suitable for smaller infants requiring VSD closure. To circumvent these access issues in smaller infants, Amin and colleagues described a perventricular approach for closure of both membranous and muscular VSDs in both an animal model and subsequently a human infant.[32,33] The cited benefits of this approach were direct access to the heart following surgical sternotomy with echocardiography-guided placement of the device across the VSD without the need for cardiopulmonary bypass or ionizing radiation. Initial complications rates were low with complete closure of all muscular defects. Residual flow was seen following membranous occlusion in three of five animals and one went on to develop aortic regurgitation. Subsequent studies followed confirming these outcomes either in isolated VSDs or when occurring in conjunction with other congenital cardiac lesions.[34-36] Of a total of 47 collective attempted procedures, a perventricular device was placed in 40 patients. Twenty-one of these patients weighed 6 kg or less at the time of the procedure. In one of these studies evaluating exclusive muscular VSD closure in small infants, residual shunting requiring pulmonary artery banding was seen in two of eight patients. Attempts at perventricular membranous VSD closure using robotically assisted surgery has also been described.[37] However, due to difficulty with device delivery and presence of residual leaks with concerns for device impingement on the aortic valve leaflets, further developments of this approach have not been reported. Experience with alternative occlusion devices, namely the CardioSEAL Occluder, have also been published, with successful deployment of the device in four of five attempted cases.[38] There was one device failure with the arms of the device protruding through the right ventricular free wall in a 4-kg neonate, necessitating surgical removal of the device.

The approach to perventricular VSD closure in the neonate is demonstrated in Figure 27-6. Good intraprocedural imaging is particularly important both prior to and during device deployment and either transesophageal or epicardial echocardiography may be used. The location and relationship of the VSD to the apex of the heart, the tricuspid valve, and the mitral valve apparatus are noted. In general, a device 1-2 mm larger than the maximum defect size measured in at least two planes using color Doppler is chosen. Measurement of the distance from the right ventricular free wall to the posterior wall of the left ventricle may also be helpful to ensure the sheath is not advanced too far with the risk of perforation of the left ventricular wall. The intended puncture site of the right ventricular free wall may vary according to VSD location. Once the device is deployed, careful evaluation for residual shunting and presence of worsening tricuspid or mitral regurgitation should be performed. Direct comparisons with surgical closure have not been carried out; however, the avoidance of cardiopulmonary bypass and its consequent effects have usually translated into immediate postprocedural extubation without the need for inotropic support and early hospital discharge. Longer term evaluation of the impact of these rigid devices on ventricular function are awaited; however, anecdotal experience has not indicated any deleterious effects to date.

Adjustable Pulmonary Artery Bands

Restriction of excessive pulmonary blood flow secondary to left-to-right shunting may be achieved by placing a surgical band around the main pulmonary artery and this strategy has been employed as a palliation for a number of congenital heart defects since its initial description in 1952.[39] Pulmonary artery banding (PAB) has also been carried out in the setting of transposition of the great arteries as a means of "retraining" the systemic ventricle prior to surgical correction.[40] This strategy in both circumstances has proved effective, although with advances in neonatal cardiac surgery, primary repair when achievable is often preferred to palliation. In cases of complex congenital cardiac defects, however, this is not possible and hence PAB remains an important therapeutic procedure in the management of these infants.

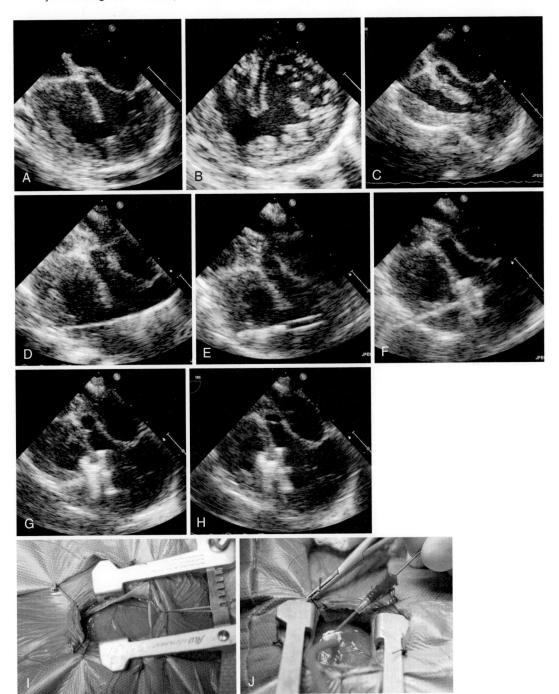

Figure 27-6 Series of images demonstrating perventricular closure of a large muscular ventricular septal defect in a 4.6-kg infant. The defect is imaged in two different planes (**A** and **B**) with the site of proposed ventricular puncture indicated by digital pressure on the right ventricular wall (**C**). Once the wire is across the defect (**D**), the sheath is advanced into the left ventricle and the device advanced through the sheath (**E**). Initially the left ventricular disc is deployed (**F**) followed by the right ventricular disk (**G**), with the device sitting in a good position across the defect following release (**H**). The surgeon's and interventionalist's view of the heart following sternotomy is seen (**I**) with advancement of the guidewire following needle puncture (**J**). (See Expert Consult site for color image.)

The main problem encountered with PAB is the difficulty in determining the appropriate "tightness" of the band to achieve a balanced circulation. Excessive restriction will lead to right-to-left shunting and cyanosis whereas the opposite approach will allow too much pulmonary blood flow with clinical heart failure and the potential for damage to the distal pulmonary vasculature. These problems are compounded by growth as the neonate may double or even triple in weight before a further procedure is required and therefore an adequate band may evolve into an overly restrictive band over the course of the first few months of life. Mathematical formulas have been reported to adapt the diameter of the PAB to the child's size; however, these formulas cannot fully encompass the varying physiological parameters controlling pulmonary blood flow in each individual. According to Poiseuille's law, flow is inversely proportional to the fourth power of the radius and therefore minute changes in vessel diameter may significantly amplify variations in blood flow.[41] In addition, variability in large artery compliance and distal resistance may exist in both the pulmonary and systemic circulations and therefore alter flow dynamics. It is in this setting that the pursuit of an adjustable pulmonary artery band evolved. In order to be effective this band would require bidirectional adjustment capabilities through noncontact means. Initial reports began in the early 1960s with more extensive reports with percutaneous adjustable bands published in the early 1980s.[42] However, each required skin incision or manipulation of a subcutaneous reservoir or screw mechanism to alter the band tightness.[43-45] A flow regulator with bidirectional functionality was subsequently described; however, attempts with devices adjustable through remote or noncontact means were initially disappointing due to device failure.[46,47] In 2002, a new telemetrically controlled device implantation was reported in a 1-month-old female with unbalanced atrioventricular septal defect.[48] This FloWatch device (Fig. 27-7) was successfully adjusted on a number of occasions in the postoperative period under echocardiographic guidance to assess effects of alterations on estimated pulmonary blood flow. The device consists of three functional parts: the box, the piston, and the counterpiece. The box is the core of the device containing a small motor and an antenna able to receive signal from the remote antenna. The motor drives the piston which compresses or decompresses the pulmonary artery. The counterpiece is closed around the pulmonary artery forming a ring. Further clinical experience with this device was reported in 2004 in 13 children aged 6 days to 11 years with a median weight of 4.2 kg.[49] The device functioned well and there were no device-related complications. A mean of 5.8 telemetric regulations to the device were required per patient to adjust tightening of the PAB according to clinical needs. The device was easily removed with spontaneous reexpansion of the pulmonary artery, which is in contrast to the fibrous restriction often induced by standard PAB. Further reports have described improved outcomes in young infants with complex atrioventricular septal defects using an adjustable banding strategy compared with standard PAB.[50] In this report, 10 of 13 patients undergoing standard PAB died. In comparison, none of the seven patients with the adjustable PAB died, and five progressed to PA debanding and surgical repair. There were no device-related complications in this cohort; however, two reports of pseudoaneurysm of the pulmonary artery following implantation of the FloWatch PAB have been reported. Although this technology is promising, further monitoring for this complication is warranted.[51,52]

Intraoperative Angiocardiography

Advancement in pediatric cardiac surgical techniques has given rise to repair of increasingly complex congenital heart lesions. This may involve complicated reconstructions and anastomoses of very small vessels. The direct and indirect hemodynamic impact of these interventions is not immediately evident to the surgeon until blood flow is restored to the heart. Vessel stenosis, due either to obstruction at the site of the suture lines or secondary to distortion of the anatomical course of the vessel may impact upon postoperative morbidity and the need for early postoperative invasive investigation and or intervention associated with overall mortality rates

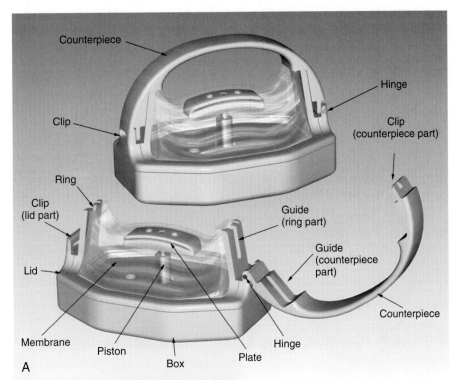

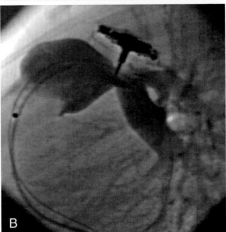

Figure 27-7 **A,** Description of the FloWatch-PAB, which comprises three distinct functional parts. The box contains a small motor, an antenna to receive the signal sent by the external antenna, and electronics to interpret the signal and drive the motor. The piston compresses or decompresses the pulmonary artery. It originates from the box through the lid and terminates with a plate that is glued to a silicone membrane. This silicone membrane is inserted and glued between the lid and a ring that goes around the device. This membrane stretches when the piston moves up and regains its original position when the piston moves down. The counterpiece is designed to close around the pulmonary artery. The dimensions of the device are 26 mm (length) × 18 mm (width) × 18 mm (height). According to Trusler's rule, the device should theoretically be suitable for PAB in patients from 3 to 10 kg of body weight. **B,** Lateral angiogram of the right ventricular outflow tract with the device seen in position providing adequate banding of the main pulmonary artery. (See Expert Consult site for color image.)

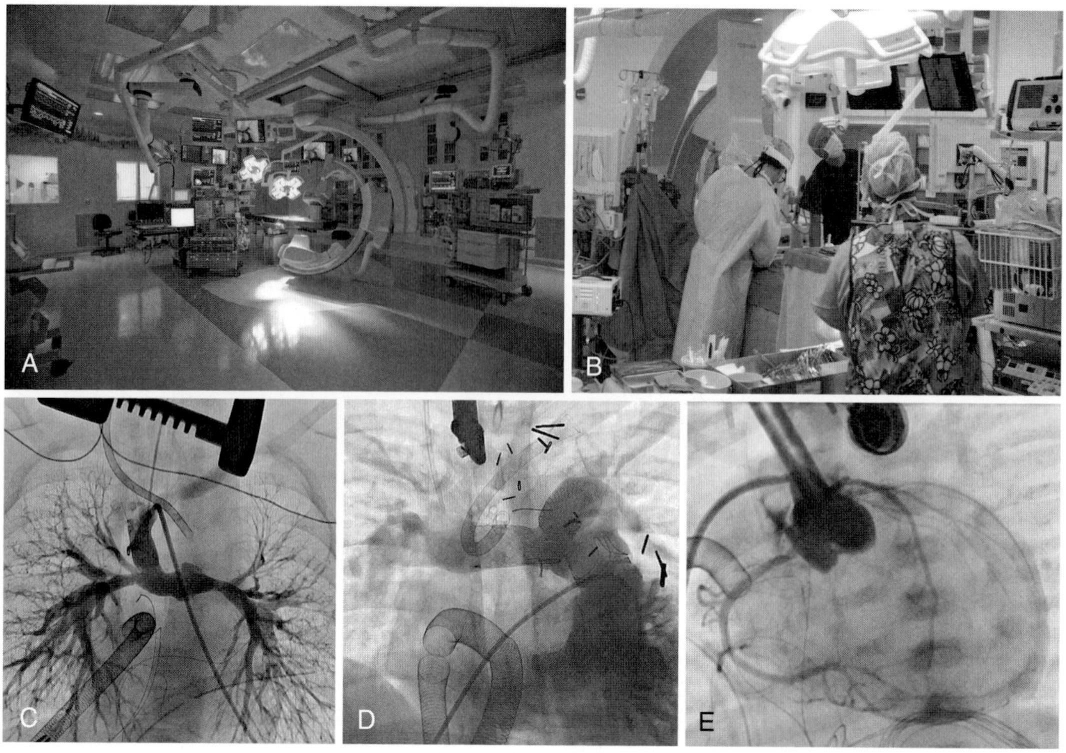

Figure 27-8   The hybrid operative suite is a perfect environment to perform intraoperative or "exit" angiograms. **A,** The Hybrid Suite at Nationwide Children's Hospital is shown with the ceiling-mounted angiographic system as an integrated component of the operative theater. The surgical and interventional teams work seamlessly in performing the exit angiogram **(B).** Exit angiograms after comprehensive stage 2 completion for hypoplastic left heart syndrome **(C),** after pulmonary valve replacement and bilateral intraoperative pulmonary artery stents **(D),** and after arterial switch for transposition of the great arteries with an intramural coronary artery **(E)** are demonstrated. (See Expert Consult site for color image.)

of over 40%.[53] Thus intraoperative evaluation of the hemodynamic impact of surgical repair may be extremely important. This has evolved from direct pressure measurement of the intracardiac chambers to the use of intraoperative (either transesophageal or epicardial) echocardiography. However, both techniques have limitations particularly when evaluating extracardiac structures such as the pulmonary arteries, aorta, and systemic veins. Other technologies, such as intravascular ultrasound, may be used to assess vessel patency; however, this may not be ideal in small infants.[54] Angiography on the other hand may complement these other techniques by identifying the exact location and extent of any residual stenoses or vessel distortion (Fig. 27-8) and the benefits of this approach after surgical or hybrid procedures have been reported.[55-56] These reports have varied in their approach, both in the location of the imaging, and the agents used to perform the intraoperative imaging. Holzer and colleagues described completion angiography on 11% of surgical procedures performed at their institution.[55] Angiography in all 32 procedures was performed in a dedicated hybrid operating suite. The benefit of this facility is a fixed ceiling-mounted C-arm, which leads to minimal disruption of both the procedure and the extensive personnel and equipment present in the hybrid suite. Unexpected or unusual pathology was identified in 56% of cases. In 28% of these procedures a change in clinical management was deemed to have occurred as a result of the data obtained from the angiography. Procedure-related adverse events were minimal with mild staining of the left pulmonary artery after angiography in one patient. Shuhaiber and colleagues described a standard mobile C-arm in the operating room to provide angiography. In their series of 18 patients, two patients had immediate reintervention in the operating room for abnormalities noted on the intraoperative angiogram.[57]

The use of a mobile C-arm in this setting requires preprocedural planning, and the availability of the interventional cardiologist, adequate space for the C-arm, ensuring sterility of the surgical field, and radiation protection require attention. Other approaches reported in congenital heart disease patients that may avoid some of these difficulties include the use of indocyanine green fluorescence angiography.[56] This imaging system emits light at wavelengths of approximately 800 nm and causes the indocyanine green contrast agent, which is administered through an existing central line, to fluoresce. The system is theoretically less cumbersome than a mobile C-arm and has been used successfully to assess patency of coronary artery bypass grafts in adult cardiac surgery.[58]

To date most reports commenting on intraoperative angiography in patients with congenital heart disease have been selective. Thus it is difficult to comment on the true incidence of potential intraoperative abnormalities and indeed interpretation of these images is somewhat subjective. Intraprocedural echocardiography is an excellent tool for imaging ventricular and valvar function and residual patch leaks and therefore intraoperative angiography may not be necessary in these more standard lesions. Suggested pathologies where angiography may be of benefit include tetralogy of Fallot repair, pulmonary artery reconstruction, cavopulmonary anastomosis, transposition of the great arteries to assess coronary artery patency, and following complex aortic arch procedures, including following Norwood surgery for HLHS. Further experience with this form of intraoperative imaging may expand on the potential applications of its use, and provide further integration between interventional cardiology and cardiac surgery which is the foundation to the hybrid approach to the treatment of congenital heart disease.

Conclusion

The hybrid approach to the treatment of the neonate with congenital heart disease represents the future of one of the most demanding but exciting medical specialties. It has come to define innovation through cooperation, removing boundaries between surgeons and interventionalists, and with the common goal of improving longer term outcomes for infants with congenital heart disease. This chapter has outlined some of the potential applications of this strategy and many more exist. Further endeavors to provide the best physiological palliation with the least invasive means possible represent the future of this approach and a challenge for future "hybrid specialists."

References

1. Norwood WI, Lang P, Hansen DD. Physiologic repair of aortic atresia-hypoplastic left heart syndrome. N Eng J Med. 1983;308:23-26.
2. Migliavacca F, Pennati G, Dubini G, et al. Modeling of the Norwood circulation: effects of shunt size, vascular resistances, and heart rate. Am J Physiol Heart Circ Physiol. 2001;280:H2076-H2086.
3. Razzouk AJ, Chinnock RE, Gundry SR, et al. Transplantation as a primary treatment for hypoplastic left heart syndrome: intermediate-term results. Ann Thorac Surg. 1996;62:1-7.
4. Sano S, Ishino K, Kawada M, et al. Right ventricle-pulmonary artery shunt in first-stage palliation of hypoplastic left heart syndrome. J Thorac Cardiovasc Surg. 2003;126:504-509.
5. Mahle WT, Spray TL, Wernovsky G, et al. Survival after reconstructive surgery for hypoplastic left heart syndrome: a 15-year experience from a single institution. Circulation. 2000;10:III136-141.
6. Stasik SN, Goldberg CS, Bove EL, et al. Current outcomes and risk factors for the Norwood procedure. J Thorac Cardiovasc Surg. 2006;131:412-417.
7. Ohye RG, Sleeper LA, Mahony L, et al. Pediatric Heart Network Investigators. Comparison of shunt types in the Norwood procedure for single-ventricle lesions. N Engl J Med. 2010;362: 1980-1992.
8. Sarajuuri A, Jokinen E, Puosi R, et al. Neurodevelopmental and neuroradiologic outcomes in patients with univentricular heart aged 5 to 7 years: related risk factor analysis. J Thorac Cardiovasc Surg. 2007;133:1524-1532.
9. Gibbs JL, Rothman MT, Rees MR, et al. Stenting of the arterial duct: a new approach to palliation for pulmonary atresia. Br Heart J. 1992;67:240-245.
10. Ruiz CE, Gamra H, Zhang HP, et al. Stenting of the ductus arteriosus as a bridge to cardiac transplantation in infants with the hypoplastic left-heart syndrome. N Engl J Med. 1993;328: 1605-1608.

27

11. Gibbs JL, Wren C, Watterson KG, et al. Stenting of the arterial duct combined with banding of the pulmonary arteries and atrial septectomy or septostomy: a new approach to palliation for the hypoplastic left heart syndrome. Br Heart J. 1993;69:551-555.

12. Gibbs JL, Uzun O, Blackburn ME, et al. Fate of the stented arterial duct. Circulation. 1999;99:2621-2625.

13. Akintuerk H, Michel-Behnke I, Valeske K, et al. Stenting of the arterial duct and banding of the pulmonary arteries: basis for combined Norwood stage I and II repair in hypoplastic left heart. Circulation. 2002;105:1099-1103.

14. Akintuerk H, Michel-Behnke I, Valeske K, et al. Hybrid transcatheter-surgical palliation: basis for univentricular or biventricular repair: the Giessen experience. Pediatr Cardiol. 2007;28:79-87.

15. Galantowicz M, Cheatham JP. Lessons learned from the development of a new hybrid strategy for the management of hypoplastic left heart syndrome. Pediatr Cardiol. 2005;26:190-199.

16. Galantowicz M, Cheatham JP, Phillips A, et al. Hybrid approach for hypoplastic left heart syndrome: intermediate results after the learning curve. Ann Thorac Surg. 2008;85:2063-2070.

17. Holzer RJ, Wood A, Chisolm JL, et al. Atrial septal interventions in patients with hypoplastic left heart syndrome. Catheter Cardiovasc Interv. 2008;72:696-704.

18. Stoica SC, Philips AB, Egan M, et al. The retrograde aortic arch in the hybrid approach to hypoplastic left heart syndrome. Ann Thorac Surg. 2009;88:1939-1946.

19. Naguib AN, Winch P, Schwartz L, et al. Anesthetic management of the hybrid stage 1 procedure for hypoplastic left heart syndrome (HLHS). Paediatr Anaesth. 2010;20:38-46.

20. Luce WA, Schwartz RM, Beauseau W, et al. Necrotizing enterocolitis in neonates undergoing the hybrid approach to complex congenital heart disease. Pediatr Crit Care Med. 2011;12:46-51.

21. Bacha EA, Daves S, Hardin J, et al. Single-ventricle palliation for high-risk neonates: the emergence of an alternative hybrid stage I. J Thorac Cardiovasc Surg. 2006;131:163-171.e2.

22. Honjo O, Benson LN, Mewhort HE, et al. Clinical outcomes, program evolution, and pulmonary artery growth in single ventricle palliation using hybrid and Norwood palliative strategies. Ann Thorac Surg. 2009;87:1885-1892.

23. Forbess JM, Cook N, Roth SJ, et al. Ten-year institutional experience with palliative surgery for hypoplastic left heart syndrome. Risk factors related to stage I mortality. Circulation. 1995;92(9 Suppl):II262-266.

24. Gaynor JW, Mahle WT, Cohen MI, et al. Risk factors for mortality after Norwood procedure. Eur J Cardiothoracic Surg. 2002;22:82-89.

25. Venugopal PS, Luna KP, Anderson DR, et al. Hybrid procedure as an alternative to surgical palliation of high-risk infants with hypoplastic left heart syndrome and its variants. J Thorac Cardiovasc Surg. 2010;139:1211-1215.

26. Ballard G, Tibby S, Miller O, et al. Growth of left heart structures following the hybrid procedure for borderline hypoplastic left heart. Eur J Echocardiogr. 2010;11:870-874.

27. Egan MJ, Hill SL, Boettner BL, et al. Predictors of retrograde aortic arch obstruction after hybrid palliation of hypoplastic left heart syndrome. Pediatr Cardiol. 2011;32:67-75.

28. Caldarone CA, Benson LN, Holtby H, et al. Main pulmonary artery to innominate artery shunt during hybrid palliation of hypoplastic left heart syndrome. J Thorac Cardiovasc Surg. 2005;130:e1-e2.

29. Wernovsky G, Ghanayem N, Ohye RG, et al. Hypoplastic left heart syndrome: consensus and controversies in 2007. Cardiol Young. 2007;17(Suppl 2):75-86.

30. Sharafuddin MJ, Gu X, Titus JL, et al. Transvenous closure of secundum atrial septal defects: preliminary results with a new self-expanding nitinol prosthesis in a swine model. Circulation. 1997;95:2162-2168.

31. Amin Z, Gu X, Berry JM, et al. A new device for closure of muscular ventricular septal defects in a canine model. Circulation. 1999;100:320-328.

32. Amin Z, Berry JM, Foker JE, et al. Intraoperative closure of muscular ventricular septal defect in a canine model and application of the technique in a baby. J Thorac Cardiovasc Surg. 1998;115:1374-1376.

33. Amin Z, Gu X, Berry JM, et al. Perventricular [correction of Periventricular] closure of ventricular septal defects without cardiopulmonary bypass. Ann Thorac Surg. 1999;68:149-153.

34. Bacha EA, Cao QL, Galantowicz ME, et al. Multicenter experience with perventricular device closure of muscular ventricular septal defects. Pediatr Cardiol. 2005;26:169-175.

35. Crossland DS, Wilkinson JL, Cochrane AD, et al. Initial results of primary device closure of large muscular ventricular septal defects in early infancy using perventricular access. Catheter Cardiovasc Interv. 2008;72:386-391.

36. Michel-Behnke I, Ewert P, et al; for the Investigators of the Working Group Interventional Cardiology of the German Association of Pediatric Cardiology. Device closure of ventricular septal defects by hybrid procedures: a multicenter retrospective study. Catheter Cardiovasc Interv. 2011;77:242-251.

37. Amin Z, Woo R, Danford DA, et al. Robotically assisted perventricular closure of perimembranous ventricular septal defects: preliminary results in Yucatan pigs. J Thorac Cardiovasc Surg. 2006;131:427-432.

38. Lim DS, Forbes TJ, Rothman A, et al. Transcatheter closure of high-risk muscular ventricular septal defects with the CardioSEAL occluder: initial report from the CardioSEAL VSD registry. Catheter Cardiovasc Interv. 2007;70:740-744.

39. Muller WH, Dammann JF. Treatment of certain congenital malformations of the heart by the creation of pulmonic stenosis to reduce pulmonary hypertension and excessive pulmonary blood flow: a preliminary report. Surg Gynecol Obstet. 1952;95:213.

40. Yacoub MH, Radley-Smith R, Maclaurin R. Two-stage operation for anatomical correction of transposition of the great arteries with intact interventricular septum. Lancet. 1977;1:1275-1278.

41. Trusler GA, Mustard WT. A method of banding the pulmonary artery for large isolated ventricular septal defect with and without transposition of the great arteries. Ann Thorac Surg. 1972;13: 351-355.

42. Shane RA, Kimmell GO, Jaques WE, et al. Adjustable prosthesis for pulmonary artery banding. Comparison with umbilical tape and teflon bands. Circulation. 1967;35:1148-1151.

43. Muraoka R, Yokota M, Aoshima M, et al. Extrathoracically adjustable pulmonary artery banding. J Thorac Cardiovasc Surg. 1983;86:582-586.

44. Solis E, Bell D, Alboliras H, et al. Left ventricular preparation with an extrathoracically adjustable balloon occluder. Ann Thorac Surg. 1987;44:58-61.

45. Higashidate M, Beppu T, Imai Y, et al. Percutaneously adjustable pulmonary artery band. An experimental study. J Thorac Cardiovasc Surg. 1989;97:864-869.

46. Schlensak C, Sarai K, Gildein HP, et al. Pulmonary artery banding with a novel percutaneously, bidirectionally adjustable device. Eur J Cardiothorac Surg. 1997;12:931-933.

47. Däbritz S, Sachweh J, Tiete A, et al. Experience with an adjustable pulmonary artery banding device in two cases: initial success—midterm failure. Thorac Cardiovasc Surg. 1999;47:51-52.

48. Corno AF, Sekarski N, von Segesser LK. Remote control of pulmonary blood flow: a dream comes true. Swiss Med Wkly. 2002;13:423-424.

49. Bonnet D, Corno AF, Sidi D, et al. Early clinical results of the telemetric adjustable pulmonary artery banding FloWatch-PAB. Circulation. 2004;110:II158-II163.

50. Dhannapuneni RR, Gladman G, Kerr S, et al. Complete atrioventricular septal defect: outcome of pulmonary artery banding improved by adjustable device. J Thorac Cardiovasc Surg. 2011;141: 179-182.

51. Michel-Behnke I, Akintuerk H, Valeske K, et al. Pseudoaneurysm of the pulmonary trunk after placement of an adjustable pulmonary artery banding device (FloWatch-PAB) in a patient with muscular ventricular septal defect. J Thorac Cardiovasc Surg. 2005;130:894-895.

52. Venugopal PS, Hayes N, Simpson J, et al. Transection with pseudoaneurysm formation of the pulmonary trunk after placement of an adjustable pulmonary artery banding device (FloWatch-PAB) in a patient with residual muscular ventricular septal defect. J Thorac Cardiovasc Surg. 2010;139: e103-e104.

53. Asoh K, Hickey E, Dorostkar PC, et al. Outcomes of emergent cardiac catheterization following pediatric cardiac surgery. Catheter Cardiovasc Interv. 2009;73:933-940.

54. Hijazi ZM, Ahmad WH, Geggel RL, et al. Intravascular ultrasound during transcatheter coil closure of patent ductus arteriosus: comparison with angiography. J Invasive Cardiol. 1998;10:251-254.

55. Holzer RJ, Sisk M, Chisolm JL, et al. Completion angiography after cardiac surgery for congenital heart disease: complementing the intraoperative imaging modalities. Pediatr Cardiol. 2009;30: 1075-1082.

56. Kogon B, Fernandez J, Kanter K, et al. The role of intraoperative indocyanine green fluorescence angiography in pediatric cardiac surgery. Ann Thorac Surg. 2009;88:632-636.

57. Shuhaiber JH, Bergersen L, Pigula F, et al. Intraoperative assessment after pediatric cardiac surgical repair: initial experience with C-arm angiography. J Thorac Cardiovasc Surg. 2010;140:e1-e3.

58. Hol PK, Lingaas PS, Lundblad R, et al. Intraoperative angiography leads to graft revision in coronary artery bypass surgery. Ann Thorac Surg. 2004;78:502-505.

59. Caldarone CA, Benson L, Holtby H, et al. Initial experience with hybrid palliation for neonates with single-ventricle physiology. Ann Thorac Surg. 2007;84:1294-1300.

60. Pizarro C, Murdison KA, Derby CD, et al. Stage II reconstruction after hybrid palliation for high-risk patients with a single ventricle. Ann Thorac Surg. 2008;85:1382-1388.

61. Pilla CB, Pedra CA, Nogueira AJ, et al. Hybrid management for hypoplastic left heart syndrome: an experience from Brazil. Pediatr Cardiol. 2008;29:498-506.

27

Index

Page numbers followed by "f" indicate figures, "t" indicate tables, and "b" indicate boxes.